PROPERTY OF LLUMC
JESSE MEDICAL LIBRARY

P9-AGN-967

VEGETARIAN NUTRITION

CRC SERIES IN MODERN NUTRITION
Edited by Ira Wolinsky and James F. Hickson, Jr.

Published Titles

Manganese in Health and Disease, Dorothy J. Klimis-Tavantzis

Nutrition and AIDS: Effects and Treatments, Ronald R. Watson

Nutrition Care for HIV-Positive Persons: A Manual for Individuals and Their Caregivers,
  Saroj M. Bahl and James F. Hickson, Jr.

Calcium and Phosphorus in Health and Disease, John J.B. Anderson and
  Sanford C. Garner

Edited by Ira Wolinsky

Published Titles

Practical Handbook of Nutrition in Clinical Practice, Donald F. Kirby
  and Stanley J. Dudrick

Handbook of Dairy Foods and Nutrition, Gregory D. Miller, Judith K. Jarvis,
  and Lois D. McBean

Advanced Nutrition: Macronutrients, Carolyn D. Berdanier

Childhood Nutrition, Fima Lifschitz

Nutrition and Health: Topics and Controversies, Felix Bronner

Nutrition and Cancer Prevention, Ronald R. Watson and Siraj I. Mufti

Nutritional Concerns of Women, Ira Wolinsky and Dorothy J. Klimis-Tavantzis

Nutrients and Gene Expression: Clinical Aspects, Carolyn D. Berdanier

Antioxidants and Disease Prevention, Harinda S. Garewal

Advanced Nutrition: Micronutrients, Carolyn D. Berdanier

Nutrition and Women's Cancers, Barbara Pence and Dale M. Dunn

Nutrients and Foods in AIDS, Ronald R. Watson

Nutrition: Chemistry and Biology, Second Edition, Julian E. Spallholz,
  L. Mallory Boylan, and Judy A. Driskell

Melatonin in the Promotion of Health, Ronald R. Watson

Nutritional and Environmental Influences on the Eye, Allen Taylor

Laboratory Tests for the Assessment of Nutritional Status, Second Edition,
  H.E. Sauberlich

Advanced Human Nutrition, Robert E.C. Wildman and Denis M. Medeiros

Handbook of Dairy Foods and Nutrition, Second Edition, Gregory D. Miller,
  Judith K. Jarvis, and Lois D. McBean

Nutrition in Space Flight and Weightlessness Models, Helen W. Lane
  and Dale A. Schoeller

Forthcoming Titles

VEGETARIAN NUTRITION

Edited by
JOAN SABATÉ

in collaboration with
ROSEMARY RATZIN-TURNER

CRC Press
Boca Raton   London   New York   Washington, D.C.

Library of Congress Cataloging-in-Publication Data

Vegetarian nutrition / Joan Sabaté, editor ; in collaboration with Rosemary Ratzin-Turner.
    p. cm.--(Modern nutrition)
ISBN 0-8493-8508-3
1. Vegetarianism. I. Sabaté, Joan. II. Ratzin-Turner, Rosemary. III. Modern nutrition
(Boca Raton, Fla.)
RM236 . V43 2001
613.2′62—dc21   00-068871
                                                          CIP

This book contains information obtained from authentic and highly regarded sources. Reprinted material is quoted with permission, and sources are indicated. A wide variety of references are listed. Reasonable efforts have been made to publish reliable data and information, but the author and the publisher cannot assume responsibility for the validity of all materials or for the consequences of their use.

Neither this book nor any part may be reproduced or transmitted in any form or by any means, electronic or mechanical, including photocopying, microfilming, and recording, or by any information storage or retrieval system, without prior permission in writing from the publisher.

All rights reserved. Authorization to photocopy items for internal or personal use, or the personal or internal use of specific clients, may be granted by CRC Press LLC, provided that $.50 per page photocopied is paid directly to Copyright Clearance Center, 222 Rosewood Drive, Danvers, MA 01923 USA. The fee code for users of the Transactional Reporting Service is ISBN 0-8493-8508-3/01/$0.00+$.50. The fee is subject to change without notice. For organizations that have been granted a photocopy license by the CCC, a separate system of payment has been arranged.

The consent of CRC Press LLC does not extend to copying for general distribution, for promotion, for creating new works, or for resale. Specific permission must be obtained in writing from CRC Press LLC for such copying.

Direct all inquiries to CRC Press LLC, 2000 N.W. Corporate Blvd., Boca Raton, Florida 33431.

Trademark Notice: Product or corporate names may be trademarks or registered trademarks, and are used only for identification and explanation, without intent to infringe.

Visit the CRC Press Web site at www.crcpress.com

© 2001 by CRC Press LLC

No claim to original U.S. Government works
International Standard Book Number 0-8493-8508-3
Library of Congress Card Number 00-068871
Printed in the United States of America 1 2 3 4 5 6 7 8 9 0
Printed on acid-free paper

SERIES PREFACE FOR MODERN NUTRITION

The CRC Series in Modern Nutrition is dedicated to providing the widest possible coverage of topics in nutrition. Nutrition is an interdisciplinary, interprofessional field par excellence. It is noted by its broad range and diversity. We trust that the titles and authorship in this series will reflect that range and diversity.

Published for a scholarly audience, the volumes in the CRC Series in Modern Nutrition are designed to explain, review, and explore present knowledge and recent trends, developments, and advances in nutrition. As such, they will also appeal to the educated general reader. The format for the series will vary with the needs of the author and the topic, including, but not limited to, edited volumes, monographs, handbooks, and texts.

Contributors from any bona fide area of nutrition, including the controversial, are welcome.

We welcome the contribution *Vegetarian Nutrition*, edited by Joan Sabaté with the collaboration of Rosemary Ratzin-Turner. There is a great deal of interest regarding vegetarianism as an alternate dietary pattern. This book discusses that issue in detail and will appeal to nutritionists, dietitians, physicians, students, and professionals in the health sciences and health services arenas.

Ira Wolinsky, Ph.D.
Series Editor
University of Houston

PREFACE

From antiquity, vegetarian diets have been followed for a variety of reasons, albeit with widely differing nutritional outcomes. As a result, numerous scientific and professional questions have arisen. Currently, professional interest in vegetarian nutrition has reached unprecedented levels. This is only partly explained by the growing number of vegetarians and the increased popularity of vegetarian diets. As disease patterns shifted away from nutrient deficiencies and toward diet-related chronic diseases, vegetarian nutrition research also changed emphasis, and the benefits of vegetarian diets have begun to emerge.

In the past 30 years, scientific endeavors in the area of vegetarian nutrition seem to have progressively shifted from investigating concerns held by nutritionists and other health professionals to a fertile area of investigation in which creative solutions for various medical conditions and preventive approaches to chronic diseases may be found.

Despite this broadening shift in the focus and study of nutrition, current knowledge regarding the relationship between vegetarian diets and human health is far from complete. However, scientific advances made during the last few decades have noticeably changed the role of vegetarian diets and other diets largely based on plant foods in human nutrition and public health. This book on vegetarian nutrition is an attempt to summarize the large body of literature accumulated on the topic.

Although most of the information presented in this book centers on the dietary practices of vegetarians, it has sweeping implications for the general population. In the past few years, scientific literature has extensively reported on the health effects of plant foods such as whole grains, legumes, vegetables, fruits, and nuts. Although they are essential components, these dietary factors are not unique to vegetarian diets. Thus, the information reviewed on plant foods and health has direct applications for all persons.

The primary focus of this volume is on the human health implications of consuming vegetarian diets. Besides personal health, however, one may follow a vegetarian diet for a plethora of reasons that may include religion, ethics, or the sustainability of our food supply. The chapters in the concluding section of this text address these issues. From a global, inclusive perspective, personal and public health are most influenced by the manner in which we treat our fellow inhabitants and the resources of our planet.

Joan Sabaté

ACKNOWLEDGMENTS

The publication of a book is never the work of a single individual. This is obviously the case in a contributed-chapter volume such as this. I am greatly indebted to each of the authors for their efforts.

I would like to acknowledge Dr. Rosemary Ratzin-Turner for initially sharing with me her idea to create a book of this nature and initiating the contact with the publisher. Her interest in the subject and desire to see this volume published have continually motivated me.

I would like to recognize the dedication of Mr. Jack Brown, who carefully assembled the several preparatory versions of the different chapters. Also, Ms. Anuradha Job, for her assistance in editing the final manuscript.

I wish to also thank every faculty member of the Nutrition Department, and many of the School of Public Health at Loma Linda University, who anonymously reviewed many chapters and offered advice and constructive criticism.

Finally, thank you to my wife, Carmen Llorca, who, 20 years ago, inspired me to study vegetarian nutrition and gave generously of her time to take care of our children while I was devoting countless hours to completing this volume.

EDITOR

Joan Sabaté is Professor and Chair of the Department of Nutrition and Professor of Epidemiology at the Loma Linda University School of Public Health. He is also Professor of Preventive Medicine at the university's School of Medicine.

A native of Barcelona, Spain, Dr. Sabaté obtained his medical degree from the Autonomous University of Barcelona. He moved to the United States with a Fulbright Scholarship to further train in Public Health Nutrition. In 1989, after completing his thesis research on the growth and anthropometric parameters of vegetarian school-age children and adolescents, he received a Dr.P.H. (Doctor in Public Health) in Nutrition from Loma Linda University.

Dr. Sabaté served as a co-investigator of the Adventist Health Study, a cohort of 34,000 Seventh-Day Adventists in California, half of whom were vegetarians, and studied the relationships between their diet and chronic diseases. He also served as the principal investigator of several nutritional studies that directly link the consumption of nuts to substantial reductions in blood serum cholesterol. He was the co-chair of the program committee for the Third International Congress on Vegetarian Nutrition.

Dr. Sabaté is a member of several scientific societies, associations, and councils including the American Society of Nutritional Sciences and its affiliate, the American Society of Clinical Nutrition, and the International Epidemiological Association.

CONTRIBUTORS

Paul Appleby, Ph.D.
ICRF Cancer Epidemiology Unit
University of Oxford
Radcliffe Infirmary
Oxford, England

Susan Barr, Ph.D., R.D.
Family and Nutritional Science
University of British Columbia
Vancouver, BC, Canada

Glen Blix, Dr.P.H.
Health Promotion and Education
School of Public Health
Loma Linda University
Loma Linda, CA

Jack Brown
Department of Nutrition
School of Public Health
Loma Linda University
Loma Linda, CA

Mark F. Carr, Ph.D.
Assistant Professor of Ethics
Faculty of Religion
Loma Linda University
Loma Linda, CA

Peter Clarys, Ph.D.
Laboratory of Human Biometry
  and Biomechanics
Faculty of Physical Education
and Physical Therapy
Vrije Universiteit Brussel
Brussels, Belgium

Winston J. Craig, Ph.D., R.D.
Andrews University
Department of Nutrition
Berrien Springs, MI

Elaine Fleming, M.P.H., R.D.
Department of Nutrition
School of Public Health
Loma Linda University
Loma Linda, CA

Ella H. Haddad, Dr.P.H., R.D.
Department of Nutrition
School of Public Health
Loma Linda University
Loma Linda, CA

**Mervyn Hardinge, M.D., Ph.D.,
  Dr.P.H.**
Brewster, WA

Marcel Hebbelinck, Ph.D
Professor Emeritus
Laboratory of Human Biometry
  and Biomechanics
Faculty of Physical Education
  and Physical Therapy
Vrije Universiteit Brussel
Brussels, Belgium

Richard W. Hubbard, Ph.D.
School of Medicine
Loma Linda University
Loma Linda, CA

Patricia K. Johnston, Dr.P.H., RD
School of Public Health
Loma Linda University
Loma Linda, CA

Tim Key, D.Phil.
ICRF Cancer Epidemiology Unit
University of Oxford
Radcliffe Infirmary
Oxford, England

Paul K. Mills, Ph.D.
Cancer Registry of Central
California
and University of California
Fresno Medical Education Program
Fresno, CA

David C. Nieman, Dr.P.H.
Department of Health, Leisure,
  and Exercise Science
Appalachian State University
Boone, NC

Laura Pinyan
Andrews University
Department of Nutrition
Berrien Springs, MI

Sujatha Rajaram, Ph.D.
Department of Nutrition
School of Public Health
Loma Linda University
Loma Linda, CA

Rosemary A. Ratzin-Turner, Ed.D.
Weight Away
Clifton, NJ

Lucas Reijnders
Department of Environmental
  Science
University of Amsterdam
Amsterdam, Netherlands

Joan Sabaté, M.D., Dr.P.H.
Department of Nutrition
School of Public Health
Loma Linda University
Loma Linda, CA

Pramil N. Singh, Dr.P.H.
Department of Epidemiology and
  Biostatistics
School of Public Health
Loma Linda University
Loma Linda, CA

Crystal Whitten, M.S., R.D.
Department of Nutrition and
  Dietetics
School of Allied Health
Loma Linda University
Loma Linda, CA

James C. Whorton, Ph.D.
Department of Medical History
  and Ethics
School of Medicine
University of Washington
Seattle, WA

Michelle Wien, R.D., C.D.E.
City of Hope National Medical Center
Department of Diabetes,
Endocrinology and Metabolism
Duarte, CA

Gerald R. Winslow, Ph.D.
Faculty of Religion
Loma Linda University
Loma Linda, CA

PROLOGUE

Editor's Note: I would like to recognize Dr. Mervyn Hardinge, a pioneer in the field of vegetarian nutrition. His work and dedication to the scientific investigation of vegetarian diets have served as an inspiration to those who have followed. To this end, Dr. Hardinge has submitted a historical prologue to this volume, for which I wish to thank him.

Historical records of ancient times reveal that each nation passes through well-defined dietary stages. When the nation is young and struggling to develop, the people are generally poor and the diet is frugal, consisting chiefly of plant foods. As the nation becomes well established and its people prosper, animal foods become more plentiful. Thus, the interest in vegetarian dietaries has waxed and waned through the centuries. Historians have noted that, in times of plenty, interest in such diets has been low, while during periods of famine, the reverse has been true. During cycles of riotous living and profligacy, non-flesh diets have been spurned only to gain favor when political and religious reforms again come into vogue.

It might be said that the era of modern nutrition was marked by the discovery by Liebig of how the level of protein in foods can be determined. Carl Voit (1870), a German physician and researcher, studied with Liebig. On returning to Munich, his home town, he determined the protein intake of 1000 hard-working coal miners and found that they consumed approximately 120 grams of protein per day. This became "Voit's standard for protein requirement." He was later supported by McCay (1912), an Englishman. Together, they recommended a daily intake of 100–150 grams of protein for an adult.

The investigations to determine the protein requirements for humans indirectly aroused an interest in vegetarian diets. Chittenden of Yale (1913) and Hindhede of Sweden (1913) challenged such intakes, maintaining that a much lower level of protein in the diet, namely, 25–55 grams per day for a adult, was more than adequate. The interest in protein requirements faded by the 1950s when Hegsted and Stare (1946) and other investigators determined that 25–35 grams per day of all plant proteins were adequate for adults.

And this is where my scientific interest in vegetarian diets began. On graduating from medicine (1942) I began teaching at Loma Linda University School of Medicine. Although raised as a life-long vegetarian (lacto-ovo), I began to wonder if sound scientific investigation would vindicate such a diet's adequacy. In the fall of 1948, I enrolled as a graduate student in the Harvard School of Public Health. Doctor Fred Stare, then chairman of the department of nutrition, became my senior professor. My doctoral research was approved, and a comparative study of the nutritional status of vegetarians versus non-vegetarians began. Three groups were evaluated, namely, adults (men and women), adolescents (boys and girls), and pregnant women. Complete vegetarians (vegans), and lacto-ovo vegetarians (use milk and eggs but no fish or fowl) were compared with non-vegetarians.

Protein was still the dominating interest. Did a vegetarian diet provide an adequate quantity of protein, and, if it did, would it provide the spectrum of essential amino acids in adequate amounts deemed essential for good nutrition? Interest in fats and carbohydrates was, at most, slight. Since the plan of study required the determination of not only the total protein intake of each subject, but also the amounts derived from both plant and animal sources (lacto-ovo-vegetarians consume milk, eggs, and products derived from them), I decided to determine the amount of fat in the diets obtained from these same two sources.

This proved to be a fortuitous decision; I had listened to a paper by the coroner's surgeon of the City of Boston 2 years earlier in which he showed evidence that cholesterol crystals could be found in atheromatous plaques. And so, while doing blood analyses, why not determine the levels of blood cholesterol?

The diets of all groups of vegetarians were found to be adequate in all the parameters studied. An obvious difference was seen in the cholesterol levels of the adult groups: the higher the intake of animal fat in the diet, the higher the blood cholesterol level. While the paper on the adequacy of vegetarian diets for adults, pregnant women, and adolescents was accepted with little comment, the paper showing the relationship of animal fat and cholesterol stirred up an unexpectedly wide interest.

The focus of nutritional research appeared to shift. What was the difference between plant and animal fat? Soon the literature and the medical and nutritional worlds were speaking of saturated, unsaturated, and polyunsaturated fats. Cholesterol was chemically taken apart, the lipids were characterized, and some were deemed good while others were bad. One thing followed another. In 1958, Stare and Hardinge published a paper showing a relationship between fiber in the diet and blood cholesterol levels. The relationship was inverse; the higher the intake of fiber, the lower the cholesterol in the blood. In time, dietary fiber became another focus of interest.

Vegetarians suddenly became sought-after "guinea pigs."

Another study, also centering at Loma Linda University School of Medicine began in the early '50s. An investigation initiated by Earnest Wynder of the Sloan Kettering Institute of Cancer Research in New York compared Seventh-Day Adventists in California with Californians who smoked. Adventists are non-smokers, and roughly one-third to one-half are vegetarians. The findings not only showed that Adventists who had never smoked had virtually no primary cancers of the lung, they also had no emphysema, chronic bronchitis, coronary heart disease, hypertension, diabetes, etc., and lived longer. Subsequent studies showed that significant differences existed in the incidences of the above entities between vegetarian and non-vegetarian Adventists, the vegetarians having the advantage.

Interest in vegetarians and their diets was established and continued to grow. The relatively recent discovery of nutraceuticals or phytochemicals and their role in human health and disease opens a vast field of exploration before the researcher and practitioner. The use of whole foods in the therapy of serious diseases, such as cancers, diabetes, heart disease and other illnesses offers an exciting future. The attitudes toward vegetarian diets have progressed through the years — from onetime ridicule and skepticism through condescending tolerance, gradual and sometimes grudging acceptance, and finally, to acclaim.

I authored a paper in the mid-'60s on non-flesh dietaries in scientific literature (1963) in which I reviewed the significant scientific publications to that date. Some years later, I hoped to publish a second paper updating the subject. To my consternation, the publications had grown exponentially. I decided to leave it to younger researchers.

This current volume is a publication whose time has come. The information on vegetarian nutrition has grown tremendously, and has become too vast for the average health professional to keep pace with. To find a single volume arranged in neat packets of timely information on the varied aspects of vegetarian nutrition should prove a gold mine to the busy nutritionist, health professional, and medical practitioner.

Mervyn Hardinge, M.D., Dr.P.H., Ph.D.
Professor Emeritus
School of Public Health
Loma Linda University

CONTENTS

I

BACKGROUND

1

VEGETARIAN DIETS: DESCRIPTIONS AND TRENDS

Joan Sabaté, Rosemary A. Ratzin-Turner, and Jack E. Brown

CONTENTS

I.   INTRODUCTION

In response to basic questions, this chapter defines who a vegetarian is and what the major forms of the vegetarian diet comprise. It also reports trends of acceptance of this dietary practice in industrialized nations as well as publication trends of vegetarian nutrition articles in the biomedical literature.

II.   DEFINITION OF TERMS

Defining terms can, at times, be a challenging task. Furthermore, once a term has been defined, its general acceptance and proper use often

0-8493-8508-3/01/$0.00+$.50
© 2001 by CRC Press LLC

constitute a greater challenge. Here is where we begin the debate with the word "vegetarian." The dictionary is quite clear in stating that a vegetarian is "one who eats a diet consisting wholly of vegetables and fruit, and sometimes eggs or dairy products."[1] However, there seems to be some confusion among the general population as well as in the scientific community as to whether this definition is sufficient. Support for this confusion can be found in the number of professed vegetarians who eat meat products in varied frequency.

In many ways, defining a vegetarian could simply be: "one who abstains from meat." However, a closer look at the various social, religious, philosophical, historical, and political influences that have affected the label and its usage over time present the reality that the term has different meanings to different people.

Weinsier addresses the issue of defining terms.[2] He presents valid concerns similar to those listed above, while stressing a fear that there are too many non-nutritional connotations present when the word vegetarian is used. While this chapter will demonstrate that the vegetarian diet and lifestyle are becoming more accepted by the mainstream, it is true that there have been, and still are to some degree, several stigmas attached to it. Weinsier reviews the attitudes of the 1940s and 1950s, when avoidance of meat was often assumed to be due to religious belief rather than for health reasons. He continues by stating that in the 1960s and 1970s, a person who chose not to eat meat was considered to be part of the anti-establishment movement. Not until the 1980s was it accepted, for the most part, that a person choosing not to eat meat was doing so for health reasons. However, Weinsier does point out that motives unrelated to health are still often suspected of those adhering to a vegetarian diet. For these reasons, he advocates that the term "vegetarian" be removed from the scientific literature and perhaps a term such as "plant-based" be adopted.

Willett also addresses the shifts in thinking that have occurred in the past decade regarding vegetarian diets.[3] He points out that there was a time when the focus was on foods, such as meat, that were excluded from the diet. However, more recently, the trend has been to focus on the benefits of certain foods such as fruits and vegetables. As this shift in attitudes continues, the definition of vegetarianism will become clearer and the stigmas attached to it will, in turn, be minimized. The terms "meatless diet" and "plant-based diet" are being used with increasing frequency. Both terms appear to have less stigma attached to them than the more-traditional "vegetarianism." Regardless of any ideological influences, the reality is that most scientific literature considers a person a vegetarian if flesh (combined frequency of meat, poultry, and fish) is eaten less than once per week.

III. TYPES OF VEGETARIAN DIETS

The eating patterns of professed vegetarians vary considerably. Persons who choose the diet for health reasons typically have more flexibility in their use of animal foods and products. On the contrary, those who choose to be vegetarians for ethical or ideological reasons may be inclined toward a complete avoidance of meat and, in some cases, all animal products. These motivations begin to explain some of the variation. Nevertheless, for the purpose of this book, unless otherwise noted, a "vegetarian" will be considered an individual who consumes no animal flesh of any kind more than once per week.

The major types of vegetarian diets are listed below. The one common characteristic of these diets is that they are all plant based. More specifically, the diets described below are based on grains, vegetables, fruits, legumes, seeds, and nuts. And, depending on the particular diet, foods of animal origin are partially or totally excluded.

Vegetarian: This term encompasses all meatless diets. It is usually qualified or further categorized by one of the following:

- Lacto vegetarian: In addition to plant foods, milk and dairy are included.
- Ovo vegetarian: Eggs are included.
- Ovo-lacto or lacto-ovo vegetarian: Both eggs and dairy are included. Approximately 90–95% of vegetarians in North America include dairy and/or eggs in their diets.[4]

Determinations of other dietary patterns somehow related to vegetarian diets follow.

- Strict vegetarian/vegan: A small but growing number of people follow this diet that excludes animal flesh (meat, poultry/fowl, fish, and seafood) and animal products (eggs and dairy). Vegans may also exclude honey from the diet and will often not wear clothing made from animal products.
- Semi-vegetarian: Occasional meat eaters who predominately practice a vegetarian diet. These include:
  - Pescovegetarian: those who include fish in the diet
  - Pollovegetarians: those who include chicken in the diet
- Fruitarian: A diet consisting of foods that do not kill the plant of origin. In practical terms, this type of diet gets reduced to fresh fruits, dried fruits such as dates and raisins, nuts and seeds, and selected vegetables.

■ Macrobiotic: This type of diet is typically classified as vegetarian, but often includes fish. The diet stems from a 10-step approach to eating that, at the highest level, is almost exclusively brown rice. Today, most macrobiotic diets still emphasize brown rice and other whole grains, but also include sea vegetables, legumes, and root vegetables.[5]

IV. HISTORICAL AND SOCIOLOGICAL PERSPECTIVES

The word "vegetarian" was first used in 1847 by the Vegetarian Society of the United Kingdom.[6] However, as other chapters of this volume show, vegetarian practices can be traced back to at least 600 B.C., with prominent figures such as Pythagoras (considered the Father of Vegetarianism), Zoroaster, Daniel, and Buddha advocating and following a vegetarian diet. Throughout history, several religious groups have followed vegetarian diets with varying degrees of adherence. However, it wasn't until the last part of the 20th century that the practice began to secure mainstream acceptance for positive health associations.

Today's vegetarians comprise a diverse group. Table 1.1 displays several demographic characteristics of the vegetarian population in the United States. From the data,[7] we can extrapolate that a greater proportion of females than males are vegetarians and, while there is no difference in socioeconomic status, vegetarians tend to be slightly more educated than the general U.S. population. Although a higher percentage of the vegetarian population is more than 40 years of age, a larger percentage is composed of young families (those with children under 18 years of age).

People choose vegetarian diets for varied reasons. These include, but are not limited to, health concerns, religious or ethical beliefs, metaphysical, ecological, and even political reasons. Table 1.2 shows the results from a 1992 U.S. survey in which individuals were polled on their reasons for choosing the vegetarian diet. These results are similar to previous polls.

V. DEMOGRAPHICS AND TRENDS

While some surveys indicate that as many as 7% of the population in the U.S. and the U.K. are vegetarian,[8] others have put the number at about 2%.[9] Many factors account for this discrepancy. Besides methodological differences in surveys, such as small sample sizes, determining how many people do not eat meat is different from determining how many define themselves vegetarian. Many people call themselves vegetarian even though they may consume some meat or meat products regularly. Survey data obtained by asking people to identify their dietary pattern by name

Table 1.1   Characteristics of the Vegetarian Population of the U.S.

	Vegetarians [%]	General Population [%]
Gender		
Female	68	52
Male	32	48
Education		
College graduate	30	25
High school graduate	45	56
No high school degree	21	18
Marital status		
Married	48	59
Single	24	22
Widowed	14	8
Divorced/separated	11	11
Have children under 18		
Yes	37	24
No	60	75
Income		
Under $35,000/yr	56	55
Over $35,000/yr	44	45
Occupation		
White collar	37	35
Blue collar	60	62
Age		
Under 40	42	49
Over 40	55	50

Adapted from Messina[23]

(i.e., vegetarian, omnivore) will yield different results from asking people to indicate how many times a week they consume various foods. Most survey data comes from the U.K. and the U.S., although there are data and anecdotal evidence to support similar trends in other industrialized nations.

Three types of surveys have been identified.

1. Surveys that capture individual philosophy or ideology concerning vegetarian diets; namely, if the individual considers himself or herself to be a vegetarian. These surveys are usually sponsored by special-interest organizations.

**Table 1.2   Reasons U.S. Individuals Chose a
Vegetarian Diet in 1992, Expressed in
Percentage**

Health	46
Animal rights	15
Family/friend influence	12
Ethics	05
Environmental issues	04
Other/no response	18

Vegetarian Times, Yankelovich Partners study, 1992[7]

2. This type of study gathers data on the frequency of food consumption, including meat, dairy, and eggs, using a variety of dietary assessments. They are often administered by a government agency or scientific investigation.

3. Surveys and marketing research analyses that are primarily industry sponsored and provide information on collective consumption, distribution, and availability of certain foods as opposed to individual food intake. Some studies or surveys combine aspects of two or more of these types.

In Britain, during World War II, 120,000 individuals registered for food rationing cards as vegetarians. At that time, this accounted for only 0.25% of the population, most of whom were in middle age or elderly.[10] The RealEat[11] polls, conducted in the U.K. over a period of 14 years (1984–1997), report that in 1984 more than 2% of the population considered themselves vegetarian. By 1997, 5.4% were self-reported vegetarians, almost a threefold increase from 1984. In 1984 an additional 1.9% of the population claimed to be avoiding red meat and in 1997, 14.3% reported this avoidance. Combined with the 5.4% of vegetarians, this data suggests that about 20% of the population of the U.K. is avoiding red meat consumption. Figure 1.1, constructed from the RealEat data, depicts two upward trends. One trend details a slow but very steady growth over time in the percentage of the population in the U.K. who define themselves as vegetarians. The second, more noticeable trend, shows an accelerated growth in the percentage of individuals who, although they are not self-defined vegetarians, are avoiding red meat.

Further analysis of data from the RealEat polls substantiates what was also found in the U.S. For example, a higher percentage of women than men are vegetarians and, while the overall vegetarian population is slightly

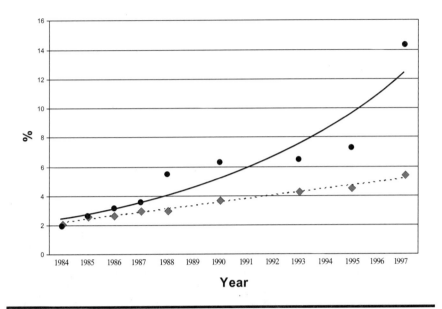

Figure 1.1   Percentage of British population who are self-reported vegetarians is represented by the ♥ symbol. The ● represents the percentage of population who are self-reported avoiders of red meat.

older than the general population, young men and women and families are increasingly becoming a larger percentage of the vegetarian and red-meat-avoiding population in the U.K.

The government-sponsored 1977–1978 Nationwide Food Consumption Survey (NFCS)[12] is recognized as the first to acknowledge the increased interest in vegetarian diets in the U.S. NFCS focused on the food use of households and the dietary intakes and patterns of individuals. These surveys have been conducted approximately every 10 years since 1935 by the U.S. Department of Agriculture's Human Nutrition Information Service (HNIS). Of the 37,135 people surveyed in 1977–1978, 1.2% defined themselves as vegetarians. However, some of these individuals reported consumption of flesh foods during the 3 days on which dietary information was gathered, so it is not clear how vegetarianism was defined to the participants.[13]

A national Zogby poll sponsored by the Vegetarian Resource Group in 1994 reported that 12.4 million or about 7% of the U.S. population were self-reported vegetarians.[8] Analysis of the respondents' answers to the survey questions showed that approximately 1% of the population were true vegetarians (those who do not eat meat, fish, or fowl). However, the same poll administered in the year 2000[14] showed that the number of self-reported and true vegetarians is on the rise. The latest Zogby survey, defining vegetarians as those who never eat meat, poultry, or fish, concluded that 2.5% of the population can be considered vegetarian. It is worth noting that all Zogby surveys found that 0.9% of the population practices a vegan/strict vegetarian diet. Over the years, these Zogby polls identified the same linear trends as the RealEat polls in England did, although the percentage of vegetarians in the U.S. population is smaller.

In the U.S., regional differences exist in the prevalence of vegetarianism. The Zogby polls found a greater proportion of individuals not eating meat or calling themselves vegetarian in the West than in the East. The racial makeup and socioeconomic status of vegetarians or those not eating meat did not differ from the general population. Finally, more females than males consider themselves vegetarians. Again, these results are consistent with what has been found in the U.K.

There are several social and economic indicators, as well as anecdotal evidence, showing a trend toward acceptance and practice of a vegetarian diet, or, at a minimum, avoidance of meat. This evidence comes from industry-sponsored polls and product marketing research. The various types of vegetarian burgers have created a market of over $300 million,[9] catering to an estimated 20–30% of the population who regularly purchased this type of food product. In many geographic regions and in most big cities, it is hard to find a restaurant that will not accommodate a customer who desires vegetarian options. This is not surprising, as a 1991 Gallup poll conducted for the National Restaurant Association found that about 20% of the population looks for a restaurant with vegetarian items when they eat out.[15] Just 8 years later, in 1999, the Vegetarian Resource Group poll found that 57% of the population sometimes, often, or always orders a meatless option when eating out.[16] Another survey by the National Restaurant Association in 1994 reported that, on any given day, almost 15% of the nation's college students selected a vegetarian option in their dining halls and 97% of college foodservices have incorporated meatless options into their daily menus.[17] At least in the U.S., these data illustrate the restaurant- and food-industry response to the growing demand and interest of many consumers for meatless/vegetarian options.

VI. PUBLICATION TRENDS IN THE SCIENTIFIC LITERATURE

Professional interest in vegetarian nutrition has reached unprecedented levels. This is only partly explained by the growing numbers of vegetarians and the increased popularity of vegetarian diets.[18] The mounting evidence of the health benefits of certain vegetarian diets as presented in biomedical literature has also impacted on the professional and scientific interest in the subject.[19,20] The number and proportion of the total articles published on a particular topic in scientific journals reflects the interest of professionals in the subject at a particular time. Historical surveys and biblio-metric analysis of the scientific literature on vegetarian nutrition may provide an appropriate indicator of changes in attitude toward vegetarian nutrition and vegetarian diets among health professionals and scientists.

Hardinge and Crook evaluated the scientific literature covering vege-tarian diets and related topics up to 1962.[21] For that review article, the authors identified fewer than 100 reports on the subject, including books and book chapters, published in the English language. They identified research reports of metabolic and physiologic studies, growth, nutrient balance, vitamin B_{12} status, and deficiency diseases of vegetarians, as well as therapeutic applications of meatless diets and their effects on serum cholesterol. The paucity of reports in the scientific literature to that time on vegetarian nutrition, meatless diets, or "diets dependent mostly on plant foods," is evidenced by the relatively low scientific interest on these subjects up to the last third of the 20th century.

Sabaté et al.[22] documented publication trends in the biomedical liter-ature between 1966 to 1995 of articles related to vegetarian nutrition, using a bibliographic database. During those three decades, the total number of articles on vegetarian nutrition indexed in MEDLINE was 1309. Of those, 401 were published in nutrition journals; the remaining 908 were published in non-nutrition, mainly medical, and basic sciences journals. The publi-cation rate of vegetarian articles increased steadily during the three decades, from an average of less than 10 per year in the late 1960s to 76 articles per year in the early 1990s.

Figure 1.2 shows the average number of vegetarian nutrition articles published per year in peer-reviewed nutrition, non-nutrition, and all journals from 1966 to 1995, by 5-year time increments. Among nutrition journals, the publication rate increased from two to 22 per year over the 30-year span of this study, representing an 11-fold increase. A similar proportional increase was observed among non-nutrition journals, from an average of 5 to 54 per year during the period studied.

A point to consider is the relevance of these increases in light of secular increases in the total number of articles published in the biomedical literature during this period. From 1966 to 1995, there was a steady, almost linear increase in the total number of articles indexed in MEDLINE annu-ally. Figure 1.3 shows the proportion of vegetarian nutrition articles relative to all articles indexed by this bibliographic database. After adjusting for the number of articles indexed in MEDLINE each year, a dramatic increase was observed in the vegetarian literature during the 1970s, reaching an oscillating plateau during the 1980s with a new surge in the early 1990s. The rate of growth during the 1970s was about 400%, from fewer than five to 20 articles on vegetarian nutrition per 100,000 articles in the biomedical literature.

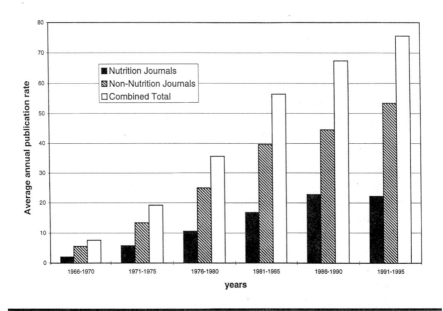

Figure 1.2   The annual average publication rate of vegetarian nutrition articles in nutrition journals, non-nutrition journals, and their combined total, 1966–1995.

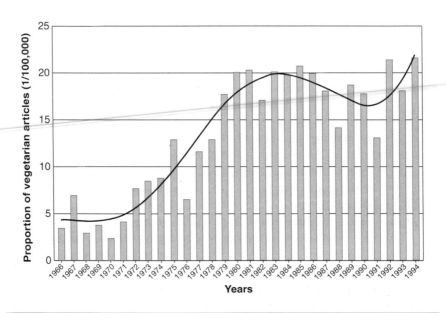

Figure 1.3   The ratio of vegetarian nutrition articles to the total number of articles indexed by MEDLINE annually between 1966 and 1995.

An interesting phenomenon is the steady decrease in the proportion of the total number of vegetarian nutrition articles published in nutrition journals compared with non-nutrition journals. Non-nutrition journals are progressively publishing a larger share of all vegetarian nutrition articles in the scientific literature. Figure 1.4 presents the proportion of vegetarian nutrition articles published in nutrition journals to those published in non-nutrition journals. The ratio shows a decreasing trend throughout the period studied, dropping from 72:1 during 1966–70 to 47:1 during 1991–95.

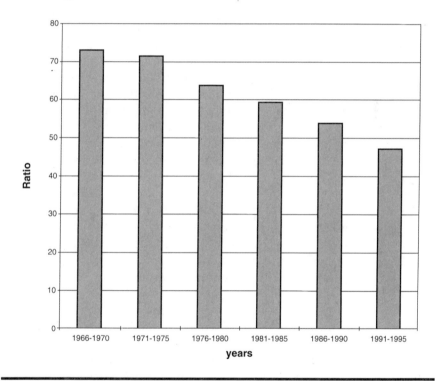

Figure 1.4 Vegetarian nutrition articles in nutrition journals as a proportion of those in non-nutrition journals.

In summary, this study documented a sharp increase in the number of vegetarian nutrition publications in the scientific literature during the last third of the last century. This increase occurred in both absolute and relative numbers and was observed in nutrition, as well as non-nutrition, journals. This increase in the publication of vegetarian nutrition articles in the scientific literature undoubtedly reflects increased professional interest in this subject over the past 30–40 years. Moreover, the number and proportion of vegetarian nutrition articles in nutritional journals relative to non-nutrition journals followed a downward trend. Non-nutrition journals are progressively publishing a larger share of all vegetarian nutrition articles in the biomedical literature. These trends can be interpreted as a growing interest in vegetarian nutrition issues among scientists and professionals of disciplines other than nutrition, a tendency for nutrition scientists to also publish in non-nutrition journals, or both.

Sabaté et al.[11] also used bibliometric techniques to quantify and assess scientific activity in the field of vegetarian nutrition. The authors attempted to evaluate the quality and tendencies of research on vegetarian nutrition on the basis of assessments of selected characteristics of the articles on the subject. Several trends emerged from these analyses. First, over the years, hard research data replaced soft data in that original research articles, the backbone of peer-reviewed professional journals, constituted the largest type of vegetarian nutrition publications in the 1990s, while letters to the editor, a less rigorous type of publication, constituted only a minority. Second, stronger study designs superseded weaker ones. Clinical trials on vegetarian diets were very common in the 1990s, whereas case reports of vegetarians were rare. The opposite was true in the 1960s. Similarly, reports in the scientific literature of epidemiological studies with longitudinal designs have now superseded in number and proportion the weaker cross-sectional designs.

A systematic tabulation of the main themes of the vegetarian nutrition articles published in the scientific literature between 1966 and 1995 are presented in Table 1.3. The proportion of topics addressed in these articles has changed throughout the period studied. Articles dealing with nutritional adequacy issues, such as nutritional status, deficiency diseases, adequacy of vegetarian diets, and growth or anthropometric indexes, prevailed (48%) in the first decade studied, but their overall frequency decreased over the years with a significant linear trend. Articles on preventive or therapeutic applications of vegetarian diets, such as the ones dealing with risk factors, chronic diseases, and other medical conditions, have increased over the years. Articles with multiple themes (any combination of the above) also increased over time, representing 9% of the total in the last decade. Thus, the main focus of vegetarian nutrition research has changed over time. While the major theme in 40% of all vegetarian nutrition articles published in the decade 1986–1995 was preventive and therapeutic applications of vegetarian diets, the nutritional adequacy of vegetarian diets was the major theme two decades earlier.

VII. CONCLUSION

The reality that there is a large and growing number of vegetarians mandates that health professionals in a variety of fields be informed of

Table 1.3 Main Themes of Published Vegetarian Nutrition Articles in the Biomedical Literature, 1966–1995

	Total	1966–1975	1976–1985	1986–1995	p-value*
	n(%)	n(%)	n(%)	n(%)	
Nutritional adequacy issues	162 (29.7)	14 (48.2)	66 (37.2)	82 (24.2)	0.001
Nutritional status	78 (14.3)	9 (31)	29 (16.4)	40 (11.8)	0.006
Deficiency diseases	32 (5.9)	2 (6.9)	16 (9)	14 (4.1)	0.058
Adequacy of vegetarian diets	41 (7.5)	3 (10.3)	16 (9)	22 (6.5)	0.241
Growth and anthropometric	11 (2)	0 (0)	5 (2.8)	6 (1.8)	0.899
Preventive and therapeutic applications	210 (38.6)	7 (24.1)	68 (38.5)	135 (40.0)	0.196
Risk factors	123 (22.6)	3 (10.3)	47 (26.6)	73 (21.6)	0.982
Chronic diseases	38 (7)	2 (6.9)	9 (5.1)	27 (8)	0.333
Medical conditions	49 (9)	2 (6.9)	12 (6.8)	35 (10.4)	0.575
Multiple themes**	40 (7.4)	0 (0)	10 (5.6)	30 (8.9)	0.044
Guidelines and recommendations	45 (8.3)	2 (6.9)	12 (6.8)	31 (9.2)	0.193
Other	87 (16)	6 (20.7)	21 (11.9)	60 (17.8)	0.367
Total	544 (100)	29 (100)	177 (100)	338 (100)	

*chi-square test for linear trends
**any combination of ≥ 2 of the above-listed themes

the health benefits and risks associated with these often diverse dietary practices. Considering the paucity of reliable data on those following vegetarian diets, more research is necessary to identify characteristics of vegetarians, their actual dietary practices and the rationale for them.

Up to 1962, fewer than 100 journal articles or book chapters were published in the scientific literature on issues related to vegetarian nutrition. However, since 1966, a phenomenal growth in the number and proportion of vegetarian nutrition articles has been documented in the biomedical literature. The sustained increases in publication rate of vegetarian nutrition articles during the last decades is both responsible for and reflects the increased professional interest in vegetarian diets and vegetarian nutrition. The types of research articles on vegetarian nutrition have evolved over the years from more observational to more analytic, paralleling similar trends in other areas of scientific endeavor. The observed progressive change in the main themes of published vegetarian nutrition articles is interpreted as a shift in the role of vegetarian diets in human nutrition. In the past 30 to 40 years, scientific endeavors in the area of vegetarian nutrition have progressively shifted from investigating concerns held by nutritionists and other health professionals to a fertile area of investigation in which creative solutions for various medical conditions and preventive approaches to chronic diseases may well be discovered.

REFERENCES

1. *Merriam Webster's Collegiate Dictionary 10th ed.*, Merriam-Webster, Inc.; Springfield, MA; 1993; 1309.
2. Weinsier R. Use of the term vegetarian, *Am J Clin Nutr* 71(5):1211-12, 2000. Letter to the editor.
3. Willett W.C. Convergence of philosophy and science: the third international congress on vegetarian nutrition, *Am J Clin Nutr* 70(3S):434S-438S, 1999.
4. Melina V., Davis B., Harrison V. *Becoming Vegetarian*, Book Publishing Co., Summertown, TN, 1995, 2.
5. Johnston P.K. Nutritional implications of vegetarian diets, in *Modern Nutrition in Health and Disease*, Shils M.E., Olson J.A., Shike M., Ross A.C., Eds., Williams & Wilkens, Baltimore, MD, 1999, 1756.
6. Vegetarian Times, Eds., *Vegetarian Times Vegetarian Beginner's Guide*, Macmillan, New York, 1996, 3.
7. The American Vegetarian: Coming of Age in the 90s – A study of the Vegetarian marketplace conducted for Vegetarian Times by Yankelovich, Skelly and White/Clancy, Shulman, Inc., 1992.
8. Stahler C. *Veg J*, 13:6-9, 1994.
9. Grande S., Leckie S. Meat avoiders & casual vegetarians. Toronto Vegetarian Association Newsletter 5/6 1997.
10. Erhard D. The new vegetarians. *Nutr Today*, 8:4-12, 1973.
11. RealEat Surveys (1984-1997). Gallup surveys into meat-eating and vegetarianism conducted for the RealEat Company Ltd. London.
12. National Research Council, Eds., *Diet and Health*, National Academy Press, Washington, D.C., 1989, 42.
13. National Research Council, Eds., *Diet and Health*, National Academy Press, Washington, D.C., 1989, 76.
14. Vegetarian Journal, Eds., How many vegetarians are there?. *Veg J*. 5/6 2000.
15. Vegetarian Journal, Eds., How many vegetarians are there?. *Veg J*. 9/10, 1997.
16. Vegetarian Journal, Eds., How many people order vegetarian meals when eating out?, *Veg J*. 9/10, 1999.
17. Growing interest in vegetarianism among campus food services, *J Am Diet Assoc*, 1994, 94:596.
18. White R., Frank E. Health effects and prevalence of vegetarianism. *West J Med* 1994;160:465-71.
19. Messina V.K., Burke K.I. Position of the American Dietetic Association: vegetarian diets. *J Am Diet Assoc* 1997;97:1317-21.
20. Messina M., Messina V., Eds., *The Dietitian's Guide to Vegetarian Diets*, Aspen Publishers, Gaithersburg, MD, 1996, 17-78.
21. Hardinge M.G., Crooks, H. Non-flesh dietaries II. Scientific literature *J Am Diet Assoc* 1963;43:550-8.

22. Sabaté J., Duk A., Lee C.L. Publication trends of vegetarian nutrition articles in biomedical literature, 1966-1995 *Am J Clin Nutr* 1999;70(S):601S-7S.
23. Messina M., Messina V., Eds., *The Dietitian's Guide to Vegetarian Diets*, Aspen Publishers, Gaithersburg, MD, 1996, 6.

2

THE PUBLIC HEALTH RISK-TO-BENEFIT RATIO OF VEGETARIAN DIETS: CHANGING PARADIGMS

Joan Sabaté

CONTENTS

I.   INTRODUCTION

Scientific advances during the last decades have noticeably changed our understanding of the role of vegetarian diets in human health and disease. Because of famines, infectious diseases, accidents, or wars, the average human life expectancy up to the beginning of the 20th century was very low. However, in the last century, populations living in industrialized

0-8493-8508-3/01/$0.00+$.50
© 2001 by CRC Press LLC

countries have experienced a sharp increase in life expectancy due to successful public health interventions. As disease patterns shifted away from nutrient deficiencies and infectious diseases toward chronic and degenerative diseases, nutrition policy and research also changed emphasis.

An adequate diet, by definition, is one that prevents nutrient deficiencies by providing sufficient nutrients and energy for human growth and reproduction. Additionally, an optimal diet promotes health and longevity, characterized by a reduction in risks for diet-related chronic diseases. The precise composition of the optimal diet is not completely known; however, scientific consensus is proposing that diets largely based on plant foods could best prevent nutrient deficiencies as well as diet-related chronic diseases.

After introducing a perspective on the health risks of vegetarian diets, this chapter presents three models depicting the expected health risks and benefits of populations following either a vegetarian diet or a meat-based diet. In a way, these models encapsulate the evolution of our scientific understanding of the overall effects of these dietary patterns on human health.

II. AN OVERESTIMATION OF THE HEALTH RISKS OF VEGETARIAN DIETS?

Compared with animal foods, plant foods generally have lower concentration and bioavailability for some essential nutrients and energy. This may represent an advantage for adult sedentary populations and the prevention of chronic diseases. However, in situations of high metabolic demand, such as in pregnancy, lactation, and during the growing years, those following a vegetarian diet are at higher risk for marginal intakes or even biochemical or clinical nutrient deficiencies than those following a meat-based diet.

A review of the early nutrition literature on vegetarian diets portrays a cornucopia of nutrient deficiencies and children with compromised physical growth in single case or case series reports.[1,2] A systematic assessment of vegetarian nutrition articles published in the biomedical literature from 1966 to 1995 documented that, 30 years ago, half of the articles dealt with nutrition adequacy issues such as deficiency diseases, nutritional status, and growth, while two decades later, the frequency of these themes decreased to 24%.[3] In contrast, articles on the preventive and therapeutic aspects of vegetarian diets followed opposite temporal trends.[3]

This early emphasis in the biomedical literature on the health risks related to the consumption of vegetarian diets could be explained by several historical, methodological, and sociological reasons. First, nutrient adequacy, rather than optimal nutrient intake, until recently was the emphasis of nutrition science and policy. In industrialized countries, nutrient deficiency diseases were much more prevalent some decades ago than currently. Nutritional science concentrated its efforts on identifying and proposing adequate nutrient intake values. The idea of meeting nutritional needs was predominant. Dietary prevention of chronic and degenerative diseases was not an issue at that time. Thus, from a historical perspective, it is not surprising that the main focus when studying vegetarian diets was to determine if they met the normative nutrient intake values.[4]

Second, nutritional science research and endeavors followed, until recently, the clinical model approach. It was easier to prepare case reports of vegetarians with medical problems coming to the clinic than to actually go to the community, identify vegetarians, follow them over time, and report on their health and disease status, as is required by the public health model approach. Moreover, most of the nutrition research done in the past was on the short-term health effects of diet. Due to its nature, the study of the health effects of diet on chronic diseases requires long-term approach methodology. The classic methods of nutritionists, such as laboratory tests, animal experiments, or human metabolic studies, were well suited to examining different aspects of the adequacy of vegetarian diets but not their effects on chronic diseases. These diseases have long latency periods and multiple causes. Nutritional epidemiology, a relatively young discipline, was needed to directly address the relationship between vegetarian diets and chronic diseases and longevity.

Finally, a cultural bias against meatless diets contributed to the publication and increased awareness of potential health risks of vegetarian diets. Up to the 1970s, those following vegetarian diets were assumed to be part of the anti-establishment underground culture or members of a religious sect, and the avoidance of meat was for reasons other than health.[5,6] Mainstream society in industrialized nations, those paying for research, were by and large non-vegetarians and scientists performing research, who probably did not perceive the cultural bias and therefore did not allow for it on this issue.

III. EARLY MODEL ON VEGETARIAN DIETS

Figure 2.1 shows an early model comparing the adequacy of vegetarian diets with diets largely based on animal foods. This model prevailed for the first part of the 20th century. In this figure, the area under each curve represents the proportion of the population for which a given diet pattern may be adequate or deficient. The basic tenet was that if a population were to follow a vegetarian diet it would be more prone to develop

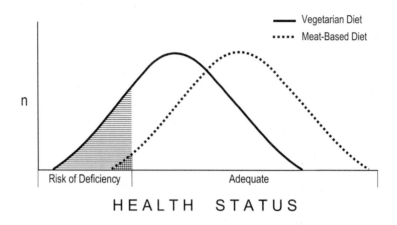

Figure 2.1   Early model on the adequacy of vegetarian diets. The area under each curve represents the proportion of individuals in a population for whom a given diet may be adequate or deficient.

nutrient deficiency diseases than if on a diet based on animal foods. This was, and still is, the case in poor countries, where the relation between diet and health, and particularly meat consumption and health, is confounded with several socioeconomic parameters.

Parenthetically, it was suggested that one practical way to decrease the probability of nutrient deficiencies for those following meatless diets was to add to the diet generous amounts of other animal products such as eggs and dairy products,[4] thus making, de facto, a mixed diet and displacing the curve to the right. This early model used a unilateral approach in the relationship of vegetarian diets to health, since it paid attention only to the health risks and did not take into account their potential benefits.

IV.   HEALTH BENEFITS OF VEGETARIAN DIETS

All types of diets have potential health risks as well as benefits associated with their consumption, both at the individual and collective level. Plant-based vegetarian diets are no exception to this rule. Nutritionists and other health professionals should be aware of the potential nutritional risks associated with vegetarian diets and suggest ways to minimize them; however, it is also important to take notice of the potential benefits associated with this diet pattern.

During the past 30 years, scores of nutritional epidemiological studies have documented important and quantifiable benefits of vegetarian and other plant-based diets, namely a reduction of risk for many chronic degenerative diseases and total mortality.[7] Such evidence is derived from the study of vegetarians as well as other populations. Vegetarians living in affluent countries enjoy remarkably good health, exemplified by low rates of obesity,[8-10] coronary diseases,[11-13] diabetes,[14] many cancers,[14-16] and increased longevity.[17] This is possibly due to the absence of meat in the diet and a greater amount and variety of plant foods.[18] While meat intake has been related to increased risk for a variety of chronic diseases such as ischemic heart disease[11] and some cancers,[17,19] an abundant consumption of essential food components of the vegetarian diet such as fruits and vegetables,[20-22] legumes, unrefined cereals,[23-26] and nuts[23,27-28] have consistently been associated with a lower risk for many chronic degenerative diseases, and, in some cases, increased longevity. Hence, foods of plant origin seem to be beneficial on their own merit for chronic disease prevention. This is possibly more definite than the detrimental effects of meats.[18] It is worth noting that epidemiological studies of diet and health among vegetarian and non-vegetarian populations have observed many more correlations between the protective effect of plant foods than the hazardous effects of animal foods such as meat and dairy products.[17]

V. PUBLIC HEALTH RISK-TO-BENEFIT RATIO OF VEGETARIAN AND MEAT-BASED DIETS

It is now well accepted that the relationship between a dietary factor and health is not linear. There is an optimal range of intake, but at both extremes there are marginal or detrimental intake ranges, and further apart are deficient or toxic intake ranges.[29] In general, the same idea may apply to the diet patterns, since they can be considered as combinations of dietary factors. Great concern exists about the potential health risks of excessive consumption of some nutrients. In answer, most of the current dietary guidelines for chronic disease prevention place caps on the consumption of many dietary factors, especially macronutrients, alcohol, and total energy intake.

A basic public health tenet is that any intervention must weigh the risks against the benefits. Whether concerning a vaccination program, the fluorination of water, or a lifestyle change, the principle should be the same. If we consider vegetarian diet patterns as a public health intervention, the increased risk for the now-rare nutrient deficiencies in most affluent nations must be weighed against the reduction of risk prevention for chronic diseases. Reciprocally, the excessively high risk for chronic diseases currently found in affluent populations following diets based on animal foods must be weighed against the clearly decreased risk for the classic nutrient deficiencies in these populations.

Figure 2.2 depicts a model that allows for the health risks and benefits of vegetarian and meat-based diets. The area under each curve represents

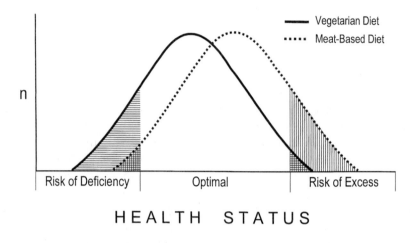

n

| Risk of Deficiency | Optimal | Risk of Excess |

Vegetarian Diet
····· Meat-Based Diet

HEALTH STATUS

Figure 2.2   Current model on the public health risks and benefits of vegetarian and meat-based diets. The area under each curve represents the proportion of individuals in a population for whom a given diet pattern may be a health risk or benefit (optimal). At both extremes of the health continuum there is risk of disease through deficiency or excess of nutrients. The area in the center represents the proportion of individuals for whom the diet is optimal or most beneficial.

the proportion of the population for which a given diet pattern may be of risk or benefit. At both extremes of this continuum there is the risk of disease, with either a deficiency or an excess of nutrients. The area in the center represents the proportion of subjects for which the diet is optimal or most beneficial. The risk–benefit ratio of a diet can easily be defined as the proportion of subjects at risk divided by the proportion of subjects benefiting. To calculate the proportion of the population at risk will obviously require the addition of both the risk of deficiency and the risk of excess. In Figure 2.2, if we add both areas with the cross-hatched lines, we will get the proportion of the population that is at risk (through deficiency or excess) by following a plant-based vegetarian diet pattern. Similarly, both areas on vertical lines represent the proportion of the population at risk by following a diet pattern largely based on animal foods.

On this rendition of the model, there is no overall difference in the risk–benefit ratio of one diet versus the other diet pattern. This version of the model (Figure 2.2) is prone to the interpretation that no overall improvements would be accomplished if the population distribution curve were to be displaced to the right or left by changing the mix of plant and animal foods in the diet. If the curves move, the same amount gained

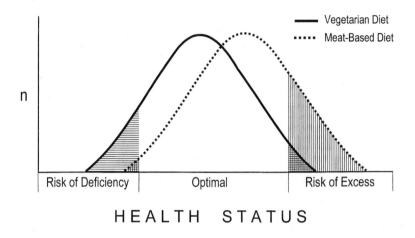

n

Risk of Deficiency | Optimal | Risk of Excess

HEALTH STATUS

Figure 2.3 Model depicting an overall lower risk–benefit ratio for the vegetarian diet than for the meat-based diet. The risk–benefit ratio of a diet pattern is defined as the proportion of subjects at risk (deficiency or excess) divided by the proportion of subjects benefiting (optimal). (See Figure 2.2 legend for more explanation.)

in one end is lost at the other. This apparent public health dilemma, the seemingly inevitable trade-off of malnutrition with over-nutrition diseases, was already described in 1979 by Olson.[30] He proposed a similar version of this model when contrasting the Asian diet, also largely based on plant foods, with the typical meat-based American diet at that time. Olson stated that if one were to change the American diet to greatly reduce animal protein and increase carbohydrate from processed grains, the nutritional status curve would move to the left, and he argued that, "for every case of coronary disease avoided, there would be a case of infant malnutrition."

However, Olson failed to recognize that, in the public health model he proposed, a trade-off in disease morbidity due to changes in the diet was not so predictable. Actually, this model shows that small displacements of the population distribution curve may yield, in one way or another, substantial differences in the risk–benefit ratio of contrasting diet patterns. This is really the case when comparing a vegetarian diet with a diet based on animal foods.

Figure 2.3 presents another version of the same public health model. This figure, however, depicts a lower risk–benefit ratio for the vegetarian diet than for the meat-based diet, thus portraying vegetarian diets more favorablly from the public health viewpoint than diets based on animal foods. In practical terms, if one were to exchange small amounts of vegetables for small amounts of dairy products or eggs on a strict vegetarian or vegan diet, the substantial reduction in risk for vitamin B_{12}

deficiency in the population will not be offset by the small increase in risk for coronary diseases. Hence, a small displacement of the vegetarian diet curve to the right results in an overall more favorable risk–benefit ratio. However, on a diet largely based on animal foods, exchanging small amounts of meat for vegetables will not noticeably move the curve to the left. Major exchanges in the meat-based diet would be required to slightly displace the curve to the left and improve the risk–benefit ratio for this diet pattern.

For most individuals in an era of abundance of foods such as in industrialized societies today, a meat-based diet can more easily exceed the optimal intake range for many nutrients and energy than a vegetarian diet can fall below the requirements for other nutrients. Additionally, according to this model, it seems that incorporating small amounts of animal products in vegetarian diets may greatly reduce the risk for acute nutrient deficiencies without much increase in risk for chronic diseases.

VI.   A PROPOSED NEW MODEL

A new paradigm is emerging. For the last 10 to 20 years, epidemiological, clinical, and basic science research on the health effects of several plant foods is greatly expanding our understanding of the role these foods have on human health and nutrition. Antioxidants abundantly present in plant foods have been postulated to prevent cardiovascular disease and many cancers, and to postpone the aging process. Anticarcinogenic properties have been described for a myriad of substances present mainly in fruits and vegetables and other plant foods.[31,32]

Plant foods, such as fruit, vegetables, legumes, nuts and whole grains, provide active substances on which human metabolism is dependent. However, only a few of these to date have been labeled as "essential nutrients." Fruits and vegetables are not only rich sources of carotenoids, ascorbic acid, tocopherols, folic acid, and dietary fiber, but also provide to the diet, indoles, thiocyanates, cumarins, phenols, flavonoids, terpenes, protease inhibitors, plant sterols, and a host of other yet unknown and unnamed phytochemicals and "non-nutrient" compounds that may protect humans from many cancers and other diseases.[22,33].

The increased risk for cancer and cardiovascular disease experienced by populations following diets largely based on animal foods as opposed to vegetarians, may be due not only to an excess of energy, total and saturated fat, and other nutrients, but also to a deficiency or very marginal intake of phytochemicals and other substances abundant in plant foods but not yet labeled as "nutrients." Accordingly, chronic degenerative diseases may also be considered deficiency diseases, as well as diseases of excess. Therefore, the contribution of diets largely based on animal

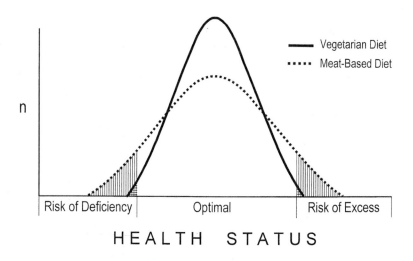

Figure 2.4   **Proposed model on the public health risks and benefits of vegetarian and meat-based diets. (See Figure 2.2 legend for more explanation.)**

foods to the causation of human diseases from excess, unbalance, or deficiency appears to be notoriously different from what was estimated earlier

Figure 2.4 presents our proposed model trying to capture the new understanding of the roles vegetarian and meat-based diets play in human health and disease in affluent societies. As in previous public health models, the area under each diet pattern curve is the same; however, the shape of the two curves varies considerably as a result of the different distribution of individuals in the population by health status. In this new model, the relative contribution to the causation and prevention of diseases through excess or deficiency is clearly unequal for the two contrasted diets, with a much more favorable risk-to-benefit ratio for the vegetarian diet.

The expanded area on risk of deficiency under the meat-based diet curve portrays the risk of diseases attributed to phytochemical deficiency due to the marginal intake of plant foods on this diet pattern. In affluent societies, this model considers the risk of phytochemical deficiency diseases — namely an unknown proportion of cancers, cardiovascular and other degenerative diseases — among those following a meat-based diet to be greater than the risk of the classic acute nutrient deficiency diseases for vegetarians.

VII. CONCLUSION

Our knowledge is far from complete regarding the relationship between vegetarian diets and human health. However, scientific advances in the last decades have considerably changed the role that vegetarian diets may play in human nutrition. Essential components of a vegetarian diet include a variety of vegetables, fruits, whole-grain cereals, legumes, and nuts. Numerous studies show important and quantifiable benefits of the different components of vegetarian diets, namely the reduction of risk for many chronic diseases and the increase in longevity. Such evidence is derived from the study of vegetarians as well as other populations. While meat intake has been related to increased risk for a variety of chronic diseases, an abundant consumption of vegetables, fruits, cereals, nuts, and legumes has been independently related to a lower risk for several chronic degenerative diseases such as ischemic heart disease, diabetes, obesity, and many cancers. Also, frequency of consumption of plant foods has been identified as a factor for increased longevity in industrialized nations. Hence, foods of plant origin seem to be beneficial on their own merit for chronic-disease prevention. This is possibly more certain than the detrimental effects of meats.

Vegetarian diets, as any other diet pattern, have potential health risks, namely marginal intake of a few essential nutrients. However, from the public health viewpoint, the health benefits of a plant-based vegetarian diet far outweigh the potential risks. The ensuing chapters are intended to further our progress in this direction.

REFERENCES

1. MacLean W.C. and Graham G.G. Vegetarianism in children. *Am J Dis Child,* 134: 513, 1980.
2. Hardinge M.G. and Crooks H. Non-flesh Dietaries II. *JADA,* 43:550-8, 1963.
3. Sabaté J., Duk A., and Lee C.L. Publication trends of vegetarian nutrition articles in biomedical literature, 1966-1995 *Am J Clin Nutr,* 70(S):601S-7S, 1999.
4. Register U.D. and Sonnenbeg L.M. The vegetarian diet. *JADA,* 62:253-261, 1973.
5. Weinsier R. Use of the term vegetarian, *Am J Clin Nutr,* 71(5):1211-12, 2000. Letter
6. Dwyer J.T., Mayer L.D., Kandel R.F., and Mayer J. The new vegetarians. *JADA,* 62(5):503-9, 1973.
7. Messina V.K. and Burke K.I. Position of the American Dietetic Association: vegetarian diets, *J Am Diet Assoc,* 11:1317-21 1997.
8. Key T. and Davey G. Prevalence of obesity is low in people who do not eat meat, *BMJ,* 313:816-817, 1996. Letter.
9. Singh P.N. and Lindsted K.D. Body mass and 26-year risk of mortality from specific diseases among women who never smoked. *Epidemiology,* 9(3):246-54, May 1998.

10. Appleby P.N., Thorogood M., Mann J.I., and Key T.J. Low body mass index in non meat eaters: the possible roles of animal fat, dietary fibre and alcohol. *Int J Obes Relat Metab Disord*, 22(5):454-60, 1998.

11. Snowdon D.A., Phillips R.L., and Fraser G.E. Meat consumption and fatal ischemic heart disease. *Prev Med*, 13:490-500, 1984.

12. Fraser G.E., Linsted K.D., and Beeson W.L. Effect of risk factor values on lifetime risk of and age at first coronary event. The Adventist Health Study. *Am J Epidemiol*, 142:746-58, 1995.

13. Thorogood M., Mann J., Appleby P., and McPherson K. Risk of death from cancer and ischemic heart disease in meat and non-meat eaters. *BMJ*, 308:1667-70, 1994.

14. Snowdon D.A. and Phillips R.L. Does a vegetarian diet reduce the occurrence of diabetes? *Am J Public Health*, 75:507-12, 1985.

15. Mills P.K., Beeson W.L., Phillips R.L., and Fraser G.E. Cancer incidence among California Seventh-day Adventists, 1976-1982. *Am J Clin Nutr*, 59(S):1136S-42S, 1994.

16. Phillips R.L., Garfinkel L., Kuzma J.W., Beeson W.L., Lotz T., and Brin B. Mortality among California Seventh-day Adventists for selected cancer sites. *J Natl Cancer Inst*, 65:1097-107, 1980.

17. Fraser G.E. Associations between diet and cancer, ischemic heart disease, and all-cause mortality in non-Hispanic white California Seventh-day Adventists. *Am J Clin Nutr*, 70(S):532S-538S, 1999.

18. Willett W.C. Convergence of philosophy and science: the Third International Congress on Vegetarian Nutrition. *Am J Clin Nutr*, 70(S):434S-438S, 1999.

19. Giovannucci E. and Willett W.C. Dietary factors and risk of colon cancer. *Ann Med*, 26:443-52, 1994.

20. Steinmetz K.A. and Potter J.D. Vegetables, fruit and cancer. I. Epidemiology. *Cancer Causes Control*, 2:325-57, 1991.

21. Block G., Patterson B., and Subar A. Fruit, vegetables, and cancer prevention: a review of the epidemiological evidence. *Nutr Cancer*, 18:1-29, 1992.

22. Rimm E.B., Ascherio A., Giovannucci E., Spiegelman D., Stampfer M.J., and Willett W.C. Vegetable, fruit, and cereal fiber intake and risk of coronary heart disease among men. *JAMA*, 275:447-51, 1996.

23. Fraser G.E., Sabate J., Beeson W.L., and Strahan T.M. A possible protective effect of nut consumption on risk of coronary heart disease. The Adventist Health Study. *Arch Intern Med*, 152:1416-24, 1992.

24. Jacobs D.R., Jr., Meyer K.A., Kushi L.H., and Folsom A.R. Whole-grain intake may reduce the risk of ischemic heart disease death in post-menopausal women: the Iowa Women's Health Study. *Am J Clin Nutr*, 68:248-57, 1998.

25. Jacobs D.R., Jr., Slavin J., and Marquart L. Whole grain intake and cancer: a review of the literature. *Nutr Cancer*, 24:221-9, 1995.

26. Kushi L.H., Meyer K.A., Jacobs D.R., Jr., Cereals, legumes, and chronic disease risk reduction: evidence from epidemiological studies. *Am J Clin Nutr*, 70(S):451S-458S, 1999.

27. Hu F.B., Stampfer M.J., Manson J.E., Rimm E.B., Colditz G.A., Rosner B.A., et al. Frequent nut consumption and risk of coronary heart disease in women: prospective cohort study. *BMJ*, 317(7169):1341-5, 1998.

28. Sabaté J. Nut consumption, vegetarian diets, ischemic heart disease risk, and all-cause mortality: evidence from epidemiologic studies. *Am J Clin Nutr*, 70(S):500S-3S, 1999.

29. Mertz W. The essential trace elements. *Science*, 213:1332-8, 1981.
30. Olson R.E. Is there an optimum diet for the prevention of coronary heart disease, in *Nutrition, Lipids, and Coronary Heart Disease*, Levy R., Rifkind B., Dennis B., and Ernst N., Eds., Raven Press, New York, 1979.
31. Bidlack W.R., Omaye S.T., Meskin M.S., and Jahner D. *Phytochemicals: A New Paradigm*, Technomic, Lancaster, PA, 1998.
32. World Cancer Research Fund/American Institute for Cancer Research. *Food, Nutrition and the Prevention of Cancer: A Global Perspective*, Washington, D.C., 1997.
33. American Institute for Cancer Research. *Dietary Phytochemicals in Cancer Prevention and Treatment: Advances in Experimental Medicine and Biology Volume 401*, Plenum Press, London, 1996.

II

VEGETARIAN DIETS AND CHRONIC DISEASE PREVENTION

3

VEGETARIANISM, CORONARY RISK FACTORS AND CORONORY HEART DISEASE

Timothy J. Key and Paul N. Appleby

CONTENTS

0-8493-8508-3/01/$0.00+$.50
© 2001 by CRC Press LLC

I. INTRODUCTION

Coronary heart disease (CHD) is the major cause of death in most Western countries, and is rapidly becoming a major cause of death in developing countries too. Lopez and Murray[1] predicted that, by the year 2020, CHD will be the leading cause of disease worldwide. Differences in the diets consumed by different populations account for much of the observed variation in CHD mortality rates, and the effect of vegetarian diets on CHD is a topic of great interest.

Vegetarian diets are defined by what they do not include and can vary enormously in terms of both foods and nutrients. The diets of affluent Western vegetarians are very different from those of poor vegetarians in developing countries. Even within Western countries, vegetarian diets vary substantially according to the degree of exclusion of animal foods and according to whether the diet is followed predominately for ethical or health reasons. In view of this, any discussion of the health effects of a vegetarian diet must take into account the type of vegetarian diet studied and, equally important, the type of diet of the non-vegetarian comparison group. In this chapter, we concentrate on studies that compare vegetarians with non-vegetarians from a similar background. Unless otherwise specified, reference to vegetarians means lacto-ovovegetarians, because relatively few data are available for vegans.

In section II, we review the established and possible risk factors for CHD and comment on their relationships with vegetarian diets. Behavioral risk factors such as smoking should be considered as potential confounding factors that are not due to diet but that could cause differences in CHD rates between vegetarians and non-vegetarians; it is important that statistical analyses adjust for such factors. In contrast, factors such as fruit and vegetable consumption and body mass index are either components of the vegetarian diet or are strongly determined by diet; such factors are not confounders and, in general, it is not appropriate to adjust for these factors in statistical analyses.

In section III, we review epidemiological studies of CHD in vegetarians and the use of a low-fat vegetarian diet in the secondary prevention of CHD. Topics requiring further research are considered in section IV and our conclusions are presented in section V.

II. VEGETARIANISM AND CORONARY RISK FACTORS

A. Established Risk Factors

1. Lipids and Lipoproteins

Serum total cholesterol concentration is the most important biochemical risk factor for CHD. There is an approximately linear relationship between serum total cholesterol and the risk of death from CHD. Most studies have underestimated the strength of this relationship because they have categorized individuals on the basis of a single measurement of serum cholesterol, which is only imperfectly correlated with the usual long-term cholesterol level of an individual. Correction for this underestimation, due to the "regression dilution bias," increases the strength of the relationship between serum cholesterol and CHD. Law et al.[2] estimated that a 0.6 mmol/l reduction in serum total cholesterol causes a 24% reduction in mortality from CHD in middle-aged men. The effect is greater at younger ages; a reduction of total serum cholesterol of 0.6 mmol/l is estimated to reduce the incidence of CHD by 54% at age 40, 39% at age 50, 27% at age 60, 20% at age 70 and 19% at age 80.[3] Importantly, the relationship between serum cholesterol concentration and CHD is observed not only in Western populations with high average serum cholesterol concentrations, but also within populations with relatively low cholesterol levels by Western standards, suggesting that reductions in cholesterol would reduce CHD rates in most populations.[4]

The association between serum total cholesterol and CHD mortality is largely due to low-density lipoprotein (LDL) cholesterol, which in Western countries typically comprises about four-fifths of total serum cholesterol. The relationship between LDL cholesterol and CHD mortality is stronger than that for total cholesterol — Law et al. estimated that a 0.6 mmol/l reduction in LDL cholesterol causes a 27% reduction in mortality from CHD.[2]

The other major component of total cholesterol is high-density lipoprotein (HDL) cholesterol that is inversely related to the risk of CHD.[5] Therefore, it is important to consider both LDL cholesterol and HDL cholesterol when discussing the effects of vegetarian diets on serum lipids and CHD risk.

Since the pioneering work of Hardinge and Stare,[6] numerous studies have established that vegetarians have lower total serum cholesterol con-

Table 3.1 Plasma Lipid Concentrations in Vegetarians and Non-Vegetarians, Adjusted for Age and Sex[a]

Diet	N	Total Cholesterol (mmol l⁻¹)		LDL-Cholesterol (mmol l⁻¹)		HDL-Cholesterol (mmol l⁻¹)	
		Mean	SE	Mean	SE	Mean	SE
Meat-eater	1198	5.31	0.101	3.17	0.091	1.49	0.035
Vegetarian	1550	4.88	0.100	2.74	0.090	1.50	0.035
Vegan	114	4.29	0.140	2.28	0.126	1.49	0.048

[a]From Thorogood et al.[7]

centrations than comparable non-vegetarians. In Britain, data on 3277 participants in the Oxford Vegetarian Study showed that total cholesterol was, on average, 0.43 mmol/l lower in vegetarians than in meat-eaters.[7] This difference was entirely due to differences in LDL cholesterol, which was also 0.43 mmol/l lower in the vegetarians (Table 3.1). Among vegans, total cholesterol was 1.02 mmol/l lower than in meat-eaters, largely due to a difference of 0.89 mmol/l in LDL cholesterol. The principal dietary determinant of total cholesterol in this population was fat intake, as summarized by the Keys score[8] calculated from the intake of saturated fatty acids, polyunsaturated fatty acids, and cholesterol.[9]

The relatively low serum total cholesterol of vegetarians has been observed in diverse populations, including white American Seventh-Day Adventists,[10,11] American commune-dwelling vegans,[12] American macrobiotic vegetarians,[13] British vegetarians,[14,15] elderly Chinese vegetarians,[16] Slovakian vegetarians,[17] West African Seventh-Day Adventists,[18] Siberian vegans,[19] German vegetarians,[20] and many others.[21] Furthermore, intervention trials have demonstrated that changing to a vegetarian diet can reduce serum cholesterol concentrations.[21,22] However, a vegetarian diet was not significantly related to plasma cholesterol concentrations among Asians from the Indian subcontinent living in London[23] or among Asian Indian physicians living in the USA.[24]

The effects of a vegetarian diet on HDL cholesterol levels are less clear. The Oxford Vegetarian Study found that HDL levels were the same in vegans, vegetarians, and meat-eaters (Table 3.1), and that the principal dietary determinant of HDL cholesterol in this population was alcohol intake.[9,25] In contrast, Fraser[11] reported that HDL cholesterol was lower in largely vegetarian Seventh-Day Adventists than in their neighbors, with the result that the ratio of total to HDL cholesterol was almost identical in the two groups. Replacement of total fat by complex carbohydrate lowers HDL cholesterol[26] and it is likely that the British vegetarians did not have lower HDL cholesterol than non-vegetarians because they did not have a low total fat intake.[9] The relatively low level of HDL cholesterol in Seventh-Day Adventists may be due to their abstinence from alcohol, because alcohol raises HDL cholesterol.[11]

In terms of coronary risk, the data on lipid levels in vegetarians imply that they are definitely at lower risk in terms of their levels of total and LDL cholesterol, but that, within some populations, part of this benefit might be offset by an accompanying reduction in HDL cholesterol levels.

The role of triacylglycerol as an independent risk factor for CHD has been uncertain, because adjustment for HDL cholesterol has tended to reduce or eliminate the association. However, a recent meta-analysis of prospective studies has shown that triacylglycerol is an independent risk factor for CHD; Austin et al.[27] found that, after adjustment for HDL cholesterol, a 1 mmol/l increase in triacylglycerol was associated with increases in cardiovascular disease risk of 14% and 37% in men and women, respectively. Some small studies have reported that vegetarians have lower plasma triacylglycerol concentrations than meat-eaters,[13,18] but other studies have not observed any difference between vegetarians and non-vegetarians.[16]

2. Hypertension

CHD is linearly related to increasing levels of systolic and diastolic blood pressure.[28] As with serum cholesterol, most epidemiological studies have underestimated the size of the effect because they used a single measurement of blood pressure for each individual. After correction for this regression dilution bias, a reduction in diastolic blood pressure of 10 mmHg was associated with a 37% reduction in the risk of CHD (and a 56% reduction in the risk of stroke).[29]

The principal diet-related determinants of high blood pressure are obesity, high alcohol intake, high sodium intake, and low potassium intake.[30,31] Most comparative studies have found that vegetarians are thinner and have a lower alcohol intake than non-vegetarians, and that they have a higher potassium intake, but there is no consistent evidence that vegetarians have a low sodium intake; some vegetarian foods are high in sodium. A number of studies have examined the association of vegetarian diets with blood pressure. Some studies comparing groups of vegetarians and non-vegetarians found lower blood pressure in the vegetarians, but other studies found no difference.[32] Randomized trials of the effects of vegetarian diets on blood pressure have shown reductions in blood pressure of around 5 mmHg that were not due to changes in sodium intake and did not appear to be explicable by changes in other relevant nutrients such as potassium.[32] Subsequent trials have attempted to establish whether the apparent hypotensive effect of a vegetarian diet could be explained by changes in nutrients such as fat and dietary fiber, but the results have been inconclusive.[32]

Some populations in rural Japan and China have semi-vegetarian diets, with a low intake of meat and dairy products and a heavy reliance on staple plant foods. These populations have a high prevalence of hypertension and high rates of stroke, but also have low cholesterol levels and low rates of CHD. The high prevalence of hypertension may be largely due to a high salt intake, but this observation demonstrates that a semi-vegetarian diet does not have a strong protective effect against hypertension. Indeed, there is some evidence from Japan that within this population, a low intake of animal protein might increase the risk for hypertension.[33]

Vegetarian diets, *per se*, do not strongly protect against the development of hypertension. To reduce the risk of developing hypertension, all diets should be low in sodium and high in potassium, alcohol intake should be low, and obesity should be avoided.

3. Hemostatic Factors

Most fatal and non-fatal myocardial infarcts are caused by coronary thrombosis, and there is evidence of an association between the long-term risk of CHD and various measures of hemostatic function.[34] Increased risks for CHD are associated with platelet hyperreactivity with high plasma levels of fibrinogen,[35] and possibly with high levels of factor VII coagulant activity (factor VII$_c$).[36]

Dietary factors influence haemostasis, but the precise nature of these relationships is not well understood.[37] Some studies, but not all, have reported lower levels of fibrinogen and of factor VII$_c$ in vegetarians than in non-vegetarians.[38-41] However, both Mezzano et al.[39] and Li et al.[41] reported that vegetarians had higher indices of platelet aggregation than controls, perhaps because of the lower levels of long chain n-3 fatty acids in the platelets of the vegetarians.

Overall, it is difficult to say whether the effects of a vegetarian diet on hemostatic factors are likely to have any important effect in relation to CHD.

4. Glucose Intolerance and Insulin Resistance

People with diabetes (both non-insulin-dependent and insulin-dependent) or with impaired glucose tolerance have a higher risk of CHD than people with normal glucose tolerance.[34] Some of this association is due to the coexistence of glucose intolerance with low HDL cholesterol, high blood pressure, and obesity, but hyperglycemia also increases CHD risk independently of these other risk factors.[42]

Vegetarian diets do not have a well-defined effect on glucose tolerance. Western vegetarian diets generally include more low glycemic index foods, such as legumes and fruit, than non-vegetarian Western diets and might therefore reduce the incidence of glucose intolerance. Snowdon and Phillips[43] found that self-reported diabetes was less prevalent among vegetarian than among non-vegetarian Seventh-Day Adventists, and that diabetes was only half as common as a cause of death among Seventh-Day Adventists, as compared with the American population as a whole. However, Asian vegetarians from the Indian subcontinent suffer a high incidence of diabetes, despite eating relatively large amounts of legumes. It is possible that a vegetarian diet high in complex carbohydrates has some protective effect against glucose intolerance and diabetes, but other factors such as energy intake, physical activity, and genotype may play more important roles in determining the risk of these conditions.

5. Obesity

Obesity has many different metabolic effects, some of which would tend to increase the risk of CHD. In particular, obesity increases serum total cholesterol while reducing HDL cholesterol, raises blood pressure, and induces glucose intolerance.[44] Data from prospective studies also indicate that obesity is an important risk factor for CHD.[45,46]

Numerous studies have consistently found that vegetarians are, on average, thinner than comparable non-vegetarians.[21,47-49] The data from four large cohorts are shown in Figure 3.1. The average body mass index (BMI) varies substantially between cohorts (higher in the Seventh-Day Adventist cohorts in California than in the European cohorts), but, on average, vegetarians in each cohort have a BMI about 1 kg/m² lower than that of non-vegetarians within the same cohort. The difference is similar in men and women, and is seen in all age groups. The lower mean BMI of vegetarians leads to a substantially lower prevalence of obesity.[47]

The reasons for this association have not been established. An analysis of data from 5,000 men and women in the Oxford Vegetarian Study suggested that the lower BMI of non-meat-eaters was partly due to a higher intake of dietary fiber and a lower intake of animal fat, and, in men only, a lower intake of alcohol. These factors, however, accounted for only one third of the observed difference in BMI.[50]

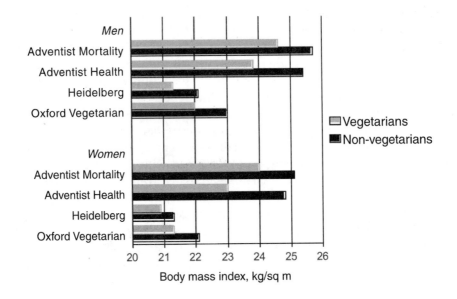

Figure 3.1   Mean body mass index in vegetarians and non-vegetarians in four large cohort studies. (Adapted from Key et al.[48])

6. Smoking

Smoking is a major cause of CHD and the risk is linearly related to the amount smoked.[51] The greater the number of cigarettes smoked, the higher the risk, with an approximately threefold higher risk in heavy smokers than in non-smokers.[34] Smoking tobacco in other forms such as cigars and pipes also increases risk.

Studies of Western vegetarians have generally shown that they have a much lower prevalence of smoking than the general population, and also a substantially lower prevalence than comparable non-vegetarians.[48] Therefore, when considering the effects of a vegetarian diet on CHD risk, it is essential to statistically adjust the results for the confounding effect of smoking.

7. Alcohol

Numerous studies have reported that CHD rates are about 30% lower in moderate alcohol drinkers than in comparable people who drink no alcohol.[34] Although non-drinkers differ in many ways from drinkers, analyses suggest that consumption of moderate amounts of alcohol probably has a protective effect against CHD. Alcohol is known to raise HDL cholesterol and to reduce fibrinogen, both of which would be expected to reduce CHD risk.

Few studies have reported on alcohol intake in Western vegetarians, but the data available suggest that their alcohol intake is relatively low.[52] In theory, this might cause a slight increase in risk of CHD relative to non-vegetarians. However, there is no evidence that alcohol reduces CHD risk among vegetarians; in the Oxford Vegetarian Study, CHD risk did not decrease with increasing alcohol intake,[53] while in the studies of Seventh-Day Adventists, alcohol intake is very low and no data on alcohol and CHD risk have been published.

8. Exercise

Physical activity reduces the risk of CHD.[34] Studies of Western vegetarians have generally shown that vegetarians take more exercise than comparable non-vegetarians,[52] and this difference would be expected to cause a moderate reduction in CHD.

B. Possible Risk Factors

1. Homocysteine

Patients with CHD have higher plasma concentrations of homocysteine than controls, and these differences have been observed in both case-control and prospective studies.[54-56] Plasma concentrations of homocysteine are inversely related to the dietary intake of folic acid, vitamin B_6, and vitamin B_{12}.[57]

Typically, vegetarians have relatively high intakes of folate and similar intakes of vitamin B_6, as compared with the general population.[58] However, vegetarians (and particularly vegans) typically have relatively low intakes of vitamin B_{12}.[59] Vitamin B_{12} is essentially absent from plant foods and is present in small amounts in dairy products (but in somewhat higher amounts in eggs). Therefore, dietary intake of vitamin B_{12} in vegetarians is low unless they consume large amounts of dairy products and eggs, or regularly consume fortified foods or vitamin supplements. For example, Hokin and Butler[60] reported that 73% of vegetarian Seventh-Day Adventist ministers in Australia had low serum vitamin B_{12} (<221 pmol/L), probably because of the limitation in food fortification with vitamin B_{12} in Australia. Similarly, Woo et al.[16] reported that 54% of elderly Chinese vegetarians had serum vitamin B_{12} below the reference range. In the general population (largely non-vegetarian), folate is an important determinant of homocysteine, whereas vitamin B_{12} is not, but vitamin B_{12} intakes are relatively high and vitamin B_{12} deficiency is rare. Vegetarians are at increased risk of vitamin B_{12} deficiency and this might cause elevated homocysteine. Indeed, a recent small study in Chile reported that 21 out of 26 vegetarians had serum vitamin B_{12} concentrations below 200 pg/ml and that mean plasma homocysteine was 41% higher in the vegetarians than in age-matched meat-eaters.[39]

2. Antioxidants

Steinberg et al.[61] proposed that LDL cholesterol is only atherogenic when it is oxidized, and that antioxidants might therefore protect against CHD. There is a considerable amount of epidemiological evidence that supports the hypothesis that dietary antioxidants such as carotenoids, vitamin C, vitamin E, selenium, and various non-nutrients may reduce CHD risk, but this effect has not been firmly established by clinical trials.[46]

Vegetarian diets are generally higher in carotene, vitamin C, and vitamin E than non-vegetarian diets. For example, in a study in New Zealand, Zino et al.[62] reported that vegetarian Seventh-Day Adventists consumed more fruits and vegetables than both non-vegetarian Seventh-Day Adventists and non-Adventist non-vegetarians who were subjected to an intervention designed to increase their intake of fruits and vegetables. Plasma concentrations of β-carotene and α-tocopherol were also higher in the vegetarians than in the other groups. Similar results have been reported in other studies.[63]

Although vegetarian diets are generally relatively rich in carotene, vitamin C, and vitamin E, they are not necessarily rich in selenium, another antioxidant nutrient. Selenium levels are high in fish and moderately high in meat, but the selenium content of plant foods is strongly determined by the selenium content of the soil. Some small studies have reported low selenium levels in vegetarians and vegans, for example, in Britain,[64] Finland,[65] and Slovakia,[66] probably reflecting the low soil selenium levels in these countries.

3. n-3 Fatty Acids

The observation that Eskimos living a traditional lifestyle had low rates of CHD despite a high total fat intake led to the hypothesis that a high consumption of fish rich in n-3 fatty acids might be protective.[67] Since then, many physiological and epidemiological studies have investigated the role of n-3 fatty acids in CHD. The majority of this work has concerned long chain n-3 fatty acids largely provided by fatty fish and fish oils, specifically eicosapentaenoic acid (EPA) and docosahexaenoic acid (DHA). Recently, however, more attention has been given to the precursor 18-carbon fatty acid α-linolenic acid, which is provided by some plant foods.

An important physiological effect of n-3 fatty acids in relation to CHD is the reduction in thrombotic tendency due to the inhibition of thromboxane production from arachidonic acid. The long chain n-3 fatty acids in fish oil are very potent in this regard, but α-linolenic acid has also been shown to be effective. Both fish oil and α-linolenic acid also have an anti-arrhythmic effect on the cardiac muscle.[68,69] Fish oils can reduce serum triacylglycerol concentrations, but α-linolenic acid does not have this effect.

A number of observational epidemiological studies, though not all, have shown that moderate fish consumption (versus very low fish consumption) is associated with a reduction in the risk of CHD.[46] In addition, one randomized secondary prevention trial found that following advice to eat fish regularly caused a 32% reduction in cardiac death[70] and another trial reported that supplementation with fish oil caused a 20% reduction in coronary deaths.[71] Fewer data are available for α-linolenic acid, but there is some evidence that it too might reduce CHD risk. Hu et al.[72] reported that women with a relatively high consumption of α-linolenic acid had a 45% reduction in mortality from CHD, perhaps because of its antiarrhythmic effect. Also, a small randomized trial, which incorporated an increase in α-linolenic acid (as well as several other dietary changes) in the treatment arm caused a 65% reduction in CHD.[73]

Vegetarian diets are generally very low in long chain n-3 fatty acids. Eggs can provide significant amounts if the chickens are fed a diet high in α-linolenic acid, but most egg production in Western countries relies on feeds such as corn, which have a very high ratio of n-6 to n-3 fatty acids and the resulting eggs are low in long chain n-3 fatty acids.[74] Dairy products contain only trace amounts of long chain fatty acids, and plant foods none (with the exception of some algae). Vegetarian diets generally provide reasonable amounts of α-linolenic acid (about 1.5 mg/day), but can also be very high in n-6 linoleic acid, which competes for the same enzymes. Tissue levels of long chain n-3 fatty acids are relatively low in vegetarians and vegans.[59,75]

III. VEGETARIANISM AND CORONARY HEART DISEASE

A. Observational Studies

The relatively low plasma cholesterol concentrations of vegetarians would be expected to reduce the risk of CHD. The first epidemiological study of CHD in vegetarians was published by Phillips et al.[76] They reported that the risk of fatal CHD was three times greater in non-vegetarian than in vegetarian Seventh-Day Adventist men aged 35–64; the difference was smaller for older men and for women, but in the same direction. The lower risk in vegetarians was partly due to differences in other risk factors, such as smoking, hypertension, and exercise, but substantial differences in mortality remained after adjusting for these risk factors.

Data on mortality rates in Western vegetarians are available from the early study reported by Phillips et al.[76] and from four other cohort studies that included a large proportion of vegetarians. Two of these studies were conducted among Seventh-Day Adventists in California, two among members of the Vegetarian Society and others in Britain, and one among the readers of vegetarian magazines in Germany. A pooled analysis of original data from these five cohort studies was published recently[48,52] and included data for 76,000 men and women (of whom 28,000 were vegetarians). Importantly, the vegetarians and the non-vegetarians in each study had a shared interest in healthy living or a similar social/religious background. All results were adjusted for age, sex, and smoking, and a random effects model was used to calculate pooled estimates of effect for all studies combined. Further adjustments for body mass index, alcohol consumption, exercise, and education level had little effect on the results. There were 2264 deaths from CHD before age 90. In comparison with non-vegetarians, vegetarians had a 24% reduction in mortality from this disease (death rate ratio 0.76, 95% confidence interval (CI) 0.62–0.94). The reduction in mortality was greater at younger ages: death rate ratios were 0.55 (95% CI 0.35–0.85), 0.69 (95% CI 0.53–0.90) and 0.92 (95% CI 0.73–1.16) for deaths from CHD at ages <65, 65–79 and 80–89 respectively. The reduction in mortality was confined to vegetarians who had followed their current diet for more than 5 years. When the non-vegetarians were divided into regular meat-eaters (who ate meat at least once a week) and semi-vegetarians (who ate fish only or ate meat less than once a week), the CHD death rate ratios compared with regular meat-eaters were 0.78 (95% CI 0.68-0.89) in semi-vegetarians and 0.66 (95% CI 0.53-0.83) in vegetarians (test for trend P<0.001) (Figure 3.2).

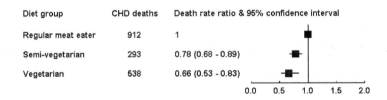

Figure 3.2   Pooled analysis of mortality in vegetarians and non-vegetarians: death rate ratios (& 95% confidence intervals) for CHD by diet group, relative to regular meat-eaters, adjusted for age, sex, and smoking, and for study using a random effects model. (Adapted from Key et al.[48])

B. Intervention Trial of a Low-Fat Vegetarian Diet

Ornish et al.[22] conducted a randomized controlled trial among 48 patients with moderate to severe CHD to compare the effects of usual care with a more intensive lifestyle change program that included a low-fat vegetarian diet. After 5 years, coronary artery percent diameter stenosis decreased in the low-fat vegetarian arm of the trial and increased in the control group. The risk ratio for any cardiac event in the control group was 2.47 (95% CI 1.48–4.20). After 1 year of intervention, LDL cholesterol had decreased by 40% in the experimental group, but had decreased by only 1% in the control group, and, although this difference diminished during further follow up, it is possible that the beneficial effects observed were due to the reduction in LDL cholesterol. It should be noted that the reductions in fat intake and in LDL cholesterol in the experimental group were much larger than the differences observed between vegetarians and meat-eaters in free-living populations.

C. Foods, Nutrients, Vegetarianism, and Coronary Heart Disease

It is likely that the reduction in CHD among vegetarians is, at least partly, due to a lower serum cholesterol concentration caused by a lower dietary intake of saturated fat and cholesterol. Unfortunately, none of the five prospective studies of mortality in vegetarians has complete information on serum cholesterol concentrations in all subjects, therefore, it is currently impossible to investigate whether the difference in CHD between vegetarians and non-vegetarians can be statistically explained by the difference in cholesterol levels.

Some data are available, however, on the relationships of various foods to CHD within the cohort studies of vegetarians. Meat intake was strongly positively associated with CHD among male Seventh-Day Adventists in the two large prospective studies in California.[49,77] There was also a positive, but weaker, association with meat intake among women in the earlier study,[77] but not in the more recent study.[49] Eggs, but not dairy products, were also associated with an increased risk of CHD among Seventh-Day Adventists.[77] In the Oxford Vegetarian Study, the frequency of meat consumption was not significantly related to mortality from CHD, but consumption of cheese, eggs, total animal fat, and dietary cholesterol were each strongly associated with CHD mortality. Compared with those who ate relatively little of these foods, the death rate ratios in those who ate the most were 2.47 (95% CI 0.97–6.26) for cheese, 2.68 (95% CI 1.19–6.02) for eggs, 3.29 (95% CI 1.50–7.21) for total animal fat and 3.53 (95% CI 1.57–7.96) for dietary cholesterol (Figure 3.3).[78] These observations might all be due to the effects of saturated animal fats on serum cholesterol.

In the Oxford Vegetarian Study, no foods that significantly reduced CHD risk were identified, but in the Adventist health study in California, eating whole-wheat bread and frequently consuming nuts were both associated with a reduction in risk.[79,80] Similar associations have been observed in non-vegetarian populations for both fiber-rich foods[81] and for nuts.[82]

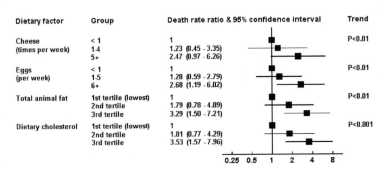

Figure 3.3   Oxford Vegetarian Study: death rate ratios (& 95% confidence intervals) for CHD by dietary factor among subjects with no evidence of preexisting disease at the time of recruitment, adjusted for age, sex, smoking, and social class. (Adapted from Appleby et al.[78])

There are currently insufficient data to establish the reasons for the reduction in risk of CHD associated with a vegetarian diet. Several mechanisms are possible, perhaps in combination.[83] In our opinion, the simplest and perhaps most likely explanation is that the low intake of animal fats in vegetarians causes a lower serum cholesterol concentration and therefore, a reduced risk of CHD. Ongoing large prospective studies of vegetarians that include both assessment of diet and measurement of serum cholesterol concentrations should allow researchers to test this hypothesis.

IV.   TOPICS REQUIRING MORE RESEARCH

A. Coronary Heart Disease in Vegans

There are few data on the long-term health of vegans. The pooled analysis of five prospective studies described above included 27,808 vegetarians, but only 753 of these subjects were vegans.[52] Compared with regular meat-eaters in these cohorts, the death rate ratio for CHD in vegans was 0.74 (95 % CI 0.46–1.21). The confidence interval for this estimate is wide, so that it is currently impossible to say whether mortality from CHD in vegans differs from that in regular meat-eaters, although the death rate ratio is similar to that observed for vegetarians compared with non-vegetarians in this analysis.

In terms of coronary risk factors, all studies have shown that vegans have a substantially lower serum total cholesterol concentration than meat-eaters (around 1 mmol/l lower) and are also thinner than meat-eaters (by 1 to 2 kg/m^2). These differences would be expected to cause a substantial reduction in mortality from CHD. No consistent differences in blood pressure or in hemostatic factors have been established. Vegan diets are often low in vitamin B_{12}, which could potentially cause raised homocysteine levels, and very low in long chain n-3 fatty acids, which could result in increased platelet aggregation (see IV.C and IV.D below).

B. Coronary Heart Disease in Vegetarian South Asians

South Asian migrants from the Indian subcontinent (Bangladesh, India, and Pakistan) have higher mortality from CHD than other ethnic groups living in the new host country.[84] Reliable population-based CHD mortality data are not available from South Asia, but mortality is probably low in rural areas and high in urban areas.[84] Many South Asians are vegetarians, which might suggest that this type of vegetarian diet does not reduce the risk for CHD. However, South Asians differ from other ethnic groups, both in many aspects of lifestyle and also genetically, and a case-control study of risk factors for CHD (specifically acute myocardial infarction) in Bangalore, India, did observe a 45% reduction in risk in vegetarians, which was partly explained by their lower blood glucose concentration and lower waist to hip ratio.[85]

C. Vitamin B_{12} and Homocysteine

Dietary intake of vitamin B_{12} can be low in both vegetarians and vegans.[58–60,86] The sources of vitamin B_{12} in a vegetarian diet are dairy products, eggs, fortified foods (especially meat analogues, soya milks, yeast extracts, and breakfast cereals) and vitamin supplements. If none of these sources of vitamin B_{12} is regularly consumed, intake of this vitamin will be low and the risk of deficiency will increase. More data are needed on current intakes of vitamin B_{12} in vegetarians, and on whether this is a determinant of homocysteine and CHD risk in these populations.

D. n –3 Fatty Acids

Vegetarian diets are, by definition, devoid of oily fish, which are rich sources of long-chain n-3 fatty acids. Dairy products contain negligible amounts of long chain n-3 fatty acids, whereas eggs may provide significant quantities of these fatty acids, depending on the diet of the hens (see II.B. 3 above). Vegetarian diets usually contain moderate quantities of n-3 α-linolenic acid, particularly from soya and rapeseed (canola) oils (linseed oil is very rich in this fatty acid but is not commonly consumed). However, vegetarian diets are also often very rich in n-6 linoleic acid, which inhibits the elongation of α-linolenic acid to the longer chain derivatives, EPA and DHA. The importance of these factors for CHD (and for other aspects of health) remains to be fully elucidated. However, current knowledge supports the recommendation that vegetarians should select their foods to provide adequate amounts of n-3 α-linolenic acid and to keep consumption of n-6 linoleic acid moderate to give an n-6 to n-3 ratio of between 4:1 and 10:1.[87,88] In practice, this implies preferring oils such as rapeseed and soya to oils such as corn and sunflower.

V. CONCLUSION

The most important, well-established, diet-related risk factors for CHD are high serum cholesterol, high blood pressure, and high BMI. Compared with non-vegetarians, Western vegetarians have a lower plasma cholesterol concentration (by about 0.5 mmol l^{-1}) and lower body mass index (by about 1 kg/m^2), and may have slightly lower blood pressure. The low cholesterol levels of vegetarians would be expected to cause an approximately 25% reduction in mortality from CHD, and a pooled analysis of prospective studies has shown that CHD mortality is 24% lower in vegetarians than in non-vegetarians.

Overall, therefore, it appears that Western vegetarian diets have an important protective effect against CHD. More research is needed on mortality in vegans and South Asian vegetarians, and on the possible adverse effects of a vegetarian diet on plasma levels of homocysteine and tissue levels of long chain n-3 fatty acids.

ACKNOWLEDGEMENT

We thank Drs. Robert Clarke and Pia Verkasalo for their comments on this chapter.

REFERENCES

1. Lopez, A.D. and Murray, C.J.L. The global burden of disease, 1990-2020. *Nature Medicine*, 4: 1241, 1998.
2. Law, M.R., Wald, N.J., Wu, T., Hackshaw, A., and Bailey, A. Systematic underestimation of association between serum cholesterol concentration and ischaemic heart disease in observational studies: data from the BUPA study. *Brit. Med. J.*, 308: 363, 1994.

3. Law, M.R., Wald, N.J., and Thompson, S.G. By how much and how quickly does reduction in serum cholesterol concentration lower risk of ischaemic heart disease? *Brit. Med. J.*, 308: 367, 1994.
4. Chen, Z., Peto, R., Collins, R., MacMahon, S., Lu, J., and Li, W. Serum cholesterol concentration and coronary heart disease in a population with low cholesterol concentrations. *Brit. Med. J.*, 303: 276, 1991.
5. Sacks, F.M. Why cholesterol as a central theme in coronary heart disease? *Am. J. Cardiol.*, 82: 14, 1998.
6. Hardinge, M.F. and Stare, F.J. Nutritional studies of vegetarians. II. Dietary and serum levels of cholesterol. *Am. J. Clinic. Nutr.*, 2: 83, 1954.
7. Thorogood, M., Carter, R., Benfield, L., McPherson, K., and Mann, J.I. Plasma lipids and lipoprotein cholesterol concentrations in people with different diets in Britain. *Brit. Med. J.*, 295: 351, 1987.
8. Keys, A., Anderson, J.T., and Grande, F. Prediction of serum cholesterol responses of man to changes in fats in the diet. *Lancet*, 2: 959, 1957.
9. Thorogood, M., Roe, L., McPherson, K., and Mann, J. Dietary intake and plasma lipid levels: lessons from a study of the diet of health conscious groups. *Brit. Med. J.*, 300: 1297, 1990.
10. West, R.O. and Hayes, O.B. Diet and serum cholesterol levels. *Am. J. Clinic. Nutr.*, 21: 853, 1968.
11. Fraser, G.E., Dysinger, W., Best, C., and Chan, R. Ischemic heart disease risk factors in middle-aged Seventh-Day Adventist men and their neighbors. *Am. J. Epidemiol.*, 126: 638, 1987.
12. Burslem, J., Schonfeld, G., Howald, M.A., Weidman, S.W., and Miller, J.P. Plasma apoprotein and lipoprotein lipid levels in vegetarians. *Metabolism*, 27: 711, 1978.
13. Sacks, F.M., Castelli, W.P., Donner, A., and Kass, E.H. Plasma lipids and lipoproteins in vegetarians and controls. *New Eng. J. Med.*, 1148, 1975.
14. Burr, M.L., Bates, C.J., Fehily, A.M., and St. Leger, A.S. Plasma cholesterol and blood pressure in vegetarians. *J. Human Nutr.*, 35: 437, 1981.
15. Thomas, H.V., Davey, G.K., and Key, T.J. Oestradiol and sex hormone-binding globulin in premenopausal and postmenopausal meat-eaters, vegetarians, and vegans. *Brit. J. Cancer*, 80: 1470, 1999.
16. Woo, J., Kwok, T., Ho, S.C., Sham, A., and Lau, E. Nutritional status of elderly Chinese vegetarians. *Age & Ageing*, 27: 455, 1998.
17. Nagyová, A., Kudlácková, M., Grancicová, E., and Magálová, T. LDL oxidizability and antioxidative status of plasma in vegetarians. *Ann. Nutr. & Metab.*, 42: 328, 1998.
18. Famodu, A.A., Osilesi, O., Makinde, Y.O., and Osonuga, O.A. Blood pressure and blood lipid levels among vegetarian, semi-vegetarian, and non-vegetarian native Africans. *Clinic. Biochem.*, 31: 545, 1998.
19. Medkova, I.L., Manchuk, V.T., Mosiakina, L.I., Polivanova, T.V., Lundina, T.A., and Koroleva-Munts, L.I. Data from an expedition to study a Siberian vegan settlement. Russian. *Voprosy Pitaniia*, 3: 3, 1998.
20. Richter, V., Purschwitz, K., Bohusch, A., Seim, H., Weisbrich, C., Reuter, W., Sorger, D., and Rassoul, F. Lipoproteins and other clinical-chemistry parameters under the conditions of lacto-ovo-vegetarian nutrition. *Nutr. Res.*, 19: 545, 1999.
21. Dwyer, J.T. Health aspects of vegetarian diets. *Am. J. Clinic. Nutr.*, 48: 712, 1988.

22. Ornish, D., Scherwitz, L.W., Billings, J.H., Gould, K.L., Merritt, T.A., Sparler, S., Armstrong, W.T., Ports, T.A., Kirkeeide, R.L., Hogeboom, C., and Brand, R.J. Intensive lifestyle changes for reversal of coronary heart disease. *JAMA*, 280: 2001, 1998.

23. McKeigue, P.M., Marmot, M.G., Adelstein, A.M., Hunt, S.P., Shipley, M.J., Butler, S.M., Riemersma, M.J., and Turner, P.R. Diet and risk factors for coronary heart disease in Asians in northwest London. *Lancet*, 2: 1086, 1985.

24. Chuang, C.Z., Subramaniam, P.N., LeGardeur, B.Y., and Lopez, A. Risk factors for coronary artery disease and levels of lipoprotein(a) and fat-soluble antioxidant vitamins in Asian Indians of USA. *Indian Heart J.*, 50: 285, 1998.

25. Appleby, P.N., Thorogood, M., McPherson, K., and Mann, J.I. Associations between plasma lipid concentrations and dietary, lifestyle, and physical factors in the Oxford Vegetarian Study. *J. Human Nutr, & Dietetics*, 8: 305, 1995.

26. Clarke, R., Frost, C., Collins, R., Appleby, P., and Peto, R. Dietary lipids and blood cholesterol: quantitative meta-analysis of metabolic ward studies. *Brit. Med. J.*, 314: 112, 1997.

27. Austin, M.A., Hokanson, J.E., and Edwards, K.L. Hypertriglyceridemia as a cardiovascular risk factor. *Am. J. Cardiol.*, 81: 7, 1998.

28. Stamler, J., Stamler, R., and Neaton, J.D. Blood pressure, systolic and diastolic, and cardiovascular risks. *Arch. Intern. Med.*, 153: 598, 1993.

29. MacMahon, S., Peto, R., Cutler, J., Collins, R., Sorlie, P., Neaton, J., Abbott, R., Godwin, J., Dyer, A., and Stamler, J. Blood pressure, stroke, and coronary heart disease. *Lancet*, 335: 765, 1990.

30. Elliott, P., Marmot, M., Dyer, A., Joossens, J., Kesteloot, H., Stamler, R., Stamler, J., and Rose, G. The INTERSALT study: main results, conclusions, and some implications. *Clinical & Experimental Hypertension — Part A, Theory & Practice*, 11: 1025, 1989.

31. Elliott, P., Stamler, J., Nichols, R., Dyer, A.R., Stamler, R., Kesteloot, H., and Marmot, M. for the Intersalt Cooperative Research Group. Intersalt revisited: further analyses of 24-hour sodium excretion and blood pressure within and across populations. *Brit. Med. J.*, 312: 1249, 1996.

32. Beilin, L.J. Vegetarian and other complex diets, fats, fiber, and hypertension. *Am. J. Clinic. Nutr.*, 59: 1130S, 1994.

33. Kihara, M., Fujikawa, J., Ohtaka, M., Mano, M., Nara, Y., Horie, R., Tsunematsu, T., Note, S., Fukase, M., and Yamori, Y. Interrelationships between blood pressure, sodium, potassium, serum cholesterol, and protein intake in Japanese. *Hypertension*, 6: 736, 1984.

34. Marmot, M.G. and Mann, J.I. Ischaemic heart disease: Epidemiology and prevention. In: *Oxford Textbook of Medicine.* Weatherall, D.J., Ledingham, J.G.G., and Warrell, D.A., Eds., Oxford University Press, Oxford, 1996, 2305.

35. Danesh J., Collins, R., Appleby, P., and Peto, R. Association of fibrinogen, C-reactive protein, albumin, or leukocyte count with coronary heart disease: meta-analyses of prospective studies. *JAMA*, 279: 1477, 1998.

36. Meade, T.W., Ruddock, V., Stirling, Y., Chakrabarti, R., and Miller, G.J. Fibrin-olytic activity, clotting factors, and long-term incidence of ischaemic heart disease in the Northwick Park Heart Study. *Lancet*, 342: 1076, 1993.

37. Vorster, H.H., Cummings, J.H., and Veldman, F.J. Diet and haemostasis: time for nutrition science to get more involved. *Brit. J. Nutr.*, 77: 671, 1997.

PROPERTY OF LLUMC
JESSE MEDICAL LIBRARY

38. Famodu, A.A., Osilesi, O., Makinde, Y.O., Osonuga, O.A., Fakoya, T.A., Ogu-nyemi, E.O., and Egbenehkhuere, I.E. The influence of a vegetarian diet on haemostatic risk factors for cardiovascular disease in Africans. *Thrombosis Res.*, 95: 31, 1999.
39. Mezzano, D., Muñoz, X., Martínez, C., Cuevas, A., Panes, O., Aranda, E., Guasch, V., Strobel, P., Muñoz, B., Rodríguez, S., Pereira, J., and Leighton, F. Vegetarians and cardiovascular risk factors: Haemostasis, inflammatory markers, and plasma homocysteine. *Thrombosis and Haemostasis*, 81: 913, 1999.
40. Pan, W.H., Chin, C.J., Sheu, C.T., and Lee, M.H. Hemostatic factors and blood lipids in young Buddhist vegetarians and omnivores. *Am. J. Clinic. Nutr.*, 58: 354, 1993.
41. Li, D., Sinclair, A., Mann, N., Turner, A., Ball, M., Kelly, F., Abedin, L., and Wilson, A. The association of diet and thrombotic risk factors in healthy male vegetarians and meat-eaters. *Europ. J. Clinic. Nutr.*, 53: 612, 1999.
42. Turner, R.C., Millns, H., Neil, H.A.W., Stratton, I.M., Manley, S.E., Matthews, D.R., and Holman, R.R. Risk factors for coronary artery disease in non-insulin dependent diabetes mellitus: for the United Kingdom Prospective Diabetes Study Group (UKPDS:23). *Brit. Med. J.*, 316: 823, 1998.
43. Snowdon, D.A. and Phillips, R.L. Does a vegetarian diet reduce the occurrence of diabetes? *Am. J. Public Hlth.*, 75: 507, 1985.
44. LaRosa, J.C., Hunninghake, D., Bush, D., Criqui, M.H., Getz, G.S., Gotto, A.M., Jr., Grundy, S.M., Rakita, L., Robertson, R.M., Weisfeldt, M.L., and Cleeman, J.I. A summary of the evidence relating dietary fats, serum cholesterol, and coro-nary heart disease. *Circulation*, 81: 1721, 1990.
45. Hubert, H.B., Feinleib, M., McNamara, P.M., and Castelli, W.P. Obesity as an independent risk factor for cardiovascular disease: A 26-year follow-up of participants in the Framingham Heart Study. *Circulation*, 67: 968, 1983.
46. Willett, W. Diet and coronary heart disease. In: *Nutritional Epidemiology.* Willett, W., Oxford University Press, Oxford, 1998, 414.
47. Key, T.J. and Davey, G. Prevalence of obesity is low in people who do not eat meat. *Brit. Med. J.*, 313: 816, 1996.
48. Key, T.J., Fraser, G.E., Thorogood, M., Appleby, P.N., Beral, V., Reeves, G., Burr, M.L., Chang-Claude, J., Frentzel-Beyme, R., Kuzma, J.W., Mann, J., and McPherson, K. Mortality in vegetarians and non-vegetarians: a collaborative analysis of 8300 deaths among 76,000 men and women in five prospective studies. *Publ. Hlth. Nutr.*, 1: 33, 1998.
49. Fraser, G.E. Associations between diet and cancer, ischemic heart disease, and all-cause mortality in non-Hispanic white California Seventh-Day Adventists. *Am. J. Clinic. Nutr.*, 70: 532S, 1999.
50. Appleby, P.N., Thorogood, M., Mann, J.I., and Key, T.J. Low body mass index in non-meat-eaters: the possible roles of animal fat, dietary fibre, and alcohol. *Int. J. Obesity*, 22: 454, 1998.
51. Parish, S., Collins, R., Peto, R., Youngman, L., Barton, J., Jayne, K., Clarke, R., Appleby, P., Lyon, V., and Cederholm-Williams, S. Cigarette smoking, tar yields, and non-fatal myocardial infarction: 14,000 cases and 32,000 controls in the United Kingdom. The International Studies of Infarct Survival (ISIS) Collabo-rators. *Brit. Med. J.*, 311: 471, 1995.

52. Key, T.J., Fraser, G.E., Thorogood, M., Appleby, P.N., Beral.V., Reeves, G., Burr, M.L., Chang-Claude, J., Frentzel-Beyme, R., Kuzma, J.W., and McPherson, K. Mortality in vegetarians and non-vegetarians: detailed findings from a collaborative analysis of five prospective studies. *Am. J. Clinic. Nutr.*, 70: 516S, 1999.

53. Mann, J., Appleby, P.N., Key, T.J., and Thorogood, M. Dietary determinants of ischaemic heart disease in health conscious individuals. *Heart*, 78: 450, 1997.

54. Stampfer, M.J., Malinow, M.R., Willett, W.C., Newcomer, L.M., Upson, B., Ullmann, D., Tishler, P.V., and Hennekens, C.H. A prospective study of plasma homocysteine and risk of myocardial infarction in U.S. physicians. *JAMA*, 268: 877, 1992.

55. Arnesen, E., Refsum, H., Bønaa, K.H., Ueland, P.M., Førde, O.H., and Nordrehaug, J.E. Serum total homocysteine and coronary heart disease. *Int. J. Epidemiology*, 24: 704, 1995.

56. McCully, K.S. Homocysteine, folate, vitamin B_6, and cardiovascular disease. *JAMA*, 279: 392, 1998.

57. Hankey, G.J. and Eikelboom, J.W. Homocysteine and vascular disease. *Lancet*, 354: 407, 1999.

58. Draper, A., Lewis, J., Malhotra, N., and Wheeler, E. The energy and nutrient intakes of different types of vegetarian: a case for supplements? *Brit. J. Nutr.*, 69: 3, 1993.

59. Sanders, T.A.B. The nutritional adequacy of plant-based diets. *Proc. Nutr. Soc.*, 58: 265, 1999.

60. Hokin, B.D. and Butler, T. Cyanocobalamin (vitamin B_{12}) status in Seventh-Day Adventist ministers in Australia. *Am. J. Clinic. Nutr.*, 70: 576S, 1999.

61. Steinberg, D., Parthasarathy, S., Carew, T.E., Khoo, J.C., and Witztum, J.L. Modifications of low-density lipoprotein that increase its atherogenicity. *New Engl. J. Med.*, 320: 915, 1988.

62. Zino, S.J.M., Harman, S.K., Skeaff, C.M., and Mann, J.I. Fruit and vegetable consumption and antioxidant status of Seventh-Day Adventists. *Nutr. & Metabol. Cardiovasc. Disease*, 8: 297, 1998.

63. Pronczuk, A., Kipervarg, Y., and Hayes, K.C. Vegetarians have higher plasma alpha-tocopherol relative to cholesterol than do non-vegetarians. *J. Am. College of Nutr.*, 11: 50, 1992.

64. Judd, P.A., Long, A., Butcher, M., Caygill, C.P., and Diplock, A.T. Vegetarians and vegans may be most at risk from low selenium intakes. *Brit. Med. J.*, 314: 1834, 1997.

65. Rauma, A.L., Torronen, R., Hanninen, O., Verhagen, H., and Mykkanen, H. Antioxidant status in long-term adherents to a strict uncooked vegan diet. *Am. J. Clinic. Nutr.*, 62: 1221, 1995.

66. Kovacikova, Z., Cerhata, D., Kadrabova, J., Madaric, A., and Ginter, E. Antioxidant status in vegetarians and non-vegetarians in Bratislava region (Slovakia). *Zeitschrift fur Ernahrungswissenschaft*, 37: 178, 1998.

67. Sinclair, H. Diet and heart disease. *Brit. Med. J.*, 2: 1602, 1977.

68. Leaf, A. Dietary prevention of coronary heart disease. *Circulation*, 99: 733, 1999.

69. Simopoulos, A.P. Essential fatty acids in health and chronic disease. *Am. J. Clinic. Nutr.*, 70: 560S, 1999.

70. Burr, M.L., Fehily, A.M., Gilbert, J.F., Rogers, S., Holliday, R.M., Sweetnam, P.M., Elwood, P.C., and Deadman, N.M. Effects of changes in fat, fish, and fibre intakes on death and myocardial reinfarction: diet and reinfarction trial (DART). *Lancet*, 2: 1450, 1989.

71. GISSI-Prevenzione Investigators. Dietary supplementation with n-3 polyunsaturated fatty acids and vitamin E after myocardial infarction: results of the GISSI-Prevenzione trial. *Lancet*, 354: 447, 1999.

72. Hu, F.B., Stampfer, M.J., Manson, J.E., Rimm, E.B., Wolk, A., Colditz, G.A., Hennekens, C.H., and Willett, W.C. Dietary intake of α-linolenic acid and risk of fatal ischemic heart disease among women. *Am. J. Clinic. Nutr.*, 69: 890, 1999.

73. de Lorgeril, M., Salen, P., Martin, J.-L., Monjaud, I., Delaye, J., and Mamelle, N. Mediterranean diet, traditional risk factors, and the rate of cardiovascular complications after myocardial infarction. *Circulation*, 99: 779, 1999.

74. Simopoulos, A.P. and Salem Jr, N. n-3 fatty acids in eggs from range-fed Greek chickens. *New Engl. J. Med.*, 321: 1412, 1989.

75. Li, D., Ball, M., Bartlett, M., and Sinclair, A. Lipoprotein (a), essential fatty acid status and lipoprotein lipids in female Australian vegetarians. *Clinical Science*, 97: 175, 1999.

76. Phillips, R.L., Lemon, F.R., Beeson, W.L., and Kuzma, J.W. Coronary heart disease mortality among Seventh-Day Adventists with differing dietary habits: a preliminary report. *Am. J. Clinic. Nutr.*, 31: S191, 1978.

77. Snowdon, D.A., Phillips, R.L., and Fraser, G.E. Meat consumption and fatal ischemic heart disease. *Preventive Medicine*, 13: 490, 1984.

78. Appleby, P.N., Thorogood, M., Mann, J.I., and Key, T.J. The Oxford Vegetarian Study: an overview. *Am. J. Clinic. Nutr.*, 70: 525S, 1999.

79. Fraser, G.E., Sabaté, J., Beeson, W.L., and Strahan, T.M. Possible protective effect of nut consumption on risk of coronary heart disease. *Arch. Int. Med.*, 152: 1416, 1992.

80. Sabaté, J. Nut consumption, vegetarian diets, ischemic heart disease risk, and all-cause mortality: evidence from epidemiologic studies. *Am. J. Clinic. Nutr.*, 70: 500S, 1999.

81. Pietinen, P., Rimm, E.B., Korhonen, P., Hartman, A.M., Willett, W.C., Albanes, D., and Virtamo, J. Intake of dietary fiber and risk of coronary heart disease in a cohort of Finnish men. *Circulation*, 94: 2720, 1996.

82. Hu, F.B., Stampfer, M.J., Manson, J.E., Rimm, E.B., Colditz, G.A., Rosner, B.A., Speizer, F.E., Hennekens, C.H., and Willett, W.C. Frequent nut consumption and risk of coronary heart disease in women: prospective cohort study. *Brit. Med. J.*, 317: 1341, 1998.

83. Fraser, G.E. Diet and coronary heart disease: beyond dietary fats and low-density-lipoprotein cholesterol. *Am. J. Clinic. Nutr.*, 59: 1117S, 1994.

84. McKeigue, P.M. Cardiovascular disease and diabetes in migrants — interactions between nutritional changes and genetic background, lessons from contrasting worlds. In: *Diet, Nutrition and Chronic Disease.* Shetty, P.S. and McPherson, K., Eds., John Wiley & Sons, Chichester, 1997, 59.

85. Pais, P., Pogue, J., Gerstein, H., Zachariah, E., Savitha, D., Jayprakash, S., Nayak, P.R., and Yusuf, S. Risk factors for acute myocardial infarction in Indians: a case-control study. *Lancet*, 348: 358, 1996.

86. Alexander, D., Ball, M.J., and Mann, J. Nutrient intake and haematological status of vegetarians and age-sex matched omnivores. *Europ. J. Clinic. Nutr.*, 48: 538, 1994.

87. Sanders, T.A.B. Essential fatty acid requirements of vegetarians in pregnancy, lactation, and infancy. *Am. J. Clinic. Nutr.*, 70: 555S, 1999.

88. FAO/WHO. Fats and oils in human nutrition (report of a joint expert consultation). FAO, Rome, 1994. (Food and Nutrition paper 57.)

4

VEGETARIAN DIETS AND CANCER RISK

Paul K. Mills

CONTENTS

0-8493-8508-3/01/$0.00+$.50
© 2001 by CRC Press LLC

I. INTRODUCTION

Interest in the relationship between dietary habits and health dates back to antiquity. There are numerous references in the Old Testament to dietary regimens thought to promote or enhance health, and most of the major world religions (both Eastern and Western) have incorporated at least some dietary recommendations, admonitions or proscriptions in their teachings for more than two millennia. Evidence of human cancer has been found in the ancient Egyptian mummies, although only in the 20th century, as life expectancy has increased and after the relative decline of infectious diseases as a cause of death, has cancer emerged as a major public health concern. Many modern-day studies of diet and cancer have focused on religious groups that advocate a vegetarian lifestyle. Vegetarian populations are useful for study because they can be compared with "external," non-vegetarian referent populations and the differences in cancer risk can be measured. They are also instructive in that internal comparisons can be made in which cancer risk by level of adherence to vegetarianism is evaluated (or within other subgroups of interest such as smokers vs. non-smokers, by body weight, etc.).

It was not until the 20th century, however, that systematic study of the diet–cancer relationship emerged. More recent interest in diet and cancer was spurred by the report of Doll and Peto (1981), who released a comprehensive analysis of avoidable cases of cancer mortality in the U.S.[1] Their analysis indicated that about 35% of cancer deaths in the U.S. were attributable to dietary practices and this estimate was second only to the impact of cigarette smoking on cancer death. However, their estimate was associated with a large degree of uncertainty (10%–70%). In 1995, Willett updated the estimate and indicated that about 32% of all cancer deaths in the U.S. may be associated with diet and this estimate ranged only from 20% to 42%.[2] Regardless of which figure is accurate, these data indicate that dietary habits may be responsible for about 177,000 cancer deaths and 394,000 new cases of cancer in the U.S. every year, thus making diet a major source of public health concern. The estimate of 32% by Willett was in reference to all types of cancer combined, but varied considerably by specific types of cancer. For prostate cancer, for example, Willett estimated that perhaps 75% of deaths were attributable to dietary habits, while for colorectal cancer, the estimate was 70%, and for both pancreas and breast cancer the estimate was 50%.

Although the relationship between diet and cancer is clearly complex, it is now more amenable to study than in the past because of the complete and accurate certification of death, the development of population-based cancer registries and because of the emergence of epidemiologic and statistical methods. Accurate measurement of diet remains problematic, however, particularly for case-control studies.

Another issue is the fact that cancer is multifactorial in etiology. In addition to diet, known causes of cancer include tobacco, 'excess consumption of alcohol, endogenous and exogenous hormones, radiation, certain occupations and some environmental chemicals, as well as genetic predisposition. The ability of scientists to "tease out" effects of diet from other lifestyle exposures is exceedingly difficult and, in reality, the concept of ceteris paribus (i.e., all other things being equal) is difficult to achieve.

The study of cancer in vegetarian populations can be instructive and indeed has indicated that, in general, vegetarians experience a lower overall risk of cancer incidence and mortality than non-vegetarians. The question remains, however, whether the lower risk of cancer in vegetarians is due to their dietary habits or because of some other lifestyle habit that is highly correlated with their avoidance of meat. Vegetarians usually do not smoke or consume alcoholic beverages with the same frequency as the general population and both of these lifestyle habits are associated with increased cancer risk. In addition, the vegetarian diet is different from non-vegetarian diets in more ways than simply the absence of meat. Vegetarians consume more fruits, vegetables, and grains as well as particular meat substitutes such as soy that may offer some cancer preventive potency. Vegetarians are also different from the general population in that they may be of higher educational or socioeconomic status and different race or ethnicity than non-vegetarians and both of these are known risk factors for cancer.

In this review, risk of cancer (both morbidity and mortality) in vegetarians is examined. Several studies of cancer death (mortality) and incidence (newly diagnosed disease) among vegetarians are reviewed. Most quantitative estimates of risk appear in the form of Standardized Mortality Ratios (SMR), which is the ratio of the number of observed cancer deaths in vegetarians to the number of expected deaths in vegetarians. Expected numbers are generated by applying the same rate of death in the general population to the person-years at risk in vegetarians. The reference value of no difference in risk is set at 1.0 (or 100). When within-group comparisons are presented, they are usually in the form of relative risks, which quantify the risk of cancer in those persons characterized by some habit (e.g., food use group) compared with persons in another category of use. Again, a reference value of 1.0 is used to denote no difference in risk.

A. Epidemiologic Studies of Cancer in Vegetarian Societies

As mentioned, interest in the relationship between dietary habits and human health has existed since antiquity. It was not until the early part of the 20th century, however, that systematic efforts to quantify the relation between human nutrition and cancer were undertaken. These studies were possible because death certification was becoming universal and reasonably complete for all causes of death and because of statistical and epidemiologic methods to conduct relatively sophisticated analyses of data. For example, studies in Britain in the early part of the 20th century evaluated death in religious orders that consumed little or no meat. These early studies found essentially no relationship between vegetarianism and cancer mortality.[3] However, elevated mortality from colorectal cancer was observed in persons with comparatively lower intakes of carrots, onions, cabbage, beets, and turnips in a separate study.[4] Subsequent studies by the same investigator revealed additional negative associations between green vegetable intake and intestinal cancer.[5]

These early studies suggested a protective impact on cancer risk of dietary regimens rich in fruits and vegetables. Subsequent observations in migrant groups to the U.S. showed a dramatic increase in cancer mortality (particularly for colon cancer) in Japanese migrants after assuming a Western diet.[6] The migrant studies pointed to dietary practices, particularly in early life, as predictive of adult cancer risk, a finding that confirmed studies in rodents[7] and more recent epidemiologic observations.[8] In addition, patterns emerged from international correlation studies that indicated that dietary practices might determine breast and colon cancers.[9] Further studies of cancer in vegetarians commenced in the middle of the 20th century, with focus on religious groups (both clerical and lay).

An example of such studies was an analysis of cancer mortality (1911–1978) conducted in two groups of British nuns, one of which consumed no meat (n = 1769) and one in which meat consumption was limited (n = 1044).[10] In this study, mortality from colorectal cancer was not lower than the general population in either group even when using mortality rates in single women for comparison. The SMR in the no-meat group was 0.99 for colon and small bowel cancer although esophagus cancer was found in excess in both no-meat and limited-meat intake groups (SMR = 1.93 and 2.04, respectively). Breast cancer was somewhat lower in the no-meat group (SMR = 0.87) and somewhat higher in the some-meat group (SMR = 1.17), although neither finding was statistically significant (Figure 4.1).

No relationship between cancer mortality and length of exposure to a no-meat diet was noted in this study, nor was there any association between breast, colorectal, or ovarian cancer mortality and estimated fat intake in the no-meat communities of nuns.

Members of the Vegetarian Society of Manchester (founded in 1847) and the Vegetarian Society of London (founded in 1888) were studied for patterns of mortality during the years 1936 to 1970. Based on 759 total deaths, only a slight reduction in lung and colon cancer mortality was found, as was an apparent excess of breast and stomach cancer.[11] Bladder

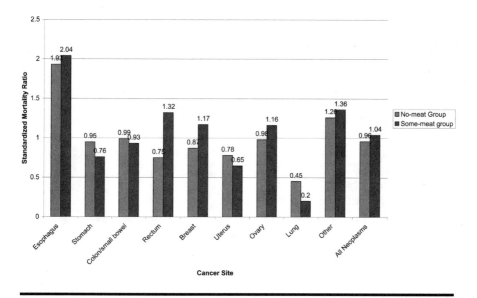

Figure 4.1   Standardized mortality ratios from cancer among British nuns consuming little or no meat, 1911–1978 (Kinlen, 1982).

cancer was found less frequently in the vegetarians as well. When the analysis was restricted to those who had been members of the vegetarian societies for >5 years or >15 years, the excess of stomach and breast cancer persisted. The authors noted that of the 23 deaths from breast cancer, 12 occurred among women who were unmarried, a high-risk group for breast cancer (Figure 4.2).

The Health Food Shoppers Study[12] in the U.K. recruited both vegetarian (n = 3790) and non-vegetarian (n = 6088) study subjects. Participants were identified via health food shops, magazines, and vegetarian societies between 1973 and 1979. Follow-up was completed by record linkage with National Health Service Central Register through 1995. SMRs were calculated based on the national mortality rates for England and Wales. For all malignant neoplasms combined, the SMR was significantly reduced in both males and females (0.50 and 0.76, respectively). Risk of stomach and colorectal cancer death was also lower, although the SMR for breast, ovary, and prostate cancers were close to 1.0 (See Figure 4.3). Death rate ratios (and 95% confidence limits) comparing vegetarians with non-vegetarians within the study were reported for stomach, colorectal, lung, breast, and prostate cancers after adjustment for age, sex, and smoking status.[14] The rate ratios were as follows: for stomach, 1.23 (0.62–2.47); for colorectal 0.90 (0.58–1.39); for lung 1.13 (0.67–1.92); for breast 1.74 (1.11–2.72); for prostate 1.31 (0.65–2.66). These data then indicate that, compared with the general population, some cancers are found less frequently in the

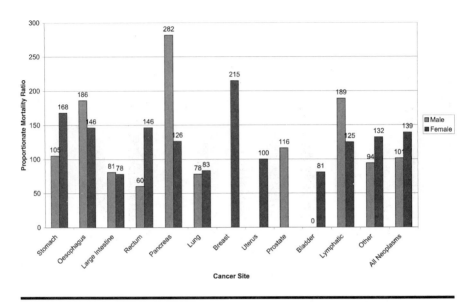

Figure 4.2 Proportionate mortality ratios for British vegetarians by sex, 1936–1970 (Kinlen, 1983).

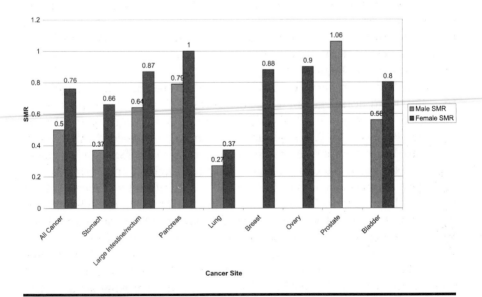

Figure 4.3 Standardized mortality ratios for the Health Food Shoppers Study, 1973–1995 (Key, 1996).

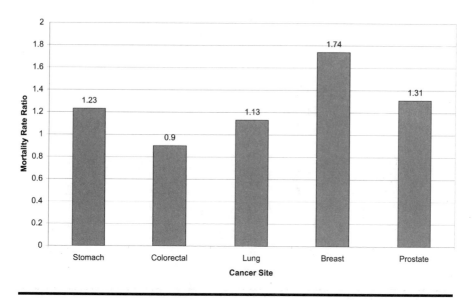

Figure 4.4   Mortality rate ratios for vegetarians compared with non-vegetarians in the Health Food Shoppers Study, 1973–1995 (Key, 1999).

vegetarians. However, there was little evidence for reduced cancer risk when the vegetarians were specifically compared with the non-vegetarians within the study cohort. For breast cancer, the data actually indicate a 74% elevated risk (see Figure 4.4).

The Oxford Vegetarian Study[15] involved 5927 vegetarians and 4912 meat eaters who were initially identified between 1980 and 1984 through advertisements in the publications of the Vegetarian Society of the United Kingdom as well as through the news media and by word of mouth. A comparison group of meat-eaters was identified by the vegetarians (including friends and relatives) and hence was thought to be similar to the vegetarian group in regard to socioeconomic status and lifestyle factors besides diet.

The SMR for all subjects in this study for all malignant neoplasms was .62 (95% C.I. 53–73) (based on 164 observed deaths and 262.5 expected). However, for meat-eaters, the SMR was .80 (89 observed, 111.2 expected) while for non-meat-eaters the SMR was lower, .50 (75 observed, 151.3 expected). The overall SMR of 62 persisted after adjusting for smoking, social class, and weight. An analysis of cancer-specific SMR in this cohort[14] revealed insignificantly lower SMRs when the vegetarians were compared with the non-vegetarians for stomach, colorectal, lung, and prostate cancer but not for breast cancer (see Figure 4.5).

In 1976, a cohort of 1904 vegetarians was identified in Germany by inserting a brief questionnaire into several vegetarian magazines. In 1978,

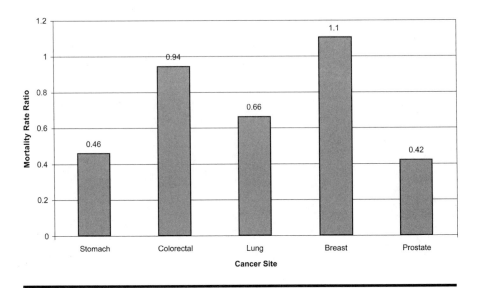

Figure 4.5 Mortality rate ratios for vegetarians compared with non–vegetarians in the Oxford Vegetarian Study, 1981–1995 (Key, 1999).

the respondents to the initial invitation completed another questionnaire concerning dietary habits, physical activity, medical history, socioeconomic information, and information about changes in lifestyle. The cohort was followed for 11 years (1979–1989) and the observed number of deaths (n = 225) was compared with the expected number, which was based on age- and sex-specific mortality rates in the Federal Republic of Germany between 1980 and 1986. The results indicated a lower risk of cancer death among both sexes in the vegetarians than in the general population for most causes of cancer death (in particular, for colon cancer), although both liver and pancreas cancers were elevated among male vegetarians (Figure 4.6). Risk of all-cause cancer mortality was reduced by almost 50% in males, whereas females experienced a more modest 26% reduction in cancer mortality. An interesting observation in this study concerned the comparison between the strict vegetarians and those who practiced a moderate dietary regimen. Those practicing the more moderate habit experienced a lower risk of cancer death than did those who practiced a strict vegetarian lifestyle.[16]

Between 1966 and 1981, a cohort study involving 122,261 Japanese men was conducted in which participants were grouped into those exhibiting "SDA-like" behaviors (e.g., those who never smoked, drank alcohol, or ate meat) were contrasted with those not exhibiting such behaviors.[17] The relative risks of death from cancer in the two groups were calculated by comparing age-adjusted death rates. The results showed the "SDA-like"

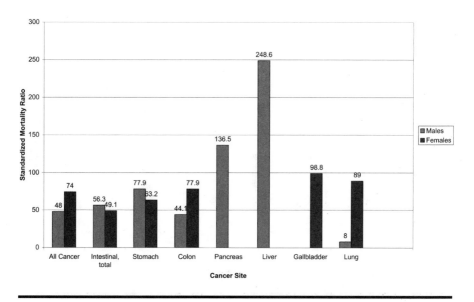

Figure 4.6   Standardized mortality ratios from the German Vegetarian Study, 1979–1989 (Frentzel–Beyme, 1994).

group to experience lower risk for most cancer sites, in particular those related to smoking (i.e. mouth, pharynx, esophagus, lung, and bladder). However, prostate cancer mortality was not decreased in the vegetarian compared with the non-vegetarian group (Figure 4.7).

B.   Studies in Seventh-Day Adventists

Seventh day Adventists (SDAs) are a conservative Christian denomination dating back to the mid-19th century in the U.S.. By religious belief, the SDA church proscribes the use of tobacco, alcohol, and pork among church members and recommends, but does not require, that members practice a vegetarian lifestyle. As a consequence, a small number (<5%) of SDAs are pure vegetarians, a substantial proportion (40–50%) practice a lacto-ovo-vegetarian lifestyle (i.e., consume no flesh products but use eggs and dairy products), while the rest consume meat to one degree or another. Due to their avoidance of tobacco and alcohol and their dietary habits, SDAs have received sustained attention from scientists and others interested in evaluating lifestyle and disease relationships. Several studies have been conducted among SDAs in both the U.S. and elsewhere. In this review, the studies among SDAs in the U.S will be separate from the non-U.S. studies.

The U.S. SDA studies involve cohort mortality and incidence studies that were initiated in the late 1950s and a prospective cancer incidence

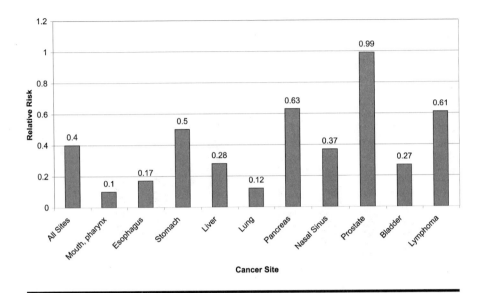

Figure 4.7 **Relative risk of cancer death in vegetarian vs. non-vegetarian Japanese males, 1966–1981 (Hirayama, 1985).**

study initiated in the early 1970s. These studies are reviewed below. However, as early as 1958, Wynder and Lemon examined cancer and heart disease in SDA hospital patients compared with non-SDA patients.[18] In this early study, based on 564 SDA and 8128 non-SDA patients admitted to eight SDA hospitals throughout the U.S., lower risk of epidermoid lung, mouth, esophagus, larynx, and bladder cancer were found in the SDAs than in the non-SDAs. Colon and rectum cancer, however, were not found less frequently in the SDA than the non-SDA comparison group, while prostate and breast cancer were found somewhat more frequently in the SDA patient series. Interviews with study subjects indicated that only 41% of the SDA patients consumed any meat, whereas 95% of the general population consumed meat.

The Adventist Mortality Study was based on a prospective study of fatal disease among 27,000 California SDAs who completed the same lifestyle questionnaire completed by approximately one million Americans as part of the American Cancer Society's Cancer Prevention Study in 1960. The population was followed up for 21 years (through 1980), although results were reported through different points in time including 1965, 1976, and 1980. Various analyses of this cohort compared cancer death rates in California SDAs to the general California population, while separate analyses compared the non-smoking SDA population with non-smoking participants in the ACS nationwide study. Further attempts were made to compare cancer mortality in the SDA population with educationally and sociodemographically similar populations.

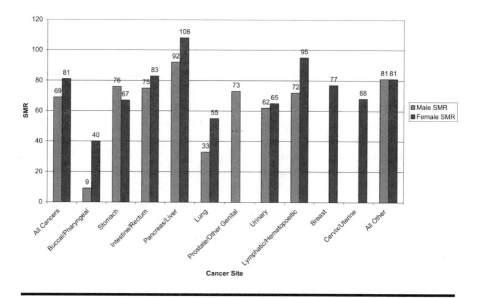

Figure 4.8   Standardized mortality ratios for cancer in California SDA, 1955–1959 (Lemon, 1964).

In 1958, approximately 47,000 SDAs in California were identified and patterns of mortality for the years 1955–1959 were reported.[19] Based on 3481 deaths, observed-to-expected ratios were calculated comparing mortality ratios in the SDA to age-comparable mortality ratios in the California general population on a sex-specific basis. The overall SMR for all cancer sites was decreased in both men (SMR = 70.6) and women (SMR = 80.1), both of which were statistically significant. In addition, buccal and pharyngeal cancer in men were significantly lower than expected (see Figure 4.8).

Between the years 1958 and 1965, an updated analysis that examined mortality in the SDA population was conducted wherein various adjustments were made to make the SDA:non-SDA comparison more valid. In particular, adjustment for educational attainment was made. Adventists were compared with non-smoking participants in the ACS Cancer Prevention study, and SDA physicians were compared with non-SDA physicians (thus controlling for education, social class, and other lifestyle characteristics).[20] After controlling for education (in addition to age and sex), the SMRs in the SDAs were closer to the reference value (i.e., 100) for all cancers combined, colorectal cancer, stomach cancer, and ovary/uterus cancer, but further from 100 for breast and prostate cancers, thus indicating a differential impact of educational adjustment by cancer site. As expected, however, when comparisons were made between SDA and non-smoking ACS participants, the SMRs for Adventists were not nearly as reduced as when using a general population comparison. The SMRs for all cancer sites combined was 54 when the general California population was used but this changed to 82 when the comparison with non-smokers was made. When the mortality experience of SDA physicians for the years 1914 to 1971 was compared with the mortality experience of physician graduates of the University of Southern California (USC), the SMRs were similar for all cancer sites combined (58 for SDA physicians, 52 for USC physicians). For colorectal cancer, the SDA physician SMR was actually considerably higher than the USC SMR (90 vs. 44).

A further follow-up of this population was completed through 1976 and Standardized Mortality Ratios were reported comparing age-adjusted mortality rates in California SDAs to the U.S. white population.[21] SMRs were reduced, in particular in males, for most cancer sites (Figure 4.9) and were substantially and significantly reduced for colorectal cancer and lung cancer. However, SMRs were not significantly reduced for breast cancer, prostate cancer, or the lymphomas in this analysis.

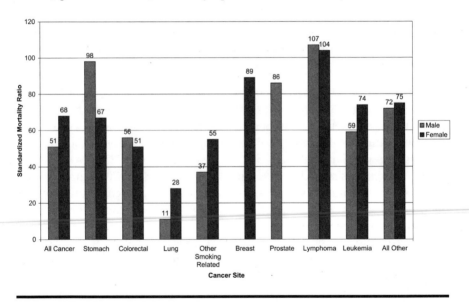

Figure 4.9   Standardized mortality ratios from the Adventist Mortality Study, 1960–1976 (Phillips, 1980).

In addition to the evaluation of fatal cancer risk through the calculation of standardized mortality ratios (using various types of reference populations), risk of cancer was evaluated within the Adventist cohort by examining relative risk of cancer death between individuals characterized by various food consumption profiles. These profiles reflected general adherence to the vegetarian lifestyle by examining consumption of several animal products including meat (or poultry), milk, eggs, and cheese.

Mortality from cancers of the colon, rectum, breast, ovary, and prostate has been evaluated in this fashion and the results of these studies are summarized in Table 4.1.

Risk of colon cancer was elevated in those in the highest meat/poultry consumption categories in males (but not females), while cheese consumption was also associated with elevated colon cancer risk in males. Rectum cancer was associated only with egg consumption.[22]

Breast cancer was not strongly associated with intake of animal products in the mortality study. After taking into account age at menarche, age at first pregnancy, age at menopause, relative weight, and education, increasing consumption of meat, milk, cheese, and eggs was unrelated to fatal breast cancer risk.[23]

Animal product consumption was more strongly associated with ovarian cancer death, however, with significant increases in risk associated with egg consumption and less strongly with meat consumption.[24]

Prostate cancer was positively associated with milk consumption (R.R = 1.5), but not so strongly associated with other animal products.[25] However, risk of fatal prostate cancer was found to be elevated threefold in those men with a combined high intake of all four animal products.

C. New Adventist Health Study

The mortality studies of SDAs in the U.S. and elsewhere were useful in comparing risk of cancer death with non-SDA populations and for examining the relationship between diet and risk of several fatal cancers. However, the mortality studies were hindered by certain limitations. First, by restricting attention only to fatal outcomes, differences in stage at diagnosis, or differences in survival may have partly explained the differences between SDA and non-SDA populations. Second, in comparing cancer mortality with the general population, the possibility of selection bias may have obscured the true relationship between diet and cancer risk. Therefore, in the early 1970s, a new study of cancer incidence in California SDAs was designed in which risk of newly diagnosed cancers was to be measured and relationships between dietary intake and cancer incidence within the SDA population was to be evaluated.

The new Adventist Health Study was launched in 1974, when a census questionnaire was mailed to every known SDA household in the state of California. In 1976, a lifestyle questionnaire was mailed to all respondents to the first questionnaire who were 25 years of age and older. The second questionnaire included a 65-item food frequency recall component designed to measure three aspects of diet: (1) current use of specific foods, (2) past intake of specific foods, and (3) current intake of major nutrients.[26]

Table 4.1   Age- and Sex-Adjusted Relative Risks for Fatal Cancer Among SDA Age >35 Years, by Selected Dietary Variables, 1960–1980

Cancer	No. of Deaths	Sex	Foods	Frequency of Consumption	Relative Risk (95%CI)	Reference
Prostate	96	M	Meat	<1/day vs. >3/wk	1.3 (p>0.1)	Snowdon, 1984[25]
	99		Milk	<1 glass/day vs. >3 glasses/day	1.5 (p<0.1)*	
	97		Cheese	<1/wk vs. >3/wk	1.4 (p>0.1)	
	97		Eggs	<1/day vs. >3/wk	1.3 (p>0.1)	
Ovary	50		Eggs	<1/wk vs. >3/wk	3.0 (1.2–7.3)	Snowdon, 1985[24]
Colon	52	M	Meat	<1/wk vs. 4/wk	1.5 (.7–3.3)	Phillips, 1985[22]
	54		Eggs	<2/wk vs. >5/wk	1.6 (.8–3.4)	
	55		Milk	<1/day vs. >3/day	0.5 (.2–1.1)	
	54		Cheese	<1/wk vs. >3/wk	1.9 (1.0–3.6)	
Colon	87	F	Meat	<1/wk vs. >4/wk	0.7 (.3–1.4)	
	88		Eggs	<2/wk vs. >5/wk	1.7 (.9–3.0)	
	91		Milk	<1/day vs. >3/day	1.1 (.5–2.2)	
	88		Cheese	<1/wk vs. >3/wk	0.8 (.5–1.4)	
Rectum	33	M/F	Meat	<1/wk vs. >4/wk	0.8 (.3–2.4)	
	33		Eggs	<2/wk vs. >5/wk	1.1 (.5–2.9)	
	33		Milk	<1/day vs. >3/day	1.2 (.6–2.7)	
	33		Cheese	<1/wk vs. >3/wk	1.0 (.5–2.2)	
Breast	142	F	Meat	None vs. >4/wk	1.15 (.53–2.53)**	Mills, 1988[23]
			Cheese	None vs. >3/wk	1.25 (.60–2.61	
			Milk	None vs. >3/wk	0.89 (.34–2.35)	
			Eggs	None vs. >3/wk	0.67 (.31–1.45)	

*Adjusted for age, education, weight and several foods.

**Adjusted for age at menarche, age at first pregnancy, age at menopause, weight, education, and for several foods.

Between 1976 and 1982, study of cancer incidence in the cohort of about 34,200 non-Hispanic white respondents to the lifestyle questionnaire was conducted by annual mailings to the study participants. Members of the cohort were asked to report any hospitalization in the previous year and study staff subsequently reviewed medical records for any evidence of a cancer diagnosis.[27]

Using an external reference population (i.e., Connecticut Tumor Registry) to generate expected numbers of cancer cases (adjusting for age, sex, and calendar year), the California SDA population was found to experience decreased cancer risk, although the reduction was more apparent in males than females. For all cancer sites combined, the standardized incidence ratio in males was 0.73, and for females it was 0.92; the result in females was of borderline statistical significance.[28] (See Figure 4.10.) For most of the major cancer sites, the SDAs experienced low cancer risk (e.g., colon, lung) although for other cancer sites, risk was not substantially different in the SDAs (e.g., breast) or even somewhat elevated (e.g., prostate, corpus uteri).

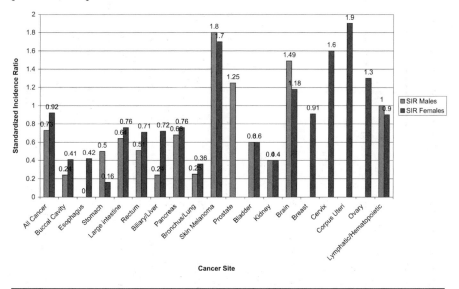

Figure 4.10   Standardized incidence ratios for selected cancer sites in California SDA, 1976–1982 (Mills, 1994).

Relationships between several foods and food groups have been examined in relation to cancer within the Adventist cohort for the years 1976 and 1982. Currently, results have been presented for breast, prostate, lung, colon, bladder, and pancreas cancer. (See Table 4.2.)

Table 4.2 Adjusted Relative Risks for Newly Diagnosed Cancers Among SDA >25 Years, By Selected Dietary Variables, 1977–1982

Cancer Site	No. Cases	Risk Enhanced	Rel. Risk	Risk Reduced	Rel.Risk	Comment	Ref.
Breast	215	Meat (never vs.>3/wk	1.33(.9–1.95)			Adjusted for several covariates*	Mills[29]
		Cheese (<2/mo. vs.>3/wk.	1.43(.99–2.06)				
		Whole Milk (never vs. daily)	0.94(.66–1.33)				
		Eggs (<1/wk vs. >2/wk)	1.07(.73–1.56)				
Lung	61	Meat (never vs.>2/wk)	1.31(.52–3.28)	Fruit (<3/wk vs.>2/day)	0.26(.1–.7)	Adjusted for age, sex, smoking	Fraser[30]
		Poultry (never vs.>1/wk)	2.20 (.84–5.77)	Green Salads (<3/wk vs.>7/wk)	0.65(.29–1.47)		
Prostate	180	Current meat (never vs.>daily)	1.41(.79–2.51)	Beans, lentils, peas (<1/mo.vs.>3/wk)	0.53(.31–.90)	Adjusted for several covariates**	Mills[31]
		Current Fish (never vs. >1/wk)	1.57(.88–2.78)	Current Tomatoes (<1/wk vs.>5/wk)	0.60(.37–.97)		
				Raisins, dates, dry fruit (<1/wk vs.>5/wk)	0.62(.36–1.06)		Jacobsen[46]
				Soy milk (>1/day vs. <1/day)	0.30(.1–1.0)		
Colon	145	Total meat (never vs.>1/wk)	1.85 (1.16–2.87)	Legumes (never vs. >2/wk)	0.53(.33–.86)	Adjusted for several covariates***	Singh[32]

Bladder	52	Red meat (never vs. >1/wk)	1.41 (.9–2.21)		
		Poultry, Fish (never vs. >1/wk)	1.46 (.86–2.48)		
		Nuts (never vs. >4/wk)	0.68 (.45–1.04)	Adjusted for multiple covariates****	Mills[33]
		Meat, poultry, fish (<3/wk vs. >3/wk)	2.38 (1.23–4.61)		
		Sweetened Fruit Juice (<1/wk vs.>1/wk)	0.34 (.11–1.11)		
		Cooked Green Vegetables (<2/wk vs. >1/day)	0.77(.41–1.43)		
Pancreas	40	Vegetarian Protein Products (<1/wk vs.>3/wk)	0.15(.03–.89)	Adjusted for several covariates*****	Mills[34]
		Beans, lentils, peas (<1/wk vs.>3/wk)	.03(.003–.24)		
		Raisins, dates, dry fruit (<1/mo. Vs. >3/wk)	0.19 9.04–.86)		

*Adjusted for age at entry, age at first pregnancy, age at menarche, menopausal status, history of benign breast disease, maternal history of breast cancer, education and weight.

**Adjusted for age, education and several other foods.

***Adjusted for age, sex, weight, physical activity, parental history of colon cancer, smoking, alcohol and aspirin use.

****Adjusted for age, sex, smoking, coffee, alcohol, urban vs. rural residence, and several other foods.

*****Adusted for age, sex, smoking and several other foods.

As with the analysis of fatal breast cancer, no strong relationship between consumption of animal products and breast cancer risk emerged from the new incidence study. After controlling for the effects of several covariates known to be associated with breast cancer risk (e.g., age at first menstrual period, age at first full-term pregnancy, and body weight), risks associated with meat intake were negligible. Comparing current use of meat, poultry and fish in those who consumed these products more than three times per week with never users, a non-significant relative risk of 1.33 was found, thus indicating that meat was only weakly associated with breast cancer in this study, if at all.[29]

When meat and poultry intake were evaluated in regard to lung cancer risk, the relative risks were somewhat elevated, though not significantly so. More noteworthy was the protective association between fruit and green salad intake and lung cancer risk. After taking into account smoking history, lung cancer risk was decreased 74% in those who frequently consumed fruit and a significant dose–response relationship was found.[30]

Prostate cancer risk bore a similar relationship to meat intake in that risk appeared to be somewhat elevated in the highest consumption categories (daily intake), yet the elevated risks were not as substantial (or statistically significant) as the protective associations seen with consumption of certain vegetables and fruits. In the prostate cancer analysis, a relative risk of 0.53 was noted for frequent consumption of beans, lentils, or peas and a relative risk of 0.60 was noted for frequent tomato consumption.[31]

For colon cancer, however, meat intake and, in particular, intake of both red meat and white meat (i.e. poultry, fish) bore significant associations with elevated risk. In addition, legumes (i.e., beans, lentils, split peas) were associated with a nearly 50% reduction in colon cancer risk. The increases in risk appeared to act synergistically in that men with high meat intake, heavy body weight, and low legume consumption experienced a threefold increase in colon cancer risk.[32]

Bladder cancer risk was also found to be positively associated with meat consumption (relative risk = 2.38) and inversely associated with fruit juice and cooked green vegetable consumption. These associations persisted after simultaneously controlling for smoking history (a risk factor for bladder cancer) as well as for all dietary variables.[33]

Pancreas cancer death was also evaluated in the incidence study. Because survival with this form of cancer is extremely poor, mortality is tantamount to incidence. When patterns of dietary intake were evaluated, risk of pancreas cancer was observed to decrease with increasing consumption of several foods commonly found in the vegetarian diet. Consumption of vegetarian protein products, legumes, and dried fruit all bore substantial reductions in risk of pancreas cancer. When meat consumption was included in the multivariate model, it was not associated with cancer risk although the vegetarian foods were all associated with decreased risk.[34]

D. SDA Studies Outside the U.S. (Denmark, Netherlands, and Norway)

As noted, several studies concerning diet and cancer risk have been conducted among SDAs in the U.S., where about 600,000 SDAs reside. The worldwide population of SDAs is approximately 3 million, and additional studies of SDAs residing outside of the U.S. have also been conducted. For example, in the Netherlands, patterns of mortality in approximately 4000 SDAs were evaluated during a 10-year study period between 1968 and 1977. Cancer of the colon and rectum (SMR = 0.43), lung (SMR = 0.45), and breast (SMR = 0.50) were all significantly lower in the SDA population than expected. (See Figure 4.11.) However, in the SDA group, pancreas cancer showed a threefold elevation that was not statistically significant.[35]

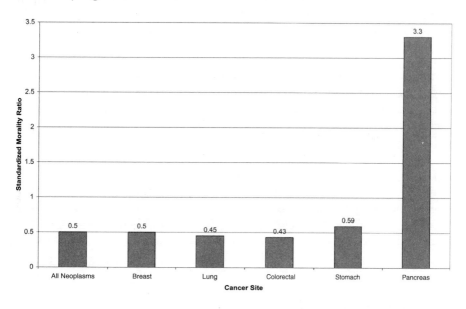

Figure 4.11   Standardized mortality ratios for cancer in Dutch SDA, 1968–1977, (Berkel,1983).

In Norway, 7253 SDAs were followed between 1961 and 1986 and monitored for cancer diagnoses. The Standardized Incidence Ratios (SIR) were divided into two groups: those under 75 years of age and those greater than 75 years of age. Only the SIR for lung cancer in those less

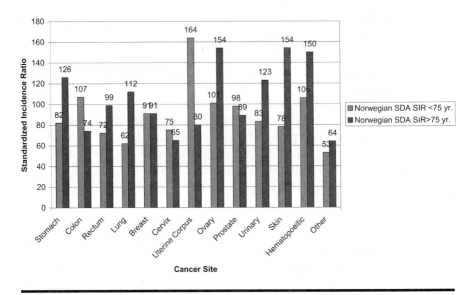

Figure 4.12   Standardized incidence ratios for Norwegian SDAs, 1961–1986, by site and age group (Fonnebo,1991).

than 75 years was significantly decreased in the SDAs, in comparison with the general Norwegian population.[36] (See Figure 4.12.) The authors note that the cancer incidence rate is quite low in the general Norwegian population and due to this low "background" risk, it may be difficult to detect further departures in cancer risk associated with lifestyle habits.

In 1983, Jensen reported on cancer morbidity in male SDA members in Copenhagen for the years 1943 to 1977. In addition, results were presented for members of other (i.e., non-SDA) temperance society members. The SIR was significantly lower in the SDAs for all cancers and for lung and colon cancer. Incidence of lymphatic and hematopoietic cancers was increased but not significantly so (see Figure 4.13). Interestingly, cancer incidence among members of the other temperance society was not substantially different from the general population.[37]

E. Analysis/Interpretation

In general, these studies of vegetarian populations have revealed lower cancer mortality (or incidence) in vegetarians than in non-vegetarians. In comparing vegetarians with the general population, in comparing vegetarians specifically with non-vegetarians, in comparing different cancer sites for different genders, ages groups, and time periods, a total of 204 SMRs or relative risks have been evaluated. More than 70% (71%) of the

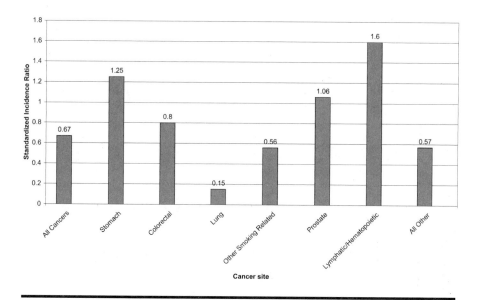

Figure 4.13   Standardized incidence ratios for selected cancer sites in SDA males age > 35 years in Copenhagen, 1943–1977 (Jensen, 1983).

SMRs or relative risks were decreased (i.e., <100 or 1.0) when comparing vegetarians with non-vegetarians.

Of the 145 SMRs or relative risks that were less than 100, 39% were deemed to be statistically significant (i.e., not due to chance). These figures varied when evaluating specific cancer sites, however. For colon cancer, out of a total of 20 studies, 19 (95%) reported an SMR/RR less than 100 (or 1.0). Six of these were statistically significant. For the other cancer sites evaluated, this figure was lower. For prostate cancer, only 55% of the SMRs reviewed were <100 (none significantly so) while for breast cancer 67% were <100, of which one was significantly less than 100 and two were significantly greater than 100. Table 4.3 summarizes the percent of SMRs and/or RRs less than the null value for all cancer sites combined as well as for colon, prostate, breast, lung, stomach, pancreas and ovarian cancer as well as for the lymphatic/hematopoietic cancers.

The difference experienced by vegetarians compared with non-vegetarians appeared to be moderated by gender. Males appeared to enjoy a stronger degree of protection from cancer mortality/incidence than females. For example, four out of six studies (67%) that evaluated colorectal cancer risk by gender revealed lower SMRs for males than females. For lung cancer, six out of six (100%) SMRs were lower in males and for all cancer sites combined, six out of six studies (100%) showed lower SMRs in males than females.

Table 4.3 Standardized Mortality (Morbidity) Ratios and Relative Risks for Vegetarian vs. Non-Vegetarian Populations for Several Types of Cancer

Study	Years	Subgroups	All Sites	Colon	Breast	Prostate	Lung	Stomach	Lymph/ Hem.	Pancreas	Ovary
Kinlen's Nuns[10]	1911–1978	No Meat	96	99	87	–	45*	95	–	–	98
		Some meat	104	93	117	–	20*	76	–	–	116
Kinlen's Vegetarians[11]	1936–1970	Males	101	81		116	78	105	189	282*	–
		Females	139*	78	215*		83	168	125	126	–
Health Food Shoppers[13]	1973–95	Males	50*	64*	–	106	27	37*	–	79	–
		Females	76*	87	88	–	37*	66	–	100	90
Health Food Shoppers[14]	1973–1995	Veg vs. Non-Veg.	–	90	174*	131	113	123	–	–	–
Oxford Vegetarians[15]	1981–1995	Both Sexes Veg. vs. Non-Veg.	50*	–	–	–	–	–	–	–	–
Oxford Vegetarians[14]	1981–1995	Non-Veg.	–	94	110	42	66	46	–	–	–
German Veg.[16]	1979–89	Males	48*	44	–	–	8*	78	–	137	–
		Females	74	78	–	–	89	63	–	–	–
SDA (U.S.)[19]	1955–59	Males	69*	75	–	73	33*	76	72	92	–
		Females	81*	83	77	–	55	67	95	108	–
SDA (U.S.)[21]	1960–76	Males	51*	56*	–	86	11	98	107/59*	–	–
		Females	68*	51*	89	–	28	67	104/54	–	–
SDA (U.S.)[28]	1976–82	Males	73*	64*	–	125	25*	50*	100	68	–
		Females	92	76*	91	–	36*	16*	87	76	129
SDA (Dutch)[35]	1968–77	Females	50*	43*	50*	–	45*	59*	–	330	–

SDA (Norway)[36]	1961–86	<75 yrs.	—	107	91	98	62*	82	106	—	101
		>75 yrs.	—	74	91	89	112	126	150	—	154
SDA (Copenhagen)[37]	1943–1977	Males	67*	80	—	106	15*	125	160	—	—
Japanese Vegetarians[17]	1966–81	Males	40*	—	—	99	12*	50*	61	63	—
%SMR< 100			.83	.95	.67	.55	.90	.76	.43	.45	.33

* SMR/RR statistically significant (p<0.05)

A possible explanation for this phenomenon is the lifestyle habits of the general population. Traditionally, the prevalence of smoking and drinking is lower among females than males in the general population. When comparisons are made between female vegetarians and female non-vegetarians, therefore, the contrast is not as dramatic as when vegetarian males are compared with non-vegetarian males, who generally consume more tobacco and alcohol than females. This may explain the apparent stronger effect of vegetarianism on cancer risk among males.

Overall, the protective association with vegetarianism seems most pronounced for colon, stomach, and lung cancer and less pronounced for ovarian, pancreatic, and the lymphatic/hematopoietic cancers.

When within-group comparisons are evaluated where dietary variation exists (e.g., within the SDA populations), several patterns emerge regarding consumption of various foods and food groups. In the SDA mortality studies in the U.S., in which high fat foods of animal origin are examined (e.g., meat, milk, eggs, and cheese), no strong consistent pattern of increasing risk of cancer attendant to increasing consumption of these foods is observed. For several cancer sites including prostate, ovary, colon, and breast cancers, relative risks are either close to the null value (i.e., 1.0) or only slightly higher (e.g., 1.3–1.8). Of the 21 relative risks evaluated in regard to cancer mortality associated with animal-product consumption in the Adventist Health Studies (Table 4.1), only 19% were >1.5, while 52% were between 1.0 and 1.5. Another 29% were actually <1.0 in value. Values of this magnitude (i.e., close to 1.0) must be interpreted cautiously, as they might be explained by misclassification, confounding, or sampling error.

Data from the SDA incidence study provided slightly more evidence for increased cancer risk with increasing meat consumption (particularly for colon and prostate cancers), but no strong evidence for a positive association with breast cancer. On the other hand, several strong reductions in cancer risk were observed in association with frequent consumption of several types of vegetables and fruits, as well as for consumption of soy-based foods, legumes, and nuts. These patterns were observed for most of the cancer sites evaluated in the incidence study including lung, prostate, colon, bladder, and pancreas.

Although initial interest in the diet–cancer relationship focused on dietary fat as a potential culprit, studies conducted among vegetarian populations during the last two decades have not, in general, supported the dietary fat hypothesis for many forms of cancer. Rather, a pronounced protective effect of fruit and vegetable consumption has emerged.

II. COMPONENTS OF VEGETARIAN DIETS THAT MAY BE ASSOCIATED WITH ALTERED CANCER RISK

The vegetarian diet differs from the non-vegetarian diet in more ways than the mere absence of meat. Some vegetarians often consume vegetarian protein products (e.g., soy) as meat substitutes and also tend to consume more fruits and vegetables and more whole wheat grains, which are rich in many micronutrients thought to offer some protection against cancer. Thus, the question that remains is whether it is something in meat itself (or perhaps the cooking of meat) or the lack of protective substances in the non-vegetarian diet that increases cancer risk in non-vegetarians. In this review, the common components of a typical vegetarian diet, including the role of soy, fiber, whole grains, fruits, and vegetables, are reviewed in reference to cancer risk.

A. Soy, Isoflavones and Breast or Prostate Cancer Risk

The observation that both breast and prostate cancers are common in the Western industrialized nations, while relatively rare in oriental countries such as China and Japan, suggests that some component of the oriental diet may include substances that protect against these cancers. In addition, studies of migrants from these low-risk countries to the U.S. revealed that risk of breast and prostate cancer increased to the level of Caucasians in the U.S. after only a few generations.

One such aspect of diet that has received recent attention is the consumption of soy-based foods such as tofu. Tofu is a major source of protein in many oriental diets, while consumption is uncommon in the U.S. (e.g., one recent study among women in Iowa found that only 2.9% of study participants reported consumption of any tofu).

Soy-based products contain isoflavones, which are thought to exhibit anticarcinogenic properties. These compounds (e.g., genistein) exhibit weak estrogenic properties that bind with estrogen receptor sites (much like tamoxifen) and compete with much more potent estrogens for these sites.[38]

Several case-control studies and one cohort study have reported on the relationship between soy intake (or indirect measures of intake) and breast cancer risk. These studies are summarized in Table 4.4. In a study in Singapore involving 200 breast cancer cases, breast cancer risk was reduced approximately 60% among women in the highest quintile of soy consumption, compared with those in the lowest quintile of soy consumption.[39] However, this relationship was observed only in premenopausal women. In a larger hospital-based study in Japan, those women consuming soy three or more times per week had approximately 20% lower risk of

Table 4.4 Summary of Epidemiologic Studies of Soy/Tofu Intake and Breast Cancer Risk

Reference	Location	Study Design	No. of Cases	Consumption	Odds Ratio or Relative risk	Comment
Lee[39]	Singapore	Case-control	200	Highest Quintile vs. Lowest Quintile	.39 (.19–.77)	Premenopausal women only
Hirose[40]	Japan	Case-control	1186	>3/wk vs. <3/wk	.81 (.65–.99)	Hospital-based study; premenopausal only
Yuan[41]	Shanghai	Case-control	534	Per 18 gram serving	0.9 (.6–1.4)	Includes both pre- and postmenopausal
Yuan[41]	Tainjin	Case-control	300	Per 18 gram serving	1.4 (.8–2.6)	Includes both pre- and postmenopausal
Wu[42]	U.S.	Case-control	597	Per 1 time/week	0.85 (.74–.99)	Asian women in the U.S.
Ingram[43]	Australia	Case-control	144	Highest Quartile of metabolite excretion vs. Lowest Quartile	0.41 (.19–.90)	Soy intake estimated by metabolite excretion. Both pre- and postmenopausal
Greenstein[44]	U.S.	Cohort	1018 cases in cohort >34,000	Any vs. none	0.76 (.50–1.18)	Postmenopausal

breast cancer than those women who consumed soy less frequently. Again, the findings of a protective relationship were restricted to premenopausal women only.[40] Two studies in China (one in Shanghai involving 534 breast cancer cases and one in Tianjin involving 300 cases) did not detect any decreased or increased breast cancer risk attendant to soy consumption in either pre- or postmenopausal women.[41] A study conducted among Asian women in the U.S., involving 597 breast cancer cases found a modest (about 15%) decrease in breast cancer risk in both pre- and postmenopausal women.[42] More recently, a study based in Australia that measured urinary excretion of soy metabolites, found a significant reduction in breast cancer risk among those women in the highest quartiles of metabolite excretion[43] and a strong dose–response relationship was observed. Similar trends were observed in both the pre- and postmenopausal groups.

A cohort study involving more than 34,000 women in Iowa evaluated soy consumption in relation to breast cancer risk. When women were dichotomized simply into those that had any soy consumption vs. those with none, the relative risk of breast cancer was 0.76 in those with any consumption after taking into account several known risk factors for breast cancer. This finding, however, was not statistically significant.[44] Therefore, although there is suggestive evidence (from both biology and epidemiology) that soy may reduce risk of breast cancer, further research is clearly warranted to investigate this relationship.

Although the biologic evidence suggesting that soy may be important in the development of prostate cancer is quite strong, only a few epidemiologic studies have evaluated this relationship. Among men of Japanese ancestry living in Hawaii, risk of prostate cancer was reduced 65% in those men who ate tofu more than five times per week, in comparison with those who ate it less than once per week. However, the number of men in the study was small and the finding was of borderline statistical significance.[45] Among Seventh-Day Adventist men, risk of prostate cancer was reduced 70% among men who consumed more than one serving of soy milk per day (R.R. = 0.3, 95% confidence interval 0.1–1.0) and a significant trend of decreased risk was observed with increased consumption.[46] A recent study among Chinese men found no significant difference between prostate cancer cases and controls in regard to soy consumption (9.9 servings/week vs. 11.7 servings/week respectively, $p = 0.16$).[47]

B. Dietary Fiber and Cancer Risk

Since the original suggestion by Denis Burkitt that dietary fiber might protect against colon cancer,[48] numerous case-control and a few cohort studies have investigated this relationship. Most, but not all, have supported the original hypothesis of a protective role for fiber in the etiology of colon cancer. A recent review reported that 11 out of 17 case-control studies found an inverse relationship between dietary fiber intake and colorectal cancer.[49] Another review and meta-analysis (based on 5255 patients with colorectal cancer) also found a significant inverse relationship between dietary fiber and colorectal cancer risk. An overall relative risk of 0.53 comparing those in the highest quintile with those in the lowest quintile was calculated; it persisted after controlling for adjustment for other nutrients and for vitamin C and beta-carotene).[50]

The few cohort studies of this question, however, have offered less convincing evidence. Although both the Iowa Women's Health Study[51] and the Nurses Health Study[52] have demonstrated some reduction in risk of colorectal cancer with increasing fiber intake (relative risks on the order of .8–.9), the Health Professionals Study found no protection after controlling for potential confounding.[53] In addition, neither a study among Dutch Civil Servants[54] nor the Hawaiian study of Japanese American men[55] found any convincing reduction in risk with increasing fiber consumption.

The conflicting results from case-control and cohort studies are difficult to reconcile. Recall bias is a serious limitation in the conduct of case-control studies, and the overall protective role of dietary fiber in colorectal cancer may be more modest than suggested by these case-control studies.

There are few studies on the relationship between dietary fiber intake and cancer risk for cancers other than colon/rectum. Studies on breast cancer show mixed results for fiber,[56–58] but a more consistent, protective role for fiber appears evident in regard to pancreas cancer.[59]

C. Whole Grains and Cancer

There is a wide range of protective substances found in whole grains that exert their effect through various mechanisms including antioxidant activity, hormonal effects, binding of carcinogens, and otherwise influencing the environment of the gut in a beneficial fashion.[60] A recent review of some 40 case-control studies (involving 20 different types of cancer) found a pooled odds ratio of 0.66 (99% confidence interval = 0.60–0.72) for high vs. low whole grain intake.[61] Most odds ratios in this review were <1 for studies of colorectal cancers (or polyps), other gastrointestinal cancers, all hormone-related cancers, and all studies of pancreas cancer. Most of the odds ratios for the various cancer sites that were reviewed were of the order of 0.5 to 0.8, although for both breast and prostate cancer the relationship was not as pronounced. The odds ratios for breast cancer studies was 0.86 and was even higher for the prostate cancer studies reviewed (odds ratio = 0.90). Overall, there appears to be a fair amount of consistency in the evidence that intake of whole grains (e.g., whole grain bread or pasta, whole meal bread, brown bread, and non-white bread) is associated with a reduced risk of a variety of different cancers.

D. Fruits and Vegetables

The term "vegetarian" implies a lifestyle characterized by a diet rich in vegetable intake. A recent review based on 206 human epidemiologic studies and 22 animal studies concluded that fruits and vegetables were effective in the prevention of several forms of cancer including stomach, esophagus, lung, oral cavity, pharynx, endometrium, pancreas, and colon.[62] Twenty cohort studies (perhaps offering the strongest type of evidence) were reviewed and indicated that fruit and vegetable consumption afforded protection against lung cancer across all studies reviewed. The 174 case-control studies that were reviewed indicated that there was "convincing" evidence for a protective role for fruits and vegetables for cancer of the lung, stomach, and esophagus and "probable" evidence for protection against cancer of the oral cavity and pharynx, colon, breast, pancreas, and bladder. In this review, prostate cancer was the one form of cancer not found to be associated with fruit and vegetable consumption. For those cancers that were associated with fruit and vegetable consumption, however, the decrease in cancer risk associated with high intake was estimated to be about 50% and the greatest degree of protection against cancers appears to be from the consumption of raw vegetables.

E. Alternative Explanations for Low Cancer Risk in Vegetarians

Vegetarians differ from non-vegetarians in many ways besides diet. Differences between the two groups may account for observed differences in cancer mortality or incidence, rather than differences in diet itself. Several aspects of lifestyle must be considered when evaluating the health and mortality experience of vegetarian and non-vegetarian populations.

Smoking: The reduction in cancer mortality (and incidence) in vegetarians appears to be stronger in men than women and the possibility that differences in alcohol and tobacco consumption in vegetarians vs. non-vegetarians must be considered as an explanation for this finding. The use of tobacco, generally lower in vegetarian populations,[12] is clearly related to cancer risk. A recent review indicated that 38% of cancer deaths among males in the U.S. could be attributed to cigarette smoking, while among women, 23% of all cancer deaths are due to cigarettes.[63] These estimates do not include the impact of cigar, pipe, or smokeless tobacco, nor do they include the influence of environmental tobacco smoke. Cancer sites that have been associated with cigarette smoking include lung, oral cavity, esophagus, larynx, bladder, pancreas, kidney, and cervix. Recent data have suggested that colon cancer may be associated with cigarette smoking (but only after a long latency period).[64,65] The more relevant question today may be which cancer sites are not associated with tobacco; the list appears to be quite short and currently includes prostate, endometrium, and breast cancer.

Alcoholic beverage consumption is also associated with increase in cancer risk for several types of cancer. Cancer of the oral cavity, pharynx, larynx, esophagus, and liver are associated with excess alcohol consumption and, in some instances, alcohol may act synergistically with tobacco in cancer initiation.[66]

Many of the epidemiologic studies reviewed, however, adjusted for smoking history or compared risk of cancer death only to a non-smoking reference population.[20] In general, those studies in which adjustments such as these were made found the reduced risk of cancer death in non-meat eaters to persist, suggesting that the reduction in cancer risk that vegetarians experience does not seem to be due to differences in tobacco use.

Screening Bias: For some forms of cancer, screening is effective in early detection. Specifically, some of the female cancers such as cervix and breast, as well as prostate cancer in men may be detected more frequently in populations that have a greater than normal degree of access to screening programs. For example, in the Adventist Health Study in which cancer incidence was monitored among SDA between 1976 and 1982, elevated incidence of skin cancer, prostate, and cervix cancers was observed.[28] These findings may not be a reflection of an actual increased biologic risk of these forms of cancer in SDAs, but an artifact of more intense screening for cancers among SDAs than in the general population. There is a strong focus on healthy lifestyles among SDAs, as well as greater access to health services among SDAs than the general public. The same phenomenon may act in the opposite direction in regard to mortality, since screening most likely is associated with early detection and better survival for many forms of cancer, which would impact mortality rates in populations with different levels of cancer screening. Specifically, if vegetarians were to enjoy greater access to screening programs than non-vegetarians, the numbers of observed cancer deaths would be lower than otherwise, which would tend to produce lower SMRs for vegetarians.

Selection: Another phenomenon that must be considered when evaluating cancer risk in vegetarian societies or religious organizations that promote a vegetarian lifestyle is the possibility of selection bias. Only a very small percentage of the general population choose to join religious groups that advocate lifestyle changes, yet a large proportion (about 50%) of the SDA church, for example, is composed of adult converts. It is possible that people who join these organizations as adults already experience lower cancer risk due to educational or socioeconomic status and lifestyle practices, and it is these conditions that explain their lowered cancer risk rather than membership in a vegetarian organization.[21]

Religiosity: Those people who are observant of a religious faith (regardless of which particular sect or denomination) enjoy lower incidence and mortality than the general population.[67] Regular attendance at church services has been associated with lowered mortality from several chronic diseases.[68] The possibility that some aspect of spiritual life or some other lifestyle highly correlated with spirituality explains the lower cancer risk in religious denominations that espouse vegetarianism must be considered.

III. PUBLIC HEALTH IMPLICATIONS

In 1996, the Board of Directors of the American Cancer society set a challenge goal of a 50% reduction in U.S. cancer mortality by the year 2015 and, in 1998, set a parallel goal of reducing cancer incidence rates by 25%.[69,70]

A recent review of the feasibility of reaching these goals indicated that, if present trends in risk factor reductions continue, cancer mortality would actually decline by 21% and cancer incidence rates will decline 13% by 2015.[71] The dietary risk factors identified in this review included low intake of fruits and vegetables as well as high fat intake, and indicated that, in 1995, 70% of Americans consumed too few fruits and vegetables and 20% of Americans consumed a diet high in fat intake. According to the estimate, if dietary habits alone (i.e., exclusive of changes in other risk factors) were modified, in the year 2015, a reduction of between 3 and 5% in cancer incidence would be achieved, as well as a reduction in cancer mortality of between 4 and 6%

The U.S. National Cancer Institute and National Research Council recommends that five servings of fruits and vegetables be consumed every day. However, data from the NHANES II survey (1976–1980) indicated that only 9% of the U.S. population consumed this amount of fruits and vegetables per day during that time.[72] More recently, however, 23% of Americans reported eating five or more servings of fruit and vegetables per day, and, in 1991, Americans consumed an average of 3.4 servings of fruits and vegetables per day. Hence, the trends appear to be encouraging.

The degree of protection against cancer afforded by a vegetarian diet might be estimated by examining the decreased risk of cancer experienced by male and female vegetarians. As noted above, the protective effect of vegetarianism in males might be explained, in part, by differences in tobacco and alcohol use in vegetarian men compared with non-vegetarian men. In women, the role of these substances may not be as pronounced and hence the true "effect" of vegetarianism on cancer risk might be reflected among female rather than male vegetarians. However, for all cancer sites combined, the alteration in cancer mortality among female vegetarians compared with female non-vegetarians ranged from a 39% increase to a 32% decrease (average reduction in mortality was 12%). For males, the reduction was substantially greater, with a decrease in mortality ranging from 31% to 60% (average reduction of 38%). Where incidence data are available, the reduction in risk among females was 8%, while for males, the average reduction was 30%. These figures suggest that, if Americans not only decreased intake of fat and increased vegetable intake (as suggested by numerous nation health organizations, both public and private), but also actually embraced a vegetarian lifestyle, the number of newly diagnosed cancers and the number of deaths from cancer would decrease substantially each year.

Current and future research (e.g., the European Prospective Investigation into Cancer and Nutrition[73]) will further our understanding of the relationship between vegetarian nutrition and cancer risk but may take many years to complete. Until then, a prudent dietary action would be to increase the daily consumption of fresh vegetables in particular and to refrain from animal product intake.

REFERENCES

1. Doll, R. and Peto, R. The causes of cancer: quantitative estimates of avoidable risks of cancer in the U.S. today. *J. Natl. Cancer Inst.*, 66:1191-1308, 1981.
2. Willett, W. Diet, nutrition, and avoidable cancer. *Environ. Health Perspect.*, 103 (Suppl 8):165-170, 1995.
3. Copeman, S.M. and Greenwood, M. Diet and Cancer. Reports on Public Health and Medical Subjects, no. 36. Ministry of Health: H.M. Stationery Office, London, 1926.
4. Stocks, P. and Karn, M.N. A comparative study of the habits, home life, dietary, and family history of 450 cancer patients and of an equal number of control patients. *Ann. Eugenics.*, 5:30-280, 1933.
5. Stocks, P. Cancer incidence in North Wales and Liverpool region in relation to habits and environment. In: *British Empire Cancer Campaign 35th annual report supplement part II.* London, 1957.
6. Haenszel, W., Berg, J.W., and Segi, M., et al. Large bowel cancer in Hawaiian Japanese. *J. Natl. Cancer Inst.*, 51:1765-1779, 1973.
7. Albanes, D. Total calories, body weight and tumor incidence in mice. *Cancer Res.*, 47:1987-92, 1987.
8. Must, A. Childhood energy intake and cancer mortality in adulthood. *Nutr. Reviews*, 57:21-24, 1999.
9. Armstrong, B. and Doll, R. Environmental factors and cancer incidence and mortality in different countries, with special reference to dietary practices. *Int. J. Cancer.*, 15:617-631, 1975.

10. Kinlen, L.J. Meat and fat consumption and cancer mortality: A study of strict religious orders in Britain. *Lancet*, 1:946-949, 1982.

11. Kinlen, L.J., Hermon, C., and Smith, P.G. A proportionate study of cancer mortality among members of a vegetarian society. *Br. J. Cancer.*, 48:355-361, 1983.

12. Burr, M.L. and Sweetnam, P.M. Vegetarianism, dietary fiber, and mortality. *Am. J. Clin. Nutr.*, 36:873-7, 1982.

13. Key, T.J.A., Thorogood, M., Appleby, P.N., and Burr M.L. Dietary habits and mortality in 11,000 vegetarians and health conscious people: results of a 17-year follow up. *BMJ*, 313:775-779, 1996.

14. Key, T.J., Fraser, G.E., and Thorogood, M., et al., Mortality in vegetarians and non-vegetarians: detailed findings from a collaborative analysis of 5 prospective studies. *Am. J. Clin. Nutr.*, 70 (suppl):516S-24S, 1999.

15. Thorogood, M., Mann, J., Appleby, P., and McPherson, P. Risk of death from cancer and ischemic heart disease in meat- and non-meat-eaters. *BMJ*, 308:1667-71, 1994.

16. Frentzel-Beyme, R., and Chang-Claude, J. Vegetarian diets and colon cancer: the German experience. *Am. J. Clin. Nutr.*, 59 (suppl):1143S-52S, 1994.

17. Hirayama, T. Mortality in Japanese with life-styles similar to Seventh-Day Adventists. Strategy for risk reduction by life-style modification. *Natl. Cancer Inst. Monogr.*, 69:143-153, 1985.

18. Wynder, E. and Lemon, F. Cancer, coronary artery disease, and smoking—a preliminary report on differences in incidence between Seventh-Day Adventists and others. *California Medicine*, 89:267-272, 1958.

19. Lemon, F.R., Walden, R.T., and Woods, R.W. Cancer of the lung and mouth in Seventh-Day Adventists: A preliminary report on a population study. *Cancer*, 17:486-497, 1964.

20. Phillips, R.L. Role of lifestyle and dietary habits in risk of cancer among Seventh-Day Adventists. *Cancer Res.*, 35:3513-3522, 1975.

21. Phillips, R.L., Garfinkel, L., Kuzma, J.W., Beeson, W.L., Lotz, T., and Brin, B. Mortality among California Seventh-Day Adventists for Selected Cancer Sites. *J. Natl. Cancer Inst.*, 65:1097-1107, 1980.

22. Phillips, R.L. and Snowdon, D.A. Dietary relationships with fatal colorectal cancer among Seventh-Day Adventists. *J. Natl. Cancer Inst.*, 74:307-317, 1985.

23. Mills, P.K., Annegers, J.F., and Phillips, R.L. Animal product consumption and subsequent fatal breast cancer risk among Seventh-Day Adventists. *Am. J. Epidemiol.*, 127:440-453, 1988.

24. Snowdon, D.A. Diet and ovarian cancer (lett). *JAMA*, 254:356-5. 1985.

25. Snowdon, D.A., Phillips, R.L., and Choi, W. Diet, obesity, and risk of fatal prostate cancer. *Am. J. Epidemiol.*, 120:244-50, 1984.

26. Phillips, R.L. and Kuzma, J.W. Rational and methods for an epidemiologic study of cancer among Seventh-Day Adventists. *Natl. Cancer Inst. Mongr.*, 47:107-112, 1977.

27. Beeson, W.L., Mills, P.K., Phillips, R.L., Andress, M., and Fraser, G.E. Chronic disease among Seventh-Day Adventists, a low-risk group. *Cancer*, 64:57-81, 1989.

28. Mills, P.K., Beeson, W.L., Phillips, W.L., and Fraser, G.E. Cancer incidence among California Seventh-Day Adventists, 1976-82. *Am. J. Clin. Nutr.*, 59 (suppl):1136S-1142S, 1994.

29. Mills, P.K., Beeson, W.L., Phillips, R.L., and Fraser, G.E. Dietary habits and breast cancer incidence among Seventh-Day Adventists. *Cancer*, 64:582-90, 1989.

30. Fraser, G.E., Beeson, W.L., and Phillips, R.L. Diet and lung cancer in California Seventh-Day Adventists. *Am. J. Epidemiol.*, 133: 683-93, 1991.

31. Mills, P.K., Beeson, W.L., Phillips, R.L., and Fraser, G.E. Cohort study of diet, lifestyle and prostate cancer in Adventist men. *Cancer*, 64:589-604, 1989.

32. Singh, P.N., and Fraser, G.E. Dietary risk factors for colon cancer in a low-risk population. *Am. J. Epidemiol.*, 148:761-74, 1998.

33. Mills, P.K., Beeson, W.L., Phillips, R.L., and Fraser, G.E. Bladder cancer in a low-risk population: results from the Adventist Health study. *Am. J. Epidemiol.*, 133:23039, 1991.

34. Mills, P.K., Beeson, W.L., Abbey, D.E., Fraser, G.E., and Phillips, R.L. Dietary habits and past medical history as related to fatal pancreas cancer risk among Adventists. *Cancer*, 61:2578-85, 1988.

35. Berkel, J. and de Waard, F. Mortality pattern and life expectancy of Seventh-Day Adventists in the Netherlands. *Int. J. Epidemiol.*, 12:455-59, 1983.

36. Fonnebo, V. and Helseth, A. Cancer Incidence in Norwegian Seventh-Day Adventists 1961 to 1986. *Cancer*, 68:666-671, 1991.

37. Jensen, O.M. Cancer risk among Danish male Seventh-Day Adventists and other temperance society members. *J. Natl. Cancer Inst.*, 70:1011-14, 1983.

38. Messina M. and Barnes, S. The role of soy products in reducing risk of cancer. *J. Natl. Cancer Inst.*, 83:541-546, 1991.

39. Lee, H.P., Gourley, L., Duffy, S.W., Esteve, J., and Day, N.E. Dietary effects on breast-cancer risk in Singapore. *Lancet*, 337:1197-2000, 1991.

40. Hirose, K., Tajima, K., Hamajima, N., Inoue, M., Takezaki, T., Kurisha, T., Yosida, M., and Tokudome, S. A large-scale, hospital-based case-control study of risk factors of breast cancer according to menopausal status. *Jpn. J. Cancer Res.*, 86:146-154, 1995.

41. Yuan J.M., Wang, Q.S., Ross, R.K., Henderson, B.E., and Yu, M.C. Diet and breast cancer in Shanghai and Tianjin, China. *Br. J. Cancer.*, 71:1353-58, 1995.

42. Wu, A.H., Ziegler, R.G., and Horn-Ross, P.L., et al. Tofu and risk of breast cancer in Asian-Americans. *Cancer Epidemiol. Biomarkers Prevention*, 5:901-906, 1995.

43. Ingram D., Sanders, K., Kolybaba, M., and Lopez, D. Case-control study of phyto-oestrogens and breast cancer. *Lancet,* 350:990-94, 1997.

44. Greenstein J., Kushi, L., and Zheng, W., et al. Risk of breast cancer associated with specific foods and food groups. *Am. J. Epidemiol.*, 145:S36 (abstract), 1996.

45. Severson, R.J., Nomura, A.M.Y., Grove, J.S., and Stemmerman, G.N. A prospective study of demographics, diet, and prostate cancer among men of Japanese ancestry in Hawaii. *Cancer Res.*, 49:1857-60, 1989.

46. Jacobson, B.K., Knutsen, S.F., and Fraser, G.E. Does high soy milk intake reduce prostate cancer incidence? The Adventist Health Study. *Cancer Causes and Control*, 9:553-57, 1998.

47. Lee, M., Wang, R.T., Hsing, A., Gu, F.L., Wang, T., and Spitz, M. Case-control study of diet and prostate cancer in China. *Cancer Causes and Control*, 9:545-552, 1998.

48. Burkitt, D.P. Epidemiology of cancer of the colon and rectum. *Cancer*, 29:3-13, 1996.

49. Potter, J.D. Nutrition and colorectal cancer. *Cancer Causes and Control*, 7:127-46.

50. Howe, G.R., Benito, E., and Castelleto, R., et al. Dietary intake of fiber and decreased risk of cancers of the colon and rectum: evidence from the combined analysis of 13 case-control studies. *J. Natl. Cancer Inst.*, 84:1887-96, 1992.

51. Willett, W., Stampfer, M., Colditz, G., Rosner, B., and Speizer, F. Relation of meat, fat and fiber intake to the risk of colon cancer in a prospective study among women. *New Eng. J. Med.*, 323:1664-72, 1990.

52. Steinmetz, K., Kushi, L., Bostick, R.M., Folsom, A., and Potter, J.D. Vegetables, fruit, and colon cancer in the Iowa Women's Health Study. *Am. J. Epidemiol.*, 139:1-15, 1994.

53. Giovanucci, E., Rimm, E.B., Stampfer, M.J., Colditz, G., Ascherio, A., and Willett W. Intake of meat and fiber in relation to colon cancer in men. *Cancer Res.*, 54:2390-97, 1994.

54. Slob, I., Lambregts, J., Schuit, A., and Kok, F. Calcium intake and 28-year gastro-intestinal mortality in Dutch civil servants. *Int. J. Cancer.*, 54:20-25, 1993.

55. Heilbrun, L., Nomura, A., Hankin, J., and Stemmerman, G.N. Diet and colorectal cancer with specific reference to fiber intake. *Int. J. Cancer.*, 44:1-6, 1989.

56. Howe, G.R., Hirota, T., and Hislop, G., et al. Dietary factors and risk of breast cancer: combined analysis of 12 case-control studies. *J. Natl. Cancer Inst.*, 82:561-69, 1990.

57. Franchesci, S., Favero, A., and DeCarli, A., et al. Intake of macronutrients and risk of breast cancer. *Lancet*, 347:1351-56, 1996.

58. Freudenheim, J.L., Marshall, J.R., and Vena, J.E., et al. Premenopausal breast cancer risk and intake of vegetables, fruits, and related nutrients. *J. Natl. Cancer Inst.*, 88:340-48, 1996.

59. Howe, G.R., Ghadirian, P., and Bueno de Mesquita, H.B., et al. A collaborative case-control study of nutrient intake and pancreatic cancer with the SEARCH programme. *Int J. Cancer* 51:365-72, 1992.

60. Slavin, J., Martini, M.C., Jacobs, D.R., and Marquant, L. Plausible mechanisms for the protectiveness of whole grains. *Am. J. Clin. Nutr.*, 70 (Suppl): 459S-63S, 1999.

61. Jacobs, D.R., Marquant, L., Slavin, J., and Kushi, L.H. Whole grain intake and cancer; an expanded review and meta-analysis. *Nutr. Cancer.*, 30:85-96, 1998.

62. Steinmetz, K. and Potter, J.D. Vegetables, fruit, and cancer prevention: A review. *J. Am Dietetic Assoc.*, 96:1027-1039, 1996.

63. Shopland, D.R. Tobacco use and its contribution to early cancer mortality with a special emphasis on cigarette smoking. *Env. Health Perspect.*, 103 (Suppl. 8):131-141, 1995.

64. Giovanucci, E., Rimm, E., and Stampfer, M.J., et al. A prospective study of cigarette smoking and risk of colorectal adenoma and colorectal cancer in U.S. men. *J. Natl. Cancer Inst.*, 86:183-191, 1994.

65. Giovannucci, E., Colditz, G.A., and Stampfer, M.J., et al. A prospective study of cigarette smoking and risk of colorectal adenoma and colorectal cancer in U.S. women. *J. Natl. Cancer Inst.*, 86:192-199,1994.

66. Jensen, O.M., Paine, L., McMichael, A.J., and Ewertz, M. Alcohol. In: *Cancer Epidemiology and Prevention*. Schottenfeld, D. and Fraumeni, J.F. (Eds.), Oxford University Press, New York, 1996.

67. Dwyer, J., Clarke, L., and Miller, M. The effect of religious concentration and affiliation on county cancer mortality rates. *J. Health Soc Behav.*, 31:185-202.

68. Hummer, R.A., Rogers, R.G., Nam, C.B., Ellison, C.G. Religious involvement and U.S. adult mortality. *Demography*, 36:273-85, 1990.

69. American Cancer Society Board of Directors. ACS Challenge Goals for U.S. Cancer Mortality for the year 2015. Proc. Bd. Dir., Atlanta: American Cancer Society, 1996.

70. American Cancer Society Board of Directors. ACS Challenge Goals for U.S Cancer Incidence for the year 2015. Proc. Bd. Dir., Atlanta: American Cancer Society, 1998.

71. Beyers, T., Mouchawar, J., and Marks, J., et al. The American Cancer Society Challenge Goals. How far can cancer rates decline in the U.S. by the year 2015? *Cancer*, 86:715-727, 1999.

72. Patterson, B.H., Block, G., Rosenberger, W.F., Pee, D., and Kahle, L.L. Fruits and vegetables in the American diet: data from the HANES II survey. *Am. J. Public Hlth.*, 80:1443-49, 1990.

73. Riboli, E., and Kaaks, R. The EPIC project: Rationale and study design. European Prospective Investigation into Cancer and Nutrition. *Int. J. Epidemiol.*, 26:S6-14, 1997.

5

VEGETARIAN DIETS AND OBESITY PREVENTION

Joan Sabaté and Glen Blix

CONTENTS

I. OBESITY AS A PUBLIC HEALTH PROBLEM

Obesity is rapidly becoming the scourge of modern society. Presently, at least 34% of the U.S. population is obese (20% or more above their ideal weight) and more than 55% weigh in excess of ideal.[1,2] This represents the highest prevalence ever recorded in the United States.[3] Nor is the

0-8493-8508-3/01/$0.00+$.50
© 2001 by CRC Press LLC

problem unique to Americans. It is estimated that there are now 250 million obese adults in the world (7% of the total population), with many more overweight.[4] At the 1998 International Conference on Obesity, the World Health Organization identified obesity as a worldwide epidemic.[5] In industrialized and developing countries alike, obesity ranks as one of the top five global health problems.[6]

One of the more sobering observations is that obesity is increasing rapidly among children and adolescents. The association between childhood obesity and obesity in adulthood indicates a strong relationship. Analysis by Serdula et al.[7] indicates that about one third of obese preschool children become obese as adults, and approximately half of obese school-age children become obese adults. The risk of adult obesity is greater for children with higher levels of obesity and for children who are obese at adolescence and beyond.

While many individuals bemoan their adiposity for aesthetic reasons, the major concern is the negative health impact that accompanies obesity. Since ancient times, it has been common knowledge that obesity is hazardous to health. It remained, however, for modern epidemiology to confirm the truth of this assumption. The list of illnesses that are attributable to, or aggravated by, overweight is a lengthy one. Some of the metabolic abnormalities and diseases linked to obesity include: atherogenic lipid profile, high fibrinogen levels, insulin resistance, hyperinsulinemia, glucose intolerance, hyperuricemia, type 2 diabetes, coronary heart disease, hypertension, stroke, angina pectoris, cholecystitis, gout, obstructive sleep apnea, uric acid nephrolithiasis, and breast cancer (in postmenopausal women).[8]

Allison et al.[9] attribute 280,000 deaths per year in the United States to excess body fat. Severely obese women are at triple the risk of having at least one major risk factor for cardiovascular disease, five times the risk of developing diabetes, and 1.5 times the risk of suffering from a herniated disk as compared with non-obese women. The risk of cardiovascular disease is even higher among obese men. Very obese men are five times more likely than non-obese men to have at least one cardiovascular risk factor. Very obese men also have five times the risk of diabetes compared with non-obese men.[10]

While there is consensus that obesity is a continuing and growing problem, intervention is notoriously ineffective. Weight loss, when it is achieved, is almost invariably followed by a gradual return to the previous corpulence. At any given time, almost two thirds of the population is engaged in some type of weight control, but follow-up data demonstrates that less than 5% are successful at maintaining weight loss over time. The sad fact remains that, of those who do reduce their weight, almost all regain it within 3 to 5 years.[11]

It has been observed that obesity is less prevalent among vegetarians than in their carnivorous counterparts.[12] Thus, a meat-free diet has been suggested as beneficial in the primary prevention of obesity and possibly effective in secondary prevention of obesity, such as in weight loss and maintenance. To address the efficacy of a vegetarian diet, as either an intervention or in the prevention of obesity, it is necessary to compare measures of adiposity such as body mass index (BMI) of those subsisting on vegetarian fare with their carnivorous counterparts.

II. ANTHROPOMETRICS OF VEGETARIANS

A. Meta-Analysis of Nutritional Studies on Vegetarians

In 1954, Hardinge and Stare[13] compared the nutritional status of strict vegetarians (vegans) and lacto-ovo vegetarians with non-vegetarians of southern California. No differences in height were reported, but vegetarians and especially vegans weighed about 10 kg less than the non-vegetarian counterparts. Since the publication of this landmark research, scores of similar small studies have been conducted comparing vegetarians from many countries with their non-vegetarian counterparts.[14] Evidence from these small-sample-size studies of vegetarians indicates that BMI values are either similar to or lower than non-vegetarians. On these types of studies, however, differences between vegetarian and non-vegetarians were most likely minimized due to the selection criteria for study participants (i.e., matching on anthropometrics, ineligibility of obese people).

Table 5.1 shows the result of a meta-analysis we have conducted using the data from 36 studies on females and 24 studies on males reported in

Table 5.1

	Vegetarian			Non-Vegetarian		
	Number of Studies	Weighted Mean (SE)	Number of Subjects	Weighted Mean (SE)	Number of Subjects	P-Value
Males						
Height (cm)	16	176.6 (1.1)	402	176.8 (.7)	422	0.48
Weight (kg)	18	68.2 (1.4)	490	75.8 (.5)	720	<.0001
BMI (kg/m^2)	24	22.6 (.2)	589	24.7 (.2)	813	<.0001
Females						
Height (cm)	28	161.9 (.5)	869	161.5 (.5)	1092	0.46
Weight (kg)	30	60.5 (.6)	928	63.8 (.8)	1350	0.006
BMI (kg/m^2)	36	23.6 (.4)	1140	25.4 (.5)	1556	0.007

Appendices D and E of *The Dietician's Guide to Vegetarian Diets* by Messina and Messina.[14] While anthropometric parameters were not often the main outcome variables of the studies, in most cases, this information was recorded and reported. Weighted mean height, weight, and BMI for males and females were calculated using the number of participants in each study. Results, which were similar for males and females, showed no significant difference in height between vegetarians and non-vegetarians. However, vegetarians had significantly lower weight and BMI scores. Overall, male vegetarians compared more favorably with male non-vegetarians than female vegetarians did with their non-vegetarian counterparts. The mean weight for male vegetarians was 7.6 kg less than non-vegetarians, while for females the difference was 3.3 kg. Vegetarians — both males and females — on average, had a two point lower BMI score than non-vegetarians.

B. Epidemiological Studies of Vegetarians

Data from the Adventist Health Study (AHS) is of interest in comparing the effects of a vegetarian diet on obesity. The Seventh-Day Adventist Church doctrine promotes a healthy life-style and includes the recommendation of a vegetarian diet for its members. This study collected diet and other life-style characteristics of some 34,000 individuals, following them for several years and recording the incidence of chronic disease and death. Data recorded in 1976 indicated that about 45% of Californian Seventh-Day Adventists were vegetarian, with the remaining 55% consuming flesh food from occasionally (less than once per week) to daily. This fact makes this a valuable study population in which to compare the differences between vegetarians and non-vegetarians, since both groups share many socio-demographic and life-style characteristics, differing primarily in diet.

In three dietary subgroups of the Adventist Health Study cohort, the prevalence of obesity at baseline between vegetarian and non-vegetarian groups was strikingly different. Table 5.2 shows age-adjusted mean BMI values for vegetarians who ate no meat whatsoever; semi-vegetarians who ate meat occasionally and non-vegetarians who ate meat foods more than once per week. For both men and women, BMI increased as the frequency of meat consumption increased. Vegetarian men and women had a two point lower BMI value than non-vegetarians. Although these results were for middle aged (45–60 years) subjects, similar results were observed for other ages.[15]

Figure 5.1 shows the proportion of vegetarian and non-vegetarian subjects of the Adventist Health Study cohort in three BMI categories (low, medium and high) according to four different age and gender groups.[16] Among Californian Seventh-Day Adventists in 1976, obese adults tended

Table 5.2   Vegetarian Status and Obesity*: The Adventist Health Study Cohort (1976)

	Vegetarians	Semi Vegetarians	Non Vegetarians	P for Trend
BMI (in kg/m**)				
Men	24.3 (24.1, 24.4)**	25.2 (25.0, 25.3)	26.2 (26.1, 26.4)	0.0001
Women	23.7 (23.6, 23.9)	24.8 (24.7, 25.0)	25.9 (25.8, 26.0)	0.0001

*For subjects aged 45–60 y; other ages showed similar trends. Vegetarians ate no meat, fish, or poultry; semi-vegetarians ate meat, fish, or poultry in total < 1 time/wk; non-vegetarians ate these foods ≥ 1 time/wk.

**Mean, adjusted for age. 95% CI in parenthesis.
Adapted from Fraser *Am. J. Clin. Nutr.* 1999;70(S) by permission.

to be non-vegetarian, while slim adults tended to be vegetarian. A remarkably consistent pattern can be observed in this population for the four gender–age categories (Figure 5.1). For both male and female middle-aged or older adults, a greater proportion of vegetarians was found among those with a low BMI, while a greater proportion of non-vegetarians resided in the obese group with higher BMI values. No difference was observed in the proportion of vegetarians to non-vegetarians in the intermediate BMI category.

Figure 5.2 shows the distribution in five categories of BMI of vegetarians and non-vegetarians from the Adventist Health Study cohort (Pramil Singh; personal communication). For both men and women, a striking inverse relationship exists between BMI values and vegetarian status. Prevalence data can be difficult to interpret and causality cannot be inferred from this cross-sectional analysis. Moreover, though, the baseline measure of meat intake has been shown to be a good estimation of usual dietary intake. However, it seems unlikely that vegetarian Adventists who develop obesity would shift to a non-vegetarian diet that they believe to be unhealthful. On the contrary, Adventists who develop obesity would most likely adopt or increase their adherence to a vegetarian diet that they believe to be healthful. If anything, this would weaken the inverse association found between obesity and vegetarian diets.

This inverse relationship has also been found in other epidemiological studies of vegetarians in Europe. Using cross-sectional data from the Oxford Vegetarian Study, Appleby et al.[17] examined the association of diet and other life-style factors with BMI. Mean BMI values were 1 to 2 points significantly lower in non-meat eaters than in meat eaters in all age groups for both men and women. Interestingly, BMI difference between the diet groups increased with increasing age among women, but not as clearly

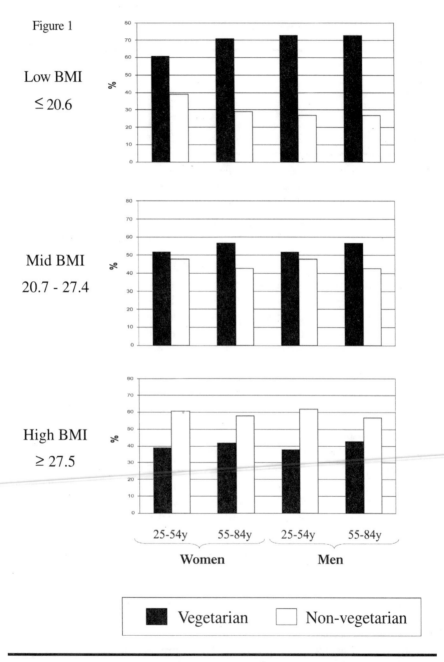

Figure 5.1   Proportion of vegetarians and non-vegetarians of the Adventist Health Study cohort (1976) in three categories of BMI by age and gender.[16]

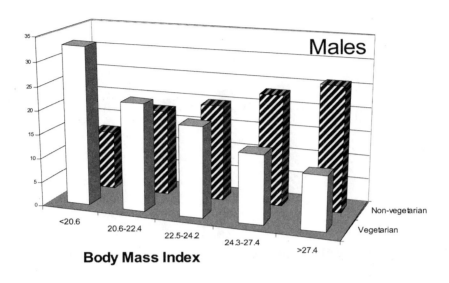

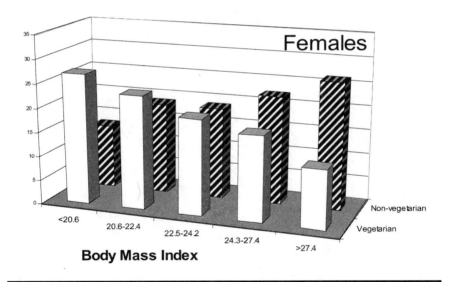

Figure 5.2 Distribution in five categories of BMI of vegetarians and non-vegetarians of the Adventist Health Study cohort.

in men (Figure 5.3). A higher proportion of meat eaters than non-meat eaters were overweight or obese (21% vs. 10% of men and 13% vs. 8% of women), whereas a lower proportion of meat eaters had a BMI < 20kg/m² (9% vs. 17% of men and 18% vs. 33% of women). No significant differences in BMI values were observed in this study between "long-term vegetarians" (5 years or more) and those who had recently given up meat.

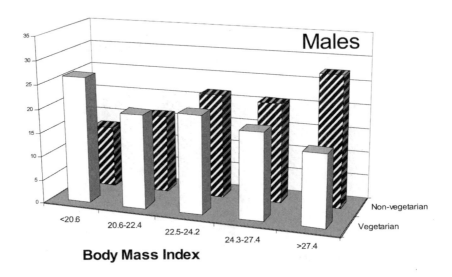

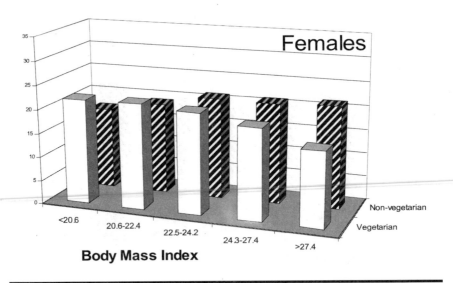

Figure 5.3   Oxford Vegetarian Study cohort. Comparison of BMI of vegetarians and non-vegetarians by gender and age.

Meat eaters consumed significantly more animal fat and alcoholic beverages and less dietary fiber than non-meat eaters. After adjusting for these dietary factors and other life-style factors, the differences in BMI between meat eaters and non-meat eaters were reduced by 33%, but were still present. Thus, these confounding factors do not fully explain the role of vegetarian diets on obesity prevention, suggesting an independent effect for low meat intake. In a cohort of about 20,000 vegetarians in Germany, an inverse relationship was also observed between BMI and vegetarian status. Strict vegetarians, those who avoided meat completely, were thinner than the occasional meat-eaters.[18]

Key & Davey[12] used data from approximately 4000 men and women collected in England for the European prospective investigation into cancer and nutrition (EPIC study) to examine the relationship between obesity and meat intake. Subjects were classified as meat eaters if they ate any meat, as fish eaters if they did not eat meat but did eat fish, as vegetarians if they did not eat meat or fish but did eat dairy products or eggs, and as vegans if they did not eat any of these four categories of food. Among both men and women, mean BMI was highest among meat eaters, lowest among the vegans, and intermediate among the fish eaters and vegetarians. These differences in body mass index are equivalent to mean differences in weight between meat eaters and vegans of 5.9 kg in men and 4.7 kg in women. In the groups that did not eat meat, mean BMI was lower among those who had adhered to their diet for 5 or more years than among those who had adhered to their diet for a shorter period. According to the authors, this association with duration of the diet patterns suggests that the differences in BMI are largely due to the qualitative differences between the diets of the four groups. Among the meat eaters, about 6.1% of the men and 9.1% of the women were clinically obese (BMI > 30). In contrast, the prevalence of obesity was about three times lower for vegans (2% for men and less than 4% for women), and for vegetarians and fish eaters the prevalence of obesity was 3% for men and 5% for women, well below the meat-eating group values.

Figure 5.4 summarizes BMI data from the four large published cohort studies of adult vegetarians.[19] These studies allow a comparison with non-vegetarian counterparts of the same cohort. Vegetarians in each study on average have 1 to 2 points lower BMI values than meat eaters within the same cohort. This difference is similarly observed in men and women. There is a substantial variation in BMI values among cohorts. USA cohorts have greater BMI than European cohorts. This can be attributed to methodological differences in data collection, geographic location, secular trends, and ethnic or genetic differences. Overall, these epidemiological data clearly suggest that meatless diets are associated with lower overall BMI scores and a low prevalence of obesity in adults.

C. Vegetarian Children and Obesity

The physical growth and development of vegetarian children and adolescents is addressed in another chapter of this volume. In general, younger vegetarian children tend to be leaner than non-vegetarians,[20] and this

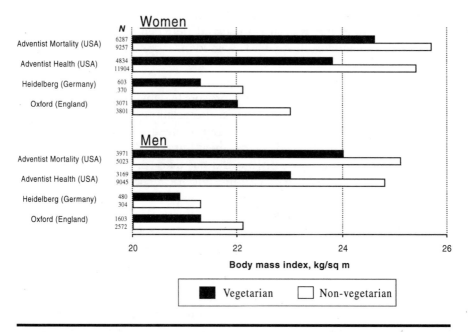

Figure 5.4   Mean BMI of vegetarians and non-vegetarians from four epidemiological studies.

attribute also tends to be present among older vegetarian children and adolescents, although limited research data are available for older children. Lousuebsakul and Sabaté[21] studied anthropometric data of 870 children aged 7 to 18 years who were attending Seventh-Day Adventist schools in California. One third of them were vegetarian. A vegetarian lifestyle was associated with lower BMI and a decreased tendency to be overweight, especially in adolescent girls. Specifically, age- and height-adjusted analysis showed that vegetarian boys and girls were, on average, 1.4 kg and 1.0 kg, respectively, leaner than their non-vegetarian classmates. Also, BMI values and skinfold measurements were lower among vegetarians. The prevalence of obesity (BMI > 75th percentile of national standards) was lower among vegetarian adolescent girls. In view of the relationship of childhood obesity to adult corpulence,[7] the adoption of a vegetarian lifestyle during the school years may not only lower the risk of obesity at adolescence, but may also actually decrease the risk of adult obesity. Moreover, data from the Harvard Growth Study indicates that being overweight during adolescence predicts adult morbidity from several chronic degenerative diseases and mortality from all causes regardless of adult body weight.[22] Thus, it is suggested that the prevention of obesity in childhood and adolescence by the adoption of a vegetarian diet may subsequently decrease a broad range of adverse health effects in adulthood.

III. WEIGHT LOSS AND VEGETARIAN DIETS

Data showing that vegetarians tend to have lower body weights and BMI scores than those who do not abstain from meat are quite consistent. There are, however, virtually no appropriate studies evaluating the use of vegetarian diets for weight loss. Nicholson et al.[23] reported that, in a very small 12-week pilot intervention study of type 2 diabetic patients, those on a low-fat vegan diet lost a mean of 7.2 kg, compared with those on a conventional low-fat diet where the weight loss averaged 3.8 kg. This study is flawed regarding its weight loss component in that the diets were not isocaloric.

A vegetarian diet may be attempted with relative frequency by those wishing to lose weight. Gilbody et al.[24] evaluated the dietary practices of 131 young adult women and found that 34.3% reported that they had used or were using a vegetarian diet. There was, however, no evaluation of the relative effectiveness of a vegetarian diet compared with a conventional weight loss intervention in terms of actual success in weight loss.

Vegetarian diets may offer the advantage of being less monotonous, and thus easier to maintain, than conventional weight loss programs. Smith et al.[25] compared young adults on weight-loss and vegetarian diets and found that those on vegetarian regimens tended to maintain their dietary style for much longer than those on conventional weight-loss dietary programs. The majority of the participants in the vegetarian group (62%) remained on their diet for more than 1 year, whereas most of the participants on the weight-loss diet (61%) maintained their program for only 1 to 3 months. While this study indicated that a vegetarian diet might be more easily maintained, it did not address the effectiveness of the diet in achieving the desired weight loss.

IV. POTENTIAL EXPLANATIONS FOR THE ANTI-OBESITY EFFECT OF A VEGETARIAN DIET

While data indicate that vegetarians may weigh less than other population subsets, it does not necessarily follow that it is their avoidance of meat that is responsible. Vegetarians are also more likely to adopt other healthy life-style habits, such as regular exercise and reduced alcohol consumption, that also impact their lack of obesity. There is some evidence, however, that eating more vegetables and abstaining from meat does play a significant role in their leaner profiles. A study by Kahn and others of 79,000 individuals followed for over 10 years showed that the one habit that seemed to prevent the development of abdominal obesity was eating vegetables. Those who consumed 19 or more servings of vegetables per week did not succumb to an increase in central girth, while those who ate meat (beef, pork, or lamb) more that seven times per week did.[26]

Vegetarian diets can be lower overall in total energy intake. Also, the macronutrient composition and sources of macronutrients tend to be different in vegetarian diets, as compared to the omnivore diet. They are overall higher in dietary fiber and complex carbohydrates and lower in protein and fat. Their nutritional differences may partially account for the potential anti-obesity effect of vegetarian diets.

A. Dietary Fiber and Total Energy Intake

The fiber intake of the average American adult amounts to around 15 gm per day,[27] while a modest 1800 kcal Western vegetarian diet contains about 45 gm of fiber. In more primitive vegetarian regimens, fiber content has been reported to be as high as 80 gm per day. Wolever and Jenkins have suggested that diets naturally high in fiber content may be beneficial in maintaining weight or preventing weight gain.[28] Since the presence of non-nutritive fiber in fruits and vegetables increases the bulk of the ingested food, a vegetarian diet may positively impact obesity due to its generally lower energy density. On a volume-for-volume basis, vegetarian fare contains fewer calories than omnivorous diets. Thus, even when the volume of food intake in a vegetarian diet is greater, the total calories ingested may be less. Levin et al.[29] compared vegetarians with omnivores and reported that the average weight of the vegetarians was significantly lower than that of the omnivores (60.8 kg vs. 69.1 kg), but that the vegetarian diet supplied a significantly greater number of calories than the non-vegetarian diet (3,030.5 cal/day vs. 2,626.8 cal/day).

Fiber apparently also affects short-term food intake. Levine et al.[30] in a study of the consequence of a high fiber breakfast indicated that fiber reduced subsequent hunger, resulting in less snacking at mid-morning breaks and a lessened food intake at lunch time. Unfortunately, data from Delargy et al.[31] reveals that most subjects consuming a high fiber breakfast compensated for these initially lower calories by eating more later in the day, so that the total daily energy intake remained unchanged. It can be speculated that including fiber-rich foods at the other meals may allow the appetite depression effect to continue throughout the day. Even small amounts (5 grams) of pectin, a soluble type of fiber found mainly in fruit, increases satiety when fed with other food.[32] This may indicate an important role for increased fruit consumption as a way to curb appetite.

Besides decreasing caloric density and curbing appetite, fiber may have an additional obesity-preventive benefit. Baer et al.[33] have demonstrated that fiber interferes with the absorption of fat and protein from the intestinal tract and, while the effect is modest (less than 4% of the energy intake), it will provide a significant advantage over time. On a 2500 kcal daily diet, this would amount to the equivalent of a 100 kcal per day reduction. During the course of a year, this means that over 36,000 kcal would be eliminated, theoretically preventing about a 10-pound (at 3500 kcal per pound) weight gain.

B. Carbohydrate Intake

Vegetarian diets tend to contain significantly more carbohydrates, particularly complex carbohydrates. A high carbohydrate meal may actually speed up the resting metabolic rate, while a high fat meal seems to have little effect on metabolism. There is some evidence that overfeeding with carbohydrates — but not with fat — provokes an insulin-mediated thermogenesis that acts to retard weight gain.[34] Toth and Poehlman[35] found that young male vegetarians had an 11% higher resting metabolic rate than non-vegetarians in spite of similar energy intakes. The major dietary difference between the two groups was an increased ingestion of carbohydrate and a reduction in fat intake by the vegetarians.

C. Protein Intake

Campbell[36] has proposed that excess protein intake may be responsible for excess weight. Vegetarian diets tend to provide a much lower protein intake than diets that include meat products. The China study, involving dietary records on thousands of Chinese, indicated that protein intake paralleled body fatness. Campbell has shown that animals on low-protein, low-fat diets burn extra energy through very slight increases in thermogenesis. The energy is thus released as heat, instead of becoming body fat. His studies in rats demonstrate that, when protein intake is low, thermogenesis increases and thus more of the ingested energy is required for heat production. Animals on a low protein, high carbohydrate diet gained less body fat even though the actual caloric intake was higher. Interestingly, animals on the low protein diet also voluntarily exercised more.

Slattery et al.,[37] in a study of over 5000 young adults, also supports a protein connection. Protein intake was positively related to BMI in all age groups, while carbohydrate ingestion showed a negative association with body fatness. Rolland-Cachera et al.[38] have shown that children who are fed high protein diets before the age of 2 are more likely to become obese in later life. Since elevated protein intake may occur more easily when meat is included in the diet, vegetarian children might have an advantage. These results are somewhat ironic, in view of the recent fad promoting high protein diets for weight loss.

D. Dietary Fat Intake

Although studies on the effect of dietary fat on obesity are somewhat equivocal, in general, a high fat diet promotes obesity to a greater extent than an isocaloric low fat intake.[39] As body fat increases, so too does the percentage of food energy reported as derived from fat.[40] When there is covert manipulation of dietary fat, subjects on a high fat program consistently eat more than those on a low fat regimen.[41] This effect may be particularly pronounced in obese subjects,[42] and extends even to children. Maffeis et al.,[41] in a study comparing obese with non-obese children, found that, in spite of a similarity in reported overall energy intake, obese children ingested significantly more fat. It is also much easier to consume extra energy on a high fat diet since fat does not induce as potent a satiety signal or produce a compensation effect on subsequent energy intake as do diets rich in carbohydrates or proteins.[44]

Restricting fat, however, is certainly not the total answer to the problem of obesity. In fact, Hervey-Bernio in a recent study indicated that those on a calorie-restricted program lose twice as much weight as those who simply restrict their fat intake.[45] The quality and type of fat may also be important. The P/S ratio of the diet may be a consideration in weight loss. A small, randomized crossover study by van Marken Lichtenbelt et al.[46] using six subjects found that the resting metabolic rate was elevated by 3.6% in subjects after a 2-week diet with a P/S ratio of 1.67, as compared with a low P/S ratio diet of 0.19.

The recent identification of the appetite regulating hormone leptin also provides some intriguing clues. Plasma concentrations of leptin tend to parallel the amount of adipose tissue, providing an inhibitory feedback that tends to reduce energy intake when body fat increases. Cha et al.[47] has documented that leptin levels (in rats at least) also respond to dietary cues, with polyunsaturated fats being more leptingenic than saturated fats. This may give vegetarians an advantage in appetite control even when dietary fat levels are similar.

V. CONCLUSION

Data demonstrate that, in general, those following a vegetarian or almost vegetarian dietary regimen tend to have lower body weights and BMI levels than their omnivorous counterparts. The exact mechanisms that produce these results have not been precisely identified. It could simply be that vegetarians have a lower total energy intake than non-vegetarians. Moreover, the lower macro-nutrient density of the vegetarian diet may allow a feeling of satiation at lower energy intake. The high fiber, low fat, and relatively low protein levels in most vegetarian diets also seem to be beneficial in preventing weight gain. While it is obvious that a vegetarian diet is not a panacea for obesity control, it does appear that it may be of use both in preventing the occurrence of obesity and perhaps in dietary intervention for weight loss. Given the documented negative outcomes of obesity and the likelihood of other positive benefits of a vegetarian regimen, it may be a prudent intervention in the epidemic of obesity now plaguing society.

REFERENCES

1. Kuczmarski, R.J. Prevalence of overweight and weight gain in the United States. *Am. J. Clin. Nutr.*, 55, 495S-502S, 1992.
2. Ammon, P.K. Individualizing the approach to treating obesity. Nurse Pract., 24(2):27-8, 31-8, 41, Feb 1999.
3. *Morb. Mortal. Wkly. Rep.* 46:199-201, 1997.
4. James, W.P. and Ralph, A. New understanding in obesity research. *Proc. Nutr. Soc.*, 58(2):385-93, May 1999.
5. The World Health Organization Report. Released at the 8th International Congress on Obesity in Paris, Aug 31, 1998.
6. Johnston, J. Doctors warn about an epidemic of obesity. www.healthscout.com, Oct 20 1998.
7. Serdula, M.K., Ivery, D., Coates, R.J., Freedman, D.S., Williamson, D.F., and Byers, T. Do obese children become obese adults? A review of the literature. *Prev. Med.*, 22(2):167-77, Mar 1993.
8. VanItallie, T.B. and Lew, E.A. Estimation of the effect of obesity on health and longevity: A perspective for the physician. In: *Obesity Theory and Treatment.* Stunkard and Wadden (Eds.), Raven Press, New York, 1993.
9. Allison D.B., Fontaine, K.R., Manson, J.E., Stevens, J., and VanItallie, T.B. Annual deaths attributable to obesity in the United States, MD. *JAMA*, 282(16):1519-1522, 1999.
10. Lean, M., et al. Effect of obesity on health and quality of life quantified. *Arch. Intern. Med.*, 159:837 843, 1999.
11. Wadden, T.A. and Sternberg, J.A., et al. Treatment of obesity by very low calorie diet, behavior therapy, and their combination: a 5-year perspective. *Int. J. Obesity*, 13(Suppl.2), 39-46, 1989.
12. Key, T. and Davey, G. Prevalence of obesity is low in people who do not eat meat, Letter, *BMJ*, 313:816-817, 1996.
13. Hardinge, M. and Stare, F. Nutritional Studies of Vegetarians. *J. Clin. Nutr.*, 2(2):73-82, 1954.
14. Messina, M. and Messina, V. *The Dietician's Guide to Vegetarian Diets: Issues and Applications.* Aspen Publishers, Gaithersburg, MD, 431-442, 1996.
15. Fraser, G. Associations between diet and cancer, ischemic heart disease, and all-cause mortality in non-Hispanic white California Seventh-Day Adventists. *Am. J. Clin. Nutr.*, 70(3):532S-538S, 1999.

16. Singh, P.N. and Lindsted, K.D. Body mass and 26-year risk of mortality from specific diseases among women who never smoked. *Epidemiology*, 9(3):246-54, May 1998.

17. Appleby, P.N., Thorogood, M., Mann, J.I., and Key, T.J. Low body mass index in non-meat eaters: the possible roles of animal fat, dietary fibre and alcohol. *Int. J. Obes. Relat. Metab. Disord.*, 22(5):454-60, May 1998.

18. Chang-Claude, J. and Frentzel-Beyme, R. Dietary and lifestyle determinants of mortality among German vegetarians. *Intl. J. Epid.*, 22(2):228-236, 1993.

19. Key, T., Fraser, G., and Thorogood, M., et al. Mortality in vegetarians and non-vegetarians: a collaborative analysis of 8300 deaths among 76,000 men and women in five prospective studies. *Pub. Hlth. Nutr.*, 1(1):33-41, 1998.

20. Jacobs, C. and Dwyer, J.T. Vegetarian children: appropriate and inappropriate diets. *Am. J. Clin Nutr.*, 48:811, 1998.

21. Lousuebsakul, V. and Sabaté, J. Dietary patterns and overweight in school-age children. *Faseb. J.*, 8(4):A166, 1994.

22. Must, A., Jacques, P.F., Dallal, G.E., Bajema, C.J., and Dietz, W.H. Long-term morbidity and mortality of overweight adolescents. A follow-up of the Harvard Growth Study of 1922 to 1935. *New Eng. J. Med.*, 5;327(19):1350-5, 1992.

23 Nicholson, A.S., Sklar, M., Barnard, N.D., Gore, S., Sullivan, R., Browning, S. Toward improved management of NIDDM: A randomized, controlled, pilot intervention using a low fat vegetarian diet. *Prev. Med.*, 29(2):87-91, Aug 1999.

24. Gilbody, S.M., Kirk, S.F., and Hill, A.J. Vegetarianism in young women: another means of weight control? *Int. J. Eat Disord.*, 26(1):87-90, Jul 1999.

25. Smith, C.F., Burke, L.E., and Wing, R.R. Vegetarian and weight-loss diets among young adults. *Obes. Res.*, 8(2):123-9, Mar 2000.

26. Kahn H.S., Tatham, L.M., Rodriguez, C., Calle, E.E., Thun, M.J., Heath, C.W., Jr. Stable behaviors associated with adults' 10-year change in body mass index and likelihood of gain at the waist. *Am. J. Public Hlth.*, 87(5):747-54, May 1997.

27. Van Horn, L. Fiber, lipids, and coronary heart disease. A statement for healthcare professionals from the Nutrition Committee, American Heart Association. *Circulation*, 95(12):2701-2704, 1997.

28. Wolever, T.M. and Jenkins, D.J. What is a high fiber diet? *Adv. Exp. Med. Biol.*, 427:35-42, 1997.

29. Levin, N., Rattan, J., and Gilat, T. Energy intake and body weight in ovo-lacto vegetarians. *J. Clin. Gastroenterol.*, 8(4):451-3, 1986.

30. Levine, A.S., Tallman, J.R., Grace, M.K., Parker, S.A., Billington, C.J., and Levitt, M.D. Effect of breakfast cereals on short term food intake. *Am. J. Clin. Nutr.*, 50(6):1303-7, 1989.

31. Delargy, H.J., O'Sullivan, K.R., Fletcher, R.J., and Blundell, J.E. Effects of amount and type of dietary fibre (soluble and insoluble) on short-term control of appetite. *Int. J. Food Sci Nutr.*, 48(1):67-77, 1997.

32. Tiwary, C.M., Ward, J.A., and Jackson, B.A. Effect of pectin on satiety in healthy US Army adults. *J. Am Coll Nutr.*, 16(5):423-8, 1997.

33. Baer, D.J., Rumpler, W.V., Miles, C.W., and Fahey, G.C., Jr. Dietary fiber decreases the metabolizable energy content and nutrient digestibility of mixed diets fed to humans. *J. Nutr.*, 127(4):579-86, 1997.

34. McCarty, M.F. The unique merits of a low-fat diet for weight control. *Med-Hypotheses.* 20(2): 183-97, 1986.

35. Toth, M.J. and Poehlman, E.T. Sympathetic nervous system activity and resting metabolic rate in vegetarians. *Metabolism*, 43(5):621-5, 1994.

36. Campbell, T.C. and Chen, J. Presented at Conference on the Role of Diet and Caloric Intake in Aging, Obesity, and Cancer, Reston, VA, October 28, 1998.

37. Slattery, M.L., McDonald, A., Bild, D.E., Caan, B.J., Hilner, J.E., Jacobs, D.R., Jr., and Liu, K. Associations of body fat and its distribution with dietary intake, physical activity, alcohol, and smoking in blacks and whites. *Am. J. Clin. Nutr.*, 55(5):943-9, 1992.

38. Rolland-Cachera, M.F., Deheeger, M., Akrout, M., and Bellisle, F. Influence of macronutrients on adiposity development: a follow up study of nutrition and growth from 10 months to 8 years of age. *Int. J. Obes. Relat. Metab. Disord.*, 19(8): 573-8, Aug 1995.

39. Alfieri, M., Pomerleau, J., and Grace, D.M. A comparison of fat intake of normal weight, moderately obese and severely obese subjects. *Obes. Surg.*, 7(1):9-15, 1997.

40. Miller, W.C., Lindeman, A.K., Wallace, J., and Niederpruem, M. Diet composition, energy intake, and exercise in relation to body fat in men and women. *Am. J. Clin. Nutr.*, 52:426-30, 1990.

41. Prentice, A.M. Manipulation of dietary fat and energy density and subsequent effects on substrate flux and food intake. *Am. J. Clin. Nutr.*, 67: 535S-541S, 1998.

42. Blundell, J.E., Lawton, C.L., and Hill, A.J. Mechanisms of appetite control and their abnormalities in obese patients. *Horm-Res.*, 39 Suppl. 3: 72-6, 1993.

43. Maffeis, C., Pinelli, L., and Schutz, Y. Fat intake and adiposity in 8- to 11-year-old obese children. *Int. J. Obes. Relat. Metab. Disord.*, 20(2):170-4, 1996.

44. Doucet, E. and Tremblay, A. Food intake, energy balance and body weight control., *Eur. J. Clin. Nutr.*, 51(12):846-55, 1997.

45. Harvey-Berino, J. The efficacy of dietary fat vs. total energy restriction for weight loss. *Obes. Res.*, 6(3):202-7, 1998.

46. van Marken Lichtenbelt, W.D., Mensink, R.P., and Westerterp, K.R. The effect of fat composition of the diet on energy metabolism. *Z. Ernahrungswiss.*, 36(4):303-5, 1997.

47. Cha, M.C. and Jones, P.J. Dietary fat type and energy restriction interactively influence plasma leptin concentration in rats. *J. Lipid Res.*, 39(8):1655-60, Aug 1998.

6

VEGETARIAN DIETS IN THE
PREVENTION OF
OSTEOPOROSIS, DIABETES,
AND NEUROLOGICAL
DISORDERS

Sujatha Rajaram and Michelle Wien

CONTENTS

0-8493-8508-3/01/$0.00+$.50
© 2001 by CRC Press LLC

I. INTRODUCTION

Epidemiological data as well as clinical experience clearly suggest that relatively unrefined vegetarian diets can provide remarkable health protection for chronic disease prevention.[1] Vegetarian diets typically contain higher amounts of whole grains, legumes, vegetables, fruits, nuts and seeds[2-4] with concomitantly decreased levels or elimination of refined foods and animal products (Table 6.1). Thus, in contrast to the omnivorous diet, the nutritional composition of the vegetarian diet is high in dietary fiber and low in saturated fat.[5] Industrialized countries face the problem of excess dietary energy and saturated fat consumption, leading to an increased incidence of chronic degenerative diseases. Not much conclusive data is available on the protective role of vegetarian diets in the prevention of osteoporosis, diabetes, and neurological disorders. However, this review summarizes the brief literature on the possible role of vegetarian dietary practice in the incidence of these three etiologically different disease conditions.

II. OSTEOPOROSIS

Osteoporosis is a multi-factorial disorder characterized by bone loss over an extended period of time. As a result of the decrease in bone density, the risk of fracture at various sites increases, making osteoporosis one of the most debilitating diseases known to mankind. Over the years, improved nutritional status and the advancements made in the field of medicine and science have caused a significant increase in the aging population and the prevalence of osteoporosis-related fractures.[6] Currently, osteoporosis is considered one of the major public health problems in the United States, affecting over 20 million people annually. The percentage of hospitalization due to osteoporotic fractures is on a steady rise and is accompanied by an escalating cost of treatment that has surpassed 10 billion dollars a year.[7-9] Considering the magnitude of the condition, it is imperative to understand the etiology and risk factors of the disease in order to develop treatment and prevention strategies. Given the complexity in the etiology of osteoporosis, a researcher in the late 1960s is quoted as having said, "The therapy of osteoporosis may lie in its prevention."[10]

The risk factors of osteoporosis include low physical activity, smoking, alcoholism, low estrogen levels, and compromised nutritional status.[11-18] The association between diet and disease incidence is established through

Table 6.1 Seventh-Day Adventist Consumption Patterns According to Vegetarian Status*

Food	Vegetarian	Semivegetarian	Nonvegetarian
		Servings/wk	
Beef	0.0	0.3	3.0
Poultry	0.0	0.1	0.7
Fish	0.0	0.1	0.6
Vegetarian meat substitutes	3.5	3.2	1.4
Soft margarine on bread	6.2	6.1	5.7
Eggs	1.3	1.7	2.2
Doughnuts	0.4	0.6	0.9
Coffee	0.3	1.2	4.8
Tomatoes	3.6	3.5	3.4
Legumes	2.4	2.0	1.3
Nuts	3.7	3.0	2.1
Green salads	4.4	4.4	4.4

*All differences were significant at $P < 0.001$, except for salads (nonsignificant). Data were adjusted for age and sex. Vegetarians ate no meat, fish, or poultry; semi-vegetarians ate meat, fish, or poultry in total <1 time/wk; nonvegetarians ate these foods ≥1 time/wk.

Adapted from Fraser, *Am. J. Clin. Nutr.*, 1999.

epidemiological studies of different populations around the world. This can be achieved by comparing disease incidence among populations with either differing diet practices (vegetarian vs. omnivorous), or by the presence or absence of specific food groups (meat, dairy, fruits, and vegetables) or specific nutrients. Certain dietary factors such as caffeine, salt, and phosphate are known to decrease bone loss associated with aging, while others like calcium, vitamin D, magnesium, and potassium may increase bone mineralization.

With respect to osteoporosis, the effect of specific nutrients on bone metabolism and in disease incidence has been previously published. Thus, in this chapter, only the studies on diet patterns, food groups that characterize these diet patterns, and their effect on the incidence of osteoporosis, risk of osteoporotic fractures, or bone mineral density (BMD) will be summarized and discussed.

A. Epidemiological Studies of Vegetarians

There are no large epidemiological studies that were designed with the primary objective of determining the incidence of osteoporosis and related fracture in populations with different diet patterns. In contrast, several large prospective cohort studies have examined the association between dietary patterns and incidence of coronary heart disease and several types of cancer.

Only within the last 5 years have secondary analyses of some of these cohorts[19,20] determined if specific animal or plant foods in the habitual diet can predict the incidence of osteoporotic fractures at different sites in men and women. These results will be discussed in the next section.

To date, about a dozen studies have been published studying the bone health of vegetarians (Table 6.2). These are cross-sectional studies with small sample sizes compared with what is typically seen in large cohort studies. The first study, published in the early 1970s,[21] compared a group of British lacto-ovo vegetarians (LOV) to non-vegetarians from the same geographical area. BMD of the third metacarpal was higher and age-related decline slower among LOV than omnivores. Similar results were observed among premenopausal[22,23] and elderly women[24] after adjusting for differences in age, height, and weight. After age 50, non-vegetarians experienced twice the rate of bone loss of LOV.[25] This suggests that vegetarian diets, particularly the LOV diet, may be protective against age-related bone loss. The influence of diet pattern on fracture risk was not assessed in any of these studies.

While lacto-ovo vegetarians include dairy products and eggs in a plant-based diet, vegans consume a plant-based diet exclusively. Some studies have shown that an exclusively plant-based diet may actually be detrimental to bone health. Bone density at the lumbar spine and femoral neck was measured using dual-photon absorptiometry in 258 postmenopausal Taiwanese vegetarian women.[26] The vegans were found to be at a higher risk of exceeding lumbar spine fracture threshold and of being classified as having osteopenia of the femoral neck. They had lower protein intake than the lacto-ovo vegetarians, suggesting that total protein intake may be an important predictor of bone density. Similar findings were reported among premenopausal vegans.[27] Vegans in this study not only had lower protein intake than LOV and non-vegetarians, but also had the lowest calcium to protein ratio among the three groups.

Not all studies comparing vegetarians distinguish between vegans and LOV. Cross-sectional comparison of spine BMD of premenopausal[28] and elderly[29] vegetarian (vegans and LOV) and non-vegetarian women demonstrated that vegetarians had a lower body mass index (BMI), percent body fat, and BMD than the non-vegetarians. In addition, the mean BMD increased by 1.1% over a year in the non-vegetarian women but not in the vegetarians. Perhaps low BMI and percent body fat has a greater role in the prevalence of low BMD in vegetarians than the diet per se.

Table 6.2 Summary of Studies on Vegetarian Population and Bone Mineral Density

Reference	Subjects	Diet practice	Outcome variable	Result
#46	Male and female 53–79 yrs	LOV/Omnivore (n = 25)	BMD of third metacarpal	LOV > Omnivore
#47	Female, premenopausal 20–79 yrs	LOV/Omnivore (n = 51)	BMC of cortical site	LOV > Omnivore
#49	Female, postmenopausal 53–87 yrs	LOV/Omnivore (n = 10)	Bone loss by 80 yrs of age	18% LOV vs. 36% Omnivore
#51	Female, postmenopausal	Vegan/LOV/Omnivore (n = 258)	BMD at lumbar spine	Vegans at highest risk of spine fracture, osteopenia of femoral neck
#52	Female, premenopausal	Vegan/LOV/Omnivore	BMD at lumbar spine	Vegan < LOV, Omnivore
#53	Female, premenopausal 20–40 yrs	Vegetarian*/Omnivore (n = 15/20)	BMD	Vegetarian < Omnivores
#54	Female, postmenopausal 70–89 yrs	Vegetarian*/Omnivore (n = 109)	BMD at hip	Vegetarian < Omnivore
#57	Female, premenopausal 28–45 yrs	Vegetarian*/Omnivore (n = 27/37)	BMD of spine	No difference
#58	Female, postmenopausal 55–75 yrs	Vegetarian*/Omnivore (n = 28)	BMD of trabecula and cortical bone	No difference
#59	Female, postmenopausal 60–98 yrs	LOV/Omnivore (n = 88/287)	BMC and BMD of mid and distal radius	No difference
#60	Female, postmenopausal 76–81 yrs	LOV/Omnivore (n = 49/140)	BMD of radius	No difference
#61	Female, postmenopausal 58–76 yrs	LOV/Omnivore (n = 144/106)	BMC	No difference

*Vegetarians include both vegan and LOV

Asian vegetarians residing in London have significantly lower serum calcium and higher parathyroid hormone than Caucasian non-vegetarians from the same city.[30] The vegetarian diet of Asians has been implicated as the cause of compromised calcium status. However, among Asian vegetarians, the prevalence of osteomalacia (a condition that is also known to decrease serum calcium levels) is rather high. An anthropological survey of pre-Hispanic burials from the Canary Islands showed a high incidence of osteoporosis.[31] Since many of the pre-Hispanics were vegetarians, the prevalence of osteoporosis was considered to be directly due to their dietary practice. However, malnutrition was very rampant among these people and it is well established that malnutrition compromises bone status. These two studies indirectly implicate a vegetarian diet in the etiology of bone loss associated with osteoporosis, but it is clear that factors beyond vegetarian diet practice may have a role in the same.

A few studies have also reported no differences in BMD among vegetarians and non-vegetarians. Carefully selected vegetarian and non-vegetarian premenopausal,[32] postmenopausal,[33,34] and free-living elderly[35,36] women were matched for age, height, weight, menarche, years of formal education, and medical histories. In spite of the many dietary differences in the two groups, no differences were observed in BMD or other aspects of bone physiology.

Thus, there are conflicting results on the association between vegetarian diet practice and incidence of osteoporosis. One of the main reasons for this inconsistency is that many of the studies did not separate vegans from LOV. The presence of dairy food in LOV may alter the risk of osteoporosis-related fractures. The two studies that did look at vegans in comparison with LOV and omnivores suggest that a vegan diet may pose a higher risk of compromised bone status than LOV and omnivore diets. Whether this is due to the low calcium to protein ratio or some other factor beyond diet is not clear from any of these studies. A large, systematically designed epidemiological study of vegans, LOV, and omnivores from the same geographical area is needed before conclusions can be drawn.

B Intake of Selected Foods and Risk of Osteoporosis

To determine the influence of a vegetarian or a non-vegetarian diet, we must consider the role of specific animal or plant foods in the diet as well. Among animal foods, the presence of meat and dairy products have been investigated with respect to incidence of osteoporosis, while among plant foods, soy products, fruits, and vegetables have been investigated. The findings from these studies are reviewed and discussed in this section.

1. Meat

In 1968, Wachman and Bernstein[10] proposed that "bone dissolution is considered as a possible mechanism to buffer the fixed acid load imposed by the ingestion of an acid ash diet in man." Animal protein, particularly from meat, is shown to increase acid load when metabolized[23] and thus has been negatively implicated in the etiology of osteoporosis. Cross-cultural variations in animal protein consumption and the incidence of hip fracture (Figure 6.1) were analyzed by comparing 34 published studies from 16 countries.[37] A strong positive association was found between animal protein intake and incidence of hip fracture that was not explained by differences in dietary calcium or caloric intakes. Although these studies did not show a causal relationship between the presence of animal protein and incidence of osteoporosis, it sparked the interest of researchers to study this association further.

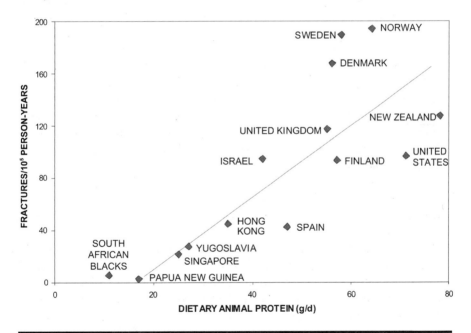

Figure 6.1   Plot of age-adjusted hip fracture incidence in women over 50 against estimated per capita dietary animal protein, by country. Adapted from Abelow et al., *Calcif. Tissue Int.*, 1992.

In the early 1970s, dietary analyses of Eskimos[38,39] revealed that they consumed high amounts of total protein (> 200 g/day) and meat in their diet. This was inferred to be the cause for the early onset and greater magnitude of bone loss observed among Eskimos compared with Caucasians residing in the U.S. Until the late 1990s, there were no other population-based studies that investigated the relationship between meat protein and bone health. Recently, secondary analyses of two large cohort studies, the Iowa Women's Health Study[19] and the Nurses' Health Study[20] were used to determine the association between animal protein intake and incidence of fracture.

The subjects in the Iowa Women's Health study[19] were postmenopausal women aged 55–69 years. About 41,000 women from the original cohort returned completed food-frequency questionnaires and were eligible for this specific study. The risk of hip fracture was not related to calcium or vitamin D intake, but was inversely associated with total protein intake. Relative risk of hip fracture decreased across increasing quartiles of animal protein intake. In contrast, the participants of the Nurses Health Study[20] were pre- and perimenopausal women aged 35–59 years. Protein intake was associated with an increased risk of forearm fracture in women who consumed more than 95 g protein per day compared with those that consumed less than 65 g per day (Table 6.3). A similar increase was observed with animal- but not vegetable-protein intake. The relative risk was higher in women who consumed red meat five or more times a week compared than in those who consumed less than once a week. No association was observed between total- or animal-protein intake and risk of hip fracture in this cohort. The opposing findings of these two cohorts suggest that the effect of animal protein on fracture risk may vary according to hormonal status and site of fracture.

It is proposed that animal protein, by virtue of its high content of sulfur amino acid, may induce bone loss by stimulating the endogenous production of acid. If meat protein produces a more acid load, one would expect a higher rate of calcium excretion[40-43] in individuals consuming higher amounts of animal products. A cross-sectional survey of middle-aged and elderly women with markedly different dietary patterns and lifestyles was conducted in five rural counties in China.[44] Urinary calcium and acid excretion were positively correlated to animal- and non-dairy animal-protein intake, but negatively associated with plant-protein intake. These findings were significant even after adjusting for age and calcium intakes. This suggests that, for free-living women, the production of endogenous acids may at least partly explain the increased loss of calcium. Although the acid load theory explains the increased loss of calcium in the urine with animal-protein intake, the effect of acid load on incidence of osteoporotic fractures is not clear.

High protein intake among free-living subjects is typically accompanied by a concomitant increase in dietary calcium that may blunt the negative effects of high protein diets on bone.[45] Comparison of women from seven

Table 6.3 Relative Risks (RR) for Forearm Fractures by Protein Consumption among U.S. Female Nurses, Nurses' Health Study

Protein Consumption	No. of Cases	Forearm Fractures			
		Age–Adjusted Model		Multivariate* Model	
		RR	95% CI	RR	95% CI
Total protein (g/day)					
<68	280	1.00**		1.00**	
68–77	317	1.10	0.94–1.29	1.11	0.94–1.30
78–85	329	1.13	0.96–1.32	1.14	0.97–1.33
86–95	340	1.14	0.97–1.34	1.16	0.99–1.36
>95	362	1.18	1.01–1.38	1.22	1.04–1.43
p trend***		0.04		0.01	
Animal protein (g/day)					
<51	280	1.00**		1.00**	
52–61	323	1.15	0.98–1.35	1.15	0.98–1.35
62–69	313	1.10	0.93–1.29	1.11	0.94–1.30
70–80	352	1.22	1.05–1.43	1.25	1.07–1.46
>80	360	1.21	1.03–1.41	1.25	1.07–1.46
p trend***		0.01		0.004	
Vegetable protein (g/day)					
<12	307	1.00**		1.00**	
12–14	323	1.02	0.87–1.19	1.01	0.87–1.18
15–16	351	1.09	0.94–1.28	1.08	0.93–1.26
17–19	336	1.03	0.88–1.20	1.01	0.86–1.18
>19	311	0.92	0.79–1.08	0.90	0.77–1.06
p trend***		0.28		0.17	

*Multivariate models were simultaneously adjusted for questionnaire time period; age; body mass index and hours of vigorous activity per week; menopausal status and use of postmenopausal hormones; cigarette smoking; use of thyroid hormone medication and thiazide diuretics; and alcohol and caffeine intakes.

**Referent group.

***Trends across quintiles of total, animal, and vegetable protein using the median value in each quintile in logistic regression models.

Adapted from Feskanich et al., *Am. J. Epidemiol.*, 1996.

countries[46] showed that the incidence of vertebral osteoporosis was highest in countries such as Japan, where the protein intake was high and the calcium intake was low. Countries such as Finland and the U.K. that reported a higher intake of both protein and calcium had lower incidence of vertebral fractures. It is therefore hypothesized that the calcium to protein ratio is a better predictor of osteoporotic fractures than the absolute amounts of these two nutrients. A longitudinal study on young adult women showed a positive association between bone gain and calcium to protein ratio.[47] The Nurses Health Study cohort also demonstrated a reduced risk of forearm fractures in women with higher protein intake accompanied by a higher calcium intake, but this reduction was small and not significant. In contrast, the Iowa women showed an inverse association between both total- and animal-protein intake and risk of hip fracture. However, this study did not determine the association between fracture risk and calcium to protein ratio. This may have provided additional information to explain the opposing findings from the two cohorts.

In summary, the association between meat protein and fracture risk is not conclusive. The opposing findings from the two cohort studies suggest that fracture risk may vary by fracture site and age at fracture incidence. In addition, the amount of calcium intake and the presence of other nutrients such as sodium, potassium, and phosphorus may alter the effect of meat protein on bone status.

2. Dairy Products

One of the main differences between a vegan and LOV diet is the inclusion of dairy products in the latter group. Dairy products are a source of both animal protein and calcium. Cross-sectional studies using FAO food availability data[48] show that hip fractures are more frequent in populations where dairy products are commonly consumed and calcium intakes are typically high (Figure 6.2). This does not implicate dairy as a causative factor, but dairy consumption may be a marker for an increased intake of animal (meat) consumption in these populations. Within the last three decades, about 52 investigator-controlled calcium intervention trials have been conducted, with six using dairy as the source of calcium.[49] These studies show that dairy consumption causes greater bone gain, decreased bone loss, or decreased fracture risk.

The relationship between lifetime milk consumption and BMD in 581 postmenopausal Caucasian women was investigated.[50] A positive and graded association between milk consumption and BMD of spine and total hip was observed. These findings were duplicated in a study of young osteoporotic patients and age-matched controls.[51] Adequate calcium intake through the consumption of dairy products in childhood and

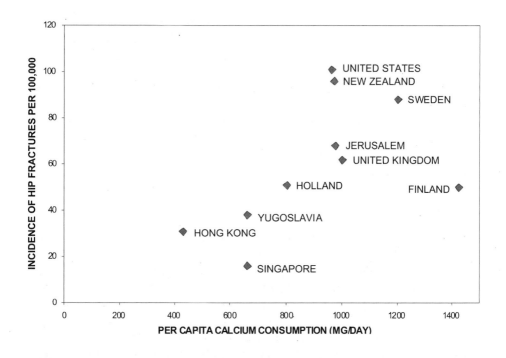

Figure 6.2   Available calcium in the food supply compared with the incidence of hip fractures in females of several nations. Adapted from Hegsted, *J. Nutr.*, 1986.

adolescent years was an important marker for attaining peak bone mass and for the prevention of osteoporosis. Osteoporotic patients had significantly lower intake of calcium and dairy products than their age-matched controls.

Alternatively, milk consumption does not seem to be associated with hip fracture risk in men. 43,063 men aged 40–75 years from the Health Professionals Follow-up Study[52] were monitored over an 8-year period for the incidence of fractures due to trauma. After controlling for confounding factors, the relative risk of forearm and hip fractures for men in the highest quintile of calcium intake compared with those in the lowest quintile was 0.98 and 1.19 respectively. Dairy product consumption per se showed a non-significant decrease in hip fracture incidence, but the use of milk, the most common dairy product, did not show a protective effect.

Another approach to understanding the importance of dairy products in preventing osteoporosis is to investigate populations with a high prevalence of lactose intolerance, since they naturally tend to avoid dairy products. Studies comparing BMD of lactose-intolerant women showed that they had lower dairy calcium intake and femoral BMD than their healthy counterparts.[53] The risk of fractures at tibia and metatarsal was elevated in the lactose-intolerant women,[54] and a high degree of correlation was observed between BMD and the percentage of calcium coming from dairy foods.[55]

A vast majority of these studies lend support to the inclusion of dairy products to maintain BMD and reduce osteoporotic fractures in women but not men. A comparison of BMD and fracture incidence among vegans and LOV after adjusting for calcium, energy, and protein intake is the next step in research, prior to confirming the importance, if any, of dairy products in reducing fracture risk associated with bone loss.

3. Soy

Incidence of osteoporotic fractures is lower among Asian women than women from most Western countries, although Asian women have lower bone mineral densities. This may be due to higher physical activity, lower intake of red meat, greater exposure to ultraviolet light, increased consumption of bony fish, or the consumption of soy products[9] — life-style habits that are commonly observed among Asians. A prospective study[56] of healthy Japanese perimenopausal women demonstrated a positive association between soybean intake and BMD even after adjusting for age and calcium intake. No other prospective studies have looked at the association between soy and other legume intake and incidence of fracture associated with bone loss.

Clinical studies using soy isoflavones, which are weak estrogens, showed positive results with respect to bone health of free-living postmenopausal women.[57] These women were fed a step I diet with either casein or varying amounts of soy protein. An increase in bone mineral content and BMD in lumbar spine was noted in the group that received the higher amount of isoflavone (2.25 mg isoflavone/g protein) suggesting that this component of soy may have a positive influence on bone status. Favorable effects were also observed on bone mineral content or biochemical markers of bone turnover after short-term consumption of soy flour[58] or isolated soy protein.[59]

Animal studies have also demonstrated the protective effects of soy and their isoflavones on bone. Although the commonly employed ovariectomized rate model does not mimic postmenopausal bone loss in women, the overall findings support the bone preserving effects of soy. Bone density of ovariectomized adult rats fed isolated soy protein was higher than in rats fed casein protein.[60] The soy isoflavones were responsible for the bone sparing effect,[61] which is mediated via stimulating bone formation rather than slowing bone resorption.[62] This suggests that to derive significant increments in bone mass, soy products have to be consumed over a reasonable length of time. In addition to stimulating bone formation, soy protein, by virtue of its low content of sulfur amino acids, may decrease calcium excretion and thus indirectly enhance bone strength.[59]

Although these preliminary human feeding studies and animal studies favor the inclusion of soy in the diet to enhance bone health, studies thus far have been of short duration and small sample size. Also, most of these studies have looked at the influence of soy on BMD but not on fracture risk per se. Therefore, long-term studies with large sample size that look at incidence of fracture as an outcome variable are needed before making any conclusions.

4. Fruits and Vegetables

Although both vegetarians and omnivores include fruits and vegetables in their diets, vegetarians typically consume higher amounts of these foods. Cross-sectional and longitudinal change in BMD was assessed among survivors of the original cohort of the Framingham Heart Study.[63] Diet and supplement use was quantified and BMD measured at hip and forearm site among these elderly subjects. Fruit and vegetable intake was positively associated with BMD in both men and women. In addition, the decline in BMD in men who consumed higher amounts of fruits and vegetables was less over the subsequent years. These associations were similar to that noted for magnesium and potassium intakes. Previously, positive association between past intake of fruits[64-67] and BMD at the spine and trochanter, after adjusting for confounders, were reported in premenopausal women. These studies suggest that the presence of specific plant foods such as fruits and vegetables may have a protective effect on BMD of both young and older adults.

Minerals such as magnesium and potassium found in higher concentration in fruits and vegetables may contribute to the protective effects of these foods on bone. In fact, magnesium supplementation to osteoporotic women for 2 years resulted in slower bone loss and fewer fractures than in a control group.[68] A diet high in potassium also tends to decrease rates of calcium excretion.[69] This effect may be due to the alkaline nature of potassium. In fact, it has been demonstrated that the highest base-forming potential is for fruits and vegetables and the highest acid-forming potential is for meat, cheese, and fish.[70] This supports the hypothesis that an alkaline load will decrease bone resorption and thus help conserve bone mineral density. However, no studies have systematically analyzed this hypothesis using animal models or by conducting human intervention studies.

Another mineral that has been implicated as having a protective role on bone health is boron. Diets rich in fruits, vegetables, nuts, and legumes provide significant quantities of boron. Although the exact mechanism by which boron affects bone health is unclear, it is thought to mediate its action via steroid hormone production and calcium metabolism.[71] Although the evidence remains limited at this time, it seems prudent to recommend increased consumption of fruits and vegetables, perhaps to maintain bone density via creating an alkaline milieu, but certainly to derive other established health benefits.

C. Public Health Implications

It was not until the early 1970s that the role of diet in the incidence of osteoporosis and related fractures was investigated. This is interesting and perplexing at the same time. Does this imply that our current knowledge in this area is lagging behind? Or is it because the role of diet per se in altering fracture risk is rather minuscule compared with other factors such as hormonal status and genetics? There are some issues that need to be addressed to answer these questions and to draw any conclusions.

The term vegetarian has not been defined consistently across the studies. Only a few distinguish between a vegan and LOV diet. This makes between-study comparisons challenging. When we consider a vegetarian diet, life-style factors such as increased physical activity and absence of smoking and drinking that are highly prevalent among vegetarians must be delineated from the diet effect per se. This is not always the case. In addition, influence of specific plant or animal foods on bone health has not been sufficiently addressed. Besides identifying the role of specific nutrients (calcium) on bone health, it is necessary to determine if the source of the nutrient (dairy vs. non-dairy) plays a role in altering bone metabolism. It is clear that multiple dietary factors are involved in regulating bone metabolism. How significant an effect they each have and how they interact with each other to modify the risk of bone loss still remains to be seen.

Osteoporosis occurs as a result of several years of accumulated damage to bone density and structure. This implies that nutrition over a period of time and not just the immediate past would be responsible for the bone loss. In many of the studies, current dietary intake and not past intake information has been reported. There is also a great extent of variability in terms of the primary outcome variable measured in the different studies. Most studies have either used biochemical markers of bone turnover or bone mineral density measured at different sites. However, very few have looked at the association of diet to the incidence of fracture, which is the more relevant clinical and public health outcome.

To enhance our understanding of how vegetarian and omnivorous diets and their food components alter risk of osteoporosis, there is certainly a need for more specific research using systematically designed studies. With the existing knowledge, one can extend a word of caution to vegans and encourage them to increase the dietary calcium to protein ratio. Given that the inclusion of plant foods such as fruits and vegetables have protective effects beyond that on bone status, it is prudent to increase consumption of these foods in the daily diet. Soy intake may be supported, but further research is warranted before conclusive recommendations can be made.

III. TYPE 2 DIABETES

Dietary surfeit is a contributing factor to the disproportionately increased incidence of type 2 diabetes seen in the U.S., and is capable of precipitating the disease onset in those who are genetically susceptible. Obesity is a major risk factor for the development of type 2 diabetes, accounting for approximately 70% of the variance in disease prevalence.[72] Therefore, plant-only and plant-based eating patterns that assist in weight management will have preventive effects in individuals at high risk for developing type 2 diabetes. Basic research and epidemiological findings are important to consider in reference to the specific components of plant-based and meat-based diets that may protect or contribute to diabetes prevalence. The research on the role of vegetarian diets in the primary and secondary prevention of type 2 diabetes will be reviewed in this section.

A. Vegetarian Diets in the Prevention of Type 2 Diabetes

Phillips et al.[3] noted that non-vegetarians consume less dietary fiber and complex carbohydrates than vegetarians. The attributes of the typical non-vegetarian diet (i.e., low-fiber and low complex carbohydrate), in concert with an excess fat intake, predominantly saturated in nature, may produce an unfavorable outcome on long-term glucose tolerance. While not yet considered causal, a correlation between dietary fat and Syndrome-X, or insulin resistance, is plausible.[73] However, not all dietary fats have been linked to diabetes incidence, and recent research provides evidence that monounsaturated fats and other fats may be beneficial[74,75] as long as total caloric intake does not exceed requirements. Thus, it is possible that non-vegetarians consume dietary components that contribute to the risk of developing type 2 diabetes, as well as lack the intake of dietary factors that confer risk protection.

The hypothesis of a vegetarian diet reducing the risk of developing diabetes is supported by findings from the cohort of 25,698 adult white Seventh-Day Adventists identified in 1960 and followed for 21 years.[76] Table 6.4 presents data on meat consumption and self-reported diabetes prevalence

Table 6. 4   Meat Consumption and the Prevalence Ratio of Self-Reported Diabetes

Meat Consumption	Prevalence Ratio Adjusted for Age and Percent Desirable Weight (95% CL)*	
	Male	Female
<1 days/wk (vegetarian)	1.0	1.0
1+ days/wk (non-vegetarian)	1.8 (1.3, 2.5)	1.4 (1.2, 1.8)
<1 days/wk	1.0	1.0
1–2 days/wk	1.3 (1.0, 1.8)	1.1 (0.9, 1.2)
3–5 days/wk	1.5 (1.0, 2.3)	1.1 (0.9, 1.2)
6+ days/wk	2.4 (1.7, 3.4)	2.1 (1.6, 2.7)
	Trend p < 0.001	Trend p < 0.001

*The reference category for each risk estimate is the group of vegetarians — those consuming meat less than 1 day per week. CL denotes confidence limits.

Adapted from Snowdon and Phillips, *Am. J. Public Hlth.*, 1985.

after adjusting for age and percent desirable weight. This data shows a moderately strong positive association between meat consumption and diabetes prevalence in both men and women. Compared with vegetarians, the prevalence ratio for diabetes among non-vegetarians was 1.8 (95% CI 1.3, 2.5) for males and 1.4 (95% CI 1.2, 1.8) for females. This prospective study also revealed that the rate of diabetes as an underlying cause of death in Adventists was approximately one-half the risk for all U.S. whites. Male vegetarian Adventists had a substantially lower risk than non-vegetarians of diabetes as an underlying contributing cause of death. It has been observed that diabetes is prevalent in beef-eating populations[77] and that animal fat consumption in individuals is positively associated with diabetes prevalence.[78] Additionally, Gear et al.[79] have shown positive association between meat consumption and blood glucose levels. These findings suggest that a vegetarian diet may reduce the risk of developing diabetes.

Salmeron et al.[80] observed that women who consumed high-glycemic-index diets were approximately 40% more likely to develop diabetes than those who consumed low-glycemic-index diets. Vegetarian diets that feature whole grains, dry beans, and soy foods confer on the glycemic index complementary effects that have a role in the prevention of type 2 diabetes mellitus.[81] Consumption of whole grains modulates the glycemic index by slowing digestion and absorption of available carbohydrate, and diminishing the postprandial blood glucose and insulin response.[82]

Several groups of investigators have observed a significant inverse association between total dietary fiber intake and the risk of developing

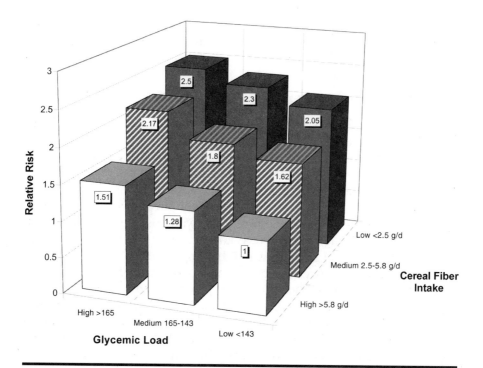

Figure 6.3 Relative risk of type 2 diabetes by different levels of cereal fiber intake and glycemic load. Adapted from Salmerón et al., *JAMA*, 1997.

type 2 diabetes.[83,84] Figure 6.3 shows the relative risk of non-insulin-dependent diabetes mellitus by different levels of cereal fiber intake and glycemic load within the Nurses Health Study cohort. The findings support the hypothesis that women consuming diets with a high glycemic load and a low cereal fiber content are at increased risk of developing diabetes.[80] In addition to the glycemic index effects, dietary fiber also enhances sensitivity to insulin.[85-87]Vegetarian lifestyles that feature the intake of beans, legumes, and soy tend to decrease the risk of type 2 diabetes incidence. Beans digest slowly and produce a low glycemic and insulin response.[88] Legumes are high in fiber, low in fat, and also have a low glycemic index. Soybeans are rich in phytates, soluble fiber, and tannins, correlate inversely with the rate of carbohydrate digestion, and produce a low glycemic index.[89,90] Gittelsohn et al.[91] studied the food consumption and preparation patterns in a Native Canadian community and observed that a high consumption of junk foods (OR = 2.40, 95% CI = 1.13 − 5.10) or bread and butter (OR = 2.22, 95% CI = 1.22 − 4.41) were associated with increased risk for diabetes and impaired glucose tolerance. In addition to these foods, methods of food preparation that involved adding fat was associated with increased risk for diabetes (OR = 2.58, 95% CI = 1.11 −

6.02). Thus, the overall dietary food pattern of individuals must be considered to assess the degree of protection plant-based foods offer in reducing the risk of developing type 2 diabetes.

1. *Proposed Mechanisms of Action*

Amino acids modulate the secretion of both insulin and glucagon, therefore, the composition of dietary protein may influence the balance of glucagon and insulin activity. Soy protein and other vegetable protein sources are higher in non-essential amino acids than most animal-derived proteins and preferentially favor glucagon production.[92] Acting on hepatocytes, glucagon promotes cAMP-dependent mechanisms that down-regulate lipogenic enzymes and cholesterol synthesis, while up-regulating hepatic low density lipoprotein receptors and production of the insulin growth factor I (IGF-I) antagonist IGF binding protein-1.[92]

The relationship between frequent meat or saturated fat consumption, both hallmarks of non-vegetarian dietary patterns, and increased diabetes incidence is supported by several plausible mechanisms. Collier and O'Dea[93] found that the co-ingestion of saturated fat (butter) with carbohydrate or protein potentiates insulin secretion. Addanki[94] suggested that saturated fat intake may alter fecal microbial enzyme activity and steroid production, which may increase the synthesis of estrogen and impair insulin sensitivity. Additionally, Helgason et al.[95] showed that N-nitroso compounds in meat may act as diabetogenic agents, as shown by steptozotocin, a nitrosamide, that induces diabetes in CD1 mice.

Many possible mechanisms and numerous loci of insulin resistance exist, however, one underlying theme emerges — the abnormal activation of catabolic body chemistry during the anabolic process of eating. Provonsha et al.[73] proposed a theme of inappropriately activated components of catabolic chemistry in the pathogenesis of type 2 diabetes based on meal-induced systemically unfavorable insulin/glucagon ratios. Clinical diabetes is a chronic catabolic state, therefore, simultaneous consumption of carbohydrate with meat and fat at meals pits insulin against glucagon, and a paradox is achieved.

Elevated blood levels of glucagon, cortisol, fatty acids, protein, and glucose can occur with meals, resulting in a multilevel, multiorgan interference with glucose handling. Hence, type 2 diabetes may be the result of the dietary activation of catabolic chemistry (consumption of body muscle and fat tissue) simultaneous to that of anabolic chemistry (mealtime protein). Since muscle protein and saturated fat are the blood messengers of catabolism ordinarily set free when insulin concentrations fall, it appears the dietary consumption of muscle and fat is creating a system-wide pseudocatabolism interfering with the carbohydrate portion of the meal.

An ideal protein source would allow for carbohydrate-induced protein sparing as meal absorption progresses, which meat protein does not appear to produce.[73]

B. Summary

Scientific data suggests that vegetarian diets may confer preventive health benefits for individuals at risk of developing type 2 diabetes. However, appropriate planning for nutritional adequacy and avoidance of a dietary surfeit are imperative to achieve beneficial outcomes. The use of a low fat vegetarian diet[96] for the secondary prevention of type 2 diabetes is gradually emerging. Further studies are needed to confirm such findings prior to recommending this dietary lifestyle to individuals with type 2 diabetes.

IV. NEUROLOGICAL DISORDERS

A. Dementia

The aging population worldwide yields concern for an increased prevalence of dementia. Hypothetical reasons exist for lifelong dietary patterns influencing the most common forms of dementia. Harman has elucidated a theory that free radicals might be involved in the onset of dementia.[97] Vegetarian diets high in antioxidants may confer protection against free radicals and thus reduce the risk of senile dementia.[98] Multi-infarct dementia may also be related to the consumption of cholesterol and different fatty acids.

Giem et al.[99] investigated the relationship between animal product consumption and evidence of dementia in two sub groups of the Adventist Health Study cohort. To ensure a wide range of dietary exposure, 272 California residents were matched for age, sex, and zip code, which included one "pure" vegetarian, one lacto-ovo vegetarian, and two heavy meat eaters in each of 68 quartets. The second sub group included 2984 unmatched subjects who resided within the Loma Linda area. Table 6.5 shows that matched subjects who ate meat (including poultry and fish) were more than twice as likely to become demented as their vegetarian counterparts (RR = 2.18) and a trend toward delayed onset of dementia in vegetarians was found in both sub groups. However, no significant difference was found in the incidence of dementia in vegetarians vs. omnivore unmatched subjects. Additional studies are warranted to validate these preliminary findings.

B. Multiple Sclerosis

In 1950, Swank first suggested that a relationship existed between the incidence of multiple sclerosis (MS) and the consumption of saturated

Table 6.5 The Occurrence of Dementia and Intake of Animal Products Among Seventh-Day Adventists, Adventist Health Study

	Demented Subjects	Nondemented Subjects	Total
Pure vegetarians and lacto-ovo-vegetarians	8	128 (740)*	136
"Heavy" (>4 X/week) meat eaters	16	120 (678)*	136
Total	24	248	272

*Mantel-Haenszel relative risk 2.18; χ^2 3.41; p = 0.065 (with 68 strata). Person years.

Adapted from Giem, Beeson, Fraser, *Neuroepidemiology*, 1993.

fatty acids of animal origin.[100] This hypothesis is supported by epidemiological studies that have established that MS is far less common in predominantly vegetarian societies and tends to correlate internationally with saturated fat intake.[100-102] Large animal fat meals are known to cause aggregation of blood cells, slowing of the circulation, and a reduction in the oxygen available to the brain.[103-106] This tendency to detain blood in micro circulation could cause acidification of surrounding areas, activate lysing enzymes, and increase the permeability of the blood–brain barrier.[107] Swank has further hypothesized that the toxic components in the plasma of normal subjects and those with MS[108,109] could permeate to the surrounding neurons and increase the tendency for their destruction.[107]

Ghadirian et al.[110] performed a case-control study of MS in Montreal and showed a protective effect with dietary patterns that included fiber, vegetable protein, vitamin C, vitamin E, thiamin, riboflavin, calcium, and potassium. These components of plant foods offer protection via regulatory processes of the nervous system or by acting as antioxidants in contrast to an increased risk with high-energy and animal-food intake. Alternatively, Sinclair has suggested that the causal factor in MS is a relative deficiency of essential fatty acids rather than consumption of an excess of saturated fatty acids.[111] Thompson and collaborators have also supported Sinclair's hypothesis.[112-114] Further, McCarty has hypothesized that a high polyunsaturate/saturate ratio of the diet or tissue lipids is the key to prevention of MS and this ratio has an impact on myelin structure such that a high polyunsaturate content somehow tends to prevent the demyelinating process. However, additional prospective studies are needed to validate these hypotheses.

REFERENCES

1. Dwyer, J. Convergence of plant-rich and plant-only diets. *Am. J. Clin. Nutr.*, 70S, 620S, 1999.

2. Fraser, G.E. Associations between diet and cancer, ischemic heart disease, and all-cause mortality in non-Hispanic white California Seventh-Day Adventists. *Am. J. Clin. Nutr.*, 70S, 532S, 1999.

3. Phillips, R.L., Snowdon, D.A., Brin, B.N. Cancer in vegetarians. In: Wynder, E.L, Leveille, G.A., Weisburger J.H., Livingston G.E., Eds. Environmental Aspects of Cancer — the Role of Macro and Micro Components of Foods. Westport, CT: Food and Nutrition Press, 1983.

4. Haddad, E.H., Sabaté J., Whitten C.G. Vegetarian food guide pyramid: A conceptual framework. *Am. J. Clin. Nutr.*, 70S, 615S, 1999.

5. West, R.O., Hayes, O.B. Diet and serum cholesterol levels: a comparison between vegetarians and non-vegetarians in a Seventh-Day Adventist group. *Am. J. Clin. Nutr.*, 21, 853, 1968.

6. Riggs, B.L., Melton, L.J., III. Involutional osteoporosis. *N. Engl. J. Med*, 314, 1676, 1986.

7. Melton, L.J. III. Hip fractures: a worldwide problem today and tomorrow. *Bone*, 14(Suppl.), S1, 1993.

8. Riggs, B.L., Melton, L.J., III. The worldwide problem of osteoporosis: insights afforded by epidemiology. *Bone*, 17(Suppl.), 505S, 1995.

9. Anderson, J.J.B. Plant-based diets and bone health: nutritional implications. *Am. J. Clin. Nutr.*, 70(Suppl.), 539S, 1999.

10. Wachman, A., Bernstein, D.S. Diet and osteoporosis. *Lancet*, 1, 958, 1968.

11. Nelson, M.E., Fiatarone, M.A., Morganti, C.M., et al. Effects of high-intensity strength training on multiple factors for osteoporotic fractures: a randomized controlled trial. *JAMA*, 272, 1909, 1994.

12. Seeman, E., Melton, L.J., III, O'Fallon, W.M., et al. Risk factors for spinal osteoporosis in men. *Am. J. Clin. Nutr.*, 75, 977, 1983.

13. Kiel, D.P., Zhang, Y., Hannan, M.T., et al. The effect of smoking at different life stages on bone mineral density in elderly men and women. *Osteoporos. Int.*, 6, 240, 1996.

14. Scharpira, D. Alcohol abuse and osteoporosis. *Semin. Arthritis Rheum.*, 19, 371, 1990.

15. Felson, D.T., Zhang, Y., Hannan, M.T., et al. The effect of postmenopausal estrogen therapy on bone density in elderly women. *N. Engl. J. Med.*, 329, 1141, 1993.

16. Dawson-Hughes, B., Dallal, G.E., Krall, E.A., et al. A controlled trial of the effect of calcium supplementation on bone density in postmenopausal women. *N. Engl. J. Med.*, 323, 878, 1990.

17. Dawson-Hughes, B., Dallal, G.E., Krall, E., et al. Effect of vitamin D supplementation on wintertime and overall bone loss in healthy postmenopausal women. *Ann. Intern. Med.*, 115, 505, 1991.

18. Heaney, R.P. Nutritional factors in osteoporosis. *Annu. Rev. Nutr.*, 13, 287, 1993.

19. Munger, R.G., Cerhan, J.R., Chiu, B.C.H. Prospective study of dietary protein intake and risk of hip fracture in postmenopausal women. *Am. J. Clin. Nutr.*, 69, 147, 1999.

20. Feskanich, D., Willett, W.C., Stampfer, M.J., et al. Protein consumption and bone fractures in women. *Am. J. Epidemiol.*, 143, 472, 1996.
21. Ellis, F.R., Holesh, S., Ellis, J.W. Incidence of osteoporosis in vegetarians and omnivores. *Am. J. Clin. Nutr.*, 25, 555, 1972.
22. Marsh, A.G., Sanchez, T.V., Mickelsen, O., et al. Cortical bone density of adult lacto-ovo-vegetarian and omnivorous women. *JADA*, 76, 148, 1980.
23. Marsh, A.G., Sanchez, T.V., Chaffee, F.L., et al. Bone mineral mass in adult lacto-ovo-vegetarian and omnivorous males. *Am. J. Clin. Nutr.*, 37, 453, 1983.
24. Sanchez, T.V., Mickelsen, O., Marsh, A.G., et al. Bone mineral mass in elderly vegetarian females. Presented at 4th Intl. Conf. on Bone Mineral Measurement, Toronto, June 1978.
25. Marsh, A.G., Sanchez, T.V., Mickelsen, O., et al. Vegetarian life-style and bone mineral density. *Am. J. Clin. Nutr.*, 48, 837, 1988.
26. Chiu, J.F., Lan, S.J., Yang, C.Y., et al. Long-term vegetarian diet and bone mineral density in postmenopausal Taiwanese women. *Calcif. Tissue Int.*, 60, 245, 1997.
27. Johnston, P.K., Makola, D., Knutsen, S., et al. Spinal bone mineral density in vegan, lacto-ovo vegetarian, and omnivorous premenopausal women. Presented at 3rd Intl. Congress on Vegetarian Nutrition, Loma Linda, California, March 1997.
28. Barr, S.I., Prior, J.C., Janelle, K.C., et al. Spinal bone mineral density in premenopausal vegetarian and non-vegetarian women: cross-sectional and prospective comparisons. *J. Am. Diet. Assoc.*, 98, 760, 1998.
29. Lau, E.M., Kwok, T., Woo, J., et al. Bone mineral density in Chinese elderly female vegetarians, vegans, lacto-vegetarians and omnivores. *Eur. J. Clin. Nutr.*, 52, 60, 1998.
30. Finch, P.J., Ang, L., Colston, K.W, et al. Blunted seasonal variation in serum 25-hydroxy vitamin D and increased risk of osteomalacia in vegetarian London Asians. *Eur. J. Clin. Nutr.*, 46, 509, 1992.
31. Gonzalez-Reimers, E., Arnay de la Rosa, M. Ancient skeletal remains of the Canary Islands: bone histology and chemical analysis. *Anthropol. Anz.*, 50, 201, 1992.
32. Lloyd, T., Schaeffer, J.M., Walker, M.A., et al. Urinary hormonal concentrations and spinal bone densities of premenopausal vegetarian and non-vegetarian women. *Am. J. Clin. Nutr.*, 54, 1005, 1991.
33. Tesar, R., Notelovitz, M., Shim, E., et al. Axial and peripheral bone density and nutrient intakes of postmenopausal vegetarian and omnivorous women. *Am. J. Clin. Nutr.*, 56, 699, 1992.
34. Tylavsky, F.A., Anderson, J.J.B. Dietary factors in bone health of elderly lacto-ovo-vegetarian and omnivorous women. *Am. J. Clin. Nutr.*, 48, 842, 1988.
35. Reed, J.A., Anderson, J.J.B., Tylavsky, F.A., et al. Comparative changes in radial-bone density of elderly female lacto-ovo-vegetarians and omnivores. *Am. J. Clin. Nutr.*, 59(Suppl.), 1197S, 1994.
36. Hunt, I.F., Murphy, N.J., Henderson, C., et al. Bone mineral content in post-menopausal women: comparison of omnivores and vegetarians. *Am. J. Clin. Nutr.*, 50, 517, 1989.
37. Hegsted, D.M. Calcium and osteoporosis. *J. Nutr.*, 116, 2316, 1986.
38. Mazess, R.B., Mather, W. Bone mineral content of North Alaskan Eskimos. *Am. J. Clin. Nutr.*, 27, 916, 1974.

39. Mazess, R.B., Mather, W.E. Bone mineral content in Canadian Eskimos. *Hum. Biol.*, 47, 45, 1975.

40. Lemann, J., Litzow, J.R., Lennon, E.J. The effects of chronic acid loads in normal man: further evidence for participation of bone mineral in the defense against chronic metabolic acidosis. *J. Clin. Invest.*, 45, 1608, 1966.

41. Lutz, J. Calcium balance and acid-base status of women as affected by increased protein intake and by sodium bicarbonate ingestion. *Am. J. Clin. Nutr.*, 39, 281, 1984.

42. Sebastian, A., Harris, S.T., Ottaway, J.H., et al. Improved mineral balance and skeletal metabolism in postmenopausal women treated with potassium bicarbonate. *N. Engl. J. Med.*, 330, 1776, 1994.

43. Breslau, N.A., Brinkley, L., Hill, K.D., et al. Relationship of animal protein-rich diet to kidney stone formation and calcium metabolism. *J. Clin. Endocrinol. Metab.*, 66, 140, 1988.

44. Hu, J., Zhao, X., Parpia, B., et al. Dietary intakes and urinary excretion of calcium and acids: a cross-sectional study of women in China. *Am. J. Clin. Nutr.*, 58, 398, 1993.

45. Heaney, R.P. Excess dietary protein may not adversely affect bone. *J. Nutr,* 128, 1054, 1998.

46. Nordin, B.E.C. International patterns of osteoporosis. *Clin. Orthop.*, 45, 17, 1966.

47. Recker, R.R., Davies, M., Hinders, S.M., et al. Bone gain in young adult women. *JAMA*, 268, 2403, 1992.

48. Nations. F. The Fourth FAO World Food Survey, Food and Agriculture Organization of the United States. Rome, 1977.

49. Heaney, R.P. Calcium, dairy products, and osteoporosis. *J. Am. Coll. Nutr.*, 19(Suppl.), 83S, 2000.

50. Soroko, S., Holbrook, T.L., Edelstein, S., et al. Lifetime milk consumption and bone mineral density in older women. *Am. J. Public Hlth.*, 84, 1319, 1994.

51. Renner, E. Dairy calcium, bone metabolism, and prevention of osteoporosis. *J. Dairy Sci.*, 77, 3498, 1994.

52. Owusu, W., Willett, W.C., Feskanich, D., et al. Calcium intake and the incidence of forearm and hip fractures among men. *J. Nutr.*, 127, 1782, 1997.

53. Honkanen, R., Pulkkinen, P., Jarvinen, R., et al. Does lactose intolerance predispose to low bone density? A population-based study of perimenopausal Finnish women. *Bone*, 19, 23, 1996.

54. Honkanen, R., Kroger, H., Alhava, E., et al. Lactose intolerance associated with fractures of weight-bearing bones in Finnish women aged 38–57 years. *Bone*, 21, 473, 1997.

55. Infante, D., Tormo, R. Risk of inadequate bone mineralization in diseases involving long-term suppression of dairy products. *J. Pediatr. Gastroenterol. Nutr.*, 30, 310, 2000.

56. Tsuchida, K., Mizushima, S., Toba, M., et al. Dietary soybean intake and bone mineral density among 995 middle-aged women in Yokohama. *J. Epidemiol.*, 9, 14, 1999.

57. Potter, S.M., Baum, J., Teng, H., et al. Soy protein and isoflavones: their effects on blood lipids and bone density in postmenopausal women. *Am. J. Clin. Nutr.*, 68(Suppl.), 1375S, 1998.

58. Dalais F.S., Rice G.E., Bell R.J. Dietary soy supplementation increases vaginal cytology maturation index and bone mineral content in postmenopausal women. *Am. J. Clin. Nutr.* 1998;68:1518S.

59. Messina, M. and Messina, V. Soyfoods, soybean isoflavones, and bone health: a brief overview. *J. Ren. Nutr.*, 10, 63, 2000.

60. Arjmandi, B.H., Alekel, L., Hollis, B.W., et al. Dietary soybean protein prevents bone loss in an ovariectomized rat model of osteoporosis. *J. Nutr.*, 126, 161, 1996.

61. Arjmandi, B.H., Birnbaum, R., Goyal, N.V., et al. Bone-sparing effect of soy protein in ovarian hormone-deficient rats is related to its isoflavone content. *Am. J. Clin. Nutr.*, 68(Suppl.), 1364S, 1998.

62. Arjmandi, B.H., Getlinger, M.J., Goyal, N.V., et al. Role of soy protein with normal or reduced isoflavone content in reversing bone loss induced by ovarian hormone deficiency in rats. *Am. J. Clin. Nutr.*, 68(Suppl.), 1358S, 1998.

63. Tucker, K.L., Hannan, M.T., Chen, H., et al. Potassium, magnesium, and fruit and vegetable intakes are associated with greater bone mineral density in elderly men and women. *Am. J. Clin. Nutr.*, 69, 727, 1999.

64. New, S.A., Bolton-Smith, C., Grubb, D.A., et al. Nutritional influences on bone mineral density: a cross-sectional study in premenopausal women. *Am. J. Clin. Nutr.*, 65, 1831, 1997.

65. Tranquilli, A.L., Lucino, E., Garzetti., G.G., et al. Calcium, phosphorus, and magnesium intakes correlate with bone mineral content in postmenopausal women. *Gynecol. Endocrinol.*, 8, 55, 1994.

66. Michaelsson, K., Holmberg, L., Maumin, H., et al. Diet, bone mass, and osteocalcin: a cross-sectional study. *Calcif. Tissue Int.*, 57, 86, 1995.

67. Angus, R.M., Sambrook, P.N., Pocock, N.A., et al. Dietary intake and bone mineral density. *Bone Miner.*, 4, 265, 1988.

68. Stendig-Lindberg, G., Tepper, R., Leichter, I. Trabecular bone density in a 2-year controlled trial of oral magnesium in osteoporosis. *Magnes. Res.*, 6, 155, 1993.

69. Lemann, J., Jr., Pleuss, J.A., Gray, R.W. Potassium causes calcium retention in healthy adults. *J. Nutr.*, 123, 1623, 1993.

70. Remer, T., Manz, F. Potential renal load of foods and its influence on urine pH. *JADA*, 95, 791, 1995.

71. Naghii, M.R., Samman, S. The role of boron in nutrition and metabolism. *Prog. Food. Nutr. Sci.*, 17(4), 331, 1993.

72. Everhart, J.E., Pettitt, D.J., Bennett, P.H., Knowler, W.C. Duration of obesity increases the incidence of NIDDM. *Diabetes*, 41, 235, 1992.

73. Provonsha, S., Wade, C., Sherma, A. Syndrome-AC: non-insulin-dependent diabetes mellitus and the anabolic/catabolic paradox. *Med. Hypothesis*, 515, 429, 1998.

74. Low, C.C., Grossman, E.B., Gumbiner, B. Potentiation of effects of weight loss by monounsaturated fatty acids in obese NIDDM patients. *Diabetes*, 45, 569, 1996.

75. Feld, C.J., Ryan, E.A., Thomson, A., Clandinin, T. Dietary fat composition alters membrane phospholipid composition, insulin binding, and glucose metabolism in adipocytes from control and diabetic animals. *J. Bio. Chem.*, 256, 11143, 1990.

76. Snowdon, D.A., Phillips, R.L. Does a vegetarian diet reduce the occurrence of diabetes? *Am. J. Pub. Hlth.*, 75, 507, 1985.

77. West, K.M. Epidemiology of Diabetes and its Vascular Lesions. New York, Elsevier North Holland, 1978.
78. West, K.M., Kalbfleisch. Influence of nutritional factors on prevalence of diabetes. *Diabetes*, 20, 99, 1971.
79. Gear, J.S., Mann, J.I., Thorogood M., Carter, R., Jelfs, R. Biochemical and haematological variables in vegetarians. *Br. Med. J.*, 1, 1415, 1980.
80. Salmeron, J., Manson, J.E., Stampfer, M.J., Colditz, G.A., Wing, A.L., Willett, W.C. Dietary fiber, glycemic load, and risk of non-insulin-dependent diabetes mellitus in women. *JAMA*, 277, 472, 1977.
81. Anderson, J., Smith, B.M., Washnock, C.S. Cardiovascular and renal benefits of dry bean and soybean intake. *Am. J. Clin. Nutr.*, 70S, 464S, 1999.
82. Slavin, J.L., Martini, M.C., Jacobs, D.R., Marquart, L. Plausible mechanisms for the protectiveness of whole grains. *Am. J. Clin. Nutr.*, 70S, 459S, 1999.
83. Salmeron, J., Ascherio, A., Rimm, E.B., Colditz, G.A., Spiegelman, D., Jenkins, D.J. Dietary fiber, glycemic load, and risk of NIDDM in men. *Diabetes Care*, 20, 45, 1997.
84. Marshall, J.A., Bessesen, D.H., Hamman, R.F. High saturated fat and low starch and fiber are associated with hyperinsulinemia in a non-diabetic population: the San Luis Valley Diabetes Study. *Diabetologia*, 40, 430, 1997.
85. Anderson, J.W., Akanji, A.O. Dietary fiber—an overview. *Diabetes Care* 1991;14:1126-1131.
86. Anderson, J.W., Ziegler, J.A., Deakins, D.A., Floore, T.L., Dillon, D.W., Wood, C.L. Metabolic effects of high-carbohydrate, high-fiber diets for insulin-dependent diabetic individuals. *Am. J. Clin. Nutr.*, 54, 936, 1991.
87. Fukagawa, N.K., Anderson, J.W., Hageman, G., Young, V.R., Minaker, K.L. High-carbohydrate, high-fiber diets increase peripheral insulin sensitivity in healthy young and old adults. *Am. J. Clin. Nutr.*, 52, 524, 1990.
88. Geil, P.B., Anderson, J.W. Nutrition and health implications of dry beans: a review. *J. Am. Coll. Nutr.*, 13, 549, 1994.
89. Jenkins, D.J., Wolever, T.M., Taylor, R.H., Barker, H., Fielden, H., Baldwin, J.M. Glycemic index of foods: a physiological basis for carbohydrate exchange. *Am. J. Clin. Nutr.*, 34, 362, 1981.
90. Liener, I.E. Implications of anti-nutritional components in soybean foods. *Crit. Rev. Food Sci. Nutr.*, 34, 31, 1994.
91. Gittelsohn, J., Wolever, T.M.S., Harris, S.B., Harris-Giraldo, R., Hanley, A.J.G., Zinman, B. Specific patterns of food consumption and preparation are associated with diabetes and obesity in a Native Canadian community. *J. Nutr.*, 128, 541, 1998.
92. McCarty, M.F. Vegetarian proteins may reduce risk of cancer, obesity, and cardiovascular disease by promoting increased glucagon activity. *Med. Hypothesis*, 536, 459, 1999.
93. Collier, G., O'Dea, K. The effect of co-ingestion of fat on the glucose, insulin, and gastric inhibitory polypeptide responses to carbohydrate and protein. *Am. J. Clin. Nutr.*, 37, 941, 1983.
94. Addanki, S. Roles of nutrition, obesity, and estrogens in diabetes mellitus: Human leads to an experimental approach to prevention. *Prev, Med.*, 10, 1981.
95. Helgason, T., Ewen, S.W., Ross, I.S., Stowers, J.M. Diabetes produced in mice by smoked/cured mutton. *Lancet*, 2, 1017, 1982.

96. Nicholson, A.S., Sklar, M., Barnard, N.D., Gore, S., Sullivan, R., Browning, S. Toward improved management of NIDDM: a randomized, controlled, pilot intervention using a low fat, vegetarian diet. *Prev. Med.*, 292, 87, 1999.

97. Harman, D. A hypothesis on pathogenesis of senile dementia of the Alzheimer's type. *Age*, 16, 20, 1993.

98. Messina, M. Health consequences of vegetarian diets. The Dietitian's Guide to Vegetarian Diets: Issues and Applications. Port Townsend, Washington: Aspen Publishers, 1996:17-78.

99. Giem, P., Beeson, W.L., Fraser, G.E. The incidence of dementia and intake of animal products: preliminary findings from the Adventist Health Study. *Neuroepidemiology*, 12, 28, 1993.

100. Swank, R.L. Multiple sclerosis: a correlation of its incidence with dietary fat. *Am. J. Med. Sci.*, 220, 421, 1950.

101. Swank, R.L., Lerstad, O., Strom, A. Multiple sclerosis in rural Norway: Its geographic and occupational incidence in relation to nutrition. *New Eng. J. Med.*, 46, 1952.

102. Alter, M., Yamoor, M., Harshe, M. Multiple sclerosis and nutrition. *Arch. Neurol.*, 1, 67, 1974.

103. Swank, R.L. Changes in the blood produced by a fat meal and by intravenous heparin. *Am. J. Physiol.*, 164, 798, 1951.

104. Cullen, C.F., Swank, R.L. Intravascular aggregation and adhesiveness of the blood elements associated with alimentary lipemia and injections of large molecular substances: effect on blood–brain barrier. *Circulation*, 9, 335, 1954.

105. Swank, R.L., Nakamura, H. Oxygen availability in brain tissues after lipid meals. *Am. J. Physiol.*, 198, 217, 1960.

106. Meyer, J.S., Waltz, A.G. Effects of changes in composition of plasma on blood flow. 9, 728, 1959.

107. Swank, R.L., Grimsgaard, A. Multiple sclerosis: the lipid relationship. *Am. J. Clin. Nutr.*, 48, 1387, 1988.

108. Bornstein, M.B., Crain, S.M. Functional studies of cultured brain tissue as related to "demyelinative disorders." *Science*, 148, 1242, 1965.

109. Wolfgram, F., Rose, A.S. The in vitro action of some organic acids on myelin. *J. Neuropathol. Exp. Neurol.*, 17, 399, 1958.

110. Ghadirian, P., Jain, M., Shatenstein, B., Morisset, R. Nutritional factors in the etiology of multiple sclerosis: a case control study in Montreal, Canada. *Int. J. Epidemiol.*, 27, 845, 1997.

111. Sinclair, H.M. Deficiency of essential fatty acids and atherosclerosis, et cetera. *Lancet,* 1, 381, 1956.

112. Thompson, R.H.S. A biochemical approach to the problem of multiple sclerosis. *Proc. Roy. Soc. Med.*, 59, 269, 1966.

113. Gul, S., Smith, A.D., Thompson, R.H.S., Zilkha, K.J. Fatty acid composition of phospholipid from platelets and erythrocytes in multiple sclerosis. *J. Neurol. Neurosurg. Psychiatry*, 33, 506, 1970.

114. Belin, J., Petet, N., Smith, A.D., Thompson, R.H.S., Zilkha, K.J. Linoleate metabolism in multiple sclerosis. *J. Neurol. Neurosurg. Psychiatry*, 34, 25, 1971.

7

DOES LOW MEAT CONSUMPTION CONTRIBUTE TO GREATER LONGEVITY?

Pramil N. Singh

CONTENTS

0-8493-8508-3/01/$0.00+$.50
© 2001 by CRC Press LLC

I. INTRODUCTION

A number of historical references have been made to populations that have purportedly experienced a greater longevity due to the low meat content of their diet.[1-17] Diets with low meat content have been described as being common among certain geographically isolated rural peoples — the Hunzakuts of the Himalayas, the Vilcabambas of Ecuador, mountain dwellers of Turkey, Russian Caucasus — who have reported ages that raise the possibility that their life expectancy may far exceed 70 years.[1-7] In a popular vegetarian food guide, these experiences were qualitatively contrasted with the estimated 40-year life expectancy of comparable (in level of technology) rural peoples — the Masai of Africa, Eskimos, Greenlanders, Lapplanders, Russian Kurgis — whose diet consists of meat as the predominant source of energy.[8] During the late 19th century, G.M. Humphry, a professor of surgery at Cambridge, identified 900 patients who were at least 90 years of age and noted that the majority of them ate little meat.[9]

At least twice in the 20th century, historical events have produced "experimental" conditions in which meat was eliminated from the diet of a large population and a subsequent decrease in the mortality rate of that population was observed. During World War I, the German occupation of Denmark created conditions in which about 3 million Danes were subjected to a severe food restriction that almost completely eliminated meat consumption. In 1920, Hindhede reported in the Journal of the American Medical Association[10] that the mortality rate in Denmark after this food restriction dropped by 2.1 deaths per 1000 — a trend that translates into 6300 lives saved per year during the period in which the Danes consumed essentially meatless diets. During World War II, the German occupation of a number of Scandinavian countries from 1939 to 1945 also resulted in a similar food restriction that substantially decreased the consumption of meats.[11-15] The mortality rate data for Norway[13,14] and Sweden[15] indicate that in both countries there was a similar decline (by about 2 deaths per 1000) in mortality rate during this period of food restriction, followed by a return to the pre-World War II rates when the food restriction was lifted in 1943–1945.

By the latter half of the 20th century, the compilation of vital statistics and food disappearance data in many developed nations provided an opportunity to relate national consumption levels of meat to national mortality rates. Using the data from 20 different countries, Stamler[16] reported a positive correlation between animal product consumption and mortality rates from coronary heart disease during the 1960s. These data identified particularly low coronary heart disease rates in Japan and Mediterranean countries — areas with a well-defined diet pattern that involved low intake of meats, particularly red meats. In addition, Nestle[17] has recently cited World Health Organization data indicating that the life expectancy of adults in Japan and certain Mediterranean countries (i.e., Greece) is up to 2 years longer than their peers in Western nations (U.S., Canada, and U.K.) in which the per capita meat intake was, until recently, substantially higher.

Does lower meat intake improve survival among humans? When considering this question, the apparently supportive, often-cited historical references and national consumption data mentioned here present a number of major methodological problems. Of particular concern is the problem of accurate determination of advanced age in rural populations and the problem of interpreting a causal effect of meat from ecologic data correlating higher national consumption levels of meat with higher national mortality rates for a given period.

In this chapter, we have therefore attempted to answer this question by focusing on two additional lines of recent evidence. First, we have summarized the most recent biochemical and clinical evidence cited in support of the plausibility of meat as a risk factor for fatal disease. Then, we have closely examined the current epidemiologic findings from 12 published prospective studies that related meat intake to all-cause mortality among 109,151 adults. Conclusions about whether low meat intake contributes to greater longevity are based on the findings from these studies.

II. MEAT AND THE PATHOLOGY OF HUMAN DISEASE

When considering whether a causative role of meat in fatal disease is biologically plausible, it is important to note that meat, as consumed in the typical human diet, contains a number of nutritional and other components that may be independently causal. Specifically, as a food group, meats can be reduced to components based on macronutrients, micronutrients, and substances present in the ingested meat due to commercial feedlot practices and methods used in the preservation, processing, handling, and cooking of meats. These components of meat and their possible relation to the development of fatal disease are summarized in Table 7.1 and discussed below.

A. Nutrient Components of Meat

1. Fat

The fat in red meats has been identified as having a very high content of saturated fat (Table 7.2). Thus, based on fat content alone, red meat could be considered an atherogenic risk factor that contributes to coronary heart disease and ischemic strokes. A number of prospective studies have linked red meat intake to higher rates of coronary heart disease and stroke.[18-22] Recent laboratory data also raise the possibility that the low polyunsaturated to saturated fat ratio in red meats (Table 7.2) increases the permeability of the cell membrane to insulin receptors and thus increases insulin resistance.[23-25] This mechanism suggests that increased red meat intake (relative to other meats or no meat intake) could potentially produce a hyperinsulinemic state that would contribute to a higher risk of diabetes, and perhaps certain cancers (prostate, colon, breast). In this context, it is noteworthy that Snowdon has reported a prospective association between red meat intake and increased diabetes risk,[26] a convincing body of evidence implicates red meat intake in colon carcinogenesis,[27] and recent evidence also links insulin-like growth factors to an increased risk of cancers of the prostate, colon, and breast.[28]

2. Protein

Ingested meat protein increases fecal nitrates among omnivores and therefore has long been implicated in the endogenous formation of carcinogenic N-nitroso compounds by the colonic flora. Recently, Bingham et al.[29] have demonstrated a threefold increase in the formation of N-nitroso compounds in a feeding trial of eight human subjects who changed from a low-meat (60 g/day of beef, lamb, or pork) to a high-meat (600 g/day of beef, lamb, or pork) diet.

Table 7.1   Nutritional and Other Components of Meat Intake as Possible Risk Factors

Component	Possible Risk Factor for:	References
Nutritional		
Meat Fat		
Saturated Fat	CVD*, Cancer	18–22
Polyunsatuarated Fat/Saturated Fat Ratio	Diabetes, Cancer	23–28
Meat Protein		
Nitrates	Cancer	29, 83
Heterocyclic Amines	Cancer, CVD	30–40
Total Energy Intake	Cancer, Aging	41–44
Iron	Cancer, CVD	45–61
Phosphorus	Osteoporosis, Fractures	62–67
Other Components		
Added to Animals in Commercial Feedlots		
Hormones (estradiol, progesterone, testosterone, trenbolone acetate, zeranol)	?	68–74
Antibiotics	Bacterial infection by Antibiotic-resistant strains	75, 76
Feed supplemented with rendered animal tissue that is infected with prion disease	Creutzfeldt-Jakob variant	77–82
Formed/Added during Preserving, Processing, and Handling		
Nitrates, Nitrites	Cancer	83
Salting, Curing	Cancer	84, 85
E. Coli	Infection	86
Salmonella	Infection	86 ,87
Trichinellosis	Infection	86
Formed/Added during Cooking**		
Benzo[a]pyrenes and other Polycyclic Aromatic Hydrocarbons	Cancer	83, 88

*CVD = cardiovascular disease
**Heterocylic amines not listed since covered under meat protein

Data indicating that the cooking of meat protein produces certain heterocyclic amines has often been cited as a possible mechanism whereby increased meat protein intake can increase risk of colon cancer and

Table 7.2 Nutrient Content of Meats and Foods that Typically Replace Meats in the Human Diet

	Meats				Foods that Typically Replace Meats in the Human Diet			
	3 oz	3 oz	3 oz	3 oz	1/2 cup	1/2 cup Pinto	1/2 cup	3 oz Veggie
	Beef	Pork	Poultry	Fish	Lentils	Beans	Tofu	Burger
Fats								
Saturated (g)	9.3	6.5	3.0	1.07	0.05	0	0.9	0.7
Polyunsaturated (g)	0.8	2.0	2.4	2.77	0.17	0.5	3.4	2.8
Calories (kcal)	264	238	187	155	114	110	94	151
Iron (mg)	1.4	0.8	1.2	0.9	3.3*	2.7*	6.7*	1.5*
Phosphorus (mg)	131	187	118	217	178	0	120	157
Calcium (mg)	6.1	8.5	9.3	12.8	18	40	138	61.2
Fiber (g)	0	0	0	0	7.8	7	1.5	5.1

*non-heme iron

perhaps cardiovascular disease.[30] Specifically, four out of the 20 known heterocyclic amines (IQ(2-Amino-3,4-dimethylimidazo[4,5-*f*]quinoline), MeIQ (2-Amino-3,4-dimethylimidazo[4,5-*f*]quinoline), MeIQx (2-Amino-3,4-imethylimidazo [4,5-*f*]quinoline), and PhiP(2-Amino-3,4-dimethylimi-dazo[4,5-*f*]quinoline)) are formed from a reaction that occurs at normal cooking temperatures between the creatinine and amino acids in all meats, including fish.

Do these four meat-derived heterocyclic amines contribute to the pathology of commonly occurring diseases? There is a growing body of evidence that suggests that the IQ, MeIQ, MeIQx, and PhiP derived from cooked meat protein have mutagenic, carcinogenic, and cardiotoxic effects.

Beginning in 1977 with the seminal work of Sugimura et al. at the National Cancer Center in Tokyo, a number of studies have documented a potent mutagenicity of IQ, MeIQ, MeIQx, and PhiP.[30,31] For example, these studies indicate that MeIQ can produce from 102 to 109 times more mutations than other well-known food-based mutagens such as aflatoxins, benzo[a]pyrene, and nitrosamines. Further suggestions that heterocyclic amines are directly causal comes from rodent models[32,33] indicating that, in tumors that were induced by MeIQ and PhiP, the mutations occurred in well-known cancer- and colon cancer-related genes (*p53*, H-*ras*, *Apc*). That heterocyclic amines might have causal effects on premalignant lesions is also supported by rodent studies that identify the carcinogenicity of IQ, MeIQ, MeIQx, and PhiP at sites in the liver, GI tract, and breast.[30,34] A few studies in rodents and primates have raised the possibility that IQ can induce mutations that contribute to cardiac myocyte hypertrophy, atrophy, and necrosis.[35-37] Such mechanisms of action raise the possibility that meat-derived heterocyclic amines may also contribute to cardiovascular disease.

When considering the possible causal effect of meat protein-derived heterocyclic amines, it is important to note that the final acetylation step in endogenous formation of these compounds is catalyzed by an enzyme, N-acetyltransferase(NAT2), that is regulated by the NAT2 gene. It has been shown that molecular variants of the NAT2 gene produce commonly occurring fast acetylator and slow acetylator phenotypes, with the former being implicated in a faster rate of production of heterocyclic amines.[38] Thus, it is reasonable to assume that the combination of fast acetylator phenotype and high meat intake might be components of a multifactorial pathology. This combination has been shown to increase the risk of colon cancer in a few recent case-control and cohort studies.[39,40]

3. Energy

The data in Table 7.2 indicate that meats can contain up to twice the calories of the equivalent serving of non-meat items (i.e., tofu, legumes) that typically replace meats in the diet. These data may explain why the prevalence of obesity appears to be substantially lower among those following meatless diets.[41] These data also raise the possibility that lower mortality rates observed among those consuming meatless diets may be attributable to the causal effect of lower energy intake.

At present, much of the data directly relating caloric restriction to greater longevity comes primarily from rodent studies[42] indicating that rodents undergoing caloric restriction experienced up to 30% increases in life span relative to those fed *ad libitum*. Also noteworthy is the data from rodents linking caloric restriction to higher cognitive performance, (i.e., spatial memory and learning tests), a possible marker for aging.[43] These findings from animal models are concordant with data from one study of an elderly population (ages > 75 years) in which an inverse relation between total energy intake and cognitive function was documented.[44] One possible mechanism of action for these effects is that caloric restriction results in fewer free radicals introduced into the body, resulting in less oxidative stress. This mechanism could specifically explain the associations with cognitive function since brain parenchyma consists of post-mitotic cells that would be more susceptible to oxidative damage.

4. Iron

The iron content of meats represents heme iron, while the iron content of plant foods is non-heme iron (Table 7.2). Data from human studies indicates that the bioavailability of heme iron (26% absorbed) is 10 times that of non-heme iron (2.5% absorbed).[45] Thus, among humans, it is reasonable to assume that increased meat intake results in increased iron *absorption* relative to plant foods.

Although absorption of an adequate amount of iron is needed for normal body function, can excess iron absorption have pathologic effects? Iron has been identified as a possible risk factor for atherosclerotic diseases due to its pro-oxidant properties. Specifically, data from animal studies indicate that, once in circulation, ionic or free iron can promote the production of free radicals that can contribute to atherosclerosis by oxidizing low density lipoproteins (LDL)[46] and also directly contribute to ischemic myocardial damage during reperfusion of the injured myocardium.[47,48] Among 847 adults, Kiechl et al. have shown a positive correlation between serum ferritin and sonographically assessed carotid atherosclerosis.[49] Also, data from a number of prospective studies implicate iron[50-52] or heme iron[53] as a risk factor for coronary heart disease, though there are some inconsistencies in the overall findings from population studies.[54]

Dietary iron that is not absorbed may also have pathologic effects. Babbs has hypothesized that an increased fecal concentration of iron can contribute to colon carcinogenesis by a mechanism whereby iron catalyzes the lumenal production of oxygen free radicals that can have a toxic and hyperproliferative effect on the colonic epithelium.[55] Recent data from animal studies has specifically implicated heme iron in increased proliferation of the colonic epithelium.[56] In this context, it is noteworthy that increased intake of red meats, a meat subtype that is high in heme iron content, has been linked to a higher risk of colon cancer[57-60] and colorectal adenomas[61] in prospective studies. Moreover, Willett has also reported a twofold increase in risk of colon cancer for high intake of liver, another meat subtype that is particularly high in heme iron content.[57]

5. Phosphorus

Meat products in the human diet contain, on average, substantially more phosphorus than calcium. The higher phosphorus-to-calcium ratio of meats as compared with plant foods (Table 7.2) raises the possibility that bone mass would be lower among meat eaters since higher phosphorus intake promotes binding and excretion of calcium that would otherwise be deposited in bone. Animal studies have shown, however, that the increased bone loss produced by an increased phosphorus intake was not entirely prevented by increasing calcium intake, but was prevented by parathyroidectomy.[62,63] These data have been used to support the presence of another causal pathway whereby the increased dietary phosphorus-to-calcium ratio of meats contributes to secondary hyperparathyroidism — a condition that could potentially contribute to loss of bone mass. Specifically, when the homeostatic balance of serum calcium and phosphorus is altered in favor of increased phosphorus, there is a compensatory release of parathyroid hormone that activates increased calcium resorption from the bone. This mechanism suggests that the high serum phosphorus levels among meat-eaters should produce chronically increased calcium resorption from bone that could decrease skeletal mass and increase risk of osteoporosis and bone fractures.

Recent data from clinical studies have shown that even short-term (1–4 weeks) maintenance of high-phosphorus, low-calcium diets among women and men can produce mild hyperparathyroidism.[64,65] In a cross-sectional study, Metz reported a significant negative correlation (R = −0.6 to −0.8) between dietary phosphorus intake and bone mineral content and bone mineral densities.[66] Teegarden et al.[67] have reported data indicating that the negative association between phosphorus and bone mineral density is complex, and may be dependent on intakes of calcium and protein. We are not aware of any large-scale prospective studies that relate phosphorus intake or meat intake to osteoporosis or bone fractures among adults.

6. Components of Meat Formed or Added During Processing, Storage, and Preparation

In developed nations, meat products in the diet have typically undergone a processing history that starts with the raising of livestock in commercial feedlots, continues with the preservation and storage of meat products obtained from that livestock, and ends with the preparation of the preserved or stored meat product as a dietary item. During this "processing history" there are commonly used methods of enhancing livestock growth and development, of prolonging the shelf-life of the meat product, and of cooking the meat product that can potentially result in the addition or formation of substances that remain in the ingested meat product. Some of these substances have been implicated in disease pathogenesis and are described in further detail in this section.

a. Exogenous Hormones, Antibiotics, and Feed Composition among Livestock

Recent media, political, and scientific attention has been given to a number of industrial practices commonly used in the raising of livestock in large commercial feedlots. These practices include the administration of hormones and antibiotic preparations to the animals, and also the supplementation of animal feed with a meat-and-bone meal that contains rendered animal tissue.

Currently, about 70–90% of cattle in feedlots in the U.S. undergo a procedure in which a hormone implant is injected below the skin of their ear flap.[68] Hormone implants have been commercialized and approved for use in livestock in the U.S. for the past 35 years. There are three naturally occurring mammalian hormones (estradiol, testosterone, progesterone) and two synthetic hormones (trenbolone acetate, zeranol) that are currently administered to cattle in the U.S. As of 1989, however, the European Union (EU) has banned use of all five hormones.[69] The widespread use of these hormones in commercial feedlots is not surprising, given that hormone-implanted cattle experience an increased rate of weight gain while depositing less fat — effects that enable faster and more efficient production of lean meat.

Does the administration to cattle of these five growth hormones result in harmful increases in the hormone content of the ingested meats? Increased estradiol levels among humans have been implicated in cancers of the breast, uterus, and prostate.[70] However, the FDA has indicated that the meat residue levels of estradiol and the two other naturally occurring hormones currently in use (progesterone, testosterone) produce a less than 1% increase in body stores of these hormones upon ingestion and thus should have little adverse effect.[68] For the two synthetic hormone implants that are not produced by the body (trenbolone acetate, zeranol), the FDA has used findings from animal toxicology studies to set maximum allowable levels of the residues of these hormones in the ingested meat products.[71] There are currently no data from large-scale population studies to support a direct causal link between the levels of these five hormones in meat and adverse health effects among humans.

When assessing the safety of meat from hormone-implanted cattle for the purpose of national and international policies, those who favor a ban on such implants often cite reports from the early 1970s that linked veal from calves treated with the growth hormone diethylstilbestrol to abnormal sexual development in infants and schoolchildren in Europe.[72,73] This hormone has since been banned from use in cattle in Europe and the U.S. Also, there are some anecdotal reports that hormone implants misapplied to the muscle areas rather than the ear flap of cattle could result in higher hormone residue levels in the resulting meat products.[74]

In addition to the hormone implants, operators of commercial feedlots also administer antibiotics to cattle, pigs, and poultry to prevent infection and, by some unknown mechanism, enhance growth on less feed. In 1999, two reports in the *New England Journal of Medicine* documented instances in which antibiotic-resistant bacterial infections in humans were linked to the consumption of meats from livestock treated with antibiotics.[75,76] In Denmark, Molbak et al.[75] linked 25 culture-confirmed cases of antibiotic-resistant Salmonella infections to a specific swine herd that had been treated with fluoroquinolones. In Minnesota, Smith et al.,[76] from the Minnesota Department of Public Health, documented a 17-fold rise in rates of quinolone-resistant *Campylobacter jejuni* infections since the 1994 FDA approval of quinolines in treating poultry infection. Taken together, these data implicate the use of livestock antibiotics in infectious human disease.

For many years, animal rendering plants have produced feed for cattle by a process of boiling down and making into feed animal tissue that usually comes from slaughterhouse scraps, dead farm animals, and animals from shelters. There is now good evidence that when cattle feed contains rendered animal tissue that is infected with a prion disease, this disease can be transmitted to the cattle that consume it.[77] Prion diseases can affect animals and humans, can be transmitted within and between species, and are characterized by an accumulation in the brain of a protease-resistant protein known as a prion protein. Transmissible prion diseases among humans include Creutzfeldt-Jakob disease (CjD) and kuru, and among animals include scrapie and bovine spongiform encephalopathy (BSE). In 1986, an epidemic of BSE, commonly known as "mad cow disease," was identified among cattle in the U.K. that has been attributed to a prion strain from the sheep scrapie in the cattle feed.[78,79] In 1996, a new variant of CjD was reported in the U.K. and has been attributed to the consumption of beef from cattle that were infected with BSE.[80] As of January 31, 1999, there have been 39 cases of CjD in the U.K. and one in France.[81] Data emerging from other European countries with similar cattle feed practices further support the possibility that contaminated feed is producing prion disease infection in livestock.[82]

b. Preservatives and Bacterial Toxins

Ingested meats have often been treated with additives to allow long-term preservation, and some of these additives have possible carcinogenic effects. Specifically, nitrates and nitrites have often been used as meat additives and these nitrosable compounds, similar to the nitrate derived from meat protein, have been implicated in colon and gastric carcinogenesis due to their contribution to endogenous formation of carcinogenic N-nitroso compounds.[83] Salting and curing of meats is prevalent in some cultures, and this process is thought to contribute to gastric cancer by a mechanism whereby the salt irritates gastric epithelium and enhances the effects of other luminal carcinogens.[84] Recent prospective evidence that links an increased risk of colon cancer to higher intake of processed meats may be identifying the independent effects of certain preservative methods.[85]

The methods of storing and handling uncooked meats in meat packing plants or by the consumer can allow for the introduction and replication of bacteria in the uncooked meat. One particular strain of the Escherichia Coli, E.coli O157:H7, can have particularly potent effects when it contaminates a meat product, and most commonly contaminates ground beef.[86] E.coli O157:H7 produces a Shiga-like toxin that severely damages intestinal epithelial cells to the point of causing hemorrhaging. This type of E. coli poisoning of uncooked meats can therefore be quite lethal among young children, the elderly, or the immune compromised. Another bacteria that even more commonly contaminates uncooked meats is Salmonella. Salmonellosis is the process by which the Salmonella-infected meat enters the intestine, replicates, and produces infection. Its severity varies and can be dependent on inoculating dose. The USDA recently reported the findings from 2 years of testing in large U.S. meat packing plants and found that the rate of Salmonella poisoning was as high as 30% for some ground meat products.[87] Finally, a much less common larval infection can occur in uncooked meats, particularly pork and wild animals, that produces trichinosis. This disease can be fatal, but current prevalence is quite low (< 2%).

c. By-Products of Cooking

Certain cooking methods have long been implicated in the formation of carcinogens and mutagens in the cooked meat product that is ingested.[83] Smoking, broiling, and grilling meats, or frying them in fat, have all been shown to produce biologically important amounts of benzo[a]pyrene and other polycyclic aromatic hydrocarbons.[88] These compounds have been shown to have both carcinogenic and mutagenic effects that are stronger than N-nitroso compounds.[30,31] Data supporting the even more potent carcinogenic and mutagenic effect of heterocyclic amines formed from cooked meat protein were summarized in the section on meat protein.

III. STUDIES RELATING VERY LOW MEAT INTAKE TO LONGEVITY

The preceding section has presented data indicating that a number of major nutritional components of meat have been linked either to higher levels of disease biomarkers or directly to a higher risk of specific fatal disease (Table 7.1). The question remains as to whether these putative effects aggregate to produce an increased overall mortality risk for meat consumption in human populations. Presently, one of the most practical methods of testing whether meat impacts survival is to conduct a prospective cohort study in which meat intake level is related to the subsequent risk of mortality. Most prospective studies that have related a dietary factor to mortality have assessed the usual dietary intake of a large population using a semi-quantitative food frequency questionnaire. Willett[89] recently reviewed the findings from a number of validation studies of food frequency questionnaires used in prospective studies and found that questionnaire-based dietary measures were good estimators of biochemical indicators of diet.

In this section, the current published evidence from prospective cohort studies in which meat intake was related to all-cause mortality is critiqued and reviewed. Previously unpublished data from California Seventh-Day Adventists, a cohort with a high prevalence of people following meatless diets, have also been included.

A. Selection of Studies

The author conducted a search of the databases of the National Library of Medicine (MEDLINE) to identify prospective cohort studies in which dietary intake was measured at baseline in a population that was then enrolled in mortality surveillance. Among those published studies that had collected these data, the author elected to summarize the studies in which the authors had published an analysis in which very low meat intake was directly related to all-cause mortality. For the purpose of this chapter, "very low meat intake" is defined as being either zero meat intake or the lowest meat intake category defined by the authors of the study. We have also chosen to summarize the studies in which the authors had used baseline data (i.e., diet scores, cluster analysis, principal components analysis) on meat intake and intake of other foods to analytically create dietary pattern variables that were then related to the subsequent risk of all-cause mortality.

B. Summary of the Studies

Based on a review of the literature and the criteria described above, 12 prospective cohort studies[90-102] of 109,151 adults that have examined the relation between very low meat intake, very low meat intake diet patterns and all-cause mortality (Table 7.3) were identified. It is noteworthy that all of the studies that examined these relations were conducted in affluent nations in which meat consumption is highly prevalent in the general population. Therefore, when examining whether very low meat intake impacts survival in these nations, there is the immediate problem that the low prevalence of very low meat intakes in these populations substantially limits statistical power, and therefore a very large sample size is needed to detect associations with very low meat intake. For example, data from

Table 7.3 Prospective Cohort Studies that Relate Very Low Meat Intake and Very Low Meat Intake Diet Patterns to All-Cause Mortality Among 109,151 Adults

Description/Name	Country/Origin	Author (Reference)	Cohort Size
Oxford Vegetarian Study	U.K.	Appleby (90)	11,000
Health Food Shoppers Study	U.K.	Key (91)	10,771
Health and Lifestyle Survey Study	U.K.	Whichelow (92)	9,003
OXCHECK Study	U.K.	Whiteman (93)	11,090
German Vegetarians	Germany	Claude-Chang (94–95)	1904
Adventist Health Study	U.S.	Fraser (96)	34,198
Adventist Mortality Study	U.S.	Kahn (97)	27,530
Dutch Civil Servants	Netherlands	Nube (98)	2820
Populations following a Mediterranean Diet:	Greece (rural)	Trichopolou (99)	182
	Greek migrants	Kouris-Blazos (100)	330
	Spain	Lasheras (101)	161
	Italians	Fortes (102)	162

random samples of the U.S. population indicate that the prevalence of zero meat intake was about 6%.[103] Based on this prevalence, a cohort of about 200,000 U.S. adults would be needed to have an 80% chance of detecting a 20% decrease in mortality risk due to zero meat intake.

In 10 of the 12 studies considered, the problem of low prevalence of meatless diets was addressed by either (1) over-sampling the "vegetarians" (Oxford Vegetarian Study[90]), (2) studying populations with a high prevalence of low meat consumers (Adventist Studies,[96,97] Health Food Shoppers Study,[91] studies that include a sizable number of subjects following a Mediterranean Diet pattern[99-102]), or (3) studying a vegetarian population and focusing on duration of adherence to a very low meat intake diet as the exposure of interest (German Vegetarians,[94,95] Adventist Studies). In the remainder of this section, the design, findings, and limitations of the 12 studies relating very low meat intake to mortality that are listed in Table 7.3 are discussed.

1. Design

a. Oxford Vegetarian Study (U.K.)

In the Oxford Vegetarian Study,[90] 6000 vegetarians, defined as those who never eat meat or fish, were recruited through the Vegetarian Society of the U.K. and announcements in the media.

A group of 5000 non-vegetarians were identified using a method whereby investigators asked the vegetarians to identify friends and relatives "of similar lifestyle and social class but who ate meat." These 11,000 subjects completed a food frequency questionnaire at baseline (1980–1984) with items on meat intake and were then enrolled in a 12-year follow-up. In a validation sub-study, conducted 2–4 years after baseline, it was found that the non-meat-eaters had significantly lower total cholesterol and LDL cholesterol levels. Thorogood et al.[90] reported the relation between very low meat intake and all-cause mortality in this study population.

b. Health Food Shoppers Study (U.K.)

In this study, a cohort of 10,771 adults was identified that consisted of either customers of health food shops and clinics, subscribers to health food magazines, subscribers to Seventh-Day Adventist publications, or members of vegetarian societies.[91] Of the total study population, 4627 (43%) indicated that they were vegetarian (not defined further on the questionnaire). In a validity sub-study, in which a detailed dietary assessment was conducted 1.5–6 years after baseline, it was found that among those classified as "vegetarian" at baseline, 66% consumed meat or fish less than once per week. Key[91] has examined the relation between baseline "vegetarian" status and the 17-year risk of all-cause mortality in this study population.

c. Health and Lifestyle Survey Study (U.K.)

During 1984–1985, the *Health and Lifestyle Survey*[92] was administered to a random sample of adults from representative areas of the U.K. (England, Scotland, and Wales). At baseline, the 9003 respondents to this questionnaire (77.5% response rate), provided data on frequency of consumption of "carcass meat" (defined as beef, lamb, pork, ham, bacon), poultry, fish, and 35 other non-meat food items. Whichelow[92] conducted a principal components analysis that identified four principal dietary components. One of these could clearly be characterized as a "low processed meat + low carcass meat + high in fruits/vegetable" component based on factor loadings. The score for this component was related to all-cause mortality.

d. OXCHECK Study (U.K.)

The OXCHECK study was a randomized trial in which 11,090 patients from five urban practices in Bedfordshire, U.K. completed a baseline survey and were followed up to 9 years.[93] The baseline questionnaire included simple food frequency items on red meat (beef, pork, lamb), poultry, fish, processed meat, and six non-meat food items. In a prospective analyses, Whiteman[93] reported the relation between specific meats, processed meats, and all-cause mortality in the OXCHECK study population.

e. German Vegetarians

In this study, the investigators identified a cohort of 1904 German vegetarians (zero or low intake of meat or fish) from the readership of vegetarian magazines.[94,95] The baseline questionnaire used in this study classified all of these subjects as either "strict vegetarian" (zero intake of meat or fish) or "moderate vegetarian" (low intake of meat or fish) and, in addition, measured duration of adherence to these meat intake patterns. Among these vegetarians, Chang-Claude et al.[94] examined the relation between duration of very low meat intake and 11-year all-cause mortality in this vegetarian study population. Chang-Claude et al. also computed standardized mortality ratios comparing the mortality of these vegetarians to the mortality of the German population.[95]

f. California Seventh-Day Adventists

The Seventh-Day Adventist Church, a Christian denomination founded in the 1850s in the U.S., currently has about 10 million members worldwide, with 760,000 of these members residing in North America. By 1900, a number of the early church doctrines had evolved into formal church proscriptions on tobacco and alcohol use and pork consumption. In addition to these guidelines, the church leaders published a set of dietary guidelines for the members that included a strong recommendation for the cessation of consumption of all meats. Dietary data collected among church members over the past four decades indicate that about one third to one half of the membership in California consumes no meat.[104]

For the purpose of two prospective cohort studies,[96,97] the population of California Seventh-Day Adventists was identified by a census taken from church membership rosters in 1958 and in 1974. The population identified in the 1958 census was used to enroll the Adventist Mortality Study, in which 27,530 non-Hispanic whites completed a baseline questionnaire (Hammond's American Cancer Questionnaire) in 1960 and were followed prospectively for 26 years. The population identified in the 1976 census was used to enroll the Adventist Health Study in which 34,198 non-Hispanic whites completed a baseline questionnaire (including a 55-item semi-quantitative food frequency questionnaire) in 1976 and were followed prospectively for 12 years. Validation studies of the Adventist Health Study cohort members indicated that the correlation between meat intake reported on the questionnaire and on 24-hour recalls was 0.83, and that 93% of those classified as weekly meat-eaters on the recalls were also classified as weekly meat-eaters on the baseline questionnaire items.[60]

The data from both cohort studies allowed the following previously unpublished analyses:

1. the relationship between very low intake of all meats and 26-year risk of all-cause mortality among adults of the Adventist Mortality Study
2. the relationship between very low intake of all meats and specific meats and 12-year risk of all-cause mortality among adults of the Adventist Health Study
3. the relationship between change in meat intake over a 17-year interval and the subsequent 17–29-year risk of all-cause mortality among adults who were cohort members of both the Adventist Mortality Study and Adventist Health Study

Fraser[96] recently reported that, among Californian Seventh-Day Adventists, vegetarians were substantially more likely to have never smoked cigarettes or used alcohol, and to have no prevalent chronic disease. To account for potential confounding by these factors, ever-smokers, alcohol users, and subjects with history of coronary heart disease, stroke, and cancer were excluded from the previously unpublished analysis of Seventh-Day Adventists given in this chapter.

g.   Dutch Civil Servants

In 1953, 2820 civil servants and spouses of civil servants from the city of Amsterdam completed a survey that included food frequency items, including items for intake of meat and fish.[98] Nube et al.[98] conducted a study in which the baseline dietary data was used to compute a ten point diet score that awarded a point for low intake of red meat and poultry and additional points for each of the following: high brown bread, low white bread, medium milk, high porridge, medium to high potatoes, high vegetables, high fish, medium to low eggs and high fruit. Meat consumption and the ten point diet score were both related to all-cause mortality.

h. Populations with a High Prevalence of Subjects Following a Mediterranean Diet Pattern

Four small prospective studies were conducted in populations of elderly subjects (at or beyond the seventh decade at baseline) with a high prevalence of adherence to a Mediterranean Diet pattern.[99-102] These study populations could be characterized as follows: rural Greeks (n = 182), Greek migrants to Australia and Australians of British origin (n = 330), Spaniards (n = 161), and Italians (n = 162). In three of the studies,[99-101] baseline data from an extensive food frequency questionnaire was used to compute an eight-point "healthy diet" score recommended by Davidson and Passmer.[104] The diet score was computed by adding one point for low meat intake and an additional point for each of the following: high monounsaturated-to-saturated fat ratio, moderate ethanol consumption, high legume consumption, high fruit consumption, high vegetable consumption and low milk or dairy-product consumption. The relationship between a one-unit increase in this score and all-cause mortality was determined for each of these studies. In the fourth study,[102] data from an extensive food frequency questionnaire were used to measure intakes of all meats and specific meat items and these exposures were then related to risk of all-cause mortality.

2. Findings

Table 7.4 and Figure 7.1 summarize the findings from the six studies that have directly related very low intake of all meats to all-cause mortality. Five out of six of these studies indicate a 12–56% decrease in risk for very low meat intake relative to higher meat consumption. The remaining study, The Health Food Shoppers Study, reported no strong association for a "vegetarian" status variable that did not specifically measure meat intake. Table 7.5 and Figure 7.2 provide the data from two studies that related duration of very low meat intake to all-cause mortality. In both studies, 30% and 29% decreases in risk were found for those indicating long-term (≥ 17 years and ≥ 20 years, respectively) adherence to a very low meat intake diet relative to those indicating short-term (< 17 years and < 20 years, respectively) adherence to a very low meat intake diet. Taken together, these data generally support a survival advantage for decreased meat consumption, and further raise the possibility that long-term maintenance of this diet pattern over about two decades or more *further reduces risk.*

A few of the studies considered also provided an analysis that related intake of specific meats to mortality; these are presented in Table 7.6. Of these, the Adventist Heath Study and a small study of elderly Italians[102] indicated a significant reduction in mortality risk for red meat and white

Table 7.4 Studies Relating Very Low Intake of All Meats to All-Cause Mortality

Cohort	Length of Follow-Up	Description of Very Low Meat Intake Group	Description of High Meat Intake Group	Adjusted Mortality Ratio (Very Low vs. High Intake Group)	Method(s) of Control for Confounding
1. Oxford Vegetarian Study (U.K.)	12 y	zero meat intake (n = 6000)	meat-eater (n = 5000)	0.80 [0.65,0.99]	age, smoking, BMI, social class
2. Health Food Shoppers Study(U.K.)	17 y	vegetarian (n = 4627)*	*non-vegetarian (n = 6144)	1.04 [0.93, 1.16]	age, sex, smoking
3. Germans	11 y	vegetarian (1904)**	general population	0.44 [0.36, 0.53] for men; 0.53 [0.44, 0.64] for women	age
4. Adventist Mortality Study (USA)	26 y	zero meat intake (n = 7918)	meat eaten once or more per week (n = 6,958)	0.88 [0.82, 0.93]	age, sex, education, and BMI by multivariate adjustment; ever-smokers, alcohol users, those with baseline chronic disease excluded from analysis
5. Adventist Health Study (USA)	12 y	zero meat intake (n = 7,191)	meat eaten once or more per week (n = 7,463)	0.85 [0.76, 0.94]	age, sex, education, BMI, physical activity by multivariate adjustment; ever-smokers, alcohol users, those with baseline chronic illness excluded from analysis
6. Italians	5 y	meat eaten less than once per week (NR)	meat eaten more than once per week (NR)	0.55 [0.28. 1.10]	age, sex, education, BMI, smoking, cognitive function, chronic diseases

* "Vegetarian" was not defined further on the questionnaire for this study. Subsequent validity studies indicated that 66% of those indicating vegetarian consumed no meat or fish.

** "Vegetarian" defined as zero or occasional intake of meat or fish as reported on a food frequency questionnaire for this study.

NR = not given in the published report

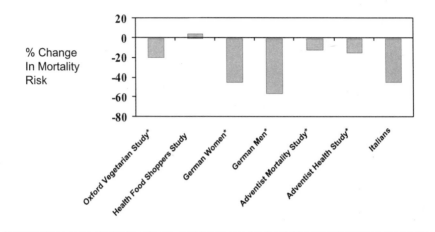

Figure 7.1   The percent change in all-cause mortality risk for very low intake of meats (zero or less than weekly) relative to higher intake of meats in five prospective studies.* p <0.05 for the change in mortality risk.

meat. It is noteworthy that the Adventist Health Study and the study of elderly Italians used a lowest meat intake category with zero or very low meat intake, while some of the studies that did not find an inverse relation with intake of specific meats had lowest meat intake categories that included those who were weekly meat consumers.

Table 7.7 summarizes the findings from five studies that have related *very low meat intake diet patterns* to all-cause mortality. A trend in the data from these studies indicating that a low meat, high plant-food diet pattern is associated with significant decreases in risk of all-cause mortality was found. Exceptions to this trend were the null findings in certain subgroups — Dutch women and Spaniards over the age of 80. This latter finding raises the possibility that associations with dietary factors attenuate with age.

3. Limitations

a. Confounding of the Associations for Very Low Meat Intake by Patterns of Intake

One of the major limitations of an analysis that relates the intake of a specific food (i.e., meats) to health outcome is that the typical human diet does not consist of intake of a single food, but rather of distinctive dietary patterns involving a number of foods. Therefore, when interpreting the findings of studies that have related intake of a single food to health outcome, it is important to note that (1) increased or decreased consump-

Table 7.5 Studies Examining the Relationship Between Duration of Very Low Intake of All Meats and the Subsequent Risk of All-Cause Mortality

Cohort	Long Duration Group	Short Duration Group	Length of Subsequent Follow-Up	Age-Adjusted Mortality Ratio [95% CI] (Long Duration vs. Short Duration Group)	Multivariate Mortality Ratio [95% CI] (Long Duration vs. Short Duration Group)
Germans with very low meat intake	Very low meat intake for ≥20 years (n = 1259)	Very low meat intake for < 20 years (n = 645)	11 years	0.69 [0.49, 0.98]	0.71 [0.49, 1.02]*
Seventh-Day Adventists with zero meat intake***	Zero meat intake for ≥17 years (n = 1906)	Zero meat intake for 17 years (n = 265)	12 years	0.64 [0.48, 0.85]	0.70 [0.51, 0.96]**

*Adjusted for age, sex, physical activity, body mass index, and adherence to vegetarianism

** Adjusted for age, sex, physical activity, body mass index by multivariate adjustment; ever-smokers, alcohol users, and those with chronic diseases at baseline were excluded.

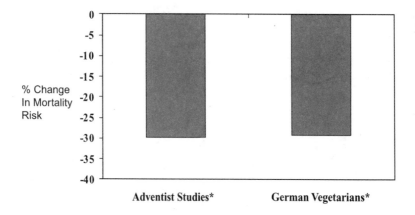

Figure 7.2   Findings from two studies for the percent change in mortality risk for long duration relative to short duration of adherence to a diet with very low intake (zero or less than weekly intake) of all meats (p* < 0.05 for both mortality comparisons). Long duration relative to short duration was defined as ≥ 20 years relative to < 20 years in the German study and ≥ 17 years relative to < 17 years in the Adventist Studies.

tion of a single food may be a marker for a specific dietary pattern, and (2) the dietary pattern may be the true causal factor rather than the single food.

When interpreting the apparently protective associations for very low meat intake given in Tables 7.4–7.6 of this chapter, it is noteworthy that many of the foods that would replace meat in the "vegetarian" diet pattern (i.e., legumes, soy products, nuts, vegetables) may be causally protective against fatal disease.[107-109] For example, among vegetarian Adventists, Kahn has reported a decreased mortality risk for green salads,[97] and Fraser has reported a decreased CHD mortality risk for higher consumption of nuts.[109] Also noteworthy is that meat has zero levels of fiber (Table 7.2) and phytochemicals. Thus, any plant food that replaces meat in the diet increases the overall intake of fiber or phytochemicals — nutritional factors that have been linked to lower risk of a wide range of chronic diseases. Taken together, these points raise the possibility that the findings in this chapter, indicating a decreased risk for very low meat intake, may be attributable, at least in part, to an increase in the health benefits of foods that typically replace meat in the human diet, rather than a reduction in the putative hazard due to meat.

Another source of confounding by patterns of intake arises when relating intake of specific meats to health outcome (Table 7.6). Specifically, an association with decreased intake of a specific meat could potentially be an indicator for the causal effects of a pattern of intake that involves increased intake of other meat types. For example, in a prospective study of diet and mortality by Whiteman,[93] low intake of fresh meats was associated with increased risk (Table 7.6). One possible explanation for this finding is that low intake of fresh meats was a marker for high intake of processed meats — a meat subtype that has been shown in a number of studies to be a possible causal factor in certain cancers.

b. Confounding by Non-Dietary Factors

A common criticism of studies that have linked very low meat intake to better health outcome is that vegetarians are likely to exhibit a number of other positive prognostic factors.[96,106] Some factors that are likely to be more prevalent among vegetarians relative to non-vegetarians include, but are not limited to, the avoidance of cigarette smoking and alcohol use, higher levels of physical activity, higher socioeconomic status, and greater awareness of personal health. Thus, when reporting the mortality ratio for very low meat intakes, adjustment for confounding by these factors is needed. In this context, it is noteworthy that the data in Tables 7.4–7.7 indicate that most studies have adjusted for some, but not all important confounders. For example, the substantial 47–56% decrease in mortality risk for German vegetarians that was adjusted only for confounding by age should be interpreted with caution since there are undoubtedly many other confounding factors that would contribute to greater longevity among the German vegetarians as compared with the total German population. In contrast, the findings from the Adventist studies that are reported here provide a unique opportunity to evaluate the causal effects of meat, since both the very low meat intake subjects and higher meat intake subjects were never-smokers, did not drink alcohol, and had no baseline history of major chronic diseases. Additionally, mortality risk for the Adventists (Tables 7.4–7.6) was further adjusted for education, body mass, and physical activity.

c. Methodological Limitations

It is important to note that all but one of the studies summarized in Tables 7.4–7.6 of this chapter related a single report of dietary intake to all-cause mortality. Thus, when interpreting the findings from these studies, there remains the possibility of bias due to changes in diet. Of particular concern is that a subject's baseline diet reflects a change in dietary pattern due to illness. In the Adventist studies, the author had the opportunity to relate two reports of diet (in 1960 and in 1976) to the subsequent risk of all-cause mortality and found that subjects who

Table 7.6 Studies Relating Very Low Intake of Specific Meats to All-Cause Mortality

Cohort	Meat Type	Length of Follow-Up	Description of Very Low Meat Intake Group	Description of High Meat Intake Group	Mortality Ratio (Very Low Intake vs. High Intake Group)	Confounder
1. Adventist Health Study (USA)	Red Meat	12 y	none (n = 8547)	meat eaten once or more per week (n = 5721)	0.88 [0.78, 0.99]	age, sex, education, and BMI by multivariate adjustment; ever-smokers, alcohol users, those with baseline chronic disease excluded from analysis
	White Meat	12 y	none (n = 8164)	meat eaten once or more per week (n = 2646)	0.81 [0.71, 0.92]	age, sex, education, and BMI by multivariate adjustment; ever-smokers, alcohol users, those with baseline chronic disease excluded from analysis
2. Italians	Red Meat + Poultry	5 y	less than once per week (n = 90)	more than once per week (n = 39)	0.50 [0.27, 0.93]	none
	Fish	5 y	less than once per week (n = 31)	once or more per week (n = 128)	1.12 [0.57, 2.17]	none
	Offal	5 y	less than once per week (n = 142)	once or more per week (n = 19)	0.85 [0.38, 1.89]	none

				less than once per week	once or more per week		
2.	Dutch Civil Servants (Holland)	Sausage	5 y	less than once per week (n = 138)	once or more per week (n = 19)	1.15 [0.49, 2.70]	none
		Red Meat + Poultry	25 y	0–300 grams per week (563 women, 536 men)	600–1800 grams per week (406 women, 563 men)	1.28 women; 1.05 men*	age
3	OXCHECK Study (UK)	Processed Meats	9 y	< one day per week (n = 6612)	4–7 days per week (n = 326)	0.95 [0.57, 1.61]	age, sex, smoking
		Fresh or Frozen Red Meat	9 y	< one day per week (n = 2247)	4–7 days per week (n = 2506)	1.41 [1.09, 1.82]	age, sex, smoking
		Fresh or Frozen Poultry	9 y	< one day per week (n = 4191)	4–7 days per week (n = 588)	1.32 [0.84, 2.08]	age, sex, smoking
		Fresh or Frozen Fish	9 y	< one day per week (n = 4874)	4–7 days per week (n = 495)	0.94 [0.63, 1.41]	age, sex, smoking

*Computed from cumulative survival estimate given in the published report.

Table 7.7 Studies Relating a Very Low Meat Intake Diet Pattern to All-Cause Mortality

Cohort	Size	Method of Determining Diet Pattern	Description of Very Low Meat Intake Diet Pattern	Adjusted Mortality Ratio	Confounders
Greeks, age >70 years	182	Diet Score*	low meat, high M/S ratio,‡ moderate ethanol, high legumes, cereals, fruits, and vegetables	0.83 [0.69, 0.99] per 1 unit increase in score	age, sex, smoking
Greek Migrants, Anglo-Australians age >70 years	330	Diet Score*	Same as above	0.83 [0.67, 1.02] per 1 unit increase in score	age, sex, smoking, ethnic origin
Spain, age 65–80 years	74	Diet Score*	Same as above	0.69 [0.43, 0.93] per 1 unit increase in score	age, sex, BMI, smoking, albumin, physical activity, baseline illness, dieting
age 80–95 years	87	Diet Score*	Same as above	1.24 [0.60, 2.53] per 1 unit increase in score	
United Kingdom	9003	Principal Components**	Component characterized by lowest processed meat, low carcass meat, highest fruit and vegetables, lowest fried foods§	0.75[0.65, 0.89] per 1 unit increase in score	age, sex, smoking, alcohol, occupation, baseline illness, region

| Dutch Civil Servants | 2820 | Diet Score | Low red meat and poultry, High vegetables, fruit, brown bread, fish, porridge | 0.83 for men; 1.11 for women¶ per 6 unit increase in score | age |

* Diet Score computed by adding points for adherence to the "very low meat intake" diet pattern described in the adjacent column

** Principal components analysis identified a component with a score (based on high factor loadings) that increases in value with greater adherence to the "very low meat intake" diet pattern described in the adjacent column

‡ Monounsaturated to saturated fat ratio

¶ $p < 0.01$ for linear trend of the score variable among men, $p = 0.54$ for linear trend of the score variable among the women reported changing from weekly meat intake in 1960 to no meat intake in 1976 experienced a non-significant 20% increase in risk relative to those who remained as weekly meat-eaters over the 17-year interval. This finding is contrary to all other findings from the Adventist populations, indicating decreased risk for very low meat intakes. One possible explanation for this unexpected effect might be that subjects may have quit consumption of meats due to an illness that was ultimately fatal. This is similar to the "sick quitter effect," shown among smokers in which those who quit smoking in response to illness were likely to have biased the protective effect of quitting the smoking habit toward the null.[111]

Measurement error of usual dietary intake of meat will have, to some extent, biased the findings from prospective cohort studies summarized here (Table 7.3). The validity studies conducted on food frequency questionnaires used in these prospective studies did indicate, however, that these instruments were good estimators of meat intake, as measured by 24-hour recall or biochemical indicators of diet.[90,92,96,99–102] Moreover, Willett[89] has reported that measurement error in dietary assessment tends to bias the effect estimate toward the null, implying that the protective associations with very low meat intake reported here may in fact be stronger.

A number of sources of bias can arise when summarizing and interpreting the findings from multiple studies. The mortality ratios for very low meat intake reported here do vary, particularly for specific meats (Table 7.6). Some of this variation may be due to the fact that some studies use a zero meat intake category, while others use a low meat intake category. If one assumes a threshold effect whereby the protective effect of very low meat intake is not evident until the diet contains zero or trace levels of the food, then these differences in methodology for determining the lowest meat intake category may contribute to important variations in the computed effect of very low meat intake. Additionally, among the "healthy volunteers" who tend to participate in medical studies, there may not be enough high meat consumption for the true harm due to the exposure to be seen. Another inevitable source of bias in our summary of the evidence is publication bias, whereby the studies described here represent the published subset of the available data from prospective investigations.

IV. SUMMARY AND CONCLUSIONS

Meat represents a major source of protein in the Western diet.[112] Thus, determining whether meat intake significantly contributes to the burden of fatal disease has important public-health and clinical implications. A summary of the published prospective cohort data from 109,151 adults revealed three major trends:

1. Five out of six studies indicated that adults who reported very low meat intake did experience 12–56% decreases in risk of death relative to those with higher meat consumption.
2. Two studies in which very low meat intake significantly decreased mortality risk provided the additional insight that among those who adhered to a very low meat intake diet, longer duration (approximately two decades or more) of adherence further contributed to a significant 30% decrease in mortality risk.
3. Five out of five studies indicated that adults who followed a low meat, high plant-food diet pattern experienced significant or marginally significant 17 to 31% decreases in mortality risk relative to other patterns of intake, though no association was found in certain subgroups.

When attempting to conclude whether these trends support a causal protective effect of low meat consumption, two major questions must be addressed. First, does confounding by the high prevalence of "healthful behaviors" among vegetarians bias the effect of low meat consumption toward greater protection? Second, is the apparent protective effect of a low meat intake diet attributable, at least in part, to the benefits obtained from plant foods that replace meats in the diet? The findings from this chapter do, to a noteworthy extent, address the first question in their indication that a significant reduction in risk for very low meat intake persists even after controlling for a number of important predictors of longevity (smoking, alcohol use, physical activity, education, body mass index) in very health conscious study populations (i.e., Adventist Studies, Oxford Vegetarian Society Study). It is not possible, however, to adequately address the second question using the current data.

Thus, the data presented in this chapter do raise the possibility that a low meat intake diet contributes to greater longevity, but more work in this area of nutritional epidemiology is needed to specifically identify the causative roles of meat and plant foods in this relation. It is important to note that, despite the unresolved questions, the findings given here, indicating a survival advantage for those following a low meat/high vegetable diet, do have immediate application when choosing the most prudent diet pattern for disease prevention. Our understanding of the hazards specifically attributable to meat will be soon be increased by the emerging data from studies that are examining the effects of metabolites of meat, enzymes involved in meat metabolism, and genetic control of these enzymes.[112] More work at the level of dietary trials to demonstrate specific biologic responses of experimental diets can also help parse out the etiologic effects of meat from the etiologic effects of plant foods that replace meats in the human diet.

REFERENCES

1. McCarrison, R. *Studies in Deficiency Diseases.* Henry Frowde and Hodder & Stoughton, London, 1921.
2. McCarrison, R. The relationship of diet to physical efficiency of Indian races. pp 90-100. The Practitioner, London, Jan 1925.
3. Mazess, R.B. Health and longevity in Vilcabamba, Ecuador. *JAMA*, 240:1781, 1978.
4. Beller, S. and Palmore, E. Longevity in Turkey. *Gerontologist*, 14(5 pt 1):373-6, Oct 1974.
5. Sachuk, N.N. A mass social-hygienic investigation of a very old population in various areas of the Soviet Union: program, procedure, results. *J. Gerontol.*, 25(3):256-61, Jul 1970.
6. Chebotaryov, D.F. and Sachuk, N.N. Sociomedical examination of longevous people in the USSR. *J. Gerontol.*, 19:435-440, 1964.
7. Georgakas, D. *The Methuselah Factors: The Secrets of the World's Longest-Lived Peoples.* Simon & Schuster, New York, 1980.
8. Strandler, M. and Strandler, N. Schocken Books, New York, New York, 1981.
9. Young, T.E. *On Centenarians.* Charles and Edward Layton, London, 1899.
10. Hindhede, M. The effect of food restriction during war on mortality in Copenhagen. *JAMA*, 76:381-382, 1920.
11. Friderica, L.S. Nutritional investigations in Denmark during the war, 1939–1945. *Proc. Nutr. Soc.*, 5:255-259, 1947.
12. Tikka, J. Conditions and research into human nutrition in Finland during the war years. *Proc. Nutr. Soc.*, 5:260-263, 1947.
13. Hansen, O.G. Food Conditions in Norway during the war, 1939–1945. *Proc. Nutr. Soc.*, 5:263-270, 1947.
14. Bang, H.O. and Dyerberg, J. Personal reflections on the incidence of ischemic heart disease in Oslo during the Second World War. *Acta. Med. Scand.*, 210:245-248, 1981.
15. Abramson, E. Nutrition and nutritional research in Sweden in the years of the war, 1939-1945. *Proc. Nutr. Soc.*, 5:271-276, 1947.
16. Stamler, J. Population studies. In: *Nutrition, Lipids, and Coronary Heart Disease.* Levy, R.I., Rifkind, B.M., Dennis, B.H., Ernst, N. (Eds.), Raven Press, New York, 1979.
17. Nestle, M. Animal v. plant foods in human diets and health: is the historical record unequivocal? *Proc. Nutr. Soc.*, 58: 211-218, 1999.
18. Kushi, L.H., Lenart, E.B., and Willett, W.C. Health implications of Mediterranean diets in light of contemporary knowledge. 2. Meat, wine, fats, and oils. *Am. J. Clin. Nutr.*, 61(6 Suppl):1416S-1427S, Jun 1995.
19. Hu, F.B., Stampfer, M.J., Manson, J.E., Ascherio, A., Colditz, G.A., Speizer, F.E., Hennekens, C.H., and Willett, W.C. Dietary saturated fats and their food sources in relation to the risk of coronary heart disease in women. *Am. J. Clin. Nutr.*, 70(6):1001-8, Dec 1999.

20. Fraser, G.E. Diet as primordial prevention in Seventh-Day Adventists. *Prev. Med.*, 29(6 pt 2):S18-23. Review, Dec 1999.

21. Menotti, A., Kromhout, D., Blackburn, H., Fidanza, F., Buzina, R., and Nissinen, A. Food intake patterns and 25-year mortality from coronary heart disease: cross-cultural correlations in the Seven Countries Study. The Seven Countries Study Research Group. *Eur. J. Epidemiol.*, 15(6):507-15, Jul 1999.

22. Campbell, T.C., Parpia, B., and Chen, J. Diet, life-style, and the etiology of coronary artery disease: the Cornell China study. *Am. J. Cardiol.*, 82(10B):18T-21T, Nov 26, 1998.

23 Field, C.J., Ryan, E.A., Thomson, A.B., and Clandinin, M.T. Diet fat composition alters membrane phospholipid composition, insulin binding, and glucose metabolism in adipocytes from control and diabetic animals. *J. Biol. Chem.*, 265(19):11143-50, Jul 5, 1990.

24 Storlien, L.H., Jenkins, A.B., Chisholm, D.J., Pascoe, W.S., Khouri, S., and Kraegen, E.W. Influence of dietary fat composition on development of insulin resistance in rats. Relationship to muscle triglyceride and omega-3 fatty acids in muscle phospholipid. *Diabetes*, 40(2):280-9, Feb 1991.

25. Joannic, J.L., Auboiron, S., Raison, J., Basdevant, A., Bornet, F., and Guy-Grand, B. How the degree of unsaturation of dietary fatty acids influences the glucose and insulin responses to different carbohydrates in mixed meals. *Am. J. Clin. Nutr.*, 65(5):1427-33, May 1997.

26. Snowdon, D.A. and Phillips, R.L. Does a vegetarian diet reduce the occurrence of diabetes? *Am. J. Public Health*, 75(5):507-12, May 1985.

27. Potter, J.D. Nutrition and colorectal cancer. *Cancer Causes Control*, 7(1):127-46, Jan 1996.

28. Giovannucci, E. Insulin-like growth factor-I and binding protein-3 and risk of cancer. *Horm Res.*, 51 Suppl 3:34-41, 1999.

29. Bingham, S.A., Pignatelli, B., Pollock, J.R., Ellul, A., Malaveille, C., Gross G., Runswick, S., Cummings, J.H., and O'Neill, I.K. Does increased endogenous formation of N-nitroso compounds in the human colon explain the association between red meat and colon cancer? *Carcinogenesis*, 17(3):515-23, Mar 1996.

30. Sugimura, T. Overview of carcinogenic heterocyclic amines. *Mutation Res.*, 211-219, 1997.

31. Sugimura, T., and Wakabayashi, K. Mutagens and carcinogens in food. In: *Mutagens and Carcinogens in the Diet.* Pariza, M.W., Aeshbacher, H.V. Felton, J.S., Sato, S. (Eds.), Wiley-Liss Inc., New York, 1990

32. Toyota, M., Ushijima, T., Kakiuchi, H., Canzian, F., Watanabe, M., Imai, K., Sugimura, T., and Nagao, M. Genetic alterations in rat colon tumors induced by heterocyclic amines. *Cancer,* 77(8 Suppl):1593-7, Apr 15, 1996.

33. Kakiuchi, H., Watanabe, M., Ushijima, T., Toyota, M., Imai, K., Weisburger, J.H., Sugimura, T., and Nagao, M. Specific 5'-GGGA-3'-->5'-GGA-3' mutation of the Apc gene in rat colon tumors induced by 2-amino-1-methyl-6-phenylimidazo[4,5-b]pyridine. *Proc. Natl. Acad. Sci. USA*, 92(3):910-4, Jan 31, 1995.

34. Adamson, R.H. and Thorgeirsson, U.P. Carcinogens in Foods: Heterocyclic Amines and Cancer and Heart Disease. In: *Nutrition and Biotechnology in Heart Disease and Cancer.* Longnecker, J.B., Kritchevsky, D., and Drezner, M.K. (Eds.), Plenum Press, New York, 1995.

35. Adamson, R.H. and Thorgeirsson, U.P. Carcinogens in foods: heterocyclic amines and cancer and heart disease. *Adv. Exp. Med. Biol.*, 369:211-20, 1995.

36. Overvik, E., Ochiai, M., Hirose, M., Sugimura, T., and Nagao, M. The formation of heart DNA adducts in F344 rat following dietary administration of heterocyclic amines. *Mutat. Res.*, 256(1):37-43, Jan 1991.

37. Thorgeirsson, U.P., Farb, A., Virmani, R., and Adamson, R.H. Cardiac damage induced by 2-amino-3-methyl-imidazo[4,5-f]quinoline in nonhuman primates. *Environ. Hlth. Perspect.*, 102(2):194-9, Feb 1994.

38. Minchin, R.F., Kadlubar, F.F., and Ilett, K.F. Role of acetylation in colorectal cancer. *Mutat. Res.*, 290(1):35-42, Nov 1993.

39. Roberts-Thomson, I.C., Butler, W.J., and Ryan, P. Meat, metabolic genotypes and risk for colorectal cancer. *Eur. J. Cancer Prev.*, 8(3):207-11, Jul 1999.

40. Kampman, E., Slattery, M.L., Bigler, J., Leppert, M., Samowitz, W., Caan, B.J., and Potter, J.D. Meat consumption, genetic susceptibility, and colon cancer risk: a U.S. multicenter case-control study. *Cancer Epidemiol. Biomarkers Prev.*, 8(1):15-24, Jan 1999.

41 Appleby, P.N., Thorogood, M., Mann, J.I., and Key, T.J. Low body mass index in non-meat eaters: the possible roles of animal fat, dietary fibre and alcohol. *Int. J. Obes. Relat. Metab. Disord.*, 22(5):454-60, May 1998.

42. Weindruch, R. and Sohal, R.S. Seminars in medicine of the Beth Israel Deaconess Medical Center. Caloric intake and aging. *New. Engl. J. Med.*, 337(14):986-94, Oct 2, 1997.

43. Algeri, S., Biagini, L., Manfridi, A., and Pitsikas, N. Age-related ability of rats kept on a life-long hypocaloric diet in a spatial memory test. Longitudinal observations. *Neurobiol. Aging*, 12(4):277-82, Jul-Aug 1991.

44. Fraser, G.E., Singh, P.N., and Bennett, H. Variables associated with cognitive function in elderly California Seventh-Day Adventists. *Am. J. Epidemiol.*, 143(12):1181-90, Jun 15, 1996.

45. Cook, J.D. Adaptation in iron metabolism. *Am. J. Clin. Nutr.*, 51:301-308, 1990.

46. Reif, D.W. Ferritin as a source of iron for oxidative damage. *Free Radic. Biol. Med.*, 12(5):417-27, 1992.

47. Zweier, J.L. and Jacobus, W.E. Substrate-induced alterations of high energy phosphate metabolism and contractile function in the perfused heart. *J. Biol. Chem.*, 262(17):8015-21, Jun 15, 1987.

48. Bolli, R., Patel, B.S., Jeroudi, M.O., Lai, E.K., and McCay, P.B. Demonstration of free radical generation in "stunned" myocardium of intact dogs with the use of the spin trap alpha-phenyl N-tert-butyl nitrone. *J. Clin. Invest.*, 82(2):476-85, Aug 1998.

49. Kiechl, S., Aichner, F., Gerstenbrand, F., Egger, G., Mair, A., Rungger, G., Spogler, F., Jarosch, E., Oberhollenzer, F., and Willeit, J. Body iron stores and presence of carotid atherosclerosis. Results from the Bruneck Study. *Arterioscler. Thromb.*, 14(10):1625-30, Oct 1994.

50. Salonen, J.T., Nyyssonen, K., Korpela, H., Tuomilehto, J., Seppanen, R., and Salonen, R. High stored iron levels are associated with excess risk of myocardial infarction in eastern Finnish men. *Circulation*, 86(3):803-11, Sep 1992.

51. Tuomainen, T.P., Punnonen, K., Nyyssonen, K., and Salonen, J.T. Association between body iron stores and the risk of acute myocardial infarction in men. *Circulation*, 97(15):1461-6, Apr 21, 1998.

52. Tzonou, A., Lagiou, P., Trichopoulou, A., Tsoutsos, V., and Trichopoulos, D. Dietary iron and coronary heart disease risk: a study from Greece. *Am. J. Epidemiol.*, 147(2):161-6, Jan 15, 1998.

53. Ascherio, A., Willett, W.C., Rimm, E.B., Giovannucci, E.L., and Stampfer, M.J. Dietary iron intake and risk of coronary disease among men. *Circulation*, 89(3):969-74, Mar 1994.

54. Corti, M.C., Gaziano, M., and Hennekens, C.H. Iron status and risk of cardiovascular disease. *Ann. Epidemiol.*, 7(1):62-8, Jan 1997.

55. Babbs, C.F. Free radicals and the etiology of colon cancer. *Free Radic. Biol. Med.*, 8(2):191-200, 1990.

56. Sesink, A.L., Termont, D.S., Kleibeuker, J.H., and Van der Meer, R. Red meat and colon cancer: the cytotoxic and hyperproliferative effects of dietary heme. *Cancer Res.*, 59(22):5704-9, Nov 15, 1999.

57. Willett, W.C., Stampfer, M.J., Colditz, G.A., Rosner, B.A., and Speizer, F.E. Relation of meat, fat, and fiber intake to the risk of colon cancer in a prospective study among women. *New Engl. J. Med.*, 323(24):1664-72, Dec 13, 1990.

58. Giovannucci, E., Rimm, E.B., Stampfer, M.J., Colditz, G.A., Ascherio, A., and Willett, W.C. Intake of fat, meat, and fiber in relation to risk of colon cancer in men. *Cancer Res.*, 54(9):2390-7, May 1, 1994.

59. Hsing, A.W., McLaughlin, J.K., Chow, W.H., Schuman, L.M., Co Chien, H.T., Gridley, G., Bjelke, E., Wacholder, S., and Blot, W.J. Risk factors for colorectal cancer in a prospective study among U.S. white men. *Int. J. Cancer.*, 77(4):549-53, Aug 12, 1998.

60. Singh, P.N. and Fraser, G.E. Dietary risk factors for colon cancer in a low-risk population. *Am. J. Epidemiol.*, 148(8):761-74, Oct 15, 1998.

61. Giovannucci, E., Stampfer, M.J., Colditz, G., Rimm, E.B., and Willett, W.C. Relationship of diet to risk of colorectal adenoma in men. *J. Natl. Cancer Inst.*, 84(2):91-8, Jan 15, 1992.

62. Anderson, G.H. and Draper, H.H. Effect of dietary phosphorus on calcium metabolism in intact and parathyroidectomized adult rats. *J. Nutr.*, 102(9):1123-32, Sep 1972.

63. Krishnarao, G.V. and Draper, H.H. Influence of dietary phosphate on bone resorption in senescent mice. *J. Nutr.*, 102(9):1143-5, Sep 1972.

64. Calvo, M.S. The effects of high phosphorus intake on calcium homeostasis. *Adv. Nutr. Res.*, 9:183-207, 1994.

65. Calvo, M.S., Kumar, R., and Heath, H. 3d. Elevated secretion and action of serum parathyroid hormone in young adults consuming high phosphorus, low calcium diets assembled from common foods. *J. Clin. Endocrinol. Metab.*, 66(4):823-9, Apr 1998.

66. Metz, J.A., Anderson, J.J., and Gallagher, P.N., Jr. Intakes of calcium, phosphorus, and protein, and physical-activity level are related to radial bone mass in young adult women. *Am. J. Clin. Nutr.*, 58(4):537-42, Oct 1993.

67. Teegarden, D., Lyle, R.M., McCabe, G.P., McCabe, L.D., Proulx, W.R., Michon, K., Knight, A.P., Johnston, C.C., and Weaver, C.M. Dietary calcium, protein, and phosphorus are related to bone mineral density and content in young women. *Am. J. Clin. Nutr.*, 68(3):749-54, Sep 1998.

68. USDA, Meat Safety and Wholesomeness, Unit 2. In: *The Livestock Industry: Production of Lean, Wholesome Meat for the Consumer, Module 1 of The Consumer's Choice Meat Education Program*. Produced by the U.S. Department of Agriculture, Extension Service.

69. Hanrahan, C. The EU's Ban on Hormone-Treated Meat. *Congressional Research Service Report RS20142*, Washington D.C., 1999.

70. Liehr, J.G. Is estradiol a genotoxic mutagenic carcinogen? *Endocr. Rev.*, 21(1):40-54, Feb 2000.

71. *Green Book — FDA Approved Animal Drug Products, 1989-2000.* Virginia Polytechnic Institute, Blacksburg, VA, 2000.

72. Loizzo, A., Gatti, G.L., Macri, A., Moretti, G., Ortolani, E., and Palazzesi, S. Italian baby food containing diethylstilbestrol: 3 years later. *Lancet,* 1(8384):1014-5, May 5, 1984.

73. Loizzo, A., Gatti, G.L., Macri, A., Moretti, G., Ortolani, E., and Palazzesi, S. The case of diethylstilbestrol treated veal contained in homogenized baby foods in Italy. Methodological and toxicological aspects. *Ann. Ist. Super Sanita.*, 20(2-3):215-20, 1984.

74. None of Us Should Eat Extra Estrogen. *Los Angeles Times*, March 24, 1997.

75. Molbak, K., Baggesen, D.L., Aarestrup, F.M., Ebbesen, J.M., Engberg, J., Frydendahl, K., Gerner-Smidt, P., Petersen, A.M., and Wegener, H.C. An outbreak of multidrug-resistant, quinolone-resistant Salmonella enterica serotype typhimurium DT104. *New Engl. J. Med.*, 341(19):1420-5, Nov 4, 1999.

76. Smith, K.E., Besser, J.M., Hedberg, C.W., Leano, F.T., Bender, J.B., Wicklund, J.H., Johnson, B.P., Moore, K.A., and Osterholm, M.T. Quinolone-resistant Campylobacter jejuni infections in Minnesota, 1992-1998. Investigation Team. *New Engl. J. Med.*, 340(20):1525-32, May 20, 1999.

77. Collinge, J. Variant Creutzfeldt-Jakob disease. *Lancet*, 354(9175):317-23, Jul 24, 1999.

78. Wilesmith, J.W., Ryan, J.B., and Atkinson, M.J. Bovine spongiform encephalopathy: epidemiological studies on the origin. *Vet. Rec.*, 128(9):199-203, Mar 2, 1991.

79. Wilesmith, J.W., Wells, G.A., Cranwell, M.P., and Ryan, J.B. Bovine spongiform encephalopathy: epidemiological studies. *Vet. Rec.*, 123(25):638-44, Dec 17, 1988.

80. Will, R.G., Ironside, J.W., Zeidler, M., Cousens, S.N., Estibeiro, K., Alperovitch, A., Poser, S., Pocchiari, M., Hofman, A., and Smith, P.G. A new variant of Creutzfeldt-Jakob disease in the U.K. *Lancet*, 347(9006):921-5, Apr 6, 1996.

81. Tan, L., Williams, M.A., Khan, M.K., Champion, H.C., and Nielsen, N.H. Risk of transmission of bovine spongiform encephalopathy to humans in the U.S. report of the Council on Scientific Affairs, American Medical Association. *JAMA*, 281(24):2330-9, Jun 23-30, 1999.

82. Ferguson, N.M., Ghani, A.C., Donnelly, C.A., Denny, G.O., and Anderson, R.M. BSE in Northern Ireland: epidemiological patterns past, present and future. *Proc. R. Soc. Lond. B. Biol. Sci.*, 265(1396):545-54, Apr 7, 1998.

83. Doll, R. and Peto, R. The Causes of Cancer. *JNCI*, 66:1191-1308, 1981.

84. Joossens, J.V. and Geboers, J. Dietary salt and risks to health. *Am. J. Clin. Nutr.*, 45(5 Suppl):1277-88, May 1987.

85. Willett, W.C. Goals for Nutrition in 2000. *CA Cancer J. Clin.*, 49: 331-352, 1999.

86. Park, S., Worobo, R.W., and Durst, R.A. Escherichia coli O157:H7 as an emerging foodborne pathogen: a literature review. *Crit. Rev. Food Sci. Nutr.*, 39(6):481-502, Nov 1999.

87. *Dow Jones Commodity Service*, March 21, 2000.

88. Lijinsky, W. and Shubik, P. Benzo[a]pyrene and other polynuclear hydrocarbons in charcoal-broiled meats. *Science*, 145:53-55, 1964.

89. Willett, W. Diet and Nutrition. In: *Cancer Epidemiology and Prevention Second Edition.* Schottenfeld, D. and Fraumeni, J.F. (Eds.), Oxford University Press, 1986.

90. Appleby, P.N., Thorogood, M., Mann, J.I., and Key, T.J. The Oxford Vegetarian Study: an overview. *Am. J. Clin. Nutr.*, 70(3 Suppl):525S-531S, Sep 1999.

91. Key, T.J., Thorogood, M., Appleby, P.N., and Burr, M.L. Dietary habits and mortality in 11,000 vegetarians and health conscious people: results of a 17-year follow up. *BMJ*, 313(7060):775-9, Sep 28, 1996.

92. Whichelow, M.J. and Prevost, A.T. Dietary patterns and their associations with demographic, lifestyle and health variables in a random sample of British adults. *Br. J. Nutr.*, 76(1):17-30, Jul 1996.

93. Whiteman, D., Muir, J., Jones, L., Murphy, M., and Key, T. Dietary questions as determinants of mortality: the OXCHECK experience. *Public Hlth. Nutr.*, 2(4):477-87, Dec 1999.

94. Chang-Claude, J., and Frentzel-Beyme, R. Dietary and lifestyle determinants of mortality among German vegetarians. *Int. J. Epidemiol.*, 22(2):228-36, Apr 1993.

95. Chang-Claude, J., Frentzel-Beyme, R., and Eilber, U. Mortality pattern of German vegetarians after 11 years of follow-up. *Epidemiology*, 3(5):395-401, Sep 1992.

96. Fraser, G.E. Associations between diet and cancer, ischemic heart disease, and all-cause mortality in non-Hispanic white California Seventh-Day Adventists. *Am. J. Clin. Nutr.*, 70(3 Suppl):532S-538S, Sep 1999.

97. Kahn, H.A., Phillips, R.L., Snowdon, D.A., and Choi, W. Association between reported diet and all-cause mortality. Twenty-one-year follow-up on 27,530 adult Seventh-Day Adventists. *Am. J. Epidemiol.*, 119(5):775-87, May 1984.

98. Nube, M., Kok, F.J., Vandenbroucke, J.P., van der Heide-Wessel, C., and van der Heide, R.M. Scoring of prudent dietary habits and its relation to 25-year survival. *J. Am. Diet. Assoc.*, 87(2):171-5, Feb 1987.

99. Trichopoulou, A., Kouris-Blazos, A., Wahlqvist, M.L., Gnardellis, C., Lagiou, P., Polychronopoulos, E., Vassilakou, T., Lipworth, L., and Trichopoulos, D. Diet and overall survival in elderly people. *BMJ*, 311(7018):1457-60, Dec 2, 1995.

100. Kouris-Blazos, A., Gnardellis, C., Wahlqvist, M.L., Trichopoulos, D., Lukito, W., and Trichopoulou, A. Are the advantages of the Mediterranean diet transferable to other populations? A cohort study in Melbourne, Australia. *Br. J. Nutr.*, 82(1):57-61, Jul 1999.

101. Lasheras, C., Fernandez, S., and Patterson, A.M. Mediterranean diet and age with respect to overall survival in institutionalized, nonsmoking elderly people. *Am. J. Clin. Nutr.*, 71(4):987-92, Apr 2000.

102. Fortes, C., Forastiere, F., Farchi, S., Rapiti, E., Pastori, G., Perucci, C.A. Diet and overall survival in a cohort of very elderly people. Epidemiology 2000; 4: 440-445.

103. Kant, A.K., Block, G., Schatzkin, A., Ziegler, R.G., and Nestle, M. Dietary diversity in the U.S. population, NHANES II, 1976-1980. *J. Am. Diet. Assoc.*, 91(12):1526-31, Dec 1991.

104. Davidson, S.S. and Passmore, R. Human Nutrition and Dietetics. Churchill Livingstone, Edinburgh, 1979.

105. Beeson, W.L., Mills, P.K., Phillips, R.L., Andress, M., and Fraser, G.E. Chronic disease among Seventh-Day Adventists, a low-risk group. Rationale, methodology, and description of the population. *Cancer*, 64(3):570-81, Aug 1, 1989.

106. Willett, W.C. Convergence of philosophy and science: the third international congress on vegetarian nutrition. *Am. J. Clin. Nutr.*, 70(3 Suppl):434S-438S, Sep 1999.

107. Messina, M.J. Legumes and soybeans: overview of their nutritional profiles and health effects. *Am. J. Clin. Nutr.*, 70(3 Suppl):439S-450S., Sep 1999.

108. Potter, J.D. and Steinmetz, K. Vegetables, fruit and phytoestrogens as preventive agents. *IARC Sci. Publ.*, (139):61-90, 1996.

109. Fraser, G.E., Sabaté, J., Beeson, W.L., and Strahan, T.M. A possible protective effect of nut consumption on risk of coronary heart disease. The Adventist Health Study. *Arch. Intern. Med.*, 152(7):1416-24, Jul 1992.

110. Singh, P.N., Tonstad, S., Abbey, D.E., and Fraser, G.E. Validity of selected physical activity questions in white Seventh-Day Adventists and non-Adventists. *Med. Sci. Sports Exerc.*, (8):1026-37, Aug 28, 1996.

111. Halpern, M.T., Gillespie, B.W., and Warner, K.E. Patterns of absolute risk of lung cancer mortality in former smokers. *J. Natl. Cancer Inst.*, 85(6):457-64, Mar 17, 1993.

112. *Designing Foods: Animal Product Options in the Marketplace.* National Research Council, National Academy Press, Washington D.C., 1988.

113. Sram, R.J. and Binkova, B. Molecular epidemiology studies on occupational and environmental exposure to mutagens and carcinogens, 1997–1999. *Environ. Hlth. Perspect.*, 108 Suppl 1:57-70, Mar 2000.

III

ADEQUACY OF VEGETARIAN DIETS THROUGH THE LIFE CYCLE AND IN SPECIAL GROUPS

8

PHYSICAL GROWTH AND
DEVELOPMENT OF
VEGETARIAN CHILDREN AND
ADOLESCENTS

Marcel Hebbelinck and Peter Clarys

CONTENTS

0-8493-8508-3/01/$0.00+$.50
© 2001 by CRC Press LLC

I.   INTRODUCTION

Human life span in the Western world is approximately 75 to 80 years. About one quarter of an individual's life span is devoted to the processes of growth and development conditioned by genetic and environmental factors. In the context of environmental factors, nutrition is paramount and of prime concern for the general good health of the growing organism. The dependency for food of infants and young children upon their parents, especially their mothers, and upon social institutions, has important links with the process of growth and development. The environmental factor is under maternal control during the gestational period and through most of infancy and childhood.

Parents practicing a vegetarian diet usually tend to raise their children on a vegetarian diet. Moreover, an increasing number of school-age children in North America and Western Europe independently decide to espouse a vegetarian diet.[1-4]

The processes of growth and development add special needs to energy and nutrition requirements. In growth studies, body height and weight, when compared with age- and sex-reference data, are considered primary indicators of health, whereas girths and skinfold measures may add information pertinent to body composition.

Concern has been expressed regarding the risk of nutrient deficiencies affecting the growth and development of young vegetarians, especially those reared on restrictive regimens such as vegan and macrobiotic diets.[5]

In this chapter, the issue of appropriateness of a vegetarian diet will be explored by examining the stages of physical growth and development from birth to adulthood. Also, this chapter will review the current literature on vegetarian regimens in children and the impact of these diets on growth and development.

To critically interpret the available research studies on the growth and development of vegetarian children and adolescents, we must consider the categories of vegetarian diets, the types of growth studies, and developmental age.

II. DEFINITIONS

A. Categories of Vegetarian Diets

Two main categories of vegetarian diets can be distinguished. Neither meat, fish, nor poultry are consumed in these categories. The most lenient of the two is the *lacto-ovo-vegetarian* (LOV) diet, which allows for milk, dairy, and egg consumption. *Lactovegetarians* (LV), on the other hand, consume milk and dairy products, but do not eat eggs. The pure or strict vegetarian diet, usually referred to as the vegan diet, contains no food derived from animals. Often, the *macrobiotic* diet is ascribed to the vegan category of diets. However, followers of this largely spiritually based regimen may occasionally use some lean fish and meat. Typical macrobiotic dietary items such as unpolished rice and other whole grain cereals, seaweeds, soya products, and miso soup are eaten regularly, whereas fresh fruit and salads are avoided or used sparsely. This explanation is important because, in the last three decades, the numerous published studies examining the growth and development of vegetarian children or children on so-called alternative diets have, in fact, dealt mainly with children following a macrobiotic diet.[6-12]

B. Types of Growth Studies

Two methods of studying child growth can be distinguished. The method of study using the same child at each age is called *longitudinal, follow-up* or *prospective*, whereas a study measuring different children at each age is called cross-sectional. In a *cross-sectional* design, since each child is measured only once, only the size at that particular age is obtained. Therefore, this does not allow for the calculation of growth velocity. Often a so-called *mixed-longitudinal* design is used, in which different cohorts of children are repeatedly examined over a relatively short period; for example, three groups of children (cohorts), one followed from 4 to 10 months, the second from 9 to 14, and the third from 13 to 18 months, may be measured simultaneously. This design covers an age range from 4 to 18 months and allows for estimates of growth velocity in a relatively short research time of 5 months. This study method requires careful sampling and special statistical techniques to get the maximum information from this data.[13]

C. Developmental Age vs. Chronological Age

To study growth, a measure of developmental age, or biological maturity, is needed; this indicates more accurately than chronological age how far a given individual has progressed along his or her road to adulthood. Differences in physical development are apparent when boys and girls of the same age are considered. However, height is not a very good measure of physical *development* since people differ in mature height.

Various methods for estimating developmental age are available, e.g., dental age (number and stage of erupted teeth), pubertal age (time of entry to the various stages of puberty), and skeletal or bone age (status of maturation of the bones of the skeleton). Only the last method, based on the radiographic examination of the successive stages of development of a specified part of the skeleton, is applicable throughout the whole period of growth.

III. REVIEW OF THE STUDIES OF GROWTH AND DEVELOPMENT OF VEGETARIAN INFANTS, CHILDREN, AND ADOLESCENTS

A. Case Studies

Reports in the medical literature of vegetarian infants suffering from malnutrition are rather exceptional. These case studies must be interpreted with caution, because they are often not typical for vegetarians as a whole. When such cases of under- or malnutrition are more closely examined, it appears that usually the infants have not been weaned into a varied balanced vegetarian diet, but rather into a more restricted vegetarian regimen.[5,14-18]

The issues of potential risks of particular restricted vegetarian or macrobiotic diets fed to children should not be ignored, but they should be placed in their proper context, with appropriate attention and respect for the dietary philosophy of the parent(s). In this respect, dietitians who are knowledgeable about balanced vegetarian regimens can play an important role in guiding parents to provide an appropriate vegetarian diet for their children.

B. Group Studies

This chapter will deal with epidemiological research studies using anthropometry related to physical growth and development of vegetarian children and adolescents.

Table 8.1. gives a comprehensive overview of these growth studies. From this table the following preliminary observations can be made:

1. **Vegetarian categories:** nine out of 23 studies deal with lacto-ovo-vegetarian (LOV) subjects,[19,21-23,25,27,28,37,38] five with vegan subjects,[20,26,39-41] three with macrobiotic (Mbiot) subjects[1,2,24,47] and six with macrobiotic and LOV subjects.[6-11]

2. **Age groups:** infants, pre-school children and primary-school-age children are the most studied age groups, whereas anthropometric data on adolescent vegetarians are scarce.[19-23]

3. **Type of study:** very few longitudinal growth studies on vegetarian children have been carried out and most followed the children for a very short period of growth.[6,10,20,21] Moreover, most of these studies apply cross-sectional statistical methods and do not really measure growth rate or velocity.

   Only the mixed-longitudinal study on macrobiotic children has specified the necessary steps to determine an appropriate statistical design.[24] Only two of the studies[9,23] considered developmental age.

4. **Anthropometry:** in all but two studies,[22,25] where only height was considered, height and weight were measured, whereas circumferences and skinfolds were also determined in many other studies. It should be pointed out, however, that height alone is a relatively poor indicator of health unless parental height is also taken into consideration. Using growth rate or velocity to monitor the health of individuals, based on frequently repeated or very short-term and accurate measurements is a better study design for observing and eventually detecting the impact of the more common ailments due to unbalanced nutrition.

5. **Sample:** all the studies, in one way or another, recruited volunteers because, since no register exists, it is very difficult, if not impossible, to choose a random sample of vegetarian children. However, in one study, practically the entire population of children in a community was examined,[26] and in another, a matched-pair design was applied.[27] The size of the samples varied a great deal, i.e., from as small as 17[28] to as large as more than 2000 subjects.[21]

In discussing the results of the studies related to the growth and development of vegetarians, one must also bear in mind that over the years, particularly in the late 1960s and early 1970s, marked changes in

Table 8.1 Synopsis of Growth Studies on Vegetarian Children

First Author (Ref)	Publication Year	Vegetarian Category	Age Group (Years)	Type of Study	Sample Size (n)	Anthropometry	Comments
Hardinge (19)	1954	LOV	13–17	cross-sect.	30	Ht, Wt	SDA, lifelong
Shull (6)	1977	LOV and Mbiot	<5	longitud.	38 LOV 34 MBiot	Ht, Wt	
Dwyer (7)	1978	LOV and Mbiot	<5	cross-sect.	119	Ht, Wt	
Dwyer (8)	1980	LOV and Mbiot	0–6	cross-sect	65 LOV 77 Mbiot	Ht, Wt	
Fulton (39)	1980	Vegan	2–5	cross-sect.	48	Ht, Wt Arm circ. Triceps and Subscap. sf.	The Farm, lifelong
Sanders (40)	1981	Vegan	1–5	cross-sect.	23	Ht, Wt, Chest-, Arm- and Head circ.	lifelong
Dwyer (9)	1982	LOV and Mbiot	0.8–8.4	cross-sect.	39	Ht, Wt	bone age on 20 Mbiot
Dwyer (10)	1983	LOV and Mbiot	0–6	longitud.	142	Ht, Wt	same subjects as in Dwyer 1980?
Hebert (38)	1985	LOV	<6	longitud.	627	Ht, Wt	all eat fish, Madras children
Staveren (11)	1985	LOV and Mbiot	0–8	cross-sect.	33 LOV 33 Mbiot	Ht, Wt	also anthroposophic diet children studied
Rona (37)	1987	LOV	6–12	cross-sect.	2506	Ht, Wt, Triceps sf.	UK children of Indian ethnicity
Sanders (20)	1988	Vegan	0–17	longitud.	39	Ht, Wt, Chest and Head circ.	

Author	Year	Diet	Age	Study type	N	Measurements	Notes
Dagnelie (47)	1988	Mbiot	0–8	cross-sect.	243	Ht, Arm circ., Triceps and Subscap. sf.	occasionally lean meat and fish
Staveren (12)	1988	Mbiot	0–8	cross-sect	300	Ht, Wt, Arm circ.	Summary of previous studies
Dagnelie (24)	1989	Mbiot	4–18 months	mixed longitud.	53	Ht, Wt, Rump length, Biiliac width, Head and Arm circ., Triceps and Subscap. sf.	occasionally lean meat and fish
O'Connell (26)	1989	Vegan	4 months – 8 years	cross-sect.; whole population	404	Ht, Wt	The Farm, lifelong
Tayter (28)	1989	LOV	11–12	cross-sect.	17	Ht, Wt, Arm circ., Triceps sf.	lifelong
Sabaté (21)	1990	LOV	6–18	longitud. (1 year)	2272	Ht, Wt	SDA
Sabaté (22)	1991	LOV	7–18	cross-sect.	1765	Ht	SDA
Sabaté (25)	1992	LOV	11–12	cross-sect.	68	Ht	SDA
Sanders (41)	1992	Vegan	5.8–12.8	longitud. (cross-sect. analysis)	20	Ht, Wt, Chest and Head circ., Biceps, Triceps and Subscap. sf.	lifelong; 15 children did not mind eating non-vegan foods
Nathan (27)	1997	LOV	7–11	longitud., matched pairs	50	Ht, Wt, Arm circ., Biceps and Triceps sf.	some subjects ate occasionally fish
Hebbelinck (23)	1999	LOV	6–18	cross-sect.	82	Ht, Wt, Triceps, Suprailiac and Calf sf.	physical fitness tests

Note: LOV, lacto-ovo-vegetarian; Mbiot, Macrobiotic; cross-sect, cross-sectional; longitud., longitudinal; Ht, Height; Wt, Weight; circ., circumference; Subscap., subscapular; sf, skinfold; SDA, Seventh Day Adventist.

attitudes, beliefs and practices of adult vegetarians took place.[29] It is likely that these changes would have an effect on child-feeding practices by vegetarian parents and in adolescent vegetarian children. Studies exploring this outcome have generated a considerable body of literature but have, however, been based on relatively few cohorts that have basically retrieved information from the same group of children (see studies of Sabaté, Dwyer, and Sanders). Many studies have been carried out on the growth of Seventh-Day Adventist (SDA)* children and adolescents, but none focused on the possible effect of a multigenerational vegetarian lifestyle. Although pertinent data on lifelong vegetarians is lacking, one may expect fewer nutritional problems from a group in which the precepts of vegetarianism and a health-oriented lifestyle are followed and often passed on through successive generations. It is possible that certain adaptive mechanisms may play a role in the final outcome with respect to the growth and development of lifetime vegetarian children and adolescents. However, until now, no study that might shed light on this issue has been carried out on lifelong vegetarians or on multigenerational vegetarian families.

C. Overview of the Studies by Dietary Category

Problems of dietary inadequacy are more likely to occur during infancy, childhood, and adolescence than in adulthood, as the requirements relative to biological growth and development are greater. The issue of growth in vegetarian children and adolescents is best dealt with by taking the category of vegetarian diet into consideration, because differences noted in growth status may reflect different food choices. The following studies of vegetarian children will be discussed by dietary category:

1. lacto-ovo-vegetarian
2. vegan
3. macrobiotic

1. Lacto-Ovo-Vegetarian (LOV) Children and Adolescents

a. SDA Studies

SDA, who are mostly LOV, show that the size of school-age children and adolescents equals[19,25,28] or exceeds[21,22] that of non-vegetarians. It should be noted that all these studies, except one,[21] are cross-sectional. Since the SDA population also adheres to other health-oriented principles such as

---

* The Seventh-Day Adventist (SDA) population is a conservative Christian group that follows a unique life-style. Over 98% of California SDA's neither smoke nor drink alcoholic beverages, and about 50% follow an LOV diet.[21]

non-smoking and avoidance of alcoholic beverages, Sabaté et al.[22] compared SDA vegetarian children with SDA omnivore children and reported that vegetarian boys and girls were slightly taller.

In a small sample (n = 17) of lacto-ovo-vegetarian children 10 to 12 years of age, Tayter and Stanek[28] reported no significant differences in group means for any of the anthropometric dimensions (height, weight, mid-arm circumference, triceps skinfold, weight-for-height index) when compared with those of an omnivore group of children of the same age and sex. Surprisingly, the weight-for-height index showed that 30% of LOV girls and 10% of omnivore girls were overweight. Because of the small sample size of this particular study, conclusions must be made cautiously. However, it indicates that vegetarian diets cannot be automatically associated with leanness. Besides energy intake, physical activity levels need to be recorded to shed light on this issue. Most studies do report energy intake but very few, if any, register energy expenditure.

In a longitudinal survey of 2272 schoolchildren and adolescents between 6 and 18 years of age, Sabaté et al.[21] found that SDA girls were significantly leaner than their counterparts in public schools and that the onset of the adolescent growth spurt occurred 1 year later in SDA school girls. Age at peak height velocity was 11 years for girls and 14 years for boys of both populations. The magnitude of the growth spurt was greater in public-school children than in SDA schoolchildren.

In a different analysis of the data from the previously mentioned SDA study, Sabaté et al.[25] noted that SDA prepubertal girls (11–12 years), tended to be slightly shorter (3 cm) than controls, suggesting that Adventist vegetarian girls have a later onset of pubertal maturation. These findings of a delayed puberty are supported by the studies of Sanchez et al.[32] and Kissinger and Sanchez,[33] who provide evidence for a significant association between a meatless diet and age of menarche. In this respect, it is important to note that risk factors for breast cancer include the early occurrence of menarche.[34-36] In the long run, this late onset of menarche in vegetarian girls may result in a health benefit.

b. Flemish Vegetarian Children, Adolescents and Young Adults Study

In a more recent study on Flemish LOV children, adolescents, and young adults,[23] no differences in height and weight were found, except that the group of adolescent vegetarians had significantly (P < 0.05) lower height and weight, as well as lower BMI than reference standards. Triceps and suprailiac skinfolds were significantly (P < 0.05) lower in the three age groups (children, adolescents, and young adults), while calf skinfold was only significantly (P < 0.05) lower in the adolescent girls. The results of puberty ratings showed that all vegetarian subjects, except for one

12-year-old girl who was clearly delayed, were within accepted normal developmental range (P3–P97). Moreover, the median menarcheal age of 13.2 years of the vegetarian girls was identical to Flemish reference data.

This study does not support the hypothesis of delayed menarche[32,22] or later physical maturation.[25] In this respect, it is suggested that studies should be made to relate diet(s) with hormone levels prior to and during early or late menarche to test the hypothesis[33] that diet can alter hormone levels associated with age at menarche.

A special feature of this study was the inclusion of physical fitness testing. Overall, the group of vegetarian children (6–12 years) was not different in physical performance compared with standards. The vegetarian adolescents did, however, score significantly lower (P < 0.05) in explosive strength (standing long-jump test) and local muscular endurance (30 sec sit-up test), whereas they performed significantly better in cardio-respiratory fitness (step test) as compared with reference values. This finding is interesting, but since the sample of vegetarian children (n = 10) and adolescents (n = 19) studied is small, the results must be interpreted cautiously. Moreover, as the authors pointed out, a confounding factor may have been the amount and pattern of sporting activity of the population studied, including a majority practicing endurance activities as contrasted to strength-related sports.

c. Longitudinal Growth Study in Northwest England

Recently, a longitudinal study compared 50 vegetarian children with 50 omnivore children, matched for age, ethnicity and sex.[27] In this study, a vegetarian diet was defined as one that may include dairy products, eggs, and occasionally fish, but no meat or meat products, and one of the criteria for selection was that the child must have followed a vegetarian diet for at least 3 months. Forty-three of the 50 subjects had not eaten meat for over 1 year, two for between 6 and 12 months and the remaining five for between 3 and 6 months. Anthropometry (height, weight, mid-upper arm circumference, and upper arm skinfold thicknesses) were taken at baseline and 1 year later. Of all the measures examined, only the predicted height increment of the vegetarians was slightly but significantly (P < 0.05) greater than that of the omnivores, after allowing for father's height, maternal smoking habit, and number of siblings. It should be noted, however, that both the vegetarian and omnivorous groups were close to the 50th percentiles of British standards for both height and weight.

Finally, two studies on Indian vegetarian children may be of interest for this section of the review on lacto-ovo-vegetarian children.

d. Indian Vegetarian Children in Britain

Within the framework of a nutritional surveillance system of primary-school children in the U.K., Rona et al.[37] studied the relation between growth status and vegetarianism in the Gujarati, Urdu, and Punjabi sub-groups of Indian ethnicity. Many of these Indian families, particularly the Gujarati, practice a vegetarian lifestyle. Vegetarian girls tended to be shorter than non-vegetarian girls in all Asian groups, although this difference was significant ($P < 0.01$) only in the Urdu group. No significant differences in weight-for-height and triceps skinfold were found between vegetarians and non-vegetarians even after adjustment for confounding variables.

e. Indian Vegetarian Children in Madras

This study was conducted longitudinally, measuring height and weight three times over a period of 15 months.[38] Children (n = 191) of 6 years and younger were selected from randomly identified households from three fishing communities in Madras that were similar for caste and socioeconomic status. On the average, the non-meat-eating children (consuming dairy products and/or fish), aged 3–6 years, were significantly taller than 123 omnivore children.

What do we learn from these findings based on studies on lacto-ovo-vegetarian children with respect to growth and development?

- The eating habits of the various lacto-ovo-vegetarian populations studied are not all alike, since some allowed for fish[37-38] and others small amounts of meat.[25]
- The results of the physical measurements showed that, even after allowing for a variety of potential confounding factors, vegetarian children grow at least as tall as omnivore children. Moreover, in the majority of studies, it is shown that vegetarian schoolchildren are leaner than their meat-eating counterparts.
- Two studies[25,28] suggest that vegetarian girls enter puberty later than omnivores, while one study[23] found that age at menarche, as well as ratings of secondary sex characteristics, fell within the normal range of reference standards.

2. Vegan Children

a. The Farm Studies

In the '80s, two studies of vegan children who lived on The Farm, a strict vegetarian commune near Summertown, Tennessee, were reported in the scientific literature.[26,39] With the exception of margarine, white sugar, infant cereal, and yeast, all foods consumed by the commune members was produced on The Farm. This all-plant diet was, however, supplemented with vitamin B_{12} after significant problems were found.

Forty-eight 2- to 5-year-old children were subjects of the first study.[39] The sample is assumed to be random. The summarized results of anthropometry can be cited as follows:

- Mean height for all age and sex groups was below national standards; of the 28 boys, five were above the 50th percentile; four were on or below the 10th percentile. All but two of the 2- and 3-year-old girls were below the 50th percentile. In interpreting these data on height it should be noted that since no measurement of the parents' stature was made, hereditary effects have not been accounted for.
- The 2-year-old girls were the only group that exceeded the average weight standards; 15 boys were above the 50th percentile for weight; and three were on or below the 10th percentile; among the girls, nine were above the 50th percentile and only two were below the 10th percentile for weight. Unfortunately, no weight-for-height relationship was calculated and therefore it is difficult to evaluate weight as such.
- Except for the values of the 4- and 5-year-old girls, mean values for triceps skinfold met or exceeded standards; the 5-year-old girls were below the standards for subscapular skinfold.
- The 4- and 5-year-old girls' arm circumference values were below standards. Moreover, arm muscle circumference of the 4-year-old boys and girls failed to meet standards, whereas mean values of the 5-year-old girls' arm muscle circumference were greater than standards.

Overall, this study provides a lot of interesting data, but the interpretation is difficult, if not impossible, because of the absence of uniform deviations and the lack of statistical inference.

A much larger study of 404 vegan children aged 4 months to 10 years in this community of plant-food eaters was conducted by researchers from the Centers for Disease Control (CDC) and The Farm.[26] Eighty-three percent of these children had been vegans after weaning, eating no animal products at all. The results of this study show that most of the height, weight, and weight-for-height data were within the 25th and 75th percentiles of the national standards. The mean height and weight, however, were slightly less than the reference median. For the different age groups, the mean height ranged from 0.2 to 2.1 cm less and the mean weight ranged from 0.1 to 1.1 kg less than the reference median. The largest height difference was observed at 1 to 3 years of age. By 10 years of age, the children averaged 0.7 cm and 1.1 kg less than the corresponding reference median. The authors consequently concluded that these children have adequately attained normal growth status, even though it was slightly less than that of the reference population. Again, also in this study, no adjustment was made for parental height and socio-economic level.

b. The U.K. Vegan Studies

Three consecutive studies by Sanders et al.[20,40,41] on growth and development of lifelong vegan children have been reported. The first study[40] consisted of a small sample of 23 vegan children (8 boys and 15 girls) aged 1 to 5 years from 17 vegan families. The main outcome of this cross-sectional study is that all children's birth weights (mean = 3.23 kg, s.e. = 0.87) fell inside the normal range; the weights for age were also inside the normal range but were generally below the 50th percentile, with five children below the 10th percentile; the heights for age were inside the normal range, except for a brother and sister whose parents were of small stature; there were more children below the 50th percentile than above. The weight-for-height relationship was within the normal range for all children, except for one girl, aged 18 months, who was on the limit for weight (P3); this child had experienced feeding difficulties owing to a series of allergic reactions. No child had a midarm circumference indicating malnutrition. Head circumferences were normal compared with reference standards and there were more values above than below the 50th percentile.

Based on these findings, the authors concluded that the growth of these lifelong vegan preschool children, with the exception of the one girl, was normal.

In 1988, Sanders et al.[20] reported on a longitudinal survey of three cohorts of lifelong vegan children (the exact number of children followed is not given; the numbers of dots plotted on the growth charts vary between 34 and 42; reference is made, however, to the 1981 survey of 23 vegan children). Heights, weights, and head and chest circumferences were inside the normal range, except for the one 13-month-old girl who was suffering from an allergic disorder (see above). Interestingly, on resurveying at age 8, the girl had caught up in height and weight (P75). Generally, the girls tended to be below the 50th percentile for weight and the boys tended to be below the 50th percentile for both height and weight.

In a third study, 20 vegan children aged 5.8 to 12.8 years were recruited from two earlier cohorts and anthropometrically examined.[41] Again, the growth and development of these lifelong vegan children were normal and their heights and weights were inside the normal range. However, there was a tendency to be lighter in weight than the standards. They were all very lean, as reflected also in their low skinfold thicknesses. It must be noted that all of the children had been breast-fed on average for 15.5 months (range: 3 months–8 years). Only three children out of the 20 received complementary feeding of a cow's-milk infant formula at 1 week, 2 years, and 5 years respectively. With regard to dental health, 19 children were registered with a dentist and 18 of these visited regularly. Compared with a reference index, the number of missing teeth, decayed teeth, and dental fillings was low (DMF index 1.2, S.E. 0.38). These latter findings corroborate the results of earlier studies on SDA children and adolescents (6–17 years old) showing lower caries prevalence in comparison with non-SDA school children living in the same area.[42-44] In two of these studies on dental health, reference is made to the Adventist educational programs emphasizing the reduction of refined carbohydrates in their diet and discouraging the excessive use of sweets and snacking between meals. This suggests that this life-style may lead to a lower prevalence of dental caries.[42,44]

From both The Farm studies and the U.K. studies on lifelong vegans, it appears that infants, children, and adolescents reared on a varied and well-planned vegan diet obtain adequate nutrients and energy to grow and develop normally. Although they tend to be leaner than omnivore children, they are within the normal ranges of the standards for height and weight. The finding that vegan infants grow more slowly and are leaner than omnivore children is probably due to the fact that vegan women tend to breast-feed their children for much longer than their average omnivorous counterparts. This slower weight increase during growth periods may be related to the factors that regulate the susceptibility to some diseases in later life.[45,46]

3. Macrobiotic Children

a. The Boston Studies (Vegetarian and Macrobiotic)

In these growth studies of preschool children, distinction was initially made between macrobiotic and non-macrobiotic vegetarians.[6] Growth (weight and length) of non-macrobiotic vegetarian children (n = 72) under 2 years of age was depressed, while boys over the age of 2 exhibited catch-up growth in weight. Moreover, macrobiotics showed significantly higher weight velocities over 2 year of age than non-macrobiotic vegetarians. The mean weight and length velocities of the macrobiotic children were not significantly different from those of the non-macrobiotics before age 2.

In a subsequent publication, Dwyer et al.[7] classified vegetarian children's diets as "extensive" with respect to avoidance of animal foods if three or more types were avoided, and as "limited" animal-food avoidance if fewer than three groups of animal foods were avoided (*sic*). Since very young infants were most often fed breast milk, all food-avoidance patterns of subjects under 6 months of age were treated separately. The results showed that more than half of subjects under 6 months of age (n = 18) — all of whom were breast fed — reached or exceeded the 50th percentiles for weight, length, and triceps skinfold, while more than half of the subjects from 6 to 17 months (n = 27) had measurements under the 50th percentiles for the same parameters. Over half of the children 18 months and over (n = 74) also had weight, length, and triceps skinfold measurements under the 50th percentiles of the standards. Head circumferences conformed closely to expected values for both vegetarian and non-vegetarian infants, except for one vegetarian whose head circumference was far below (<2sd) the mean. With regard to adherence to the type of diet, the data suggest that the non-breast-fed older macrobiotic infants fed on an extensive animal-food-avoidance diet were the smallest and leanest of all subjects. Forty-five percent (n = 22) of these subjects were extremely lean (< 3rd percentile for triceps skinfold). Taking into account parental height, the smaller subjects still fell below the 10th percentile in more than half of the vegetarian infants (87% of these being macrobiotics).

In a relatively small sample (n = 39) of preschool children who consumed different types of vegetarian diets, Dwyer et al.[9] found that, as a group, vegetarian children (0.8 to 8.4 years) were shorter, even when adjusted for parental height, and lighter than national standards. Bone age was determined on 20 (75%) of the macrobiotic children and mean bone age was 43.2 months, while mean chronological age was 51.7 months. The authors concluded that in a quarter (n = 5) of the macrobiotic subjects retarded skeletal age was present, while the majority (n = 14) of these subjects were within the normal range, and one was advanced in skeletal age. The pertinent question that arises relates to how far results from these small samples can be generalized. The authors themselves are aware of these limitations, stating that, unfortunately, it was not possible to match vegetarian and non-vegetarian children or subgroups of vegetarian children for age and sex, so that firm conclusions on anthropometric findings cannot be drawn. Also, the significance of retarded bone age among macrobiotic children is weakened by the absence of data for other groups of vegetarians, who may have been retarded in this parameter.[9]

In 1983, Dwyer et al.[10] reported the results from a larger sample of 142 vegetarian children ranging from a few weeks to 6 years. It should be noted that the children were classified according to the extent of animal-food restriction in their diet, but this time, the investigators set the limits for categorizing the subjects on the avoidance of four or more, or fewer than four of the five animal food groups, respectively labeled as "extensive" and "limited." The authors did not explain why the limits of animal food avoidance had been moved from three (cf. their previous study) to four (present study).

Length and weight measurements were fitted to growth curves using the Jenss-Bayley curve fitting techniques. The growth curves of vegetarian children were from 0.5 to 1.0 kg and 1 to 2 cm lower than curves for reference populations. Moreover, macrobiotic children's growth curves for length and weight were more depressed than those of other vegetarian children. Differences in growth curves were most pronounced after weaning and most apparent among macrobiotics who breast-fed their infants the longest. The latter finding once more indicates that there is a good deal of heterogeneity in growth velocity within vegetarians that is related to the type of vegetarian diet consumed.

b. Dutch Children on Alternative Diets

In a preliminary study, length and weight of 92 children aged 1 to 3 years raised on alternative diets (33 vegetarian, 26 anthroposophic, and 33 macrobiotic*) were compared with a control group of 50 omnivore children.[11] The children fed vegetarian and anthroposophic diets were somewhat lighter and smaller than their omnivore counterparts, but their measurements were within normal ranges. However, the macrobiotic children were significantly ($p < .05$) lower in weight and shorter in length than the control group, while the weight-for-height relationship was within the normal range.

In 1988, van Staveren et al.[12] published a review of four studies with children on the three alternative diets (ecological, anthroposophic, macrobiotic). They confirmed that growth (height and weight) in macrobiotic children (8 months–8 years; n = 300) was stunted, especially after 5 months of age. In contrast to a study by Dwyer,[10] there was no indication

---

* It is appropriate to note that in this study the criteria for grouping children on alternative diets is different from the usual classification with respect to vegetarian diets. For instance, children were classified as vegetarian if they "eat meat or poultry less than twice a week" (*sic*); "the anthroposophic diet is not vegetarian by principle, but in practice products of dead animals are seldom used"; the macrobiotic diet" approximates a vegan-like food pattern, with virtually no animal food consumed after an infant has been weaned from the breast," The latter statement is contradicted by the fact that the authors reported that, in 32 macrobiotic children, one consumed meat, fish and sea foods, eggs and diary products, six excluded meat and meat products, seven excluded meat and fish, nine excluded meat, fish and eggs, and nine excluded meat, fish and seafoods, eggs and dairy products from their diet.[47]

of catch-up growth. Interesting to note is the fact that, in a selected subsample (n = 43; age 4–6 years), intelligence was tested and showed no abnormal mental development among the group of macrobiotic children.

The same year, Dagnelie et al.[47] reported the results of a cross-sectional study on 243 lifetime macrobiotic children (aged 0 to 8 years). Birth weight was 150 g lower than the Dutch reference standards, and was positively related to the consumption frequency of fish and dairy products. From 6 to 8 months, a marked decline for weight, height, and arm circumference was observed in comparison with the reference curves; this depression was more marked in girls than in boys. A minimum level of 1 to 1.5 standard deviations below the 50th percentile of the reference was reached at the age of 18 months. Between 2 and 4 years, a partial catching-up toward the 50th percentile occurred for arm circumference and, in boys only, for weight and triceps skinfold, but not for height.

In a mixed longitudinal growth study on 53 macrobiotic infants (4 to 18 months) compared with a matched control group, Dagnelie et al.[24] cited the following outcome. Between 4 and 18 months of age, mean values for all anthropometric parameters were significantly lower in the macrobiotic subjects. In macrobiotic infants from birth to 4 months, weight gain was less than that in the control group. The growth rate in weight, length, and arm circumference was lowest between 8 and 14 months of age. During the same growth period, increase in arm muscle mass was only half that of the control group. From 14 months of age, growth stabilized at the 10th percentile of the Dutch norms. The authors expressed the opinion that both the low energy and protein content of the macrobiotic weaning diet were responsible for the observed growth decline after 6 months of age, and concluded that growth and development were far below optimal in this macrobiotic cohort. In fact, the macrobiotic group was significantly retarded in gross motor (not in fine motor) development, and, to a lesser degree, in speech and language development. However, the retardation in gross motor and language development was only temporary and in tests at the ages of 4 to 6 years no apparent delay in mental development was shown.

After a more profound analysis of the potential deficiencies in macrobiotic nutrition for infants, Dagnelie and van Staveren[48] attributed the observed differences in growth and development between the macrobiotic and omnivorous groups to differences in diet, thus corroborating the results of the Boston investigators,[6-10] who also observed multiple nutrient deficiencies in the macrobiotic infants studied. Subsequently, the authors made practical recommendations for improving the macrobiotic diet for infants and children in order to remediate the observed delay in growth and development.

The findings from both the Boston and Dutch studies clearly show that growth and development in children on macrobiotic diets is delayed and catching-up of growth is not always self evident unless certain adaptations in the macrobiotic diet are made to render it nutritionally adequate.

IV. SUMMARY AND CONCLUSIONS

This chapter reviewed the multiple studies on growth and development of children and adolescents on various vegetarian diets. Case studies of malnutrition in children on various alternative diets have not been discussed, because it is evident that these are incidental and do not necessarily represent ubiquitous nutritional deficiencies in these various types of vegetarian populations.

To ensure a practical approach based on type of diet, the multiple investigations on vegetarian children have been assembled in three groups of studies, i.e., Seventh-Day Adventist children, studies on vegan children, and studies on macrobiotic children.

SDA vegetarian children are generally lacto-ovo-vegetarians or lacto-vegetarians and the results of these studies show no marked differences in physical growth and development when compared with standard references or with non-vegetarian SDA children. We can therefore conclude that a lacto-(ovo)-vegetarian diet generally results in normal growth.

Of course, as Dwyer et al.[49] also pointed out, the patterns of animal food avoidance in vegetarians may vary considerably from group to group. This is true within a particular category of vegetarians, such as lacto-ovo-vegetarians, as well as between the different types. A pure vegetarian or vegan diet does not seem to preclude optimal growth and development, provided a well-planned and balanced plant-based diet is followed with appropriate supplements of fortified foods. Even with careful balance, both the parents and the physician should be aware that growth might be slower than expected. This, however, does not mean that this slow growth can be equated per se with poor health.

A macrobiotic diet is far more restrictive than a lacto-ovo-vegetarian, or even a vegan diet, particularly when the most desirable degree of macrobiotic regimen is followed. The most severe cases of malnutrition among infants following unconventional dietary practices seem to have been associated with macrobiotics.[14] The macrobiotic studies cited in the present review confirm potential nutritional problems with regard to growth and development of infants and children fed on a macrobiotic diet. It seems unlikely, in contrast to vegetarianism, that children raised on a higher level of macrobiotic regimen can thrive well.

REFERENCES

1. Growing interest in vegetarianism among campus food services. *J. Am. Diet. Assoc.*, 94: 596, 1994.
2. The Realeat Survey 1984-1995. *Realeat*, London, 1995.
3. Vegetarian Society U.K. Trends in vegetarianism among adults and young people, Vegetarian Society. Altrincham (U.K.), 1991.
4. Psyma Onderzoeksbureau, *Onderzoeksverslag over vegetariërs* (Research report on vegetarians), The Netherlands, 1989.
5. Jacobs, C. and Dwyer, J. T. Vegetarian children: appropriate and inappropriate diets. *Am. J. Clin. Nutr.*, 48: 811, 1988.
6. Shull, M. W., Reed, R. B., Valadian, I., Palombo, R., Thorne, H., and Dwyer, J. T. Velocities of growth in vegetarian preschool children. *Pediatrics*, 60: 410, 1977.
7. Dwyer, J. T., Palombo, R., Thorne, H., Valadian, I., and Reed, R. B. Preschoolers on alternate life-style diet. *J. Am. Diet. Assoc.*, 72: 264, 1978.
8. Dwyer, J., Andrew, E. M., Valadian, I., and Reed, R. B. Size, obesity, and leanness in vegetarian preschool children. *J. Am. Diet. Assoc.*, 77: 434, 1980.
9. Dwyer, J. T., Dietz, W. H., Andrews, E. M., and Suskind, R. M. Nutritional status of vegetarian children. *Am. J. Clin. Nutr.*, 35: 204, 1982.
10. Dwyer, J. T., Andrews, E. M., Berkey, C., Valadian, I., and Reed, R. B. Growth in new vegetarian preschool children using the Jenss-Bayley curve fitting technique. *Am. J. Clin. Nutr.*, 37: 815, 1983.
11. van Staveren, W. A., Dhuyvetter, J. H. M., Bons, A., Zeelen, M., and Hautvast, G. A. J. Food consumption and height/weight status of Dutch preschool children on alternative diets. *J. Am. Diet. Assoc.*, 85: 1579, 1985.
12. van Staveren, W. A., and Dagnelie, P. C. Food consumption, growth, and development of Dutch children fed on alternative diets. *Am. J. Clin. Nutr.*, 48: 819, 1988.
13. van 't Hof, M.A., Roede, M. J., and Kowalski, C. J. A mixed longitudinal data analysis model. *Hum. Biol.*, 49: 165, 1977.
14. MacLean, W. C., and Graham, G. G. Vegetarianism in children. *Am. J. Dis. Child*, 134: 513, 1980.
15. Langley, G. *Vegan Nutrition*. The Vegan Society, St. Leonards-on-Sea (U.K.), 1991, 14.
16. Sanders, T. A. B. and Reddy, S. Vegetarian diets and children. *Am. J. Clin. Nutr.*, 59 (suppl): 1176S, 1994.
17. Dagnelie, P. C., Vergote, F. J., van Staveren, W. A., van den Berg, H., Dingjan, P. G., and Hautvast, J. G. A. J. High prevalence of rickets in infants on macrobiotic diets. *Am. J. Clin. Nutr.*, 51: 202, 1990.
18. Roberts, I. F., West, R. J., Ogilvie, D., and Dillon, M. J. Malnutrition in infants receiving cult diets: a form of child abuse. *Brit. Med. J.*, 1: 296, 1979.
19. Hardinge, M. G. and Store, F. J. Nutritional studies of vegetarians: Nutritional, physical, and laboratory studies. *Am. J. Clin. Nutr.*, 2: 73, 1954.
20. Sanders, T. A. B. Growth and development of British vegan children. *Am. J. Clin. Nutr.*, 48: 822, 1988.
21. Sabaté, J., Lindsted, K. D., Harris, R. D., and Johnston, P. K. Anthropometric parameters of schoolchildren with different life-styles. *Am. J. Dis. Child.*, 144: 1159, 1990.

22. Sabaté, J., Lindsted, K. D., Harris, R. D., and Sanchez, A. Attained height of lacto-ovo vegetarian children and adolescents. *Eur. J. Clin. Nutr.*, 45: 51, 1997.

23. Hebbelinck, M., Clarys, P., and De Malsche, A. Growth, development and physical fitness characteristics of Flemish vegetarian children, adolescents and young adults. *Am. J. Clin. Nutr.*, 70: 3(suppl), 579S, 1999.

24. Dagnelie, P.C., van Staveren, W. A., Vergote, F. J., Burema, J., van't Hof, M.A., van Klaveren, J.D., and Hautvast, J.G.A.J. Growth and psychomotor development in infants aged 4 to 18 months on macrobiotic and omnivorous diets: a mixed-longitudinal study. *Eur. J. Clin. Nutr.*, 43: 325, 1989.

25. Sabaté, J., Llorca, M. C., and Sanchez, A. Lower height of lacto-ovo-vegetarian girls at preadolescence: an indicator of physical maturation delay? *J. Am. Diet. Assoc.*, 1263: 1992.

26. O'Connell, J. M., Dibley, M. J., Sierra, J., Wallace, B., Marks, J. S., and Yip, R. Growth of vegetarian children: The Farm study. *Pediatr.*, 84: 475, 1989.

27. Nathan, I., Hackett, A. F., and Kirby, S. A longitudinal study of the growth of matched pairs of vegetarian and omnivorous children, aged 7-11 years, in the Northwest of England. *Eur. J. Clin. Nutr.*, 51: 20, 1997.

28. Tayter, M. and Stanek, K. L. Anthropometric and dietary assessment of omnivore and lacto-ovo-vegetarian children. *J. Am. Diet. Assoc.*, 89: 1661, 1989.

29. Freeland-Graves, J. H., Greninger, S. A., Graves, G. R., and Young, R. K. Health practices, attitudes, and beliefs of vegetarians and non-vegetarians. *J. Am. Diet. Assoc.*, 86: 913, 1986.

30. Slonacker, J. R. *The Effects of a Strictly Vegetable Diet on the Spontaneous Activity, the Rate of Growth, and the Longevity of the Albino Rat.* Stanford University Publications, Stanford (CA), 1912.

31. Tanner, J. M. *Fetus into Man: Physical Growth from Conception to Maturity.* Harvard University Press, Cambridge, Massachusetts, 1990.

32. Sanchez, A., Kissinger, D. G., and Phillips, R. J. A hypothesis on the etiological role of diet on age of menarche. *Med. Hypotheses*, 7: 139, 1981.

33. Kissinger, D. G. and Sanchez, A. The association of dietary factors with the age of menarche. *Nutr. Res.*, 7: 471, 1987.

34. Miller, A. B. and Bulbrook, R. O. The epidemiology and etiology of breast cancer. *New Engl. J. Med.*, 303: 1246, 1980.

35. Kelsey, J. L. and Hildreth, N. G. *Breast and Gynecological Cancer Epidemiology.* CRC, Boca Raton, 1983.

36. De Waard, F., and Trichopoulos, D.A. A unifying concept of the aetiology of breast cancer. *Int. J. Cancer*, 41: 666, 1988.

37. Rona, R.J., Chinn, S., Dugal, S., and Driver, P. Vegetarianism in Urdu, Gujarati, and Punjabi children in Britain. *J. Epid. Commun. Health*, 41: 233, 1987.

38. Hebert, J. R. Relationship of vegetarianism to child growth in South India. *Am. J. Clin. Nutr.*, 42: 1246, 1985.

39. Fulton, J. R., Hutton, C. W., and Stitt, K. R. Preschool vegetarian children. *J. Am. Diet. Assoc.*, 76: 360, 1980.

40. Sanders, T.A.B. and Purves, R. An anthropometric and dietary assessment of the nutritional status of vegan preschool children. *J. Hum. Nutr.*, 35: 349, 1981.

41. Sanders, T.A.B. and Manning, J. The growth and development of vegan children. *J. Hum. Nutr. Diet.*, 5: 11, 1992.

42. Downs, R.A., Dunn, M.M., and Richie, E.L. Report of dental findings of Seventh Day Adventist students. *Bull. Am. Assoc. Pub. Health Dent.*, 18: 19, 1958.

43 Donnelly, C. J. Comparative study of caries experience in Adventist and other children. *Publ. Hlth. Reports*, 76: 209, 1961.

44. Glass, R. L. and Hayden, J. Dental caries in Seventh-Day Adventist children. *J. Dent. Child.*, 33: 22, 1966.

45. Ross, M. H. Nutrition, disease and length of life, in *Diet and Bodily Constitution*, CIBA Foundation, Study Group No. 17, Wolstenholme, G.E.W. and O'Connor, M., Eds., J.&A. Churchill, London, 1964, 90.

46. Ross, M. H., Lustbader, E., and Bras, G. Dietary practices and growth responses as predictors of longevity. *Nature (London)*, 262: 548, 1976.

47. Dagnelie, P. C., van Staveren, W. A., Klaveren, J. D., and Burema, J. Do children on macrobiotic diets show catch-up growth? *Eur. J. Clin. Nutr.*, 42: 1007, 1988.

48. Dagnelie, P. C. and van Staveren, W. A. Macrobiotic nutrition and child health: results of a population-based, mixed-longitudinal cohort study in the Netherlands. *Am. J. Clin. Nutr.*, 59 (suppl): 1187S, 1994.

49. Dwyer, J.T., Mayer, L.D.V.H., Dowd, K., Kandel, R.F., and Mayer, J. The new vegetarians: The natural high? *J. Am. Diet. Assoc.*, 65: 529, 1974.

9

VEGETARIAN DIETS IN PREGNANCY AND LACTATION

Patricia K. Johnston

CONTENTS

0-8493-8508-3/01/$0.00+$.50
© 2001 by CRC Press LLC

I.   INTRODUCTION

Pregnancy and lactation are recognized as times of increased nutritional vulnerability with implications for both the mother and her offspring. Few studies have undertaken comprehensive evaluations of vegetarians during these important times in the lifecycle. The growing interest in and adoption of vegetarian* diets, especially by young women, necessitate a careful assessment of their adequacy, particularly during pregnancy and lactation. In addition, the heightened awareness of the long term implications of maternal dietary practices and nutritional intake adds impetus to this concern.[1] The purpose of this chapter is not to provide a comprehensive discussion of nutrition during pregnancy and lactation, but to address the issues of particular relevance to the pregnant or lactating vegetarian.

II.   DIETARY PATTERN AND PREGNANCY OUTCOME

The first comprehensive study of pregnant vegetarians, including dietary intake, nutritional status and health history, was reported by Hardinge et al. in 1954.[2] Although vegans were included in the larger study of which this was a part, none was pregnant; consequently, comparisons were made between lacto-ovo-vegetarians (LOVs) and omnivores. There was no difference in height, weight, or weight gained during pregnancy and there were no serious delivery complications in either group. Birth weights and lengths were not significantly different.

    Nearly 20 years passed before Thomas and Ellis compared pregnancy outcome in 14 vegans (28 pregnancies) with 18 controls (41 pregnancies) in England.[3] There were no significant differences in live births, still births, toxemia of pregnancy, or infant birth weight. More recently, a tendency toward lower birth weight in term infants was reported in British vegans.[4]

---

* "Vegetarian" as used in this chapter includes all types of vegetarian diets that may or may not include animal products. LOV refers to lacto-ovo-vegetarian diets, which include milk, dairy products, and eggs. Vegan refers to diets that exclude all animal products. Macrobiotic diets emphasize whole grains—especially brown rice—sea vegetables, legumes and other vegetables. If included, fruit is locally grown; dairy products and meat are not recommended; limited amounts of white fish may be included.

Vegetarian diets have long been practiced in the U.K., which remains a fruitful source for studies of vegetarians. A comprehensive evaluation of nutrient intake and pregnancy outcome in British LOVs was recently reported.[5] No differences were found among the LOVs, fish-eaters, and non-vegetarians in length of gestation, birth weight, birth length, or head circumference. Others reported no difference in birth weight among LOVs in the U.S. compared with omnivores.[6,7]

Other studies in England reported lower birth weight in infants born to Hindu vegetarian women compared with infants born to Muslim or European women.[8,9] This difference remained even after adjusting for a variety of factors, including gestational age, sex of infant, parity, smoking, maternal age and height.[9]

Dagnelie et al. reported that the proportion of low birth weight among Dutch macrobiotics was more than twice the proportion found in the general population in the Netherlands.[10] After excluding those with low birth weight, the mean birth weight in the remaining macrobiotic infants was ~200g lower than the Dutch reference.[11] The authors found a strong positive relationship between birth weight and the frequency of consumption of dairy products and fish.[10] Adjusted birth weight was 350g greater in families consuming dairy products three or more times per week compared with families consuming them less than once per month. If fish was consumed at least once per week, adjusted birth weight was 180g greater than in families consuming fish less than once per month. No significant relationship was found between birth weight and the length of time a macrobiotic diet had been followed, and the authors concluded that the composition of the diet during rather than before pregnancy was the important factor in determining birth weight.[10] They further noted that the high educational level of the macrobiotic parents would have been expected to result in higher rather than lower average birth weights. Studies in the U.S. have also reported lower birth weight among macrobiotics.[12,13] The birth weight of vegetarians in general was similar to reference values, however, more than half the infants with birth weights ≤2500 gm were restrictive macrobiotics.[13] Another small study found that infants of vegetarians weighed about 200 gm more than infants of omnivores even though the vegetarians had gained about 2 kg less.[6] None of the 11 vegetarian infants weighed <3 kg, whereas two of six omnivore infants weighed about 2.75 kg.

The lower birth weights in some vegetarian populations is thought, with considerable certainty, to be due to diet; however, the precise nutritional factors remain to be clarified.[14] Essential fatty acid status was investigated, but the researchers were unable to demonstrate a significant relationship to birth weight in the population under study.[4] Inadequate status of iron, folate, or vitamin B_{12} have been suggested as possible factors.[15] Nonetheless, energy intake is thought to play the major role in low birth weight.[14]

The significance of the slightly lower birth weight found in some infants of vegetarians is not known; however, attention has been called to the evidence that lower birth weight may be associated with long term consequences and increased risk of developing chronic disease later in life.[1,15] Attention should be given to assuring that all pregnant vegetarians understand the importance of optimizing their dietary intake during pregnancy.

III. ENERGY INTAKE

Vegetarians may be similar in weight to the general populace or weigh somewhat less.[16] This is particularly true of vegans, who may weigh as much as 10–20% less than omnivores or LOVs.[2,17] This may, in part, be due to dietary factors such as the higher intake of plant foods, which contain much more fiber and are usually less energy dense than animal food products, as well as the somewhat lower fat intake. Thus, some vegetarians may enter pregnancy at a lower weight for height and may need more careful monitoring of weight status. Birth weight among macrobiotic infants was positively associated with maternal weight gain in pregnancy, as it was in the recent study of LOVs.[5,18]

Although studies have reported birth weight of infants born to vegetarians, little is known about maternal energy intake and gestational weight gain in such populations. Energy intake was reported to be low in Hindu vegetarian women; however, there was no evidence that it was lower than in Muslim women.[14] Weight gain was not reported. The lower birth weight in macrobiotic infants has been related to lower energy intake and weight gain during pregnancy, as well as to specific foods.[10,18,19] Energy intake in LOVs during pregnancy has been reported to be similar to, greater, or less than omnivores.[2,5,6] One study of vegan women in the U.S. found weight gain somewhat greater than the reference population.[20] The vegan women entered pregnancy 10 pounds less than the reference population, but there was no difference in birth weight.

The limited available data suggest that energy intake and weight gain among vegetarians are quite variable. Those following more restrictive diets are at greater risk of inadequate energy intake. More concentrated energy sources may need to be consumed by some vegetarians during pregnancy than are found in their usual diets. This is especially true if the woman enters pregnancy at a lower weight for height. Pregnant vegetarians should strive to achieve an adequate intake of all nutrients, including enough energy to support an appropriate weight gain.

IV. NUTRIENT ISSUES

Well-planned vegetarian diets can meet the energy and nutrient needs of pregnancy and lactation.[21] If, however, a diet becomes limited in the kinds or amounts of foods that are consumed, there is greater risk for inadequacy — and the greater the restriction, the greater the risk. Because the increase in need for nutrients during pregnancy is greater than the increase in need for energy, care must be taken to choose nutrient-rich foods to meet energy needs.

A. Protein

The need for protein in pregnancy increases about 20%, to 60 gm per day, to support the maternal and fetal tissue growth and blood volume expansion. The recommended protein intake in pregnant or lactating LOV women is readily achieved.[6,22] Protein intake is generally lower in vegans compared with either LOVs or omnivores, both in total amount consumed and as a percentage of total calories.[16] Further, it is entirely from plant sources. However, a well-planned vegan diet can be adequate in protein and supply all the essential amino acids needed during pregnancy and lactation.[21]

Adequacy of protein intake does become a concern when energy intake is compromised or when there is a major reliance on fruits with minimal intake of grains and legumes. When intake from carbohydrates and fats does not meet energy needs, a portion of the protein will be used to meet those needs and therefore will be unavailable for tissue synthesis. Increasing energy intake will spare the protein for its intended use.

The requirement for protein is really a requirement for essential amino acids as well as nonspecific nitrogen to support the synthesis of other important nitrogen-containing compounds.[23] The contribution that a given food makes to the body's protein needs depends on the concentration and availability of the essential amino acids and nitrogen it contains in relation to the physiologic requirements.[23] Amino acid scores are one way of evaluating the protein adequacy of a given food. The amino acid score compares the concentration of the limiting amino acid in a given food with the concentration of that same amino acid in a reference pattern.[23]

The concept of complementary proteins arose from the recognition that different plant foods contain different limiting amino acids. An amino acid that is low in one food can be "complemented" by that same amino acid from another food. In general, lysine is the limiting amino acid in cereals, nuts, and seeds; the sulfur-containing amino acids are limiting in legumes. Combinations of cereals and legumes can supply all the essential amino acids and increase the protein quality over either food alone because one type contains generous amounts of the amino acid that is limiting in the other.

At one time, it was thought necessary to eat the foods supplying the complementary amino acids within one meal. It is now recognized that this is not necessary; they may be eaten over the course of the day.[23] The one exception to this is young children and infants, who may need to consume the complementary proteins within a shorter period of time. Young provides a discussion of the physiologic support for these conclusions.[23]

Vegetarian diets, particularly those that include no animal products, should include regular consumption of legumes (dried peas and beans). Soybeans are an especially rich plant source of amino acids, as well as other essential nutrients, and may be consumed in various forms. These include cooked dried or green soybeans, tofu, tempeh, soy milk, and commercial meat analogs. A variety of whole-grain products, vegetables, nuts, seeds, and nut butters, as well as milk, dairy products, and eggs — for those who use them – contribute to meeting protein needs.

B. Essential Fatty Acids

Linoleic (18:2n-6) and α-linolenic (18:3n-3) acid give rise to the two series of essential fatty acids and their metabolites. The parent fatty acids are primarily supplied by plant foods; however, they each undergo elongation and desaturation in human as well as animal tissues to produce long-chain polyunsaturated fatty acids (LCP).[24] Linoleic acid is metabolized to arachidonic acid (20:4n-6, AA); the chief end product of α-linolenic acid is docosahexaenoic acid (22:6n3, DHA). The two classes of essential fatty acids compete for the desaturase enzymes that are necessary to produce the LCP.[25]

Although humans can make DHA from a-linolenic acid, high intakes of linoleic acid interfere with that conversion, as do trans fatty acids.[24] Thus, diets that are high in processed foods or vegetable oils, such as corn, safflower, and sunflower, can inhibit the production of DHA. Further, diets that are very low in fat may not supply enough α-linolenic acid.

1. Fatty Acids in Vegetarian Diets

Vegetarian diets may include fewer trans fatty acid-containing processed foods; however, when compared with omnivorous diets, they typically contain higher amounts of vegetable oils containing the n-6 fatty acids. This is especially true of vegan diets. The amount of n-3 fatty acids in vegetarian diets strongly depends on the type of cooking oil used and is generally similar to or slightly greater than the amount found in omnivorous diets.[24] Preformed DHA is absent from vegan diets and absent or low in other vegetarian diets, depending primarily on the inclusion of egg yolks, which contain small amounts. Thus, the ratio of n-6 to n-3 fatty acids is generally higher in vegetarian diets, especially those that exclude all animal products.[24]

2. Essential Fatty Acids in Pregnant Vegetarians and Their Newborns

AA and DHA are selectively transported by the placenta to the fetus during the last trimester of pregnancy. They accumulate in the fetal brain and retina and this continues during the first months of life. Evidence suggests that, although the fetus and newborn have the ability to form DHA from its precursor, that ability is limited.[26] Therefore, a dietary supply may be of particular importance.[26] This is particularly true of preterm infants.[24]

Reddy et al. compared the essential fatty acid status of infants born to vegetarian women with that of infants born to omnivores.[9] The vegetarian women consumed a greater proportion of energy as linoleic acid and had a higher dietary ratio of 18:2n-6 to 18:3n-3. They consumed no preformed DHA. The proportion of DHA was about 30% lower in cord plasma and artery phospholipids in the vegetarians.[15] Others demonstrated increased levels of DHA in plasma and red blood cells in newborns of women who were supplemented with n-3 fatty acids during the last trimester of pregnancy.[27] The amount of DHA in the infants' plasma and red blood cells was related to the amount consumed by the mother. This suggests that maternal dietary intake during pregnancy can affect the DHA status of the newborn. The difference in the proportion of DHA found in vegetarians was suggested to reflect the lack of preformed DHA in the diet, high intakes of 18:2n-6, and the limited capacity to synthesize DHA.[9]

3. Breast-Fed Infants and Essential Fatty Acids in Human Milk

DHA is found in human milk, but the amount varies by dietary pattern and it can be increased by maternal supplementation with DHA.[24,28,29] DHA in the milk of LOVs was not different from that of omnivores in Britain; it was nearly two-thirds less in the milk of vegans.[4,15] No difference was found among the three groups in the U.S.[30] It was suggested that this may be due to a greater consumption of α-linolenic acid from soybean oil in the U.S. or, in the case of macrobiotics, who may consume fish, of preformed DHA.[24]

Erythrocyte lipids of infants born to and breast-fed by vegan mothers had only one-third the proportion of DHA compared with infants who were breast-fed by omnivores.[4] The significance of these differences is not yet known. However, there is growing evidence that term infants receiving breast milk have higher levels of DHA and better neuronal functioning than infants fed commercial infant formulas, which in the U.S. do not yet include this fatty acid.[31-33] Some, but not all, studies show better visual function in infants fed breast milk or DHA-supplemented formula than in infants fed non-supplemented formula.[9,24,26,28,32] Others reported better problem solving ability in 10-month-old infants who were fed infant formula supplemented with DHA and AA than in infants receiving formula without these LCPs.[31] Problem solving scores at this age correlate with IQ and vocabulary scores at 3 years of age.

4. Implications for Vegetarians

Fat and fatty acid content of breast milk varies with dietary pattern.[22] The proportion of AA in blood, tissue lipids, and breast milk is similar in vegetarians, vegans, and omnivores.[24] Therefore, it appears that vegetarians can synthesize AA adequately and do not require it in their diet.[24] Infants breast-fed by vegetarian mothers should receive adequate amounts of this essential fatty acid.[24]

Researchers have concluded that both AA and DHA are necessary for the optimal development of the brain and eye.[26] Concern has been expressed for the lower proportion of DHA found in breast milk, as well as in blood and tissue lipids of vegans and vegetarians.[15,24] High intake of linoleic acid, as may be found in vegetarian diets, may interfere with the production of DHA due to the competition between n-6 and n-3 fatty acids for the desaturase enzymes. Because of this competition, it was suggested that there may be an optimal balance between n-3 and n-6 fatty acids for infant diets.[26]

Vegetarians should strive to achieve adequate but not excessive intakes of 18:2n-6 and 18:3n-3. The physiologic consequences of a deficiency or imbalance of the essential fatty acids have been described.[24,25,29] It is suggested that the ratio of linoleic acid to α-linolenic acid should be no more than 10:1 and preferably around 4:1.[24] Table 9.1 provides suggestions for achieving a balanced intake of the essential fatty acids.

C. Iron

Adequate iron intake is necessary in pregnancy to support the increase in maternal blood volume and provide for the growing fetus. There is currently debate regarding whether iron supplements are justified during pregnancy.[34] Data suggest that there is increased risk of prematurity and low birth weight if iron stores are low in the first trimester.[15,35] Although iron supplementation during lactation does not appear to increase the amount of iron in the breast milk, it can help to rebuild the maternal

Table 9.1   Guidelines to Achieve an Optimal Ratio of Essential Fatty Acids in the Diet

1. Do not overly restrict fat in the diet.
2. Consume a good source of α-linolenic acid every day.
3. Limit intake of foods very high in linoleic acid, such as safflower, sunflower, and corn oils.
4. Replace oils rich in linoleic acid with canola, soy, and flaxseed oils which are rich in α-linolenic acid and with monounsaturated-rich oils like olive oil.
5. Replace hard margarine with soft margarine and limit intake of processed foods.

stores. Regardless of dietary pattern, attention should be given to assuring an adequate intake of iron during these important periods.

Concern is frequently expressed regarding the iron status of vegetarians, particularly those who are pregnant. This may be because food sources in vegetarian diets provide the non-heme form of iron, which is less available than the heme form found in flesh foods. A recent review described various substances found in plant foods that can enhance or inhibit the absorption of non-heme iron.[36] Those that enhance iron uptake include ascorbic acid, and citric, malic, lactic, tartaric, and other organic acids. Fermentation products of soybeans also increase iron availability. Inhibitory substances include phytates, which are commonly found in whole grains, soy products, and bran, oxalates found in spinach and rhubarb, tannins in tea, polyphenols in coffee, and some plant foods. Eggs, milk, and high intakes of zinc or calcium may also inhibit iron availability.[36,37] A greater proportion of the iron will be absorbed when iron stores are low or when there is increased need, as in pregnancy.

1. Iron Intake in Vegetarian Females

Because iron status reflects long-term intake, it is appropriate to examine studies of vegetarian females as well as those who are pregnant. Compared with omnivores, female LOVs were reported in several studies to consume similar or greater amounts of dietary iron.[17,38–41] Vegans were reported to consume more iron than LOVs or omnivores, although this was not always the case and the differences were not always significant.[5,36,38,40,41] Vegetarians, especially vegans, also often consume more ascorbic acid, which improves the availability of non-heme iron.[5,17,39–41] However, intake of inhibitory substances, such as phytates, may also be greater in vegetarian, and especially vegan, diets.[42]

The few studies describing pregnant vegetarians reported that iron intake was similar to or greater than in pregnant omnivores.[2,5,6] Intake of ascorbic acid was significantly greater in the vegetarians.[2,5,6]

2. Iron Status in Vegetarian Females

Vegetarians generally do not have a greater incidence of iron deficiency anemia, although they do have lower iron stores.[36,38,43] Iron deficiency anemia has been reported in Asian vegetarians in the U.K. and North America, especially in those who rely on rice rather than wheat.[15]

In 14–19-year-old females in Canada, 29% of LOVs vs. 17% of omnivores had low iron stores as determined by plasma ferritin.[44] However, there were no significant differences in mean plasma ferritin values between the groups, nor were mean hemoglobin or hematocrit values different. The LOVs and omnivores consumed similar amounts of iron, but the LOVs consumed significantly more phytate. Others reported that vegetarian females had significantly lower mean serum ferritin concentration than omnivores, even though intake of iron was significantly greater in the vegetarians.[38] Similar proportions in both groups had low ferritin values. In England, both Caucasian and Asian vegetarian females of childbearing age had lower serum ferritin concentrations than omnivores.[43] Concern was expressed that the physiologic stress of pregnancy could induce iron deficiency anemia in those with low iron stores.[43,44]

3. Iron Status in Pregnant Vegetarians

Few studies have reported iron status in pregnant vegetarians. Hemoglobin and hematocrit values were similar in 26 pregnant LOVs and 28 omnivores; however, of the seven pregnant women with hemoglobin levels < 11g/dL, five were LOVs, and the only one with a value < 9g/dL was an LOV.[2] Although Thomas et al. reported anemia in 12.5% of 24 vegan pregnancies vs. 5.5% of the 36 control pregnancies, they stated this difference was not significant.[3] Only 21% of the vegans vs. 66% of the controls took iron supplements. In a recent study in England, 26% of 34 LOVs reported being told by a physician or midwife that they were anemic during pregnancy compared with only 11% of 81 omnivores.[5] This difference approached significance at p = 0.057. Caution was expressed because no data were available to validate these reports. Other studies of pregnant vegetarians did not report indices of iron status.

4. Recommendations for Iron Intake in Pregnancy

There appears to be an increased likelihood that iron stores may be low in vegetarian females, with those on more restricted diets at increased risk of Fe deficiency. It has been said that iron stores can vary over a wide range without any apparent impairment of body function.[36] Nonetheless, reduced iron stores are associated with increased risk of iron deficiency.[36,43]

Because of the increased demands of pregnancy and because low iron status in the first trimester may increase the risk for a low birth weight or premature infant, it is important to assure an adequate iron intake in pregnant vegetarians, as in all pregnant women. Further, it has been suggested that infants of women with low iron stores will be born with lower iron stores, and if they are breast-fed for a prolonged period of time, which is more likely to occur in vegetarians, they may be at greater risk of developing iron deficiency anemia.[15]

It should not be assumed that all pregnant vegetarians are at risk of iron deficiency. However, as in all pregnant women, it is appropriate to assess iron status. All pregnant women should be encouraged to follow a balanced diet that includes a generous intake of iron-rich foods, as well as concurrent ingestion of ascorbic acid-containing foods. This dietary advice is appropriate regardless of whether they take a daily supplement of 30 mg ferrous iron, which is often recommended during pregnancy.

D. Zinc

There are very few studies of zinc status in pregnant vegetarians. Thus, including selected results from studies of other vegetarians provides a context for evaluating the status in pregnancy. Some studies report that LOV females consume lower amounts of zinc than omnivores, while others report a similar intake in the two groups.[17,38,40,41,44] Zinc intake of vegans is often less than LOVs or omnivores.[17,38,40,41]

Freeland-Graves et al. reported that mean zinc intake in LOV females was less than two thirds the RDA and in vegans it was less than one third the RDA.[17] The very low intake of zinc in some subjects appeared to result from diets that consisted primarily of fruits, salads, and vegetables.[17] They found no significant differences in serum concentrations of zinc comparing both male and female vegetarians with omnivores, however, hair zinc was significantly less in the vegetarians. Serum zinc concentration was lower in vegan subjects than in LOVs and omnivores, but the difference was not significant. They also evaluated zinc in salivary sediment and found that it was significantly lower in both LOVs and vegans than in omnivores, with the amount in vegans about half that in omnivores.[17] They found an inverse relationship between salivary zinc and intake of crude fiber. The LOVs consumed twice as much, and the vegans four times as much crude fiber as the omnivores. The zinc status appeared to be further compromised, in addition to the low intake, by the high intake of crude fiber.

Zinc status was evaluated in young female vegetarians and omnivores.[44] No significant differences were found between the groups in zinc intake, zinc density of the diet, serum- or hair-zinc concentration, serum alkaline phosphatase concentration, or taste acuity. Inverse relationships were seen between the dietary phytate:zinc molar ratio and serum zinc concentrations.

Zinc intake in pregnant LOVs was significantly less than in pregnant omnivores in two studies, one in England and one in the U.S.[5,6] Zinc nutrient density was also lower in the LOVs, and their mean plasma zinc concentration was significantly less than the omnivores.[6] It was recently suggested that typical LOV diets probably contain 10–30% less zinc than omnivorous diets.[42] In addition to the lower zinc content of vegetarian diets, concern was expressed because of the lower zinc bioavailability due to the higher fiber and phytic acid content.[42] Low energy intake, poor food choices, and reliance on fruits and vegetables increase the risk for inadequate zinc intake.[17] Many foods consumed by vegetarians supply good amounts of zinc. These include legumes, soy products, whole grains, cereals, nuts, seeds, sprouts, brewer's yeast, and hard cheeses for LOVs.[45]

Vegetarians should be sure to include generous amounts of these foods on a regular basis to assure an adequate intake of zinc.

E. Calcium

Remarkable adaptations take place in calcium metabolism during pregnancy and lactation. In recognition of this, the most recent recommendations for calcium intake are age-dependent rather than pregnancy- or lactation-dependent.[46] That is, no increase in calcium intake is recommended beyond that for a given age. It is important to recognize, however, that the usual reported intake in women of childbearing age is below the recommendations.[47]

1. Calcium Intake in Vegetarians

Studies of LOVs compared with omnivores generally have not found significant differences in intake, although some have reported a greater intake in the LOVs.[5,6,48, 52] Calcium intake in vegans appears to be considerably less than that of either LOVs or omnivores.[16] Young female vegans reported consuming 300–450 mg/d less than LOVs or omnivores.[38,40] Some plant foods are rich sources of calcium, but they may not be consumed in large enough quantities to provide the recommended amount of this nutrient.[48,49]

2. Calcium Intake and Vitamin D Status in Lactation

Specker[50] reported calcium intake was 486 mg/d and 340 mg/d in lactating and nonlactating macrobiotic women, respectively, compared with 1038 mg/d and 681 mg/d in lactating and nonlactating omnivores. Although the macrobiotic diet is not always vegan, dairy products are discouraged.[51] Serum levels of 1,25-dihydroxy vitamin D, the biologically active form, which is elevated when calcium intake does not meet needs, were used to evaluate calcium status in macrobiotic women.[53] Generally, increased concentrations are not seen in lactation unless it has continued beyond 6 months or twins are being nursed.[53] Elevated levels of 1,25-dihydroxy vitamin D were found in both lactating and non-lactating macrobiotic vegetarians compared with lactating and non-lactating omnivores, suggesting that an adaptation to enhance calcium absorption was occurring in the macrobiotics.[53] This adaptation is expected to occur when there is increased calcium need. The investigators suggested that the low calcium intake among the macrobiotic women might have caused the increased 1,25-dihydroxy vitamin D concentrations. There was no difference in calcium concentration in the milk of the vegetarians compared with the omnivores.[50] Whether there was an effect on bone was not known.

Other recent studies suggest that changes in calcium metabolism during lactation are not influenced by the mother's intake of calcium.[54] However, since the number of subjects was small, the mean calcium intake was > 1300 mg/d and the studies were of much shorter duration than usual lactation in vegetarians, caution was expressed that the results should not be generalized to women who consume less calcium than used in the studies.[54] On the other hand, it was noted that calcium supplements did not affect the bone mineral content in Gambian women, who had a very low calcium intake (283 mg/d).[54] Another recent study found that calcium supplementation resulted in slightly less bone loss in lactating women and it slightly enhanced the increase in density of the lumbar spine after weaning.[55] It was suggested that recovery of bone loss after weaning may be influenced by calcium intake.[55]

3. Calcium and Bone Status in Vegetarians

There is no simple test to determine adequacy of calcium intake and status. Serum levels are maintained through homeostatic mechnisms involving the skeleton, which serves as a very large calcium reserve, and other issues. However, if calcium intake is chronically inadequate, bone mineral density (BMD) may be compromised.[56]

Some studies reported greater BMD in LOVs than in omnivores at some measurement sites, while others found no significant difference.[57-61] Marsh et al. first reported the tendency among the few vegans in their study to have lower BMD.[62] No significant difference was found in BMD comparing 15 premenopausal LOVs and 8 vegans, while the vegetarian groups combined tended to have lower BMD than the omnivore controls.[63] Postmenopausal Taiwanese women who were long-term vegans were at significantly greater risk of exceeding the lumbar spine fracture threshold and of being classified as having osteopenia of the femoral neck compared with LOVs and omnivores.[64] A recent study reported significantly lower BMD in young vegan women compared with LOVs.[65] Although the BMD in the LOVs was greater than in the omnivores, the difference was not significant, nor was the lower BMD in the vegans compared with the omnivores. Bone status was also recently evaluated in adolescents who had followed a vegan-type macrobiotic diet during childhood.[66] The early diet was characterized by low intake of calcium and vitamin D. Bone mineral content adjusted for age, bone area, weight, height, percent lean body mass, and puberty was significantly lower in the former vegans compared with omnivore controls. This was particularly true at the spine and femoral neck.

Although up to 80% of peak bone mass is determined by genetics and calcium intake as well as physical activity, which plays a major role, other dietary factors are also important.[56] It has been suggested that a calcium intake < 500mg/d may be adequate if protein and sodium intakes are also low.[67] Animal protein is thought to exert a negative effect on calcium balance and it was proposed that a lower intake from such sources was protective of bone loss.[57,68] On the other hand, too little protein has been associated with poor bone status in the elderly and protein supplements have resulted in dramatic improvements in osteoporotic patients.[69,70] It was noted that low protein intake is always detrimental to bone.[71] Concern has been expressed whether calcium intake in vegans is adequate to achieve optimal bone status in spite of the fact that all the protein in vegan diets is from plant sources.[48,49]

4. Calcium and Blood Pressure in Pregnancy

Besides its role in skeletal health, calcium has other important functions. A recent meta analysis of randomized controlled trials of calcium supplementation in pregnancy found supplements resulted in significantly lower systolic and diastolic blood pressures.[72] In addition, the calcium supplements were associated with 70% lower risk of pregnancy-induced hypertension; preeclampsia was reduced by 60% and prematurity by 30%.[72] Pregnant women 20 years of age or younger benefited more than older pregnant women. It was suggested that this demonstrated the greater calcium need of young women to meet both their own needs for skeletal growth and the needs of the fetus.[73] Others showed that calcium supplementation had no effect on preeclampsia if the women were already consuming 980 mg/d calcium.[74]

5. Recommendations

In view of its role in maintaining bone health as well as its potential for improving blood pressure status during pregnancy, it appears prudent to encourage a calcium intake approaching recommendations, regardless of dietary pattern.[16] The bioavailability of food sources of calcium acceptable to vegans has been described.[48,49]

F. Vitamin D

Vitamin D is intimately involved with calcium absorption and metabolism. Low calcium intake may be further compromised by low intake of this vitamin. The very few natural food sources of vitamin D are of animal origin, although it is now added to many different foods. With adequate sun exposure, dietary sources are not essential.

Vitamin D intake in pregnancy was reported to be significantly lower in vegetarians (11 LOVs and 1 vegan) compared with omnivores.[6] Serum concentration of 25(OH)D, an indicator of vitamin D status, was lower in lactating macrobiotic women.[50] Vitamin D deficiency or rickets has been reported in macrobiotics and in vegetarians and vegans, particularly those with darker skin or who lived where sunlight was limited.[16]

The latest recommended intake for vitamin D during pregnancy is double that for nonpregnant women.[46] The amount in breast milk is low and levels in breast-fed infants vary with exposure to sunshine.[50] Vegetarians should be sure to identify appropriate sources for this vitamin both for themselves and their infants.

G. Vitamin B$_{12}$

Vitamin B$_{12}$ is of particular interest to vegetarians, especially vegans, because the only non-fortified practical food sources are of animal origin. It is also of special interest because the effects of a deficiency may be irreversible and because cases of infants with a deficiency continue to be reported.[75,76] In some cases, the deficiency was identified by routine neonatal screening, suggesting extremely low stores at birth.[77] The affected infants were born to mothers who had used no animal products for some time; in addition, the infants were exclusively breast-fed.

1. Dietary Vitamin B$_{12}$ Deficiency in Infants

Vitamin B$_{12}$-deficient infants share certain characteristics. Their early development is normal for varying lengths of time; problems can emerge from 3–8 months of age.[76] They become irritable and apathetic; they experience developmental regression and diminished socialization; their growth may fall off, including head circumference; they may refuse solid food. They may also experience involuntary movements.[76,78] In some cases, they have progressed to coma.[78,79]

The mothers of the vitamin B$_{12}$-deficient infants have shown no symptoms of a deficiency. However, testing often reveals low serum or milk concentrations of the vitamin.[75,80] In addition, elevated concentrations of methylmalonic acid (MMA) in the mothers' urine provide evidence of a functional deficiency.[81,82] Specker et al.[81,82] reported that low vitamin B$_{12}$ concentrations in the milk were related to low concentrations in the mothers' serum and to elevated MMA in the infants' urine. The vitamin B$_{12}$ concentration in the milk was also inversely related to the mothers' urinary MMA concentrations.[82]

Recent reports are of particular interest. The first is an adolescent male who experienced severe vitamin B$_{12}$ deficiency as an infant less than 9 months of age.[78] Treatment with vitamin B$_{12}$ resulted in rapid clinical improvement, but neurological recovery was incomplete at 18 months of age. Follow-up at 12 years of age revealed borderline retardation.[75] At age 14, his physicians said he was "physically strong and healthy," but "clearly needs some assistance with his educational progress."[83]

The second case describes an infant who presented at 18 months of age.[76] He had been exclusively breast-fed until about 3 weeks before admission when, because of concern for his condition, some dairy products and eggs had been added to his diet and he had been placed on soy milk. He had experienced no developmental progress during the prior 6 months. At 20 months of age he was thought to be functioning at the 6-month level.[76]

Adolescents who had been strict (vegan) macrobiotics until 6 years of age were recently assessed.[84] They had subsequently switched to other vegetarian dietary practices or become omnivores. Nevertheless, they currently consumed dairy products, meat, chicken, and eggs, significantly less often than the controls. Only consumption of fish was more frequent in the former macrobiotics. They also consumed significantly less vitamin B$_{12}$ from all dairy products.

Significantly lower serum vitamin B$_{12}$ concentrations and significantly higher concentrations of MMA were found in the 73 former macrobiotics than in the 94 controls.[84] Elevated concentrations of MMA, indicative of a functional B$_{12}$ deficiency, were found in 21% of the former macrobiotic subjects. Previously, vitamin B_{12} deficiency and elevated MMA had been reported in macrobiotic infants.[85]

The researchers roughly estimated that the former macrobiotic females and males were presently consuming respectively, on average, 1.2 μg/d and 1.5 μg/d or 67% and 81% of the Dutch recommended intake for vitamin B_{12}. This study indicates that a strict macrobiotic diet in infancy and early childhood can result in impaired status of vitamin B_{12} in adolescence and that moderate intake of animal products over 6–7 years was not able to restore and maintain normal vitamin B_{12} function.[84] Studies evaluating the cognitive and psychomotor development of these subjects are now under way.

These and other reports illustrate the importance of vitamin B_{12}. An adequate intake of this vitamin, whether from food sources or a supplement, will prevent such outcomes in otherwise healthy individuals. A dietary deficiency of vitamin B_{12} is extremely rare, yet the number of cases reported in vegan infants suggests that there is need for a good deal of education.

2. Sources of Vitamin B_{12}

There is some confusion about sources of vitamin B_{12}. Some analytical methods used to evaluate vitamin B_{12} content of foods do not differentiate between inactive analogs and the active form of the vitamin.[86,87] Thus, the content listed on some food items may not be correct. Newer radio assays show that seaweed, spirulina, and fermented products such as tempeh may not contribute significant amounts of this vitamin.[86] Appropriate sources that are acceptable to vegans include fortified foods, Red Star nutritional yeast, and supplements.

Pregnancy is an opportune time to educate the pregnant woman on many topics relating to diet and health. This should include information about developmental milestones of her infant and the need to investigate deviations from those milestones. It is imperative that those who choose not to include any animal products in their diet be aware of the need for this vitamin, particularly as it impacts the long-term neurologic health of their infants.[80]

H. Other Nutrient Issues

Many protective nutrients are found in greater amounts in vegetarian diets, including folate, vitamin C, and beta carotene.[16] The ability of folate to protect against neural tube defects when consumed in adequate amounts before and during early pregnancy is recognized.[88]

Iodine: Lightowler et al. recently reviewed studies that included an evaluation of iodine intake or status in vegans.[89] Mean intake in female vegans was considerably less than recommendations and, where available, the biochemical data substantiated the dietary intake.

Iodized salt has largely eliminated a deficiency of this nutrient in the U.S., however, in England, only a very small percentage of salt is iodized.[89] The food products from which iodine may be obtained, including meat products, fish, milk, and dairy products, are unacceptable to vegans. In addition, they might not use iodized salt, relying instead on sea salt, which may not contribute appreciable amounts of iodine. Although high levels of iodine can be found in seaweed, it is generally not consumed in quantities that would provide the necessary amount.[89] Further, processed foods, which can contribute significant amounts through the additives and preservatives they contain, may not be acceptable to vegans.

Iodine deficiency during pregnancy can produce devastating effects.[90] It is appropriate to evaluate intake in vegans to assure needs are being met.

V.   COUNSELING THE VEGETARIAN MOTHER

A recent report found that LOVs felt that they did not receive useful dietary advice from health professionals.[5] This may occur because health professionals do not have good information regarding vegetarian diets. This, in fact, appeared to be the case in a study of midwives in England where two-thirds reported that they were concerned about their knowledge of vegetarian diets.[91]

The lack of appropriate advice may also occur because vegetarian diets have often been regarded with suspicion as to their nutritional adequacy. Such concerns have been supported by case studies of persons with nutritional problems apparently caused by the vegetarian diet they followed. Short-term studies of the availability of nutrients, especially trace minerals, and understanding of the effects of certain plant food constituents that may limit uptake of nutrients, e.g., fiber or phytate, have led to questions regarding the adequacy of vegetarian diets. Questions relating to the nutritional adequacy of dietary intake are of special concern during pregnancy and lactation, as well as periods of growth.

Current evidence supports the position of the American Dietetic Association that a well-planned vegetarian or vegan diet can provide the nutrients needed for a successful pregnancy.[21] Pregnant vegetarians should receive that assurance along with advice regarding sources for the nutrients usually obtained from any food groups they do not consume. This implies that the health professional will be knowledgeable or will refer the woman to a dietitian who is knowledgeable about alternative nutrient sources that are acceptable to various vegetarian philosophies.

Dietary intake is known to affect the concentration of many nutrients in human milk, whereas others appear less affected.[22,92,93] A very high percentage of vegetarian mothers breast-feed their infants and they do so for extended periods of time.[94] Protein concentration was observed to decrease in the milk of macrobiotic women with increasing stage of lactation and, after adjustment for stage of lactation, it contained less calcium, magnesium, vitamin B_{12}, and saturated fatty acids and more polyunsaturated fatty acids.[94] In keeping with other studies, milk from the macrobiotic mothers contained lower concentrations of contaminants.

Because of the great likelihood that vegetarians will breast-feed their infants for extended periods of time, it is important that they are provided with the appropriate dietary guidance to assure an adequate nutrient intake over the entire period of lactation. Particular nutrients of concern have been identified and suggestions have been made for obtaining them. As diets become more restrictive, there is increasing potential for inadequacies unless greater care is taken to assure an adequate intake. Usual assessment tools can be used to identify potential problem areas. Dietary patterns for different ages and energy levels have been suggested and a vegetarian food guide pyramid has been developed.[95,96] Sources for nutrients more likely to be at risk in some vegetarian diets have been provided.[97]

The pregnant vegetarian is as deeply committed to providing for her developing fetus as is the omnivore. Vegetarians, however, are also often deeply committed to their dietary practices. Thus, health care professionals must use tact and sensitivity along with their nutrition knowledge in counseling the pregnant vegetarian. What to the vegetarian is very enjoyable food may be quite different from the usual food choices of the health professional who is providing the dietary guidance. A nonjudgmental attitude, reinforcement of beneficial dietary practices, and acceptance of the mother as a person provide an essential foundation for continuing communication.[98]

Complete information about actual dietary practices and foods that are proscribed, regardless of what a person calls their diet, is an essential foundation for meaningful guidance. Although the quality of the usual diet may be very good, in order to evaluate nutritional adequacy it is also important to know the frequency and amounts of foods that are usually consumed.[98] A dietitian knowledgeable in the nutrient contributions of various types of plant foods will be helpful in identifying acceptable sources for nutrients at risk.

A recent report described toxic effects in two infants caused by large consumption of herbal tea mixtures by their lactating mothers.[99] The clinical conditions improved within 24–36 hours of discontinuing the beverage. These cases illustrate the potential negative consequences of so-called natural foods, which may be more likely to be used by some vegetarians. In light of the growing use of unconventional therapies, health care professionals need to understand the potential consequences of such practices and to develop sensitive methods to determine if they are being used.

VI. CONCLUSION

Increasing numbers of individuals, particularly young women, are adopting various kinds of vegetarian diets. While their dietary practices may differ from the American norm, vegetarians need to be assured that well-planned vegetarian diets can meet the nutrient needs of pregnancy and lactation. As more food types are eliminated from the diet, greater care must be taken to achieve nutritional adequacy. Nonetheless, nutrient needs can be met in many different ways and, with creativity and adaptability, vegetarian diets can meet the needs of different stages of the lifecycle. It is the responsibility of the health care professional to be informed and prepared to meet the varying dietary practices encountered today.[100]

REFERENCES

1. Barker, D.J.P. *Mother, Babies and Health in Later Life.* 2nd edition, Churchill Livingstone, Edinburgh, 1998.
2. Hardinge, M. G. and Stare, F. J. Nutritional studies of vegetarians. I. Nutritional, physical and laboratory studies. *J. Clinic. Nutr.,* 2: 73, 1954.
3. Thomas, J. and Ellis, F. R. The health of vegans during pregnancy. *Proc. Nutr. Soc.,* 36: 46A, 1977.
4. Sanders, T.A.B. and Reddy, S. The influence of a vegetarian diet on the fatty acid composition of human milk and the essential fatty acid status of the infant. *J. Pediatr.,* 120: S71, 1992.
5. Drake, R., Reddy, S., and Davis, J. Nutrient intake during pregnancy and pregnancy outcome of lacto-ovo-vegetarians, fish-eaters and non-vegetarians. *Vegetarian Nutrition: An International Journal,* 2: 45, 1998.
6. King, J. C., Stein, T., and Doyle, M. Effect of vegetarianism on the zinc status of pregnant women. *Am. J. Clin. Nutr.,* 34: 1049, 1981.
7. Abu-Assal, M.J. and Craig, W.J. The zinc status of pregnant women. *Nutr. Rep. Int.,* 29: 485, 1984.
8. McFadyen, I. R., Campbell-Brown, M., Abraham, R., North, W. R. S., and Haines, A. P. Factors affecting birthweight in Hindus, Moslems and Europeans. *Br. J. Obstet. Gyn.,* 91: 968, 1984.
9. Reddy, S., Sanders. T. A. B., and Obeid, O. The influence of maternal vegetarian diet on essential fatty acid status of the newborn. *Euro. J. Clin. Nutr.,* 48: 358, 1994.
10. Dagnelie, P. C., van Staveren, W. A., van Klaveren, J. D., and Burema, J. Do children on macrobiotic diets show catch-up growth? *Euro. J. Clin. Nutr..,* 42: 1007, 1988.

11. Dagnelie, P. C. and van Staveren, W. A. Macrobiotic nutrition and child health: results of a population-based, mixed-longitudinal cohort study in The Netherlands. *Am. J. Clin. Nutr.*, 59: 1187S, 1994.
12. Shull, M. W., Reed, R. B., Valadian, I., Palombo, R., Thorne, H., and Dwyer, J. T. Velocities of growth in vegetarian preschool children. *Pediatrics*, 60: 410, 1977.
13. Dwyer, J. T., Palombo, R., Thorne, H., Valadian, I., and Reed, R. B. Preschoolers on alternate life-style diets. *J. Am. Diet. Assoc.*, 72: 264, 1978.
14. Sanders, T.A.B. and Reddy, S. Vegetarian diets and children. *Am. J. Clin. Nutr.*, 59: 1176S, 1994.
15. Sanders, T.A.B. and Reddy S. Nutritional implications of a meatless diet. *Proc. Nutr. Soc.*, 53: 297, 1994.
16. Messina, M. and Messina V. *The Dietitian's Guide to Vegetarian Diets.* Aspen, Gaithersburg, MD, 1996.
17. Freeland-Graves, J. H., Bodzy, P. W., and Eppright, M. A. Zinc status of vegetarians. *J. Am. Diet. Assoc.*, 77: 655, 1980.
18. Dagnelie, P. C, van Staveren, W. A., Vergotte, F.J.V.R.A., Burema, J., van't Hof, M. A., van Klaveren, J. D., and Hautvast, J.G.A.J. Nutritional status of infants aged 4 to 18 months on macrobiotic diets and matched omnivorous control infants: a population-based mixed-longitudinal study, II. Growth and psychomotor development. *Euro. J. Clin. Nutr..*, 43: 325, 1989.
19. Dagnelie, P.C., van Dusseldop, M., van Staveren, W.A., Hautvast, J.G.A.J. Effects of macrobiotic diets on linear growth in infants and children until 10 years of age. *Euro. J. Clin. Nutr.*, 48: S103, 1994.
20. Carter, J. P., Furman, T., and Hutcheson, H.R. Preeclampsia and reproductive performance in a community of vegans. *South Med. J.*, 80: 692, 1987.
21. Messina, V. and Burke, K. Position of the American Dietetic Association: Vegetarian diets. *J. Am. Diet. Assoc.*, 97: 1317, 1997.
22. Finley, D. A., Lönnerdal, B., Dewey, K. G., and Grivetti, L. E. Breast milk composition: fat content and fatty acid composition in vegetarians and non-vegetarians. *Am. J. Clin. Nutr.*, 41: 787, 1985.
23. Young, V. R. and Pellett, P. L. Plant proteins in relation to human protein and amino acid nutrition. *Am. J. Clin. Nutr.*, 59: 1203S, 1994.
24. Sanders, T.A.B. Essential fatty acids in pregnancy, lactation and infancy in vegetarians. *Am. J. Clin. Nutr.*, 70: 555S, 1999.
25. Simopoulos, A. P. Omega-3 fatty acids in health and disease and in growth and development. *Am. J. Clin. Nutr.*, 54: 438, 1991.
26. Birch, E. E., Hoffman, D. R., Uauy, R., Birch, D. G., and Prestidge, C. Visual acuity and the essentiality of docosahexaenoic acid and arachidonic acid in the diet of term infants. *Pediatric Res.*, 44: 201, 1998.
27. Conner, W. E., Lowensohn, R., and Hatcher, L. Increased docosahexaenoic acid levels in human newborn infants by administration of sardines and fish oil during pregnancy. *Lipids*, 31: S-183, 1996.
28. Gibson, R. A., Neumann, M. A., and Makrides, M. Effect of increasing breast milk docosahexaenoic acid on plasma and erythrocyte phospholipid fatty acids and neural indices of exclusively breast-fed infants. *Euro. J. Clin. Nutr.*, 51: 578, 1997.
29. Conquer, J. A. and Holub, B. J. Docosahexaenoic acid (omega-3) and vegetarian nutrition. *Vegetarian Nutrition: An International Journal*, 1:42, 1997.

30. Specker, B. L., Wey, H. E., and Miller, D. Differences in fatty acid composition of human milk in vegetarian and nonvegetarian women: Long-term effect of diet. *J. Pediatr. Gastroent. Nutr.*, 6: 764, 1987.

31. Willatts, P., Forsyth, J. S., DiModugno, M. K., Varma, S., and Colvin, M. Effect of long-chain polyunsaturated fatty acids in infant formula on problem solving at 10 months of age. *Lancet*, 352: 688, 1998.

32. Uauy, R., Peirano, P., Hoffman, D., Mena, P., Birch, D., and Birch, E. Role of essential fatty acids in the function of the developing nervous system. *Lipids*, 31: S167, 1996.

33. Life Sciences Research Office, LSRO Report: Assessment of nutrient requirements for infant formulas, 1999.

34. U.S. Preventive Services Task Force, Routine iron supplementation during pregnancy: Policy statement. *JAMA*, 270: 2846, 1993.

35. Scholl, T. O., Hediger, M. L., Fischer, R. L., and Shearer, J. W. Anemia vs. iron deficiency: increased risk of preterm delivery in a prospective study. *Am. J. Clin. Nutr.*, 55: 985, 1992.

36. Craig, W. J. Iron status of vegetarians. *Am. J. Clin. Nutr.*, 59: 1233S, 1994.

37. Dwyer, J. T. Nutritional consequences of vegetarianism. *Ann. Rev. Nutr.*, 11: 61, 1991.

38. Alexander, D., Ball, M. J., and Mann, J. Nutrient intake and haematological status of vegetarians and age-sex matched omnivores. *Euro. J. Clin. Nutr..*, 48: 538, 1994.

39. Shultz, T. D. and Leklem, J. E. Dietary status of Seventh-day Adventists and nonvegetarians. *J. Am. Diet. Assoc.*, 83: 27, 1983.

40. Janelle, K. C. and Barr, S. I. Nutrient intakes and eating behavior scores of vegetarian and nonvegetarian women. *J. Am. Diet. Assoc.*, 95: 180, 1995.

41. Draper, A., Lewis, J., Malhotra, N., and Wheeler, E. The energy and nutrient intakes of different types of vegetarians: a case for supplements? *Br. J. Nutr.*, 69: 3, 1993.

42. Hunt, J. R., Matthys, L. A., and Johnson, L. K. Zinc absorption, mineral balance, and blood lipids in women consuming controlled lactoovovegetarian and omnivorous diets for 8 wks. *Am. J. Clin. Nutr.*, 67: 421, 1998.

43. Reddy, S. and Sanders, T. A. B. Haematological studies on pre-menopausal Indian and Caucasian vegetarians compared with Caucasian omnivores. *Br. J. Nutr.*, 64: 331, 1990.

44. Donovan, U. M., and Gibson R. S. Iron and zinc status of young women aged 14 to 19 years consuming vegetarian and omnivorous diets. *J. Am. Coll. Nutr.*, 5: 463, 1995.

45. Freeland-Graves, J. H., Ebangit, M. L., and Bodzy, P. W. Zinc and copper content of foods used in vegetarian diets. *J. Am. Diet. Assoc.*, 77: 648, 1980.

46. Institute of Medicine, Dietary reference intakes of calcium, phosphorus, magnesium, vitamin D, and fluoride, National Academy Press, Washington, D.C., 1997.

47. Alaimo, K., McDowell, M. A., Briefel, R. R., et al. U.S. Department of Health and Human Services. Dietary intake of vitamins, minerals, and fiber of persons ages 2 months and over in the United States: Third National Health and Nutrition Examination Survey, Phase 1, 1988-91. *Advance data from vital and health statistics, no. 258*, National Center for Health Statistics, Hyattsville, MD, 1994.

48. Weaver, C. M. and Plawecki, K. L. Dietary calcium: adequacy of a vegetarian diet. *Am. J. Clin. Nutr.*, 59: 1238S, 1994.

49. Weaver, C. M., Proulx, W. R., and Heaney, R. Choices for achieving adequate dietary calcium within a vegetarian diet. *Am. J. Clin. Nutr.*, 70: 543S, 1999.

50. Specker, B. L. Nutritional concerns of lactating women consuming vegetarian diets. *Am. J. Clin. Nutr.*, 59: 1182S, 1994.

51. Kushi, M., and Jack, A. *The Book of Macrobiotics: the Universal Way of Health, Happiness, and Peace.* Japan Publications, Boston, 1987.

52. Finley, D. A., Dewey, K. G., Lönnerdal, B., and Grivetti, L. E. Food choices of vegetarians and nonvegetarians during pregnancy and lactation. *J. Am. Diet. Assoc.*, 85: 678, 1985.

53. Specker, B. L., Tsang, R. C., Ho, M. L., and Miller, D. Effect of vegetarian diet on serum 1,25-dihydroxy vitamin D concentrations during lactation. *Obstet. Gynecol.*, 70: 870, 1987.

54. Allen, L. H. Women's dietary calcium requirements are not increased by pregnancy or lactation, editorial. *Am. J. Clin. Nutr.*, 67: 591, 1998.

55. Kalkwarf, H. J., Specker, B. L., Bianchi, D. C., Ranz, J., and Ho, M. The effect of calcium supplementation on bone density during lactation and after weaning. *N. Engl. J. Med.*, 337: 523, 1997.

56. Heaney, R. P. Bone biology in health and disease: a tutorial, in *Modern Nutrition in Health and Disease* 9th ed, Shils, M. E., Olson, J. A., Shike, M., and Ross, A. C., Eds., Williams & Wilkins, Baltimore, 1998, chap. 83.

57. Marsh, A. G., Sanchez, T. V., Mickelsen, O., Keiser, J., and Mayor, G. Cortical bone density of adult lacto-ovo-vegetarian and omnivorous women. *J. Am. Diet. Assoc.*, 76: 148, 1980.

58. Tylavsky, F. A. and Anderson, J. J. B. Dietary factors in bone health of elderly lactoovovegetarian and omnivorous women. *Am. J. Clin. Nutr.*, 48: 842, 1988.

59. Lloyd, T., Schaeffer, J. M., Walker, M. A., and Demers, L. M. Urinary hormonal concentrations and spinal bone densities of premenopausal vegetarian and nonvegetarian women. *Am. J. Clin. Nutr.*, 54: 1005, 1991.

60. Hunt, I. F., Murphy, N. J., Henderson, C., Clark, V. A., Jacobs, R. M., Johnston, P. K., and Coulson, A. H. Bone mineral content in postmenopausal women: comparison of omnivores and vegetarians. *Am. J. Clin. Nutr.*, 50: 517, 1989.

61. Tesar, R., Notelovitz, M., Shim, E., Kauwell, G., and Brown, J. Axial and peripheral bone density and nutrient intakes of postmenopausal vegetarian and omnivorous women. *Am. J. Clin. Nutr.*, 56: 699, 1992.

62. Marsh, A. G., Sanchez, T. V., Michelsen, O., Chaffee, F. L., and Fagal, S. M. Vegetarian lifestyle and bone mineral density. *Am. J. Clin. Nutr.*, 48: 837, 1988.

63. Barr, S. I., Prior, J. C., Janelle, K. C., and Lentle, B. C. Spinal bone mineral density in premenopausal vegetarian and nonvegetarian women: Cross-sectional and prospective comparisons. *J. Am. Diet. Assoc.*, 98: 760, 1998.

64. Chiu, J.-F., Lan, S.-J., Yang, C.-Y,, Wang, P.-W., Yao, W.-J., Su, I.-H., and Hsieh, C.-C. Long-term vegetarian diet and bone mineral density in postmenopausal Taiwanese women. *Calcif. Tissue Int.*, 60: 245, 1997.

65. Johnston, P. K., Makola, D., Knutsen, S., Haddad, E. H., dos Santos, H., Kuehl, K., and Schultz, E. Spinal bone mineral density in vegan, lacto-ovovegetarian and omnivorous premenopausal women. 3rd International Symposium on Nutritional Aspects of Osteoporosis, May 20-29, 1997, Lausanne, Switzerland.

66. Parsons, T. J., van Dusseldorp, M., van der Vliet, M., van de Werken, K., Schaafsma, G., and van Staveren, W. A. Reduced bone mass in Dutch adolescents fed a macrobiotic diet in early life. *J. Bone Miner. Res.*, 12: 1486, 1997.

67. Heaney, R. P. Nutrition and osteoporosis, in, *Primer on the Metabolic Bone Diseases and Disorders of Mineral Metabolism*, 3rd ed., Favus, M. J., Ed., Lippincott-Raven, Philadelphia, 1996, chap 48.

68. Zemel, M. B. Calcium utilization: effect of varying level and source of dietary protein. *Am. J. Clin. Nutr.*, 48: 880, 1988.

69. Bonjour, J.-P., Rapin, C.-H., Rizzli, R., Tkatch, L., Delmi, M., Chevalley, T., Nydegger, V., Slosman, D., and Vasey, H. Hip fracture, femoral bone mineral density, and protein supply in elderly patients, in *Nutrition of the Elderly*, Munro, H. and Schlierf, G., Eds., Nestle Nutrition Workshop Series, vol 29, Vevey/Raven Press, New York, 1992, 151.

70. Porter, K. H., and Johnson, M. A. Dietary protein supplementation and recovery from femoral fracture. *Nutr. Rev.*, 56: 337, 1998.

71. Heaney, R. P. Excess dietary protein may not adversely affect bone. *J. Nutr.*, 128: 1054, 1998.

72. Bucher, H. C., Guyatt, G. H., Cook, R. J., Lang, J. D., Cook, D. J., Hatala, R., and Hunt, D. L. Effects of dietary calcium supplementation on pregnancy-induced hypertension and preeclampsia, a meta-analysis of randomized controlled trials. *JAMA.*, 275: 1113, 1996.

73. McCarron, D. A. Dietary calcium and lower blood pressure, we can all benefit, editorial. *JAMA.*, 275: 1128, 1996.

74. Levine, R. J., Hauth, J. C., Curet, L. B., Sibai, B. M., Catalano, P. M., Morris, C. D., DerSimonian, R., Esterlitz, J. R., Raymond, E. G., Bild, D. E., Clemens, J. D., and Cutler, J. A. Trial of calcium to prevent preeclampsia. *N. Engl. J. Med.*, 337: 69, 1997.

75. Graham, S. M., Arvela, O. M., and Wise, G. A. Long-term neurologic consequences of nutritional vitamin B12 deficiency in infants. *J. Pediatr.*, 121: 710, 1992.

76. Gratten-Smith, P. J., Wilcken, B., Procopis, P. G., and Wise, G. A. The neurological syndrome of infantile cobalamin deficiency: developmental regression and involuntary movements. *Movement Disorders*, 12: 39, 1997.

77. Michaud, J. L., Lemieux, B., Ogier, H., and Lambert, M. A. Nutritional vitamin B12 deficiency: two cases detected by routine newborn urinary screening. *Eur. J. Pediatr.*, 151: 218, 1992.

78. Wighton, M. C., Namson, J. I., Speed, I., Robertson, E., and Chapman, E. Brain damage in infancy and dietary vitmain B_{12} deficiency. *Med. J. Aust.*, 2: 1, 1979.

79. Higginbottom, M. C., Sweetman, L., and Nyhan, W. L. A syndrome of methylmalonic aciduria, homocystinuria, megaloblastic anemia and neurologic abnormalities in a vitamin B_{12}-deficient breast-fed infant of a strict vegetarian. *N. Engl. J. Med.*, 299: 317, 1978.

80. Kühne, T., Bubl, R., and Baumgartner, R. Maternal vegan diet causing a serious infantile neurological disorder due to vitamin B_{12} deficiency. *Eur J. Pediatr.*, 150: 205, 1991.

81. Specker, B. L., Miller, D., Norman, E. J., Greene, H., and Hayes, K. C. Increased urinary methylmalonic acid excretion in breast-fed infants of vegetarian mothers and identification of an acceptable dietary source of vitamin B_{12}. *Am. J. Clin. Nutr.*, 47: 89, 1988.

82. Specker, B. L., Black, A., Allen, L., and Morrow, F. Vitamin B_{12}: low milk concentrations are related to low serum concentrations in vegetarian women and to methylmalonic aciduria in their infants. *Am. J. Clin. Nutr.*, 52: 1073, 1990.

83. Manson, J. I., Personal communication, 1991.

84. Van Dusseldorp, M., Schneede, J., Refsum, H., Ueland, P. M., Thomas, C. M. T., de Boer, E., and van Staveren, W. A. Risk of persistent cobalamin deficiency in adolescents fed a macrobiotic diet in early life. *Am. J. Clin. Nutr.*, 69: 664, 1999.

85. Schneede, J., Dagnelie, P. C., van Staveren, W. A., Vollset, S. E., Refsum, H., and Ueland, P. M. Methylmalonic acid and homocysteine in plasma as indicators of functional cobalamin deficiency in infants on macrobiotic diets. *Pediatr. Res.*, 36: 194, 1994.

86. Herbert, V. Vitamin B-12: plant sources, requirements, and assay. *Am. J. Clin. Nutr.*, 48: 852, 1988.

87. Herbert, V. Staging vitamin B-12 (cobalamin) status in vegetarians. *Am. J. Clin. Nutr.*, 59: 1213S, 1994.

88. Butterworth, Jr., C. E. and Bendich A. Folic acid and the prevention of birth defects. *Annu. Rev. Nutr.*, 16: 73, 1996.

89. Lightowler, H. J., Davies, G. J., and Trevan, M. D. Iodine in the diet: perspectives for vegans. *J. Roy. Soc. Hlth.*, Feb: 14, 1996.

90. Hetzel, B. S., Potter, B. J., and Dulberg, E. M. The iodine deficiency disorders: nature, pathogenesis and epidemiology. *Wld. Rev. Nutr. Diet.*, 62: 59, 1990.

91. Mulliner, C. M., Spiby, H., and Fraser, R. B. A study exploring midwives' education and attitudes to nutrition in pregnancy. *Midwifery*, 11: 37, 1995.

92. Finley, D. A., Lonnerdal, B., Dewey, K. G., and Grivetti, L. E. Inorganic constituents of breast milk from vegetarian and nonvegetarian women: relationships with each other and with organic constituents. *J. Nutr.*, 115: 772, 1985.

93. Worthington-Roberts, B. S. Human milk composition and infant growth and development, in *Nutrition in Pregnancy and Lactation*, 6th ed., Worthington-Roberts, B. S. and Williams, S. R., Eds., Brown & Benchmark, Madison, WI, 1997, chap 12.

94. Dagnelie, P. C., van Staveren, W. A., Roos, A. H., Tuinstra, L. G. M. Th., and Burema, J. Nutrients and contaminants in human milk from mothers on macrobiotic and omnivorous diets. *Eur. J. Clin. Nutr.*, 46: 355, 1992.

95. Haddad, E. H. Development of a vegetarian food guide. *Am. J. Clin. Nutr.*, 59: 1248S, 1994.

96. Haddad, E. H., Sabate, J., and Whitten C. G. Vegetarian food guide pyramid: a conceptual framework. *Am. J. Clin. Nutr.*, 70: 615S, 1999.

97. Johnston, P. K. and Haddad, E. H. Vegetarian and other dietary practices, in *Adolescent Nutrition: Assessment and Management*, Rickert, V. I., Ed., Chapman & Hall, New York, 1996, chap 4 and p 637.

98. Johnston, P. K. Counseling the pregnant vegetarian. *Am. J. Clin. Nutr.*, 48: 901, 1988.

99. Rosti, L., Nardini, A., Bettinelli, M. E., and Rosti, D. Toxic effects of a herbal tea mixture in two newborns, letter. *Acta. Pediatr.*, 83: 683, 1994.

100. Johnston, P. K. Vegetarians among us: implications for health professionals. *Top Clin. Nutr.*, 10: 1, 1995.

10

WOMEN'S REPRODUCTIVE FUNCTION

Susan I. Barr

CONTENTS

0-8493-8508-3/01/$0.00+$.50
© 2001 by CRC Press LLC

I. INTRODUCTION

The purpose of this chapter is to assess the adequacy of vegetarian diets in maintaining normal reproductive function in women throughout their life-span. At the outset, this topic may appear simplistic: vegetarian women, like omnivorous women, pass through puberty, some bear children, then pass through menopause. Yet, nutrition-related variables have the potential to exert either subtle or profound influences on reproductive capacity, and whether these differ between vegetarian and omnivorous women has received relatively little systematic study.

For each segment of women's reproductive lives (the pubertal transition, the years between menarche and menopause, and the menopausal transition), the normal physiology and endocrinology will be briefly reviewed. The potential influence of various dietary factors will then be described, and this will be followed by a discussion of the available data comparing vegetarians and omnivores. It should be noted that references to reproductive hormones will relate to reproductive function, per se, rather than to potential links between reproductive hormone levels and chronic diseases (e.g., breast cancer, heart disease, osteoporosis), addressed in other chapters in this volume.

II. THE PUBERTAL TRANSITION AND MENARCHE

Menarche, the first menstrual bleeding, is understood by many to signal the onset of a woman's reproductive life. Yet, as will be described herein, the pubertal transition takes place over several years, with menarche occurring not at the onset, but relatively late in the process. Moreover, in most cases, women are not fertile (i.e., capable of becoming pregnant) until some period of time after menarche. This section will examine whether vegetarianism affects the pubertal transition, first by describing the transition itself, followed by an assessment of whether nutrition-related variables influence it. Finally, the available data comparing the age at menarche between vegetarians and omnivores will be evaluated.

A. The Pubertal Transition

In girls, the onset of puberty is marked by breast budding and the development of pubic and axillary hair. Both breast and pubic hair development progress through characteristic stages, described by Tanner as Stages 1 through 5, with Stage I representing prepubertal characteristics and Stage 5, full maturity.[1] The age at which pubertal changes begin and their rate of progression vary considerably among individuals, although on average in North America, the pubertal transition begins at age 10–11 years (range 8–13).[2] Initiation of breast development usually occurs first, and is followed by initiation of pubic hair development, peak height velocity, and menarche, respectively. Menarche usually occurs at a Tanner Stage of 3–4 for breast development. The first menstrual bleedings, however, are not usually associated with ovulatory cycles, and the establishment of regular ovulatory cycles does not occur for several years. For example, only 15% of cycles are ovulatory in the first year after menarche, 58% in the fourth year, and 74% in the sixth year.[3]

The outwardly visible external changes associated with puberty reflect the exposure of sensitive tissues to the gonadal hormones, particularly estrogen. Increased release of estrogen from the ovaries is stimulated by increases in the pulsatile release of the pituitary gonadotrophic hormones, luteinizing hormone (LH) and follicle-stimulating hormone (FSH). The increase in LH is particularly large, with mean daytime LH levels rising 60-fold between prepuberty and early puberty.[3] In turn, the increased LH and FSH release result from the increased release of gonadotropin-releasing hormone (GnRH) from the hypothalamus.

The initiation of puberty does not appear to depend on the gonads' or pituitary's reaching a certain level of maturity, as both tissues are capable of responding to hormonal stimulation much earlier than normally occurs. For example, pulsatile administration of exogenous GnRH to very young female monkeys will initiate ovulatory menstrual cycles.[4] Similarly, exogenous GnRH administration to young women with anorexia nervosa and delayed puberty will also induce the onset of pubertal changes and menarche.[5] The causes of the increased activity of the GnRH pulse generator at the onset of puberty are not, however, known with certainty.[3]

B. Factors Associated with Pubertal Onset and Menarche

There is abundant evidence that overall nutritional status, especially the balance between energy intake and expenditure (often reflected by height, weight, or body composition) is an important modulator of the onset of puberty.[6-8] As reviewed by Bongaarts,[7] several lines of evidence are available to support this relationship in humans. On average, puberty occurs earlier in well-nourished than in poorly nourished girls,[9] and in those who have a higher weight-for-height at a given age. Since the end of the last century, mean age at menarche has decreased by about 3 years, and this has been associated with both improved diets and an increase in body size. Finally, age at menarche and socioeconomic status (SES) are negatively related in many countries, with differences observed between urban and rural populations and between high- and low-income groups.[7]

1. Body Size Variables

Although the data relating age at menarche to height and weight are convincing and relatively consistent at the population level, these variables are poor predictors at the individual level. A prospective study of 633 prepubertal girls, initially aged 8–10 years, obtained data on growth (height and weight measured at monthly intervals), exact age, height, and weight at menarche, health status, age at menarche of mother and sisters, adult height and weight of both parents, and SES.[10] The girls, most of whom were Caucasian and middle-class, had heights and weights that were similar to U.S. norms. The most striking finding from this study was the extreme variability in the results. Mean age at menarche was 12.8 ± 1.2 years (range 9.1–17.7 years), mean height was 156.6 ± 6.4 cm (range 135.9–177.8 cm) and mean weight was 47.3 ± 6.9 kg (range 31.3–81.6 kg). There was also great variability in relative weight: mean Body Mass Index (BMI) was 19.3 ± 0.8 kg/m^2, and ranged from about 13.5–29.7 kg/m^2. Although a significant association between age at menarche and relative weight was observed (higher relative weights in those who were younger at menarche), the proportion of the variance accounted for by this association was just over 7%.[10]

2. Diet Composition

As is evident from the above discussion, although associations exist between body size variables and age at menarche, much of the variability remains unexplained. Accordingly, it has been hypothesized that diet composition and, in particular, a high-protein, high-fat diet, may contribute to an earlier age at menarche.[11] For example, rats reared on a high-fat diet grew more rapidly and reached estrus earlier and at a lower weight than those reared on a low-fat diet.[12]

The available human evidence for an effect of diet composition is not as direct as that provided by the animal data, and it is sometimes difficult to separate effects of diet composition from those of energy intake, which in turn is associated with body size variables. However, suggestive evidence is provided by a study of 233 Slovenian girls for whom the exact date of menarche was known.[13] In this study, published in 1956, the mean age at menarche was 13.6 ± 1.2 years. The 45 girls who consumed a "proteinaceous" diet were significantly younger at menarche than the 75 who consumed a "mixed" diet (12.6 ± 0.9 vs. 13.4 ± 1.2 years), who in turn were significantly younger than the 110 girls who consumed primarily "carbohydratic" food (14.1 ± 1.6 years). Unfortunately, no data on actual nutrient intakes were obtained, and the girls classified their diets themselves. The authors attempted to address the effects of body size by observing the girls in gym class and classifying their body type as "baroque" (heavy), "renaissance" (medium) and "gothic" (thin). Direct measurements of height and weight, however, were not conducted. As expected, menarcheal age was youngest in the girls classified as heavy and oldest in those classified as thin. However, differences associated with diet persisted even when body type was considered. For example, among girls classified as heavy, menarche occurred at 12.4 ± 0.9 years and 13.9 ± 1.4 years for those consuming high-protein and high-carbohydrate diets, respectively. For girls classified as having medium body builds, the comparable ages were 12.9 ± 0.8 years and 13.8 ± 0.8 years.

Other data cited in support of this hypothesis are those of Burrell et al.,[14] who studied approximate age at menarche in South African Bantu girls. Almost 50,000 girls aged 10–18 living in Transkei were asked whether menarche had occurred, and were assessed according to whether their home conditions were "poor" or "not poor." Mean age at menarche was 15.4 years for the "poor" girls, significantly older than the mean of 15.0 years for those who were "not poor." The authors suggest that differences in diet, in particular, animal protein, may have contributed to their observations. The "not poor" girls received a fermented milk drink daily and ate beef and poultry weekly, whereas "poor" girls consumed very little animal protein. Unfortunately, because height and weight for the two groups were not reported, it cannot be determined whether these dietary differences were also associated with differences in body size.

More recently, results have been reported from prospective cohort studies that included assessment of height and weight. A cohort of 2299 fifth-grade girls completed three 3-day diet records and was followed to determine when menarche occurred. No associations were found between intakes of any nutrient and age at menarche.[15] Similarly, in a study of 213 premenarcheal girls whose diets were assessed using a semiquantitative food-frequency questionnaire, no associations between age at menarche and macronutrient intakes were observed.[16] These studies did not assess the intakes of animal vs. plant proteins, but in the latter study, saturated fat intake was nonsignificantly associated with later age at menarche, suggesting that high intakes of animal products were not a determinant of early menarche.[16]

C. Studies of Age at Menarche of Vegetarians and Omnivores

As alluded to by the above discussion, although much remains to be learned about determinants of age at menarche, the overall plane of nutrition appears to be an important factor. Accordingly, when examining studies that compare age at menarche of vegetarians and omnivores, it is important to assess whether long-term energy balance is similar. The available data on the growth of vegetarian children are further examined in other chapters in this volume. Taken together, however, studies suggest that, given similar socioeconomic conditions, the heights and weights of vegetarian children do not differ substantially from those of omnivorous children. Thus, to the extent that growth variables modulate pubertal development, one would not anticipate differences between similarly nourished vegetarians and omnivores. If differences were observed, the inference would be that diet composition is a determinant of pubertal progression.

Few data are available that compare age at menarche between vegetarians and omnivores. Perksy et al. studied 35 vegetarian and 40 non-vegetarian teenage girls.[17] The vegetarian girls were students at a Seventh-Day Adventist boarding school where a lacto-ovo-vegetarian diet was provided, and the non-vegetarians were students at a private boarding school in the same city. The diets of the two groups were similar in energy content, but the vegetarians' diets were significantly lower in total fat (33.7 vs. 39.7% of energy), saturated fat (12.3 vs. 15.5% of energy) and protein (13.0 vs. 15.1% of energy). Vegetarian girls also had higher intakes of starch and fiber, and lower intakes of sucrose and caffeine. Vegetarian girls were 2 inches shorter than non-vegetarians (P < 0.05), but the groups did not differ in weight, and means for BMI were very similar (22.8 ± 3.8 and 22.2 ± 4.2 kg/m² for vegetarians and non-vegetarians, respectively), as were physical activity levels. More of the vegetarians were Hispanic (34.3% vs. 2.5%); whether this difference in ethnicity may have contributed to the observed height difference was not reported, but the possibility should be considered. Self-reported mean age at menarche was 12.4 ± 1.3 years in both the vegetarian and the omnivorous girls. Thus, in this group with different diets but apparently similar energy balance, differences in age at menarche were not observed.

Age at menarche was also compared between vegetarians and omnivores in an earlier cross-sectional study of acne conducted by Hardinge et al.,[18] available only in abstract form, with additional details provided in an article by Sanchez et al.[11] The 481 girls, all of whom were students at private schools, included 325 non-vegetarians and 156 vegetarians. Age at menarche was reported to the nearest 0.5 year, and was classified as early (<11.5 years), average (11.5–13.5 years) or late (>13.5 years). Among non-vegetarians, 20% had an early menarche and 21% had a late menarche. In contrast, only 13% of vegetarians had an early menarche, and 28% had a late menarche. The difference in distributions was significant (P < 0.05). Unfortunately, whether this difference reflects the influence of a vegetarian diet, or of differences in energy balance, cannot be ascertained, since data on heights and weights of these groups were not provided.

The above studies have compared age at menarche between American vegetarians and non-vegetarians. This issue has also been explored in southern India, in a study of 1267 girls aged 9–18 years from three schools differing in SES.[19] All schools included both vegetarian and non-vegetarian subjects, and diets of all girls were primarily based on rice and wheat. Among vegetarians, these staples were supplemented with vegetable side dishes, whereas non-vegetarians also included mutton, fish, eggs, or fowl about 3–5 times per week. In this study, age at menarche was 12.86 years for girls at the school with the highest SES and 14.08 years for those at the poorest school. No effect of diet was observed, nor was there an interaction between diet and school. Conversely, another study from India reported that vegetarian girls had a significantly later age at menarche than non-vegetarians (13.7 ± 1.2 vs. 13.0 ± 1.2 years, P < 0.01).[20] In that study, however, higher SES was also associated with earlier age at menarche, and it was not reported whether vegetarian and non-vegetarian girls had similar SES, nor were heights and weights reported. Accordingly, the results were potentially confounded by differences in SES or body size.

In summary, the available data suggest that, when food is freely available, age at menarche does not differ between vegetarians and non-vegetarians.

III. THE REPRODUCTIVE YEARS

The time between menarche and menopause, during which reproduction is possible, spans a period of almost 40 years in women. Although the presence of menstrual bleeding is often equated with the ability to conceive, establishing a pregnancy actually depends on the presence of a normal ovarian cycle (i.e., a normal ovulatory menstrual cycle). If vegetarianism affected women's reproduction, it would necessarily affect the characteristics of the ovarian cycle. To provide background information for an examination of this issue, the normal ovarian cycle will be described, as will subclinical and clinical disturbances of the cycle and their potential impact on reproduction. This will be followed by a discussion of the effects of various dietary and non-dietary factors on cycle characteristics, and finally, by a review of the available literature assessing whether differences exist between vegetarians and non-vegetarians.

A. Characteristics of the Normal Ovarian Cycle

The ovulatory menstrual cycle reflects a complex interplay of hormones.[21] During menstrual flow, the onset of which defines the first day of the cycle, circulating levels of both estradiol and progesterone are low. Absence of feedback inhibition allows GnRH from the hypothalamus to stimulate the release of low levels of FSH and LH from the anterior pituitary. As a result of FSH stimulation, a number of ovarian follicles begin to mature and secrete estrogen. Then, estrogen levels gradually rise during the follicular phase of the cycle. The increasing estrogen levels inhibit FSH secretion and, consequently, all but the most mature of the follicles (the "dominant" follicle) undergo atresia. The dominant follicle releases large amounts of estrogen, which in turn appear to stimulate a major surge of LH at about mid-cycle (typically, days 12–14). Consequences of the LH surge include inhibition of estrogen production by follicular cells, initiation of changes leading to ovulation (rupture of the dominant follicle and release of the ovum), and transformation of the ruptured follicle to the corpus luteum, which synthesizes both estrogen and progesterone during the luteal phase of the cycle. If the ovum is not fertilized, estrogen and progesterone levels begin to fall and the corpus luteum undergoes luteolysis 10–16 days after its formation. The decline in ovarian hormones results in the shedding of the thickened uterine lining as menstrual flow, beginning the next cycle. The cycle averages 28 days in length, with a normal range from 21 to 35 days.

B. Ovulatory Disturbances

The normal ovulatory cycle described above does not invariably occur between menarche and menopause. Disturbances of cycle length and characteristics are most common in the years following menarche and preceding menopause,[22] but can occur at any time in response to physiological or psychosocial triggers. These disturbances represent a continuum, ranging from a subtle decrease in progesterone secretion during the luteal phase (luteal phase defects) to frank amenorrhea (absence of menstrual flow for at least 6 months in a nonpregnant woman).

1. Subclinical Disturbances

The least severe disturbances in the cycle are clinically silent; that is, they can occur within cycles of normal length and are not evident to women unless cycles are being monitored by techniques such as serial hormone measurements in blood or saliva. These disturbances include luteal phase defects (low progesterone levels during the luteal phase), a short luteal phase (< 10 days in duration) and anovulation (a cycle in which an ovum is not released).

Subclinical disturbances of the cycle are not uncommon. Data collected by Vollman,[22] from Swiss women in the 1950s and 1960s indicated that 3% of cycles in mature women were anovulatory, and that an additional 14.6% of cycles had short luteal phases. More recently, in a study in which women were prescreened to have two consecutive normal ovulatory cycles, only 13 of 66 women consistently had normal ovulatory cycles over the subsequent year.[23] The remaining women had one or more cycles that were either anovulatory (n = 13) or had a short luteal phase (n = 40). Examining the data another way, 29% of all cycles analyzed over the year had a short luteal phase or were anovulatory. However, only 3% of cycles analyzed fell outside the normal range for cycle length. Other studies have also documented a moderately high prevalence of subclinical disturbances in apparently healthy women.[24,25]

Anovulatory cycles are obviously associated with the inability to conceive, and cycles with luteal phase defects or a short luteal phase may also lead to reduced fertility. In the latter case, progesterone levels may not remain elevated long enough to allow the zygote to implant before the uterine lining is shed.

2. Clinical Disturbances

Oligomenorrhea (36–180 days between menses) and amenorrhea (absence of menses for at least 180 days in nonpregnant women) represent cycle disturbances that are apparent to women because of the absence or irregularity of menstrual flow. These disturbances occur less frequently than subclinical disturbances, with estimates of amenorrhea ranging from a 1-year incidence of 0.7% in Swedish women aged 18–45 years, to a 5%

incidence in selected groups such as young college students.[26,27] Accurate data on the occurrence of oligomenorrhea are more difficult to obtain, especially since the term is usually used to refer to a pattern of long, irregular cycles rather than to the occurrence of one long cycle. Nevertheless, Vollman reported that approximately 15% of the cycles of Swiss women in their early 20s were longer than 36 days, and that this decreased to fewer than 5% of cycles in women aged about 30–45.[22]

Long cycles are often anovulatory, although this is not always the case. Clearly, however, fertility would be considerably reduced in women with oligomenorrhea or amenorrhea.

C. Effects of Dietary Components on the Ovarian Cycle

In this section, studies that have assessed the effects of various dietary components on the ovarian cycle will be described. It should be noted that there is relatively abundant literature on the effects of many of these components on serum hormone levels, some of which is presented elsewhere in this volume, but this review will focus on studies that have assessed or inferred effects on the ovarian cycle, per se. Because of the overwhelming influence of energy availability on the menstrual cycle, a brief overview of this topic will also be provided.

1. Energy

Either inadequate or excessive energy availability can lead to menstrual disturbances. Because the relative weights of vegetarians and non-vegetarians may differ, it is important that studies assessing the prevalence of menstrual cycle disorders in these groups ensure that any differences in relative weight are considered.

At one extreme, starvation and emaciation are almost always associated with amenorrhea, but dieting can induce missed cycles or irregularities even before substantial weight loss occurs.[28,29] Even very short-term, acute energy shortages can interfere with LH pulsatility and may thereby affect ovarian function.[30,31]

At the other extreme, cycle disturbances also occur in association with obesity. Almost 50 years ago, before anorexia nervosa became common, a higher prevalence of obesity was observed among amenorrheic women.[32] More-recent literature suggests that anovulatory cycles are more common among obese women,[33,34] and that weight loss in these individuals results in improved ovulation and ability to become pregnant.[35]

2. Fat

The effect of diets containing 40% and 20% energy as fat on the menstrual cycle was assessed in 30 healthy premenopausal women.[36,37] Diets were similar in energy, protein, the amount of meat provided and the ratio of polyunsaturated to saturated fatty acids (P/S), but the low-fat diet contained about 37% more crude fiber. Each woman consumed both the high- and low-fat diets for four menstrual cycles. Compared with the 40% diet, the 20%-fat diet significantly increased cycle length and duration of menstrual flow.[36] The increased cycle length was due to an increase in the follicular phase length.[37]

The effect of diets high and low in fat was also assessed in another study of six lacto-ovo-vegetarian women.[38] Diets containing 46% and 25% fat, and similar in protein, energy, P/S and fiber were provided to women for 1 month each in a crossover design. No changes in menstrual cycle length or in the lengths of the follicular or luteal phases were observed. Although this study was well controlled, the small number of subjects studied and the short duration of the intervention may have limited the potential to detect differences.

A low-fat diet intervention was also assessed in women with cystic breast disease.[39] Sixteen women whose habitual diets contained about 35% fat were counseled on a low-fat diet, and reduced dietary fat to about 21% of energy. Serum hormones and gonadotropins were assessed before the intervention, as well as 2 and 3 months later. Specific data on the menstrual cycle were not reported, although the authors stated that the intervention had no discernable effects on the women's menstrual cycles.[39]

3. Fiber

The effects of doubling dietary fiber from approximately 15 to 30 g per day was assessed in 62 premenopausal women whose baseline diets contained at least 25% energy as fat and less than 25 g fiber per day.[40] Women were randomly assigned to receive a corn, oat, or wheat bran supplement (provided as muffins) for 2 months. Fat intake as a percentage of energy did not change during the intervention, and body weight was maintained. Data on menstrual cycle characteristics were not provided, but in the discussion, the authors suggest that changes did not occur.[40]

4. Fat and Fiber

The combined effects of diets low in fat and high in fiber have also been studied, although data on menstrual cycle characteristics are not always available. In the study of Woods et al.,[41] 17 premenopausal women were first fed a "typical Western diet" with 40% energy as fat and 12 g dietary fiber for one menstrual cycle. They were then fed a diet containing 25% energy as fat and 40 g dietary fiber for two menstrual cycles. No specific results pertaining to menstrual cycle length were provided.

In the study of Goldin et al.,[42] a larger number of women (n = 48) was studied using a similar protocol, and cycle length, follicular phase length, and luteal phase length were assessed. No significant changes were observed, although it is reported that increasing dietary fiber from 12 g to 40 g per day was associated with an increase in follicular phase length of 0.69 days (P = 0.27), and that decreasing fat from 40% to 20–25% was associated with an increased follicular phase length of 0.51 days (P = 0.47).

5. Meat

The effect of diets' containing or not containing meat was assessed in studies conducted by Hill et al.[43,44] In the first study, 16 Caucasian women were switched from their usual meat-containing diets (with an average of 38% energy from fat) to a diet containing no meat or meat products (with an average of 33% energy from fat and no change in P/S, but presumably more fiber). Weight was maintained during the 2-month intervention. The vegetarian diet significantly decreased cycle length from 30.4 ± 0.6 days to 26.6 ± 0.4 days, and this was associated with a significant decrease in follicular phase length.[43] In the same study, nine black South African women who customarily ate a vegetarian diet were provided with 150 g of cooked lean meat on a daily basis for 2 months. Whether fat or fiber intakes changed was not stated, but body weight was maintained. The meat-containing diet significantly increased cycle length and follicular phase length.[43]

These authors also compared the effects of a meat supplement and an isocaloric supplement of soybeans in 16 black South African women who habitually consumed a meat-free diet.[44] Body weight was maintained during the 2-month intervention. Menstrual cycle length increased from 26.5 ± 0.9 to 29.7 ± 0.8 days (P < 0.01) when women received meat, and this was due to an increase in follicular phase length. No changes occurred in women who consumed the soybean supplement.

6. Phytoestrogens

Isoflavones and lignans are two classes of phytogestrogens that are found in unusually high concentrations in soy and flaxseed, respectively. Phipps et al.[45] assessed the effects on the menstrual cycle of adding 10 g flaxseed powder to the diets of 18 healthy premenopausal women. Each woman consumed her usual diet for 3 months and the flaxseed-enriched diet for 3 months in a randomized, cross-over design. During flaxseed supplementation, mean luteal phase length was significantly longer (12.6 ± 0.4 vs. 11.4 ± 0.4 days, P = 0.002), with no difference in follicular phase length.

Results virtually opposite to those of Phipps were found by Cassidy et al.,[46,47] who assessed the effects of adding soy protein containing about 45 mg isoflavones per day to the diets of six healthy women. During soy supplementation, follicular phase length increased (17.5 ± 0.9 vs. 15.0 ± 0.4 days, P < 0.01), with no change in luteal phase length, and follicular phase serum estradiol levels also increased significantly. No changes were observed in women who consumed a soybean product from which the isoflavones had been chemically extracted.[47]

In another intervention study, six women were studied during a month on a metabolic ward, during which time they consumed soy milk that provided about 200 mg isoflavones, daily.[48] Cycle length tended to increase during the month on soy milk (P = 0.06); however, this was largely due to a 12-day increase in one woman, compared with modest changes in the other five (including a 2 day decrease in 1 woman). Although cycle phase lengths were not reported, serum estradiol levels were significantly lower throughout the cycle, in contrast to Cassidy's finding of increased follicular phase serum estradiol.[46] Serum progesterone levels were also lower with soy supplementation, and, in two of the six subjects, were consistent with anovulatory cycles.[48]

In contrast to studies assessing effects of acute interventions, associations between habitual soy product use and the menstrual cycle were assessed in a cross-sectional study of Japanese women.[49] Fifty healthy premenopausal women reported consuming a mean of 37.9 ± 26.1 g per day from nine soy products during the past year. Although soy product use was inversely correlated with estradiol levels, there was no association with menstrual cycle length (r = –0.13, P = 0.45). Length of the follicular and luteal phases was not assessed.

In summary, the available data on the effects of various dietary components on the characteristics of the menstrual cycle are inconsistent. For example, in the study of Reichman et al.,[37] a low-fat diet increased follicular phase length, but in Hill's study,[43] in which dietary fat decreased in association with the removal of meat from the diet, follicular phase length decreased. Adding soy to the diets of black South African vegetarian women had no effect on cycle characteristics,[44] while adding meat increased follicular phase length.[44] In contrast, adding soy to the diets of Caucasian women increased follicular phase length.[46] Finally, phytoestrogens from soy increased follicular phase length,[46] and increased[46] or decreased[48] follicular phase estradiol levels, whereas phytoestrogens from flaxseed increased luteal phase length.[45]

In addition to the discrepancies among studies, it is important to remember that there may not be consistent differences in the fat or fiber contents of vegetarian and omnivorous diets,[50] and that changes may occur in combination (for example, diets might have increased amounts of both soy products and flaxseed). Although additional research is warranted to assess the effects of individual dietary components on the menstrual cycle, whether differences exist between vegetarians and omnivores can only be assessed by studying free-living populations consuming their habitual diets.

D. Effects of Nutrition-Related Cognitive Variables on the Ovarian Cycle

Because the human female ovarian cycle is controlled at the level of the hypothalamus, it can be affected by psychological, as well as by physiological variables.[29,51] Stressors such as grief, travel, and moving are known to affect the menstrual cycle, but no data could be located to indicate whether these occur differentially between vegetarians and non-vegetarians. Stressors related to nutrition and food intake, however, could conceivably differ between these groups with different dietary patterns.

One such variable is cognitive dietary restraint. This is the perception that food intake is constantly being limited in an effort to control body weight, and it can be assessed using the restraint scale of the Three-Factor Eating Questionnaire.[52] That dietary restraint is "cognitive" is reflected, at least in part, by findings that women with high and low restraint scores have similar values for BMI and report similar energy intakes.[24,53-55]

In at least three studies, women with high restraint scores were found to have a higher prevalence of subclinical menstrual disturbances than women with low restraint scores,[24,54,55] despite values for BMI that were generally similar. It is possible that stress associated with monitoring food intake in women with high restraint scores leads to increased secretion of corticotropin-releasing hormone (CRH) and cortisol. CRH has been shown to inhibit gonadotropin secretion,[56] and could thereby disturb menstrual function.

Whether levels of cognitive dietary restraint differ between vegetarians and omnivores may depend on the motivation for vegetarianism. Some women with high levels of cognitive dietary restraint may adopt a vegetarian diet as a means of limiting food intake. Supportive evidence is provided by studies of women with anorexia nervosa, a condition characterized by very high levels of restraint. Among consecutive cases in two patient series, 45% and 54% were vegetarian.[57,58] And in a survey of 158 healthy women, those who had high restraint scores and were high in feminist values were more likely to be vegetarian.[59] The authors of that study speculate that women high in feminist values may view dieting for weight loss as socially unacceptable, and for these individuals, becoming vegetarian may represent an attempt to conceal dieting behavior from others.[59]

In contrast, in a study of carefully selected vegetarians and omnivores (the inclusion criteria included being weight-stable and of normal body weight, maintaining chosen dietary pattern for at least 2 years, and no history of an eating disorder), vegetarian women had significantly lower scores for dietary restraint than did omnivores.[50] Thus, levels of cognitive dietary restraint, and possibly the prevalence of eating disorders, may differ between vegetarians and omnivores, making it important to assess these variables in studies comparing menstrual function between these groups.

E. Studies of the Ovarian Cycle in Vegetarians and Omnivores

In the 1980s, several published reports suggested that menstrual disturbances were more common among vegetarian women than among omnivores.[60-62] In 1984, Brooks et al.[60] reported on the diets of 11 amenorrheic and 15 regularly menstruating runners. Nine of the amenorrheic runners were "vegetarian" (defined as eating less than 200 g meat per week), compared with only two runners with regular cycles. In another study reported the same year, Slavin et al.[61] found that the prevalence of amenorrhea was 31% among athletes who avoided meat, compared with only 4% among those who reported consuming all food categories. Other evidence was provided by a weight-loss intervention study in which normal-weight women were assigned to lose about 1 kg per week on either a vegetarian or an omnivorous diet.[62] Although the amount of weight lost was similar between groups, only two of nine women assigned to the vegetarian diet had normal ovulatory cycles, compared with 7 of 9 women on the omnivorous diet. None of these studies, however, was specifically designed to assess whether the prevalence of menstrual disturbances differed between vegetarians and omnivores, and their results could have been confounded by other variables (e.g., prevalence of eating disorders).

One of the first studies designed to address this question was that of Pedersen et al.[63] Vegetarian and non-vegetarian women, recruited through newsletters and newspaper advertisements, provided self-report data on whether they had regular cycles (11–13 menses per year), irregular cycles (three–10 menses per year), or were amenorrheic ($\leq$ two menses per year). Compared with omnivores, a higher proportion of vegetarian women reported irregular cycles or amenorrhea (26.5% vs. 5.9%, $P < 0.01$).

Inferences from this study are limited, however, as a recruitment bias may have existed: If the study had been described as trying to determine whether menstrual disturbances were more common among vegetarians, vegetarian women with menstrual disturbances might have been more likely to volunteer. Furthermore, the current use of oral contraceptive agents (OCA) was not listed as an exclusion criterion, and OCA had been used for a significantly longer period of time by omnivores than vegetarians. Because OCA use results in "regular" cycles, this could have contributed to the higher prevalence of regular cycles among omnivores. Finally, it was not stated whether women with an eating disorder, or history of an eating disorder, were excluded. In a subsequent study by this group,[64] in which OCA use during the previous 3 months was an exclusion criterion, irregular menses or amenorrhea was observed in four of 27 vegetarians and none of the non-vegetarians (P <0.05). Although the groups of women were well matched in many characteristics, the possibility of a recruitment bias remained, and history of an eating disorder did not appear to have been assessed.

The study the author and co-workers conducted was designed to attempt to avoid possible confounding variables.[24] It was reasoned that if clinical menstrual disturbances were more common among vegetarians, subclinical differences would also be more common. Accordingly, the study was controlled for a recruitment bias by including only women who reported "regular" menstrual cycles. Other recruitment criteria included:

- age 20–40 (to reduce the likelihood of subclinical disturbances of the cycle that often occur in the years following menarche or preceding menopause)
- no OCA use for at least 6 months
- weight stable with normal BMI
- no history of an eating disorder
- nulliparous (the menstrual cycle may be more stable following childbirth)
- drinking ≤ 1 alcoholic beverage daily
- exercising ≤ 7 hours weekly

Women had been following their current dietary patterns for at least 2 years. Records of daily basal body temperature were kept for 6 months, and used to classify cycles as normally ovulatory, with a short luteal phase, or anovulatory.[65] In this group of highly selected women, vegetarians had longer luteal phase lengths (11.2 ± 2.6 vs. 9.1 ± 3 days, P < 0.05) and fewer anovulatory cycles (4.6% vs. 15.1% of cycles, P < 0.01). Vegetarians in this study also had significantly lower levels of cognitive dietary restraint, which might have contributed to the findings.

Although the results of the preceding study suggest that vegetarianism, per se, is not associated with an increased prevalence of menstrual disturbances, this finding cannot be generalized to the population level. As mentioned earlier, some women adopt a vegetarian diet because of concerns about body weight, and such women would likely have been excluded from participating in the study. Population studies are needed to address this issue at the broadest level.

IV. THE MENOPAUSAL TRANSITION

Menopause signals the end of child-bearing capacity, and is also associated with changes in susceptibility to various chronic diseases, including breast cancer, heart disease, and osteoporosis.[66] Differences in age at menopause between vegetarian and omnivorous women, should they exist, could be associated with differences in chronic disease patterns between these groups. Furthermore, some women experience unpleasant symptoms during menopause (vasomotor symptoms such as night sweats and hot flushes, mood swings, insomnia, weight gain, headaches, and fatigue),[67] and these symptoms have been observed to differ among women in different cultures.[67,68] Whether dietary variables contribute to these differences in symptom experiences has not been clearly established, but there is speculation that they could.[68-70] Some of these dietary differences may also exist between vegetarian and omnivorous women. Accordingly, after defining and describing the menopausal transition, available research on variables associated with age at menopause will be reviewed, and the question of whether age at menopause differs between vegetarians and omnivores will be examined. The effect of plant components on menopausal symptoms will also be discussed.

A. Definition and Description

Research on the menopausal transition has been complicated by a lack of consistency in definitions. "Menopause" is not an event that occurs at a single point in time, but instead, is a complex endocrinological transition that occurs over a period of years.[71] The World Health Organization[72] defines the perimenopause as "the period immediately before the menopause (when the endocrinological, biological, and clinical features of approaching menopause commence) and the first year after menopause." "Menopause" is defined here as the final menstrual period, which can only be retrospectively assessed after 12 months without flow.[72] Because of the problems associated with this retrospective identification, and because hormonal changes continue during the year after the last period occurs, menopause has also been defined as beginning when a year without flow has elapsed.[71]

The entire transition may occur over a period of up to 6 years, and has been described as occurring in five phases.[71] In the first and second phases, menstrual cycles are regular but may have ovulatory disturbances, may be shorter than normal for a given woman, and may occur with either normal or increased flow. Premenstrual symptoms increase, with increased breast symptoms, cramping, and headaches. At this time, vasomotor symptoms first appear, usually as early morning night sweats at mid-cycle or before the onset of flow. FSH levels are normal or intermittently elevated, and estradiol levels may be moderately elevated. During the third and fourth phases, cycles become irregular, first with alternating short and long cycles, and then progressing to more frequent periods of oligomenorrhea. Flow may be either very high or reduced, and this often alternates. Premenstrual symptoms decrease, but vasomotor symptoms intensify and occur more often during the daytime. FSH levels are persistently elevated, and estradiol levels alternate between normal and high. Finally, the last phase represents the 12 months after the last menstrual flow. Vasomotor symptoms often increase in frequency and intensity, but may disappear in some women who experienced them earlier. FSH remains high and estradiol levels decrease, but may be intermittently high.

B. Factors Associated with Age at Menopause

Epidemiological studies have assessed the impact of various factors on age at natural menopause, and it is important to review this literature briefly, especially since the potential exists for some of these variables to confound the assessment of differences between vegetarians and omnivores.

1. Reproductive Variables

a. Age at Menarche

Based on differences between populations in mean age at menarche and menopause, Frisch[73] postulated that an early menarche was associated with a later menopause, particularly among well-nourished populations. As discussed earlier, the age at menarche in well-nourished vegetarians appears similar to that of well-nourished omnivores, so differences in age at menopause between these groups are unlikely to be confounded by differences in age at menarche. Furthermore, data obtained from individual women, rather than populations, do not support Frisch's hypothesis. For example, no association between age at menarche and menopause was observed in a prospective study of 3756 Dutch women, categorized according to whether their menopause occurred early or late.[74] The mean age at menarche was 13.88 years in 1267 women who experienced an early menopause (mean = 45.0 years), very similar to the mean of 13.94 years in the 1144 women who experienced a late menopause (mean = 54.6 years). Similarly, age at menarche was not associated with age at menopause in Scottish and British women studied cross-sectionally.[75] Thus, an individual's age at menarche does not appear to influence her age at menopause.

b. Frequency of Ovulation

The oocyte depletion hypothesis for menopause suggests that differences in the rate of depletion of oocytes lead to differences in ovarian depletion and thus age at menopause.[76] Accordingly, factors that prevent ovulation, including oral contraceptive use, pregnancy, and lactation, would lead to a later age at menopause. Supportive evidence for this hypothesis is provided by observations of a later age at menopause in women who have used oral contraceptives,[66,74,77] and an earlier age in women who are nulliparous.[66,74,75,78] Also consistent with this hypothesis is the finding that women who reported a history of irregular menstrual cycles between the ages of 20 and 35 had a later age at menopause.[79]

2. Lifestyle Variables

a. Tobacco, Alcohol and Caffeine Use

Smoking is consistently associated with an earlier age at menopause, in both retrospective and prospective studies.[74,75,78-81] Data on other life-style practices are less consistent. For example, alcohol use was associated with a later age at menopause in a cross-sectional study of almost 1500 45–49-year-old Scottish and British women conducted by Torgerson et al.[75] These results were confirmed in a subsequent 2-year prospective follow-up of the 1227 women who were not menopausal during the original study.[81] Another 11-year prospective study of Danish women, however, found no association with alcohol use.[80] Similarly, consuming coffee was associated with a later age at menopause in a cross-sectional study of 4186 Japanese women,[78] but no associations were observed in the prospective Danish study.[80]

b. Dietary Practices

Few studies have related age at menopause with dietary differences. The cross-sectional study of Torgerson et al.[75] found that the Odds Ratio for being postmenopausal was 0.25 (95% CI 0.10–0.65) among women who ate meat or poultry once a day, relative to those who reported never eating meat or poultry (P < 0.01). However, in the follow-up study conducted 2 years later with the women who were initially premenopausal, no association was observed with meat intake. Compared with those who never ate meat, the Odds Ratio for being postmenopausal among those eating meat more than once a day was 1.07 (95% CI 0.94–1.22, P = 0.28).[81] In Nagata's cross-sectional study of Japanese women, intakes of soy products were significantly higher among postmenopausal than premenopausal women after controlling for age (P<0.001),[78] but this association has not been demonstrated in a prospective study.

3. Body Size Variables

Body size does not appear to be a significant determinant of age at menopause. No associations with BMI were detected in the cross-sectional study of Scottish and British women,[75] which also assessed self-reported body weight at ages 20, 30, and 40 years. Similarly, BMI did not differ between women who became menopausal or remained premenopausal in the 11-year prospective Danish study[80] or in the 7–9-year prospective study of 3756 Dutch women,[74] despite considerable variability in BMI among the samples. Although the cross-sectional Japanese study of Nagata et al. reported that mean BMI was significantly lower among postmenopausal women, the absolute difference was small (22.2 vs. 22.5 kg/m^2).[78]

In summary, although some associations with several different types of variables and age at menopause have been observed, in many cases these associations are inconsistent or weak. For example, the large prospective study of Dutch women assessed age at menarche, number of siblings, age at first childbirth, parity, BMI, smoking, oral contraceptive use and SES. For the total sample, the multiple regression model (including all variables) predicted only 2.3% of the variance in age at menopause.[74]

C. Studies of Age at Menopause in Vegetarians and Omnivores

Surprisingly few data are available comparing age at menopause between vegetarians and omnivores. One study, reported only in abstract form,[82] retrospectively compared age at menopause in 80 Seventh-Day Adventist lacto-ovo-vegetarians and 280 omnivores who were not Adventists. Median age at menopause was 48 years among vegetarians and 50 years among omnivores, a significant difference. The difference was not explained by smoking, since no Adventists smoked, by differences in body weight (mean BMI was higher among vegetarians), or by differences in other variables for which data were available. However, the abstract did not state whether oral contraceptive use had differed between groups. The data cited earlier on dietary practices (e.g., cross-sectional studies reporting that the use of meat was associated with later menopause and the use of soy products with earlier menopause) appear to provide weak support for this study's observation, but additional research is clearly warranted.

D. Can Plant Components Replace Hormone Therapy?

At the time of menopause, some women choose to take hormone therapy to reduce the severity of menopausal symptoms such as vaginal dryness, hot flushes, and mood swings.[83] Others, however, prefer not to use hormones, and seek dietary or herbal treatments for their symptoms. The use of hormones is also suggested to modulate the risk of several chronic diseases.[66] That topic, however, is beyond the scope of this review, which will focus on the effect of plant components on symptoms associated with the menopausal transition.

1. Phytoestrogens

It has been noted that menopausal symptoms appear to occur less frequently and less intensely in women from countries such as Japan and China.[68-70] Because phytoestrogen-rich soy products are dietary staples in these areas, it has been speculated that the estrogenic actions of these compounds may explain the differences in menopausal symptomatology.

This hypothesis has been evaluated in several open trials with varying results. Brzezinski et al.[84] randomized symptomatic, early menopausal women to a phytoestrogen-rich diet that provided about 25% of daily calories as tofu, soy drink, miso, and flax seed (n = 78), or to maintain their usual omnivorous diets and avoid soy products and flax seed (n = 36). Measurements conducted at baseline and after 12 weeks on the diet included serum hormone and phytoestrogen levels and an assessment of the severity of menopausal symptoms (vaginal dryness, hot flushes, night sweats, palpitations, headache, depression, urinary discomfort, decreased libido, and insomnia). Serum phytoestrogen concentrations increased dramatically in the treatment group, confirming their adherence to the diet. In this open trial, menopausal symptom scores decreased substantially and similarly in both groups, from 10.65 ± 0.60 to 5.31 ± 0.45 in the treatment group, and from 9.23 ± 0.87 to 4.79 ± 0.71 in the control group. When symptoms were analyzed separately, however, the treatment group had greater decreases in the hot flushes and vaginal dryness scores.

In another open trial, Baird et al.[85] compared the responses of women at least 2 years postmenopause to a control (usual) diet (n = 25), and to a soy diet in which approximately 33% of energy was provided as soy products (n = 66). Urinary phytoestrogens were monitored, and the vaginal maturation index was assessed as an index of estrogenicity. After 4 weeks on the diet, urinary phytoestrogen excretion had increased substantially (an average of more than 100-fold) in the soy group, but there was no significant difference in the maturation index between groups (P = 0.40). The authors suggest that more time might have been needed to detect differences.[85]

A randomized double-blind trial was conducted by Murkies et al.,[86] with outcome measurements that included the number of hot flushes, a subjective assessment of menopausal symptoms, and the vaginal maturation index. Postmenopausal women experiencing at least 14 hot flushes per week were randomized to diets supplemented with 45 g of either soy flour (n = 28) or wheat flour (n = 30) per day for a period of 12 weeks. Urinary phytoestrogen measurements substantially increased in women in the soy group. The number of hot flushes and the menopause symptom score improved significantly in both groups, and although the improvements were slightly greater in the soy group, there were no differences between treatment groups (P = 0.82 and P = 0.90 for hot flushes and symptom scores, respectively). The vaginal maturation index was unchanged in both groups.

A randomized, double-blind trial was also conducted by Albertazzi et al.[87] Postmenopausal women, experiencing at least seven moderate to severe hot flushes per day during the prestudy period, consumed 60 g isolated soy protein (n = 40) or 60 g casein placebo (n = 39) daily for 12 weeks. In addition to recording the number of hot flushes, they completed an index that scored the severity of a variety of menopausal complaints (hot flushes, abnormal sensations such as numbness, prickling or tingling, insomnia, nervousness, depression, balance disturbances, weakness, joint pain, headaches, and palpitations). The number of hot flushes decreased significantly in both groups: at 12 weeks, there was a 45% decrease in the soy group, compared with a 30% reduction in the placebo group. The reduction in hot flushes was significantly greater in the soy group, but no improvements or differences between groups were noted in the menopausal index scores.[87] Moreover, the decrease in hot flushes did not correlate with the increase in serum or urine phytoestrogen levels.[88]

A number of trials that may provide more definitive results are currently under way in this area. Presently, however, it appears that there is a substantial placebo response to interventions. Although modest differential effects of soy phytoestrogens may exist for hot flushes, other menopausal symptoms do not appear to be affected.

2. Herbal Remedies

In addition to phytoestrogens, various herbal preparations have been used by women to relieve menopausal symptoms.[89] Although little systematic research has been conducted in North America, in other parts of the world, herbal remedies are more widely recognized. The best available data on safety and efficacy is probably produced by Germany's Commission E, which was established in 1978 to review more than 1400 herbal drugs. Commission E has recognized eight herbal remedies as being effective for various menopausal symptoms: balm, black cohosh, chasteberry, gingko, ginseng, passion flower, St. John's wort and valerian.[89] In some cases, however, the Commission placed caveats on the use of these remedies, such as limiting ginseng use to no more than 3 months or black cohosh to no more than 6 months. Other herbal remedies recommended in the lay press for the treatment of menopausal symptoms may be dangerous: for example, scullcap and life root have been found to be hepatotoxic, and dong quai to contain a carcinogen.[89] Once again, additional placebo-controlled research is warranted.

V. SUMMARY AND CONCLUSIONS

The purpose of this chapter was to assess the adequacy of vegetarian diets in maintaining normal reproductive function in women throughout their life-span. Taken together, the available data suggest few, if any, differences in reproductive function between vegetarians and omnivores, although several questions remain unanswered.

Based on the literature available, the following conclusions can be reached:

1. Provided that adequate energy is available to support normal growth, vegetarian diets do not appear to affect the pubertal transition, particularly as reflected by the age at menarche.
2. Whether vegetarian women experience a higher frequency of menstrual disturbances during adult life requires additional study:
    a. Early studies suggesting that menstrual disturbances were more common among vegetarians, were generally not designed to assess this question, and were not adequately controlled.
    b. Available data on the impact of dietary components such as phytoestrogens, fiber, and fat, intakes of which may differ between vegetarians and non-vegetarians, are not consistent.
    c. The motivation for adopting a vegetarian diet may be important, as some women may become vegetarian in the process of developing an eating disorder, with attendant menstrual disturbances. Furthermore, high levels of cognitive dietary restraint are associated with subclinical menstrual disturbances. Accordingly, the subpopulation of women who become vegetarian for reasons related to body weight issues may be at increased risk.

d. Nevertheless, in a sample of carefully screened vegetarian and non-vegetarian women, subclinical menstrual disturbances were not more common among vegetarians.

3. Almost no data are available to determine whether age at menopause differs between vegetarians and omnivores. This area requires additional study.

4. Soy phytoestrogens may reduce the frequency of menopausal hot flushes slightly in comparison to placebo, but do not appear to affect the severity of other menopausal symptoms.

REFERENCES

1. Tanner, J. M. *Growth at Adolescence.* 2nd ed., Oxford, Blackwell Scientific Publications, 1962.
2. Emans, S. J. Menarche and beyond — do eating and exercise make a difference? *Pediatr. Ann.*, 26(2): S137, 1997.
3. Apter, D. Development of the hypothalamic-pituitary-ovarian axis. *Ann. NY Acad. Sci.*, 816: 9, 1997.
4. Wildt, L., Marshall, G., and Knobil, E. Experimental induction of puberty in the infantile female rhesus monkey. *Science*, 207: 1373, 1980.
5. Marshall, J. C. and Kelch, R. P. Low dose pulsatile gonadotropin-releasing hormone in anorexia nervosa: a model for human pubertal development. *J. Clin. Endocrin. & Metab.*, 49: 712, 1979.
6. Cameron, J. L. Nutritional determinants of puberty. *Nutr. Rev.*, 52(2): S17, 1996.
7. Bongaarts, J. Does malnutrition affect fecundity? A summary of evidence. *Science*, 208: 564, 1980.
8. Frisch, R. E. and McArthur, J. W. Menstrual cycles: fatness as a determinant of minimum weight for height necessary for their maintenance or onset. *Science*, 185: 949, 1974.
9. Frisch, R. E. Weight at menarche: similarity for well-nourished and undernourished girls at differing ages, and evidence for historical constancy. *Pediatrics*, 50(3): 445, 1972.
10. Zacharias, L., Rand, W. M., and Wurtman R. J. A prospective study of sexual development and growth in American girls: the statistics of menarche. *Obstet. Gynecol. Survey*, 31(4): 325, 1976.
11. Sanchez, A., Kissinger, D. G., and Phillips, R. I. A hypothesis on the etiological role of diet on age of menarche. *Medical Hypotheses*, 7: 1339, 1981.
12. Frisch, R. E., Hegsted, D. M., and Yoshinga, K. Carcass components at first estrus of rats on high-fat and low-fat diets: body water, protein, and fat. *Prod. Nat. Acad. Sci. USA*, 74: 379, 1977.
13. Kralj-Cercek, L. The influence of food, body build, and social origin on the age at menarche. *Hum. Biol.*, 28(4): 393, 1956.
14. Burrell, R. J. W., Healy, M. J. R., and Tanner, J. M. Age at menarche in South African Bantu schoolgirls living in the Transkei reserve. *Human Biol.*, 33: 250, 1961.
15. Moisan, J., Meyer, F., and Gingras, S. Diet and age at menarche. *Cancer Causes and Control*, 1: 149, 1990.

16. Maclure, M., Travis, L. B., Willett, W., and MacMahon, B. A prospective cohort study of nutrient intake and age at menarche. *Am. J. Clin. Nutr.*, 54: 649, 1991.

17. Persky, V. W., Chatterton, R. T., Van Horn, L. V., Grant, M. D., Langenberg, P., and Marvin, J. Hormone levels in vegetarian and non-vegetarian teenage girls: potential implications for breast cancer risk. *Cancer Res.*, 52(3): 578, 1992.

18. Hardinge, M. G., Sanchez, A., Waters, D., Ghale, M., Bartholomew, E., Yahiku, P., Hoehn, G., and Scharffenberg, J. A. Possible factors associated with the prevalence of acne vulgaris. *Federation Proc.*, 30: 300, 1971.

19. Roberts, D. F., Chinn, S., Girija, B., and Singh, H. D. A study of menarcheal age in India. *Ann. Human Biol.*, 4(2): 171, 1977.

20. Ghosh, D., Kochhar, K., and Khanna, S. D. The study of puberty and after in 557 Indian school girls at Poona. *J. Obstet. Gynecol. India*, 23: 716, 1973.

21. Fritz, M. C., and Speroff, L. Current concepts of the endocrine characteristics of normal menstrual function: the key to diagnosis and management of menstrual disorders. *Clin. Obstet. Gynecol.* 26: 647, 1983.

22. Vollman, R. F. *The Menstrual Cycle.* Philadelphia, W. B. Saunders, 1977.

23. Prior, J. C., Vigna, Y. M., Schechter, M. T., and Burgess, A. E. Spinal bone loss and ovulatory disturbances. *N. Eng. J. Med.*, 323: 1221, 1991.

24. Barr S. I., Janelle, K. C., and Prior, J. C. Vegetarian vs. non-vegetarian diets, dietary restraint, and subclinical ovulatory disturbances: prospective 6-mo study. *Am. J. Clin. Nutr.*, 60: 887, 1994.

25. De Souza, M. J., Miller, B. E., Loucks, A. B., Luciano, A. A., Pescatello, L. S., Campbell, C. G., and Lasley, B. L. High frequency of luteal phase deficiency and anovulation in recreational women runners: blunted elevation in follicle-stimulating hormone observed during luteal-follicular transition. *J. Clin. Endocrin. & Metab.*, 83: 4220, 1998.

26. Pettersson, F., Fries, H., and Nillius, S. J. Epidemiology of secondary amenorrhea. I. Incidence and prevalence rates. *Am. J. Obstet. Gynecol.*, 117: 80, 1973.

27. Singh, K. Menstrual disorders in college students. *Am. J. Obstet. Gynecol.*, 3: 299, 1981.

28. Schweiger, U., Laessle, R., Pfister, H., Hoehl, C., Schwingenschloegel, M., and Schweiger, M. Diet-induced menstrual irregularities: effects of age and weight loss. *Fertility and Sterility*, 48: 746, 1987.

29. Schweiger, U., Laessle, R., Schweigher, M., Herrmann, F., Riedel, W., and Pirke, K.-M. Caloric intake, stress and menstrual function in athletes. *Fertility and Sterility*, 49: 447, 1988.

30. Loucks, A. B., and Heath, E. M. Dietary restriction reduces luteinizing hormone (LH) pulse frequency during waking hours and increases LH pulse amplitude during sleep in young menstruating women. *J. Clin. Endocrin. & Metab.*, 78: 910, 1994.

31. Loucks, A. B., Verdun, M., and Heath, E. M. Low energy availability, not stress of exercise, alters LH pulsatility in young women. *J. Appl. Physiol.*, 84: 37, 1998.

32. Rogers, J. and Mitchell, J. W. The relationship of obesity to menstrual disturbances. *N. Eng. J. Med.*, 247: 53, 1952.

33. Pasquali, R. and Casimirri, F. The impact of obesity on hyperandrogenism and polycystic ovary syndrome in premenopausal women. *Clin. Endocrin. (Oxford)* 39: 1, 1993.

34. Guzick, D. S., Wing, R., Smith, D., Berga, S. L., and Winters, S. J. Endocrine consequences of weight loss in obese, hyperandrogenic, anovulatory women. *Fertility and Sterility*, 61: 598, 1994.
35. Clark, A., M., Ledger, W., Galletly, C., Tomlinson, L., Blaney, F., Wang, X., and Norman, R. J. Weight loss results in significant improvement in pregnancy and ovulation rates in anovulatory obese women. *Human Reproduction*, 10: 2705, 1995.
36. Jones, D., Judd, J., Taylor, P., Campbell, W., and Nair, P. Influence of dietary fat on menstrual cycle and menses length. *Human Nutr. Clin. Nutr.*, 41C: 341, 1987.
37. Reichman, M. E., Judd, J. T., Taylor, P. R., Nair, P. P., Jones, Y., and Campbell, W. S. Effect of dietary fat on length of the follicular phase of the menstrual cycle in a controlled diet setting. *J. Clin. Endocrin. & Metab.*, 74: 1171, 1992.
38. Hagerty, M. A., Howie, J., Tan, S., and Shultz, T. D. Effect of low- and high-fat intakes on the hormonal milieu of premenopausal women. *Am. J. Clin. Nutr.*, 47: 653, 1988.
39. Rose, D. P., Boyar, A. P., Cohen, C., and Strong, L. E. Effect of a low-fat diet on hormone levels in women with cystic breast disease. I. Serum steroids and gonadotropins. *J. Natl. Cancer Inst.*, 78: 623, 1987.
40. Rose, D. P., Goldman, M., Connolly, J. M., and Strong, L. E. High-fiber diet reduces serum estrogen concentrations in premenopausal women. *Am. J. Clin. Nutr.*, 54: 520, 1991.
41. Woods, M. N., Gorbach, S. L., Longcope, C., Goldin, B. R., Dwyer, J. T., and Morrill-LaBrode, A. Low-fat, high-fiber diet and serum estrone sulfate in premenopausal women. *Am. J. Clin. Nutr.*, 49: 1179, 1989.
42. Goldin, B. R., Woods, M. N., Spiegelman, D. L., Longcope, C., Morrill-LaBrode, A., Dwyer, J. T., Gualtieri, L. J., Hertzmark, E., and Gorbach, S. L. The effect of dietary fat and fiber on serum estrogen concentrations in premenopausal women under controlled dietary conditions. *Cancer* 74: 1125, 1994.
43. Hill, P. B., Barbaczewski, L., Haley, N., and Wynder, E. L. Diet and follicular development. *Am. J. Clin. Nutr.*, 39: 771, 1984.
44. Hill, P. B., Garbaczewski, L., Daynes, G., and Gaire, K. S. Gonadotrophin release and meat consumption in vegetarian women. *Am. J. Clin. Nutr.*, 43: 37, 1986.
45. Phipps, W. R., Martini, M. C., Lampe, J. W., Slavin, J. L., and Kurzer, M. S. Effect of flax seed ingestion on the menstrual cycle. *J. Clin. Endocrin. & Metab.*, 77: 1215, 1993.
46. Cassidy, A., Bingham, S., and Setchell, K. D. Biological effects of a diet of soy products rich in isoflavones on the menstrual cycle of premenopausal women. *Am. J. Clin. Nutr.*, 60: 333, 1994.
47. Cassidy, A., Bingham, S., and Setchell, K. Biological effects of isoflavones in young women: importance of the chemical composition of soyabean products. *Br. J. Nutr.*, 74: 587, 1995.
48. Lu, L.-J. W., Anderson, K. E., Grady, J. J., and Nagamani, M. Effects of soya consumption for 1 month on steroid hormones in premenopausal women: implications for breast cancer risk reduction. *Cancer Epidemiology, Biomarkers and Prevention*, 5: 63, 1996.

49. Nagata, C., Kabuto, M., Kurisu, Y., and Shimizu, H. Decreased serum estradiol concentration associated with high dietary intake of soy products in premenopausal Japanese women. *Nutrition and Cancer*, 29: 228, 1997.

50. Janelle, K. C. and Barr, S. I. Nutrient intakes and eating behavior scores of vegetarian and non-vegetarian women. *J. Am. Dietetic Assoc.*, 95: 180, 1995.

51. Harlow, S. D. and Matanoski, G. M. The association between weight, physical activity, and stress and variation in the length of the menstrual cycle. *Am. J. Epidemiol.*, 133: 38, 1991.

52. Stunkard, A. J. and Messick, S. The three-factor eating questionnaire to measure dietary restraint, disinhibition and hunger. *J. Psychosomatic Res.*, 29: 71, 1985.

53. Tepper, B. J., Trail, A. C., and Shaffer, S. E. Diet and physical activity in restrained eaters. *Appetite*, 27: 51, 1996.

54. Schweiger, U., Tuschl, R. J., Platte, P., Broocks, A., Laessle, R. G., and Pirke, K.-M. Everyday eating behavior and menstrual function in young women. *Fertility and Sterility*, 57: 771, 1992.

55. Barr, S. I., Prior, J. C., and Vigna, Y. M. Restrained eating and ovulatory disturbances: possible implications for bone health. *Am. J. Clin. Nutr.*, 59: 92, 1994.

56. Barbarino, A., De Marinis, L., Tofani, A., Della Casa, S., D'Amico, C., Mancini, A., Corsello, S. M., Sciuto, R., and Barini, A. Corticotropin-releasing hormone inhibition of gonadotropin release and the effect of opiate blockade. *J. Clin. Endocrin. & Metab.*, 68: 523, 1989.

57. Bakan, R., Birmingham, C. L., Aeberhardt, L., and Goldner, E. M. Dietary zinc intake of vegetarian and non-vegetarian patients with anorexia nervosa. *Int. J. Eating Disorders*, 13: 229, 1993.

58. O'Connor, A. M., Touyz, S. W., Dunn, S. M., and Beumont, P. J. Vegetarianism in anorexia nervosa? A review of 116 consecutive cases. *Med. J. Aus.* 147: 540, 1987.

59. Martins, Y., Pliner, P., and O'Connor, R. Restrained eating among vegetarians: does a vegetarian eating style mask concerns about weight? *Appetite*, 32: 145, 1999.

60. Brooks, S. M., Sanborn, C. F., Albrecht, B. H., and Wagner, W. W. Jr. Diet in athletic amenorrhoea. *Lancet*, 1: 559, 1984.

61. Slavin, J., Lutter, J., and Cushman, S. Amenorrhoea in vegetarian athletes. *Lancet* 1: 1474, 1984.

62. Pirke, K. M., Schweiger, U., Laessle, R., Dickhaut, B., Schweiger, M., and Waechtler, M. Dieting influences the menstrual cycle: vegetarian vs. non-vegetarian diet. *Fertility and Sterility*, 46: 1083, 1986.

63. Pedersen, A. B., Bartholomew, M. J., Dolence, L. A., Aljadir, L. P., Netteburg, K. L., and Lloyd, T. Menstrual differences due to vegetarian and non-vegetarian diets. *Am. J. Clin. Nutr.*, 53: 879, 1991.

64. Lloyd, T., Schaeffer, J. M., Walker, M. A., and Demers, L. M. Urinary hormonal concentrations and spinal bone densities of premenopausal vegetarian and non-vegetarian women. *Am. J. Clin. Nutr.*, 54: 1005, 1991.

65. Prior, J. C., Vigna, Y. M., Schulzer, M., Hall, J. E., and Bonen, A. Determination of luteal phase length by quantitative basal temperature methods: validation against the midcycle LH peak. *Clin. Invest. Med.*, 13: 123, 1990.

66. Sowers, M. R. and La Pietra, M. T. Menopause: its epidemiology and potential association with chronic diseases. *Epidemiol. Rev.*, 17: 287, 1995.

67. Sturdee, D. W. Clinical symptoms of estrogen deficiency. *Current Obstet. Gynecol.*, 7: 190, 1997.
68. Lock, M. Ambiguities of aging: Japanese experience and perceptions of menopause. *Culture Med. & Psych.*, 10:23, 1986.
69. Adlercreutz, H., Hamalainen, E., Gorbach, S., and Goldin, B. Dietary phyto-oestrogens and the menopause in Japan. *Lancet*, 339: 1233, 1992.
70. Lock, M. Contested meanings of the menopause. *Lancet*, 337: 1270, 1991.
71. Prior, J. C. Perimenopause: the complex endocrinology of the menopausal transition. *Endocrine Rev.*, 19(4): 397, 1998.
72. WHO Scientific Group. Research on the menopause in the 1990s. A report of the WHO Scientific Group, World Health Organization, Geneva, Switzerland, volume 866: 1, 1996.
73. Frisch, R. E. Body fat, menarche, fitness and fertility. *Human Reproduction*, 2: 521, 1987.
74. Van Noord, P. A. H., Boersma, H., Dubas, J. S., te Velde, E., and Dorland, M. Age at natural menopause in a population-based screening cohort: the role of menarche, fecundity, and lifestyle factors. *Fertility and Sterility*, 68: 95, 1997.
75. Torgerson, D. J., Avenell, A., Russell, I. T., and Reid, D. M. Factors associated with onset of menopause in women aged 45–49. *Maturitas*, 19: 83, 1994.
76. Gougeon, A. Regulation of ovarian follicular development in primates: facts and hypotheses. *Endocrine Rev.*, 17: 121, 1996.
77. Stanford, J. L., Hartge, P., Brinton, L. A., Hoover, R. N., and Brookmeyer, R. Factors influencing the age at natural menopause. *J. Chronic Dis.*, 40: 995, 1987.
78. Nagata, C., Takatsuka, N., Inaba, S., Kawakami, N., and Shimizu, H. Association of diet and other lifestyle with onset of menopause in Japanese women. *Maturitas*, 29: 105, 1998.
79. Bromberger, J. T., Matthews, K. A., Kuller, L. H., Wing, R. R., Meilahn, E. N., and Plantinga, P. Prospective study of the determinants of age at menopause. *Am. J. Epidemiol.*, 145: 124, 1997.
80. Nilsson, P., Moller, L., Koster, A., and Hollnagel, H. Social and biological predictors of early menopause: a model for premature aging. *J. Intern. Med.*, 242: 299, 1997.
81. Torgerson, D. J., Thomas, R. E., Campbell, M. K., and Reid, D. M. Alcohol consumption and age of maternal menopause are associated with menopause onset. *Maturitas*, 26: 21, 1997.
82. Baird, D. D., Tylavsky, F. A., and Anderson, J. J. B. Do vegetarians have earlier menopause? *Am. J. Epidemiol.*, 128: 907, 1988.
83. Belchetz, P. Hormonal treatment of postmenopausal women. *N. Eng. J. Med.*, 330: 1062, 1994.
84. Brzezinski, A., Adlercreutz, H., Shaol, R., Rosler, A., Shmueli, A., Tanos, B., and Schenker, J. G. Short-term effects of phytoestrogen-rich diet on postmenopausal women. *Menopause*, 4: 89, 1997.
85. Baird, D. D., Umbach, D. M., Lansdell, L., Hughes, C. L., Setchell, K. D. R., Weinberg, C. R., Haney, A. F., Wilcox, A. J., and McLachlan, J. A. Dietary intervention study to assess estrogenicity of dietary soy among postmenopausal women. *J. Clin. Endocrin. & Metab.*, 80: 1685, 1995.
86. Murkies, A. L., Lombard, C., Strauss, B. J. G., Wilcox, G., Burger, H. G., and Morton, M. S. Dietary flour supplementation decreases post-menopausal hot flushes: effect of soy and wheat. *Maturitas*, 21: 189, 1995.

87. Albertazzi, P., Pansini, F., Bonaccorsi, G., Zanotti, L., Forini, E., and De Alyosio, D. The effect of dietary soy supplementation on hot flushes. *Obstet. Gynecol.*, 91: 6, 1998.
88. Albertazzi, P., Pansini, F., Bottazzi, M., Bonaccorsi, G., De Aloysio, D., and Morton, M.S. Dietary soy supplementation and phytoestrogen levels. *Obstet. Gynecol.*, 94: 229, 1999.
89. Israel, D. and Youngkin, E.Q. Herbal therapies for perimenopausal and menopausal complaints. *Pharmacotherapy*, 17(5): 970, 1997.

11

A VEGETARIAN DIET: HEALTH ADVANTAGES FOR THE ELDERLY

Richard W. Hubbard and Elaine Fleming

CONTENTS

I. INTRODUCTION

The most rapidly growing population group in the United States of America consists of people more than 85 years of age.[1] The number of people over 65 years of age has also significantly increased since 1900. This trend has been even more pronounced since 1980, so that by the year 2000,

0-8493-8508-3/01/$0.00+$.50
© 2001 by CRC Press LLC

some 38 million people are over the age of 65. Actual evidence that improved nutritional status contributes to an increased life span in humans is difficult, at best, to prove. However, it would appear that improved nutrition is a contributing factor to the increased number of people who have approached the maximum life span, as well as the improved life expectancy of the general population. Increased life expectancy began with the decline in infant and child mortality in the 20th century with a doubling of survival of infants to celebrate their first birthday, and the elimination of many childhood diseases. In addition, readily available food supplies and improved medical technology have allowed more people to reach the age of 65.

A medical challenge of today is to overcome the barriers preventing the majority from attaining a potential life span of 120 years.[2] This chapter summarizes evidence that supports the concept that mortality rates from nearly all causes of death can be reduced by the vegetarian diet. To attain maximum life span, dietary changes away from the Western omnivore diet will be the major part of this attainment. Indeed, in spite of high technology, chronic degenerative diseases remain firmly entrenched in our world. The omnivore diet appears to be the major reason for more than half of the leading causes of death in the U.S. and the northern European countries.[3]

Minimizing aging is of interest to all ages, for the young to maintain their youth, then for the elderly to reduce the rate of aging. It has been 40 years since aging studies embraced the free radical theory and the human bodies redox balance state.[4] The use of supplemental antioxidants has resulted in extending the mean life span of experimental rats.[5] Cellular activity at the mitochondrial level must be maximal to markedly improve mitochondrial electron transport complex activity.[6] A thiol donor, such as N-acetylcysteine or other specialized compounds, appears to be necessary to directly build up supplies of glutathione, the main redox-controlling compound in the mitochondria.[7]

Living vertebrates require a continuous dietary source of antioxidants. In human subjects, these would have to come from the regular intake of multiple helpings of fruits, vegetables, and certain mineral supplements. Actual data of plasma antioxidant increase ($p < 0.05$) from foods was demonstrated by adding 10 servings of fruit and vegetables for a 15-day period, which increased plasma antioxidant levels of subjects on a omnivore diet.[8] Oxygen radical absorptive capacity (ORAC) plus alpha-tocopherol concentrations provided the antioxidant values. Mean values from day one to 16 in ORAC units were statistically significant at the $p < 0.0005$ level. Interestingly, the group of 60- to 80-year-old subjects had significantly greater ($p < 0.01$) alpha-tocopherol levels both before and after the study period compared with those in the 20 to 40 age group.[8] Indeed, the high correlation between elevated antioxidant levels and older aged subjects is shown by Mecocci et al.,[9] whose work indicated that centenarians had higher vitamin A and E levels (p < 0.0001) and higher enzymatic antioxidant activity than younger subjects.

II. PROTEIN DIFFERENCES BETWEEN OMNIVORES AND VEGETARIANS OR VEGANS

The recommended daily allowance for dietary protein intake appears to be the same for the elderly as for young adults, at 0.75 g/kg of body weight for both age groups.[10] This is surprising, because the protein content of the adult body diminishes with age, with apparent exchanges of fat for muscle. Changes in muscle mass are related to whole-body protein turnover and changes in the rate of protein synthesis. The recent work by Campbell et al.,[11] recommends 1.0 gm/kg of protein daily to maintain nitrogen balance in the elderly. Stressful physical and psychological stimuli in the elderly can induce a negative nitrogen balance.

The percentage of calories contributed by protein in human diets, from vegan to omnivore, can vary from 8 to 18%, with approximately 2 to 10% greater intake of protein by the omnivore subjects vs. the vegetarians. The lowest level of protein intake is in vegans.[12] Animal protein is considerably higher in essential amino acids and sulfur amino acid content and promotes a higher rate of growth in a growing animal than will any single dietary plant protein. When two or more dietary plant proteins are combined in a single meal or meals for the day, however, this potential for growth difference is offset in growing children.[13,14]

The adult vegans in the Haddad et al. dietary study[15] had higher serum albumin levels than the omnivore controls, which demonstrated vegan dietary protein adequacy. The vegans demonstrated this while maintaining lower blood urea nitrogen values. Long term, this pattern aids in the reduction of the incidence of chronic renal failure.

Animal protein contains considerably more sulfur as methionine and cysteine. These amino acids cause a higher acid load with the omnivore diet, which appears to be partially retained as a major component of the pathogenesis of bone disease and muscle wasting in aging.[16] This helps to explain the improved mineral balance and skeletal metabolism in postmenopausal women treated orally with potassium-bicarbonate.[16] Also, lipid peroxidation is enhanced with decreasing extracellular pH. Acidic pH releases iron from "safe" binding sites where this free iron then enhances free radical activity.[17] Thus, the lower sulfur and phosphorus intake on an all-plant diet appears to provide a significant longevity advantage for elderly subjects.

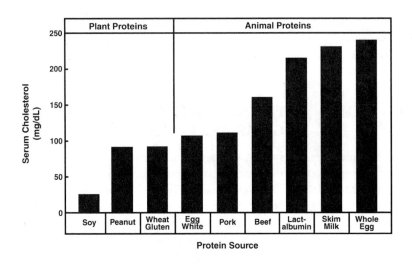

Figure 11.1 Serum cholesterol is lower in rabbits fed plant proteins compared with animal proteins. Adapted from Sanchez and Hubbard.[19]

Additional advantages from the decrease or elimination of animal protein for the elderly can be seen in the lower serum lipid levels of vegetarians or vegans. The type of dietary protein, animal or plant, is the primary factor in the effect of proteins on serum cholesterol levels. Thus, the amino acid composition of the protein is a controlling factor for serum cholesterol levels.[19] Sixteen references in this cited paper indicate that the lysine:arginine ratio in proteins explains the effect of proteins on the level of serum cholesterol and, in turn, atherogenesis.[19] Figure 11.1 shows the relationship between animal and vegetable protein on serum cholesterol levels. Soy protein from the soybean is a plant protein source that has been successfully used in long-term studies to decrease the level of serum cholesterol in hypercholesterolemic subjects. A high saturated fat intake however, can mask the soy protein effect.[20] As the level of cholesterol in serum is decreased, the plasma levels of arginine, glycine, serine, and threonine are significantly increased while lysine, leucine, valine, phenylalanine, tyrosine, and histidine are decreased. In this regard, the index interpretation of the leucine:arginine ratio change appears to be similar and just as significant as the lysine:arginine ratio.[19]

Glucagon secretion responds to arginine levels.[21] The secretion of insulin is in response to leucine.[19,22] Massive doses of arginine, however, cause the secretion of both glucagon and insulin.[23] Following the feeding of soy protein, mild increases in plasma arginine levels and, in turn, mild increases in glucagon, inhibit HMG CoA reductase, the rate limiting enzyme

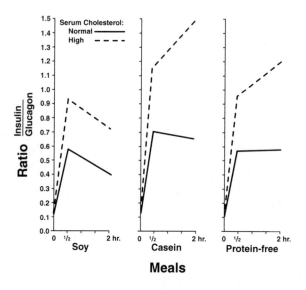

Figure 11.2   Plasma insulin/glucagon ratio in normocholesterolemic and hyper-cholesterolemic men after ingesting a single protein-free meal or one containing soy protein or casein. From Hubbard, et al.[26]

in cholesterol biosynthesis.[24] Leucine is a secretagogue of insulin[22] and insulin in turn activates HMG CoA reductase.[25]

Utilizing test meals containing animal protein as casein from cow's milk, and soy protein from the soybean, while keeping the lipid and carbohydrate in the test meals constant, demonstrated that normocholesterolemic vs. hypercholesterolemic subjects showed lower responses in insulin:glucagon ratios with both test meals. The soy protein significantly (p < 0.001) lowered this ratio in contrast to the effect of casein for the hypercholesterolemic subjects.[26] Figure 11.2 shows these differences plotted as the ratio of insulin:glucagon. High levels of insulin are recognized as a possible risk factor in coronary heart disease[27] and diabetes.[28] Recent reports suggest that Type 2 diabetes is probably preventable by reducing insulin secretion by the use of dietary plant protein during the growth and early adult years.[29] This, plus a consistent exercise program throughout life, is highly likely to protect the elderly from NIDDM.[30,31]

Increased thyroid activity is evident from the higher resting metabolic rate of vegans[32] and of the elevated thyrotropin levels in vegans.[33] This serves to explain why vegans are, on the average, leaner with lower body mass indexes (BMI).[32] Also, the immune status in vegans is elevated compared with omnivore subjects in terms of significantly elevated cytokine 2 and gamma interferon levels.[34]

Additionally, Parkinson patients also benefit from the low-leucine vegan diet because the low-leucine intake decreases the competition with their oral DOPA intake, so they can use lower amounts of DOPA medication to suppress their Parkinson disease symptoms without undesirable side effects from the higher DOPA intake.[35]

A recent complication in assessing the adequacy of dietary protein intake has been that a major proportion of our well-fed population demonstrates an inability to absorb dietary protein. This can be particularly severe in the elderly. Plasma amino acid patterns show an excess of alanine and urinary amino acids show low alanine, isoleucine, leucine, tyrosine, phenylalanine and lysine values.[36] This indicates Cori-cycle gluconeogenesis[37] or skeletal muscle breakdown, demonstrating inadequate protein intake related to decreased amino acid absorption from digested protein. Successful treatment of this condition with n-6 essential fatty acids from evening primrose oil or borage oil as a source of gamma-linolenic acid reduces or eliminates the evidence of skeletal muscle breakdown[36] with regain of lost weight. This topic is covered in more detail relative to fatty acids in the lipid section that follows. Obviously malnourished elderly subjects, of course, need to be treated promptly with protein and energy supplements to activate nitrogen kinetics.[38]

A varied diet based on plant proteins is adequate, yielding growth and body maintenance results equivalent to a diet based on meat protein.[39] The lower incidence of obesity, constipation, lung cancer, hypertension, coronary artery disease, type 2 diabetes, gallstones, reduced risk of breast cancer, diverticular disease, colon cancer, calcium kidney stones, and osteoporosis appear to be obvious advantages —particularly of the well balanced vegan diet — for the elderly.[3,39,40] Key et al.,[40] (Table 11.1) show the protective effect of daily fresh fruit intake in ischemic heart disease, cerebrovascular disease, and lung cancer, and daily raw salad protection for ischemic heart disease. They also presented a higher incidence of breast cancer in the vegetarian women, but the confidence interval was broad. The smokers in their study population demonstrated a higher rate of ischemic heart disease, cerebrovascular disease, and, of course, lung cancer, to emphasize the disease problems associated with smoking.

III. LIPID DIFFERENCES BETWEEN OMNIVORES AND VEGETARIAN OR VEGANS

The elderly vegetarian, particularly the elderly vegan, is in a protective life-style that minimizes ischemic damage, plaque formations, and lipid depositions involved in atherosclerotic disease, hypertension, stroke, or rheumatic heart disease. Plant dietary protein minimizes endogenous

Table 11.1 Mortality Ratios (95% Confidence Interval) for Smoking and Six Dietary Factors After Adjustment For Age and Sex and For Age, Sex and Smoking (4336 Men and 6435 Women)

Factor	All Cause Mortality Age and Sex	Ischemic Heart Disease Age and Sex	Cerebro-vascular Disease Age and Sex	Lung Cancer Age and Sex	Colorectal Cancer Age and Sex	Breast Cancer (Women) Age and Sex
Current Smoker	1.52 (1.34 to 1.73)**	1.43 (1.11 to 1.84)**	1.53 (1.02 to 2.20)*	5.43 (3.22 to 0.14)**	0.92 (0.45 to 1.87)	1.01 (0.50 to 2.02)
Pipe or cigars only	1.22 (0,96 to 1.55)	1.49 (1.02 to 2.18)*	1.44 (0.72 to 2.91)	1.96 (0.67 to 5.73)	0.72 (0.17 to 3.05)	*
1–14 cigarettes/day *	1.39 (1.15 to 1.69**	1.42 (0.97 to 2.09)	1/05 (0.53 to 2.06)	3.70 (1.68 to 8.15)**	1.21 (0.48 to 3.01)	1.25 (0.57 to 2.74)
15 cigarettes/day	2.00 (1.66 to 2.42)**	1.36 (0.87 to 2.12)	2.42 (1.36 to 4.31)**	11.28 (6.26 to 20.28)**	0.68 (0.17 to 2.79)	0.60 (0.16 to 2.30)
Vegetarian	0.98 (0.88 to 1.10)	0.82 (0.66 to 1.02)	0.91 (0.66 to 1.27)	0.79 (0.46 to 1.35)	0.79 (0.47 to 1.33)	1.64 (1.01 to 2.67)*
Whitemeal bread daily	0.83 (0.75 to 0.98)*	0.82 (0.66 to 1.02)	1.02 (0.72–145)	0.76 (0.45 to 1.28)	1.08 (0.63 to 1.86)	1.08 (0.65 to 1.81)
Bran cereals, daily	0.97 (0.86 to 1.10)	0.98 (0.78 to 1.24)	0.91 (0.63 to 1.31)	0.40 (0.19 to 0.84)*	1.05 (0.61 to 1.81)	0.68 (0.37 to 1.24)
Nuts or dried fruit	0.93 (0.83 to 1.04)	0.86 (0.79 to 1.07)	0.76 (0.54 to 1.06)	0.53 (0.29 to 0.95)	0.75 (0.44 to 1.27)	1.40)0.86 to 2.29)
Fresh fruit daily	0.74 (0.66 to 0.84)**	0.73 (0.58 to 0.93)**	0.63 (0.44 to 0.91)*	0.40 (0.24 to 0.68)**	0.73 (0.41 to 1.30)	0.75 (0.42 to 1.34)
Raw salad daily	0.87 (0.789 to 0.97)*	0.72 (0.58 to 0.89)**	1.15 (0.83 to 1.59)	0.67 (0.39 to 1.16)	0.79 (0.48 to 1.33)	1.15 (0.71 to 1.88)

*Two tailed p < 0.05, **p < 0.01. Categories: nonsmoker, pipe or cigars only; 1–14 cigarettes/day, ≥ 15 cigarettes/day, ***includes current cigarette smokers, (8 men and 13 women). **** The 33 women who smoked pipe or cigar only were included in the category 1–14 cigarettes/day along with the 13 women who did not declare how much they smoked. Adapted from Key, T.J.A., Thorogood, M., Appleby, P.N., and Burr, M.I. Dietary habits and mortality in 11,000 vegetarians and health conscious people: results of a 17-year follow up. *BMJ*, 313, 775, 1996. With permission from the BMJ Publishing Group.[40]

cholesterol and triacylglycerol production as previously discussed. Exogenous plant dietary fat supplies a dominance of unsaturated to saturated fatty acids to minimize not only the atherosclerotic diseases, but also several of the rheumatoid states, the mineral problems of osteoporosis, and possibly several types of cancer by the inclusion of polyunsaturated fatty acids (PUFA).[3,40,41] This protective diet combined with adequate exercise inhibits the initiation of these diseases before they reach the lipid deposition stages by decreasing the initial free radical attack with antioxidants. For example, in coronary artery disease (CAD), the vegetarian or vegan diet supplies the antioxidant vitamins and minerals from a high content of grains, fruits, vegetables, nuts, and seeds.[3,40,41] The high anti-oxidant intake of this diet for the elderly appears in detail in the accessory growth factor section that follows.

The dominance of unsaturated fat to saturated fat of the vegetarian diet lowers total cholesterol and LDL-C levels. The saturated fatty acids (SFA) lauric (C12:O), myristic (C14:O), and palmitic (C16:O) are very hypercholesterolemic. Palmitic acid is the dominant fatty acid synthesized in the human body from excess calories that are converted to fat.[42] Thus, the elderly vegetarian on a plant protein diet does not synthesize large amounts of palmitic acid. The SFA, stearic acid (C18:O), has no effect on blood lipoproteins and is considered neutral, with moderate amounts of dietary carbohydrate.[43] Of all the added dietary fats, the most hypercholesterolemic are palm-kernel, coconut, and palm oils, and butter. SFA raise LDL-C by decreasing LDL receptor synthesis and activity. All fatty acids will lower fasting triglycerides if they replace carbohydrates in the diet.[44] The most significant way to lower LDL-C and raise HDL is to replace carbohydrate with linoleic acid (C18:2), the predominant omega-6 polyunsaturated fatty acid (PUFA). This is most dominant on an all-plant diet where less than 30% of the kilocalories of the diet is fat, and one half to two thirds of that 30% are MUFA (monounsaturated fatty acid) and PUFA.[45] Decreasing SFA, however, is twice as effective in lowering serum cholesterol levels as increasing PUFA.[46] The PUFA:saturated fat ratio average is approximately 0.64 in the omnivore population, and 1.36 with a vegan population.[47–49]

Mediterranean-type diets have significant health benefits, supposedly because of the MUFA, namely oleic acid, in olive oil. MUFA substitution for SFA in diets of 23 healthy Northern European males significantly lowered LDL cholesterol concentrations ($p = 0.01$) along with postprandial factor VII activation, but postprandial triacylglycerols were significantly greater ($p = 0.003$).[50] A similar study of Southern Europeans[51] showed plasma triacylglycerol concentrations were much greater during the early postprandial phase and returned to near-fasting concentrations much earlier than in the Northern Europeans.[50] Diets high in olive oil appear to promote gastrointestinal secretions and stimulate stomach emptying, which could translate to faster lipid absorption.[52] The previous higher exposure to olive oil by the Southern Europeans may, however, invalidate the short period of 6 to 8 weeks of these experiments.[51] When omega-3 fatty acid supplements are added to an olive oil regimen, the triacylglyerols can be significantly lowered.[53]

The phyto-compounds in olive oil may also play a role in decreased platelet aggregation. A study comparing the effects of two monounsaturated fatty acid-rich oils, extra virgin olive oil (EVOO) and high oleic sunflower oil (HOSO), compared platelet aggregation in 14 postmenopausal women in their 60s who all had high-fat dietary intake habits. Both oils had approximately 76% oleic acid, but the content of palmitic and linoleic acids and other minor constituents were significantly different. These oils were used as the only culinary fats during two 28-day periods and represented approximately 62% of the total lipid intake (46% of total energy consumption). Other dietary components were very closely matched. Platelet aggregation was significantly lower after the EVOO diet than after HOSO (p < 0.05). Here, where every effort was made to have equal amounts of oleic acid between the EVOO and the HOSO diets, there was a significant difference in platelet aggregation values. The authors felt that other phyto-compounds present in the oils, aside from the fatty acids, probably played an important role in modulating platelet aggregation in this study.[54,55]

The PUFA are divided into omega-3, omega-6 and omega-9 groups. The omega-3 and omega-6 PUFA groups contain the two essential fatty acids — linoleic acid, an omega-6 fatty acid, and alpha-linolenic acid, an omega-3 fatty acid (Figure 11.3).[42] Underlying the necessity of meeting the alpha-linolenic acid requirement are the demonstrated effects of omega-3 fatty acids in suppressing carcinogenesis, allergic hyperactivity, thrombotic tendency, apoplexy, hypertension, hypertriglyceridemia, and aging in animals. The suppression of allergic hyperactivity is a suppression of the immune system, particularly marked with fish oils as the source of the omega-3 fatty acids, as a combination of alpha-linolenic, eicosapentaenoic (EPA) and docosapentaenoic acids (DHA) fatty acids.[56] Fish oils can improve the conditions of patients involved in overactive immune responses, particularly rheumatoid arthritis.[57] Overall, omega-3 fatty acids are protective against the lipid peroxide insult in aging, carcinogenesis, and chronic diseases. An equal or marginal excess of omega-6 to omega-3 fatty acid intake is recommended.[58] An excess of omega-3 to omega-6 in dietary intake decreases the phospholipid content of omega-6 fatty acids with a rapid responsive exchange in cell membrane phospholipid fatty acid content.[59]

Well-known plant sources of alpha-linolenic acid, the shortest of the omega-3 fatty acids, are the oils of canola, flaxseed, walnut, and soy. Animal sources for alpha-linolenic acid are fish and seal oils, which also contain significant amounts of EPA and DHA. Dietary inclusion of alpha-linolenic acid can provide excellent therapeutic properties to lower elevated body triacylglycerol levels. Large doses of alpha-linolenic acid over months, particularly from fish oils, significantly increases bleeding time, somewhat akin to taking several aspirin tablets per day.[60] Marine-origin omega-3 fatty acids lower systolic blood pressure and triacylglycerols, but raise LDL cholesterol, while plant source alpha-linolenic, also an omega-3 fatty acid, has no effect on LDL.[61] The essential fatty acids — gamma-linolenic acid (GLA), an omega-6 fatty acid, and EPA, an omega-3 fatty acid — have strong anticarcinogenic properties.[62]

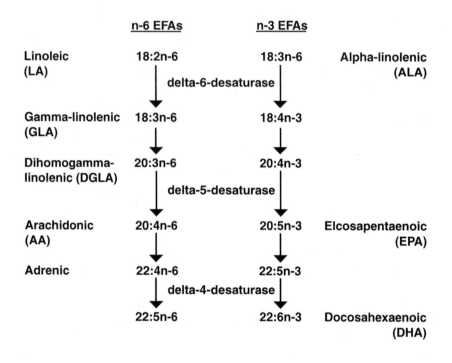

Figure 11.3 Outline of the metabolism of the omega-6 and omega-3 essential fatty acid series. Adapted from Horribin.[72]

IV. TRANS FATTY ACIDS

Elderly vegetarians will probably receive an adequate amount of omega-3 fatty acids in their diet, and the omega-6 fatty acid supply as LA will be high enough to sustain as high as a 20:1 or more of omega-6/omega 3 fatty acid ratio.[62] The ratio should ideally be at 3:1 or lower. The ability of the LA to convert to gamma-linolenic acid may, however, be blocked by a common dietary component used freely in processed foods, namely hydrogenated oils. Hydrogenated oils or partially hydrogenated oils contain the unnatural trans fatty acids (TFA). The cis fatty acid form is the natural fatty acid. These TFA can impair biosynthesis of long-chain polyunsaturated fatty acids, in turn impairing maintenance and synthesis of a variety of body skeletal protein.[62,63] Dietary TFA and also the adipose stored TFA are a major factor in a variety of diet-caused chronic degenerative diseases. Indeed, there is a strong association of data that TFA are stored in adipose tissue and that this is a causal factor in postmenopausal breast cancer.[63,64] Also, trans monounsaturated fatty acids increase LDL and decrease HDL cholesterol levels,[64,65] indicating increased risk of CHD after adjustment for age and total energy intake; the intake of trans isomers of fatty acids were directly related to risk of CHD.[65,66] It has been proposed that dietary TFA found in partially hydrogenated fats impair lipoprotein receptors during energy demands, leading to hypercholesterolemia, atherogenesis, obesity, and insulin resistance.[66,67]

The impact of dietary TFA in adult onset diabetic subjects, where lipid metabolism is impaired by the diabetic state, is further impaired by these abnormal dietary fatty acids.[67,68] The studies of Horrobin,[69] express the previously known[62] impaired biosynthesis of gamma-linolenic acid from linoleic acid, due to the disruption of delta-6-desaturase, which was shown to be a slow and rate-limiting enzyme. The direct effect of hydrogenated oils to decrease delta-6-desaturase activity is particularly emphasized by the work of Mahfouz et al.,[70] and, more recently, by Wahle and James.[71]

Horrobin's work related to gamma-linolenic acid supplementation, using evening primrose oil as a therapeutic source for this fatty acid,[72] emphasizes the effectiveness of such treatment for atopic eczema, diabetic neuropathy, rheumatoid arthritis, and other forms of inflammation, systemic sclerosis, gastrointestinal disorders, viral infections, and post-viral fatigue syndrome, endometriosis, schizophrenia, alcoholism, Alzheimer's disease, and other forms of dementia, cardiovascular disease, renal disease, cancer, and liver disease. Our own work[36] has shown the treatment efficacy of evening primrose oil (EPO) for children with untreatable seizures, adults with chronic fatigue syndrome and multiple sclerosis (MS), and the elderly with failure to maintain their body weight and energy levels. Swank,[73] studying multiple sclerosis, came to the same conclusions for treating MS patients, namely using EPO and a vegan diet with noteworthy remission results. Recent studies in elderly subjects on omnivore, vegetarian, or vegan diets have shown evidence of failure to thrive, as demonstrated by skeletal muscle breakdown, in 48 of 50 subjects, including some representatives of all three diet types.[74]

V.   CARBOHYDRATE DIFFERENCES BETWEEN OMNIVORES AND VEGETARIANS OR VEGANS

Starch or complex carbohydrates, and both soluble and insoluble fiber, are carbohydrate molecules made up of the monosaccharide glucose. Free sugars of glucose, fructose, and sucrose (a disaccharide made up of glucose and fructose), along with starch, are the main source of energy in human diets, accounting for some 40 to 80% of human energy intake.[75] In the starches and the fibers, the alpha- and beta-linkages at the glycoside carbon largely regulate whether the human digestive tract can digest them down to molecules of glucose. The indigestible carbohydrates are those that predominate with beta-linkages like the celluloses, and related polysaccharides (hemicelluloses, pectin, gums, and mucilages). These become the indigestible bulk of the stool. The free sugars of fruits are accompanied by protein, a small amount of lipid, minerals, a variety of accessory food factors including vitamins, and the soluble and insoluble fiber fraction.[76,77] Elderly vegetarians or vegans have a high amount of fiber as a natural part of their dietary intake. This contrasts to the omnivore diet, which is either deficient in fiber or requires fiber supplements to obtain adequate stool bulk.

Glucose is the major energy source for brain function. In the non-fed or fasting state, glucose levels are normally maintained from liver glycogen. In longer fasting periods or fasts combined with high-level energy expenditure, glucose levels are depleted and skeletal muscle breakdown occurs to supply glucose (gluconeogensis). Alanine, along with lactate and pyruvate, are released in high amounts to maintain blood glucose levels, and to supply pyruvate to the citric acid cycle to maintain energy levels.[37,77] In wasting disease, particularly in the elderly, this process can be fatal unless treated aggressively and early. Much of the literature on wasting disease and cachexia offers little or no real helpful therapy to supply a cure for the problem.[78] This wasting disease, with the inability to maintain muscle mass and normal energy levels, can often be treated with oral supplements of omega-6 source EPO, which contains gamma-linolenic acid as well as linoleic and oleic acids.[36] The wasting disease is insidious in its progression, with symptoms similar to numerous ailments. The gradual wasting process can suddenly become acute when it is accompanied by major stress. Weight and energy depletion may then become suddenly acute. This omega-6 deficiency plays no dietary category favorites, as our recent studies have found this disturbance in omnivores, LOVs, and vegans, who are all breaking down skeletal muscle at an accelerated rate.[74] A source of gamma linolenic acid, taken with meals at 2 to 2.5 gm per day, slowly brings the weight and energy back up to normal working levels.[36]

The mechanism of muscle wasting should be investigated, but no other effective way of improving nitrogen balance in a catabolic state has been demonstrated.[79] It appears that muscle degradation in wasting individuals is due to the lack of absorption of dietary protein to the point that the skeletal muscle breaks down to form glucose and the energy donating compounds of pyruvate and lactate directly feed the citric acid cycle. The lack of dietary protein absorption probably occurs because of the presence of interleukin-6 (IL-6). The lack of a controlling prostaglandin, most likely because of gamma-linolenic acid deficiency, appears to be the key for this lack of dietary protein absorption capability. The use of gamma-linolenic acid from EPO as a meal supplement reversed the wasting six subjects to weight-gain subjects in 6 weeks' to 6 months' time, with an increase in muscle mass and energy capability.[36] Gamma-linolenic acid is the product of the very fragile enzyme delta-6-desaturatase, which is subject to rate impairment from diene, but apparently not from monene trans fatty acids in the diet.[70]

Our observations of the incidence of involuntary weight loss find a higher incidence in the elderly. It can, however, be found at any age. Some glucose or related sugar should be a part of the diet to minimize the burning of fat to make glucose, since glucose is needed for brain energy. Increasing protein intake alone will not help. Sugar substitutes, such as aspartame, further complicate this energy problem as they lead to an excessive intake of aspartic acid from aspartame, a neuronal excitor that can be toxic for the tired or hypoxic brain.[80] The same is true for the use of glutamic acid as a flavor enhancer, commonly used as monosodium glutamate.

VI.   ACCESSORY GROWTH FACTORS

While the diet of an older vegetarian may not contain all nutrients in sufficient quantities, it does contain a greater dietary variety compared with those elderly subjects on the omnivore diet who appear to be lacking in many B vitamins and the antioxidant fat soluble vitamins.[81] However, there are two obvious exceptions to this generality for the vegetarian or vegan that deserve special emphasis.

The first of these is vitamin B_{12}, and the second is vitamin D, which acts as a hormone rather than a vitamin.[39] To provide the proper conditions for vitamin B_{12} absorption, the elderly vegetarian should be tested for adequate iron stores,[82] as prolonged iron deficiency damages the gastric mucosa and promotes gastric atrophy, including loss of gastric acid and intrinsic factor (IF), with diminished vitamin B_{12} absorption.[83] It is highly recommended that screening should be done every 5 years beginning at the age of 55 because there is a gradual loss of absorbance capability of vitamin B_{12} in a genetic- and age-related pattern. In particular, the measurement of holotranscobalamin II (holoTCII) is a measure of inadequate vitamin B_{12} delivery to cells that synthesize DNA. This can show a low or partially deficient total serum vitamin B_{12} level before clinical symptoms ever occur.[84,85] Active vitamin B_{12} can be destroyed by megadoses of vitamin C. This is particularly true in the presence of high serum iron values, where iron plus high vitamin C levels become an iron-catalyzed free radical species that can attack vitamin B_{12} and IF.[84] The use of serum homocysteine levels to predict vitamin B_{12} deficiency appears to be adequate but it must be remembered that folic acid deficiency also elevates homocysteine levels.

Vitamin D is actually not a vitamin at all, but a vital hormone of our endocrine system.[86] Supplementation of vitamin D has been practiced in the American milk supply for more than a half century. Humans can usually synthesize vitamin D by the action of UV light from the sun on the skin.[87] Around the age of 60, however, the capacity of the skin to synthesize vitamin D decreases to about 25% of its capacity at age 40.[88] Recognition of this possible vitamin D deficiency has prompted a recommended vitamin D supplementation in liquid milk for the elderly.[89] The plea for more vitamin D for the elderly can be found in the recent literature.[92] Adequate vitamin D levels must accompany calcium to combat bone loss. Excess vitamin D can, however, be toxic.[90] The resulting anemia following an overdose of vitamin D has probably been even less understood.[91] The actual amount of vitamin D required is probably small in the elderly, at 400–800 IU/week. Vitamin D involvement in the intestine, kidney, and skin is very well regulated.[93] Vitamin D deficiency affects lipid composition and calcium transport in basolateral membranes in the intestine.[94] The mechanism of primary hyperparathyroidism, along with the relationship of the parathyroid in calcium metabolism and vitamin D receptor abnormalities, has been well described.[95] The relationship between hypercalcaemia and primary hyperthyroidism and malignancy has also been described as a health risk relative to the overuse of supplemental calcium.[96]

VII.   MINERALS AND THE ELDERLY VEGETARIAN OR VEGAN

Mineral metabolism in human nutrition still remains a subject that requires extensive study. Even routine mineral evaluation methods are lacking, particularly as an inexpensive sampling technique that will answer adequacy or deficiency questions of whole body content. For the elderly vegetarian or vegan, this chapter will confine the discussion on minerals to a short presentation on calcium metabolism, while placing the emphasis on magnesium and selenium because of their major importance and frequently low intake in the elderly.

The high animal protein intake of the omnivore diet, with its high sulfur content, produces hypercalcuria and a negative calcium balance. Women on a cereal-based food plan have a daily calcium requirement of around 300 mg/day, while the U.S. female omnivore requires five times more at 1500 mg/day. Animal protein is also accompanied by high phosphate levels. This causes a hypocalcemic activity of phosphate on the parathyroid hormone (PTH), which causes a PTH-dependent renal tubular reabsorption of calcium. The increased PTH activity appears to lead to increased bone resorption, postulated as a risk factor for increased bone loss.[3] The high animal protein intake of the omnivore diet causes a high acid load that contributes to both bone and muscle wasting in aging.[16,18] The elderly vegan subject avoids this acid load. The LOV use of milk and eggs increases the sulfur load. If vitamin D intake is maintained by supplementation, the elderly vegan should more than maintain bone density, compared with LOVs or omnivores.[3]

The elderly vegetarian or vegan has a significant advantage for dietary sources of magnesium because seeds, nuts, legumes, unmilled cereal grains, and dark green vegetables are high in magnesium, while diets high in refined foods or dairy products are low in magnesium.[97] The potential for mineral deficiencies and toxicities in the elderly are well studied.[98] Pharmacological doses of vitamin D increase magnesium absorption in both the deficient and replete vitamin D subject, but significantly increased vitamin D above normal requirements, increases urinary magnesium excretion. Magnesium absorption, independent of vitamin D action, appears to be the more desirable and usual process.[99]

Chel et al.[100] present the dynamic possibilities of increasing ultraviolet light exposure for the elderly or supplementing with vitamin D. A variety of diseases are related to magnesium deficiency where the clinical complications appear to be due to perturbation of magnesium-requiring enzyme systems.[101] Magnesium concentrations affect parathyroid hormone (PTH) secretion qualitatively similar to calcium.[102] Hypocalcemia is a common manifestation of moderate to severe magnesium deficiency in humans. Magnesium therapy alone restores the serum calcium to normal; while calcium or vitamin D therapy are not effective.[103]

Over the last 5 years, Durlach et al.[104] have shown that magnesium depletion is relative to neurodegenerative and neuromuscular disease, asthma, and mitral valve prolapse, which are reminders of the importance of maintaining magnesium levels in the elderly. For the elderly with Type 2 diabetes, the problem of magnesium depletion is very common, and the need to routinely establish a selective administration of magnesium to improve glycemic control and prevent chronic complications of diabetes is very important.[105]

The elderly vegan has an optimal diet for magnesium content. The risk of trauma however, such as brain injury, is a risk for all people in all dietary groups, and even with a high continuous magnesium intake, the rapid decline of magnesium levels will require magnesium salt administration for satisfactory neurologic outcome.[106] Caution should be used with magnesium therapy in subjects with any degree of renal failure because hypermagnesmia may develop, which could result in acute renal failure.[107]

The many functions of selenium at pharmacological levels include: sparing effect for vitamin E-deficient animals against liver necrosis, as a selenoenzyme in glutathionine peroxidase (GSH-Px), as selenomethionine or selenocysteine in proteins. The GSH-Px in a variety of forms regulates eicosanoid metabolism, arachidonic acid, and lipid peroxidation. Also, type I iodothronine 5' diodinase is a selenoprotein.[97]

Dietary intake of selenium depends on the soil and water content of selenium. Many areas of the world contain soils that are selenium-deficient. Dietary selenium intake of the vegetarian is dependent on Brazil nuts, wheat germ, molasses, sunflower seeds, and whole wheat bread.[97] Eggs and milk products are too low in selenium to be considered as sources. A recommended daily allowance for the elderly would be from 60 to 70 micrograms/day. Absorption efficiency improves with deficiency. Prediagnostic levels of selenium can be made from toenail samples. When matched case-control data were analyzed, higher selenium levels were associated with a reduced risk of advanced prostate cancer.[108] A study by Clark et al.[109] revealed that prostate cancer incidence was reduced by two thirds among those in the selenium-supplemented group compared with the placebo group. The synergistic relationship between vitamin E and selenium may be a major factor in this reduced prostate cancer rate.[110] Selenium deficiency produces general depression of immune cells by three mechanisms. First, selenium upregulates the expression of the T-cell high affinity IL2 receptor. Second, it prevents oxidative-stress-induced damage to immune cells. Third, it alters platelet aggregation by decreasing the ratio of thromboxane to leukotriene production.[111] The selenoprotein GSH-Px level affects the sensitivity of human tumor cell lines to n-3 fatty acids.[112] The higher GSH-Px levels increase this sensitivity, the more toxic n-3 essential fatty acids are to cancer cells. Also, there appears to be a protective effect of selenium from UV radiation on human skin cells.[113] There is a cancer chemopreventive effect of selenium on the effect of GSH-Px. It is most likely thiol oxidation and free radical generation, which occur when selenium is present to cause toxicity to cancer cells.[114]

VIII. SUMMARY

This chapter has emphasized that a plant protein diet will give the elderly an advantage in reducing meal insulin response, which in turn decreases fat synthesis (cholesterol and triacylglycerols). The inclusion of casein from milk as an animal protein represents a disadvantage to those on the LOV diet. The inclusion of plant fat in the diet significantly aids in keeping the body content of cholesterol and triacylglycerols at a low level. A plant diet is higher in complex carbohydrate than the omnivore diet. The higher antioxidant intake of the vegetarian or vegan diet, as part of every meal, appears to promote a longer life-span for elderly subjects.[9] The necessity of supplemental vitamin B_{12} and vitamin D for the elderly vegetarian or vegan might be construed as a problem, but less so than for the elderly omnivore, who has a longer list of required supplemental vitamins and minerals. The mineral advantage, in terms of a lower calcium requirement for elderly vegans, is possibly the biggest advantage of all, if they also have supplemental vitamin D.

Table 11.2 Examples of Age-Related Changes in Body Composition and Physiologic Function that Influence Nutrient Requirements

Changes in Body Composition or Physiologic Function	Impact on Nutrient Requirement
Decreased muscle mass (sarcopenia)	Decreased need for calories
Decreased bone density (osteopenia)	Increased need for calcium, vitamin D
Decreased immune function	Increased need for vitamins B_6 and E, zinc
Increased gastric pH (atrophic gastritis)	Increased need for vitamins B_{12} folic acid, calcium, iron, zinc
Decreased skin vitamin D synthesis	Increased vitamin D need
Increased parathyroid production	Increased vitamin D need
Decreased calcium bioavailability	Increased need for calcium and vitamin D
Decreased hepatic retinal uptake	Decreased need for vitamin A
Decreased efficiency of pyridoxal	Increased need for pyridoxal
Increased oxidative stress	Increased need for β-carotene and vitamins C and E
Increased levels of homocysteine	Increased need for folate, vitamins B_{12} and B_6

Adapted from the work of J. Blumberg,, Nutritional needs of seniors. *J. Am. Coll. Nutr.* 16, 6, 517, 1997. With permission of the J. Am. Coll. Nutr.[116]

A life-style health advantage can be rated relative to improved mortality of those in other life-styles. Certainly, we must also relate to improved quality of life, or as reduced morbidity. Vegetarians, as health-conscious people, have reduced mortality from ischaemic heart disease, cerebrovascular disease, and all causes combined.[40,41] More specifically, they experience reduced morbidity and mortality due to obesity, constipation, lung cancer, hypertension, Type II diabetes, and gallstones compared with omnivores.[40] Diet and immune function are a very important part of the reduced mortality

Table 11.3   Numbers of Cases and Controls, Odds Ratio (OR), Adjusted OR and 95% Confidence Interval (CI) of Colorectal Carcinomas *in Situ* According to the Levels of Serum Lipids and Fasting Plasma Glucose

Variables (mg/dL)	Category	Cases	Controls	OR(95% CI)	Adjusted. OR (95%CI)*
Total Cholesterol	< 170	23	55	1.0 (referent)	1.0 (referent)
"	171–195	39	81	1.2 (0.6–2.1)	1.1 (0.6–2.1)
".	196–220	29	64	1.1 (0.6–2.1)	1.2 (0.6–2.5)
"	221+	38	58	1.6 (0.8–3.0)	2.0 (1.0–4.1)
"	Trend			p = 0.17	p = 0.03
Triglycerides	<70	23	67	1.0 (referent)	1.0 (referent)
"	71–110	39	92	1.2 (0.7–2.3)	1.1 (0.6–2.2)
"	111–150	28	61	1.3 (0.7–2.6)	1.3 (0.6–2.7)
"	151+	39	38	3.0 (1.6–5.7)	3.0 (1.4–6.4)
"	Trend			p = 0.0003	p = 0.0008
Glucose	<95	52	103	1.0 (referent)	1.0 (referent)
"	96–105	43	95	0.9 (0.5–1.5)	1.0 (0.6–1.7)
"	106–115	14	38	0.7 (0.4–1.5)	0.7 (0.3–1.5)
"	116+	20	22	1.8 (0.5-3.6)	2.0 (0.9–4.4)
"	Trend			p = 0.12	p = 0.11

*Adjusted for age, sex, body mass index as classified into the quartile category (<21.5, 21.6–23.4, 23.5–25.1, $25.2 +$ kg/m^2), cigarette smoking (non-smokers, 1–15, 16–30, 31 + cigarettes/day), and alcohol consumption (non-drinkers, 1–20, 21–40, 41 + g/dat). From the work of Yamada et al. Relation of serum total cholesterol, serum triglycerides and fasting plasma glucose to colorectal carcinoma *in situ*. *Int. J. Epid.* 27, 794, 1998. With permission from the Int. J. Epid.[119]

of the vegetarian or vegan lifestyles,[115] and the vegan elderly have been noted to have elevated immune capability vs. omnivores.[15,34]

Dietary guidelines for the elderly emphasize consumption of high-quality, nutrient-rich foods.[116] Table 11.2 illustrates the recognition that age-related changes in body composition and physiology change the elderly subjects' nutrient requirements.[116] The elderly vegan can, for the most part, meet these demands with supplemental vitamin D and B$_{12}$. The elderly LOV should meet dietary adequacy for vitamin D from dairy products, but will require supplemental B$_{12}$, calcium and magnesium. The omnivore will likely be in need of supplemental calcium, magnesium, folate, and the B vitamins. Recent studies indicate that essential fatty acid intake for the elderly must be considered in instances of clinically obvious loss of body weight or loss of energy attainment norms.[36,74] Anemia is not part of normal aging if iron stores are normal, however, any anemic condition must be evaluated and not automatically treated as iron deficiency. Consistent exercise programs enhance the health of the elderly.[117,118] The concept of a relation of cholesterol and triacylglycerol levels to colorectal carcinoma greatly enhances the elderly vegetarian's or vegan's healthy status.[119] The high level of significance of this is shown in Table 11.3. Clearly, the elderly vegan, in particular, can keep low serum lipids levels. Further study is needed to define the relationship between the consistent antioxidant dosage of the elderly vegetarian or vegan relative to the degenerative neuromuscular and neurological diseases, and, in particular, Alzheimer's disease.[120]

REFERENCES

1. Campion, E.W. The oldest old. *N. Engl. J. Med.*, 330, 25, 1819, 1994.
2. Olshansky, S.K., Carnes, B.A., and Cassel, C. In search of Methuselah: estimating the upper limits to human longevity. *Science*, 250, 634, 1990.
3. Hubbard, R.W., Mejia, M.S., and Horning, M.C. The potential of diet to alter disease processes. *Nutr. Res.*, 14, 12, 1853, 1994.
4. Beckman, K.B. and Ames, B.N. The free radical theory of aging matures. *Physiol. Reviews*, 76, 2, 547, 1998.
5. Kumari, M.V., Yoneda, T., and Hiramatsu, M., Effect of "beta catecchin" on the life span of senescence accelerated mice (SAM-P8 strain). *Biochem, Mol. Biol. Int.*, 41, 1005, 1997.
6. Harman, D. The aging process. *Proc. Natl. Acad. Sci. USA*, 78, 7124, 1981.
7. Satog, K. and Sakagami, H., Effect of cysteine, N-acetyl-L-cysteine and glutathione on cytotoxic activity of antioxidants. *Anticancer Res.*, 17, 2175, 1997.
8. Cao, G., Booth, S.L., Sadowski, J.A., and Prior, R.L. Increases in human plasma antioxidant capacity after consumption of controlled diets high in fruit and vegetables. *Am. J. Clin. Nutr.*, 68, 1081, 1998.
9. Schafer, F.Q. and Buettner, G.R. Acidic pH amplifies iron-mediated lipid peroxidation in cells. *Free Radical Biol. & Med.*, 28, 1175, 2000.
10. Protein and amino acids. In: *Recommended Dietary Allowances*. 10th ed., National Academy Press, Washington, D.C., 1989, chap 6.
11. Campell, W.W., Crim, M.C., Dallas, G.E., Young, V.R., and Evans, W.J. Increased protein requirements in elderly people: new data and retrospective reassessments. *Am. J. Clin. Nutr.*, 60, 501, 1994.
12. Messina, M. and Messina, V. Issues and applications, *The Dietitian's Guide to Vegetarian Diets*. Aspen Inc., Gaithersburg, 1996, Appendix A.
13. Sabate, J., Lindsted, K.D., Harris R.D., and Johnston, P.K. Anthropometric parameters of school children with different life-styles. *Amer. J. Diseases Child*, 144, 1159, 1990.
14. Taylor, M. and Stanek, K.L. Anthropometric and dietary assessment of omnivore and lacto-ovo-vegetarian children. *J. Am. Diet. Assoc.*, 89, 1661, 1989.
15 Haddad, E.H., Berk, S.L., Kettering, J.D., Hubbard, R.W., and Peters, W.R. Dietary intake and biochemical and immune status of vegans compared with non-vegetarians. *Amer. J. Clin. Nutr.*, 70(suppl),:586S, 1999.
16. Sebastian, A. and Renee, R. *NCRR Reporter*, September/October 9, 1997.

17. Mecocci, P., Polidori, C.M., Trojano, L., Cherubini, QA., Cecchetti, R., Pini, G., Straatman, M., Monti, D., Stahl, W., Sies, H., Franceschi, C., and Senin, U. Plasma antioxidants and longevity: a study on health centenarians. *Free Radical Biol. & Med.,* 28, 1243, 2000.

18. Sebastian, A., Harris, S.T., Ottaway, J.H., Todd, K.M., and Morris, R.C. Improved mineral balance and skeletal metabolism in postmenopausal women treated with potassium bicarbonate. *N. Engl. J. Med.,* 330, 25, 1776, 1994.

19. Sanchez, A. and Hubbard, R.W. Dietary protein modulation of serum cholesterol: the amino acid connection. In: *Absorption and Utilization of Amino Acids.* Friedman, M.(Ed.), CRC, Boca Raton FL, Vol II, 1989, chap 16.

20. Grundy, S.M. and Abrams, J.J. Comparison of actions of soy protein and casein on metabolism of plasma lipoproteins and cholesterol in humans. *Am. J. Clin. Nutr.,* 38, 245, 1982.

21. Assan, R., Efendie, S., Luft, R., and Cerasi, E. Dose-kinetics of pancreatic glucagon responses to arginine and glucose in subjects with normal and impaired pancreatic B-cell function. *Diabetologia,* 21, 452, 1981.

22. Reaven, G. and Grecaberg, R.E. Experimental leucine-induced hypoglycemia in mice. *Metabolism,*14, 615, 1965.

23. Palmar, J.P., Walter, R.M., and Ensink, J.W. Arginine stimulated acute phase of insulin and glucagon secretion in normal man, *Diabetes,* 24, 735, 1975.

24. Nepokroeff, C.M., Lakshmanan, M.R., Ness, G.C., Dugan, R.E., and Porter, J.W. Regulation of the diurnal rhythm of fatty liver hydroxymethylglutaryl coenzyme A reductase activity by insulin, glucagon, cyclic AMP and hydrocortisone. *Arch. Biochem. Biophys.,* 160, 387, 1974.

25. Ingebritsen, T.S., Geelen, M.J.H., Parker, R.A. Evenson, K.J., and Gibson, D.M. Modulation of hydroxymethylglutaryl CoA reductase activity, and cholesterol synthesis in rat hepatocytes in response to insulin and glucagon. *J. Biol. Chem.,* 254, 9986, 1979.

26. Hubbard, R.W., Kosch, C.L., Sanchez, A., Sabate, J., Berk, L., and Shavlik, G. Effect of dietary protein on serum insulin and glucagon levels in hyper- and normocholesterolemic men. *Atherosclerosis,* 76, 55, 1989.

27. Pyorala, D., Savolainen, E., Kaukola, S., and Haapaloski, J. Plasma insulin as a coronary heart disease risk factor in relationship to other risk factors and predictive value during 9-year follow up of the Helsinki Policemen study population. *Acta. Med. Scand.,* 701(Suppl), 38, 1985.

28. Fajans, S.S., Floyd, J.C., Knopf, R.F., and Conn, J.W. Effect of amino acids and protein on insulin secretion in man. *Recent Progr. Horm. Res.,* 123, 617, 1967.

29. Sprietsma, J.E. and Schuitemaker, G.E. Diabetes can be prevented by reducing insulin production. *Med. Hypoth.,* 42, 15, 1994.

30. Eriksson, K.F. and Lindgarde, F. Prevention of type 2 (non-insulin-dependent) diabetes mellitus by diet and physical exercise, the 6-year Malmo feasibility study. *Diabetologia,* 34, 891, 1991.

31. Goldberg, R.B. Prevention of type 2 diabetes. *Med. Clin. North Am.,* 82, 804, 1998.

32. Toth, M.J. and Poehlman, E.T. Sympathetic nervous system activity and resting metabolic rate in vegetarians. *Metabolism,* 43, 621, 1994.

33. Hubbard, R.W., Berk, L., Tan, S., and Haddad, E. Significance of elevated thyrotropin levels in vegans? *FASEB J.,* 9 (Abstr.), 3381, 1995.

34. Berk, L., Hubbard, R.W., Haddad, E., Kettering, J.D., Peters, W.R., Blix, G.G., and Tan, S. Basal fasting cytokine levels in vegans and omnivores. *Amer. J. Clin. Nutr.*, 61, 904 (Abstr.74), 1995.

35. Hubbard, R.W. and Wan, L. Dietary protein type as an aid to lower DOPA medication in Parkinson Disease. *FASEB J.*, 10(Abstr.), 2803, 1996.

36. Hubbard, R.W. and Horning, M. Daytime gluconeogenesis in the young and old apparently caused by essential fatty acid deficiency. *FASEB J.*, 10(Abstr.), 935, 1997.

37. Mayes, P.A. Gluconeogenesis and control of the blood glucose. In: *Harpers Biochemistry*, 24th ed. Murray, R.K., Granner, D.K., Mayes, P.A., and Rodwell, V.W. (Eds.) Appleton and Lange, Stamford, CN, 1996, chap 21.

38. Bios, C., Benamouzig, R., Bruhat, A., Roux, C., Mahe, S., Valensi, P., Gaudichon, C., Ferriere, F., Rautureau, J., and Tome, D., Short-term protein and energy supplementation activates nitrogen kinetics and accretion in poorly nourished elderly subjects. *Am. J. Clin. Nutr.*, 71, 1129, 2000.

39. Walter, P. Effects of vegetarian diets on aging and longevity. *Nutr. Rev.*, 55, S61, 1990.

40. Key, T.J.A., Thorogood, M., Appleby, P.N., and Burr, M.I. Dietary habits and mortality in 11,000 vegetarians and health conscious people: results of a 17-year follow up. *BMJ*, 313, 775, 1996.

41. Rosenberg, I.H. and Miller, J.W. Nutritional factors in physical and cognitive functions of elderly people. *Am. J. Clin. Nutr.*, 55, 1237S, 1992.

42. Mayes, P.A. Gluconeogenesis and control of the blood glucose. In: *Harpers Biochemistry*, 24th ed. Murray, R.K., Granner, D.K., Mayes, P.A., and Rodwell, V.W. (Eds.) Appleton and Lange, Stamford, CN, 1996, chap 23.

43. Grundy, S.M. Influence of stearic acid on cholesterol metabolism relative to other long-chain fatty acids. *Am. J. Clin. Nutr.*, 60 (Suppl), 986S, 1994.

44. Katan, M.B., Zock, P.L., and Mensink, R.P. Effects of fats and fatty acids on blood lipid in humans: An overview. *Am. J. Clin. Nutr.*, 60 (Suppl), 1017S, 1994.

45. Nydahl, M.C., Gustafsson I.B., and Vessby, B. Lipid lowering diets enriched with monounsaturated or polyunsaturated fatty acids but low in saturated fatty acids have similar effects on serum lipid concentrations in hyperlipidemic patients. *Am. J. Clin. Nutr.*, 59, 115, 1994.

46. Kris-Etherton, P.M., Krummel, D., Russell, M.E., Dreon, D., Mackey, S., Borcher, J., and Wood, P.D. The effect of diet on plasma lipids, lipoproteins, and coronary heart disease. *J. Am. Diet. Assoc.*, 88, 1373,1988.

47. Denke, M.A., Sempos, G.T., and Grundy, S.M. Excess body weight. An under recognized contributor to dyslipidemia in white American women. *Arch. Intern. Med.*, 154, 401, 1994.

48. Melby, C.L., Goldflies, D.G., and Toohey, M.L. Blood pressure differences in older black and white long-term vegetarians and non-vegetarians. *J. Am. Coll. Nutr.*, 12, 262, 1993.

49. Janelle, K.C. and Barr, S.I. Nutrient intakes and eating behavior scores of vegetarian and non-vegetarian women. *J. Am. Diet. Assoc.*, 95, 180, 1995.

50. Roche, H.M., Zampelas, A., Knapper, J.M.E., Webb, D., Brooks, C., Jackson K.G., Wright, J.W., Gould, B. J., Kafatos, A., Gibney, M.J., and Williams, C.M. Effect of long-term olive oil dietary intervention on postprandial acyglycerol and factor VII metabolism. *Am. J., Clin. Nutr.*, 68, 552, 1998.

51. Zampelas, A., Roche, H., Knapper, J.M., Jackson, K.G., Tornaritis, M., Hatzis, C., Gibney, M.J., Kafatos, A., Gould, B.J., Wright, J., and Williams, C.M. Differences in postprandial lipemic response between northern and southern Europeans. *Atherosclerosis*, 139, 83, 1998.

52. Kafatos, A. and Comas, G.E. Biological effect of olive oil in human health. In: *Olive oil.* Kiritsakis, A. (Ed.), American Oil Chemists Society, Champaign, IL, 1990, 57.

53. Sirtori, C.R., Gatti, E., Tremoli, E., Galli, C., Gianfranceschi, G., Framcescjomo, G., Colli., S., Madenra, P., Marangoni, F., Perego, P., and Stragliotto, P. Olive, corn oil, and n-3 fatty acids differently affect lipids, lipoproteins, platelets, and super-oxide formation in type II hypercholesterolemia. *Am. J. Clin. Nutr.*, 56, 113, 1992.

54. Sanchez-Muniz, F.J., Oubina, P., Benedi, J., Rodenas, S., and Cuesta, C. A preliminary study on platelet aggregation in postmenopausal women consuming extra-virgin olive oil and high-oleic acid sunflower oil. *JAOCS*, 75, 217, 1998.

55. Howell, T.J., MacDougall, D.E., and Jones, P.J.H. Phytosterols partially explain differences in cholesterol metabolism caused by corn or olive oil feeding. *J. Lipid Res.*, 39, 892, 1998.

56. Maki, P.A. and Newberne, P.M. Dietary lipids and immune function. *J. Nutr.*, 122, 610, 1992.

57. Fortin, P.R., Lew, R.A., Liang, M.H., Wright, E.A., Beckett, L.A., Chambers, T.C., and Sperling, R.I. Validation of a meta-analysis: the effects of fish oil in rheumatoid arthritis. *J. Clin. Epidemiol.*, 48, 1379, 1995.

58. Okuyama, H. Minimum requirements of n-3 and n-6 essential fatty acids for the function of the central nervous system and for the prevention of chronic disease. *Proc. Soc. Exp. Biol. Med.*, 200, 174, 1992.

59. Lands, W.E.M., Libelt, B., Morris, A., Kramer, N.C., Prewitt, T.E., Bowen, P., Schmeisser, D., Davidson, M.H., and Burns, J.H. Maintenance of lower proportions of (n-6) eicosanoid precursors in phospholipids of human plasma in response to added dietary (n-3) fatty acids. *Biochimica et Biophysica Acta*, 1180, 147,1992.

60. Sinclair, H.M. Prevention of coronary heart disease: the role of essential fatty acids. *Postgrad. Med. J.*, 56, 579, 1980.

61. Kestin, M., Clifton, P., Belling, G.B., and Nestel, P.J. n-3 fatty acids of marine origin lower systolic blood pressure and triglycerides but raise LDL cholesterol compared with n-3 and n-6 fatty acids from plants. *Am. J. Clin. Nutr.*, 51, 1028, 1990.

62. Jiang, W.G., Bryce, R.P., and Horrobin, D.F. Essential fatty acids: molecular and cellular basis of their anti-cancer action and clinical implications. *Crit. Rev. Oncol. Hematology*, 27, 179, 1998.

63. Koleltzko, B. Trans fatty acids may impair biosynthesis of long-chain polyunsaturates and growth in man. *Acta Paediatr.*, 81, 302, 1992.

64. Kohlmeier, L., Simonsen, N., Veer, P.V., Strain, J.J., Martin-Moreno, J.M., Margolin, B., Huttunen, J.K., Navajas, F.C., Martin, B.C., Alwin, M.T., Kardinall, F.M., and Kok, F.J. Adipose tissue trans fatty acids and breast cancer in the European community multicenter study on antioxidants, myocardial infarction, and breast cancer. *Cancer Epid. Biomarkers and Prev.*, 6, 705, 1997.

65. Mensink, R.P., Temme, E.H.M., and Hornstra, G. Dietary saturated and trans fatty acids and lipoprotein metabolism. *Annals of Med.*, 26, 461, 1994.

66. Willet, W.C., Stampfer, M.J., Manson, J.E., Colditz, G.A., Speizer, F.E., Rosner, B.A., Sampson, L.A., and Hennekens, C.H. Intake of trans fatty acids and risk of coronary heart disease among women. *Lancet*, 341, 581, 1993.

67. Mann, G.V. Metabolic consequences of dietary trans fatty acids. *Lancet*, 343, 1268, 1994.

68. Simopoulos, A.P. Omega-6/Omega-3 fatty acid ratio and trans fatty acids in non-insulin-dependent diabetes mellitus. *Lipids and Syndromes of Insulin Resistance of: Annals New York Acad. Sci.*, 827, 327, 1997.

69. Horrobin, D.F. Fatty acid metabolism in health and disease: the role of delta-6-desaturase. *Am. J. Clin. Nutr.*, 57(suppl), 732S, 1993.

70. Mahfouz, M.M., Smith, T.L., and Kummerow, F.A. Effect of dietary fats on desaturase activities and the biosynthesis of fatty acids in rat liver microsomes. *Lipids*, 19, 214, 1984.

71. Wahle, K.W.J. and James, W.P.T. Isomeric fatty acids and human health. (Review), *Eur. J. Clin. Nutr.*, 47, 828, 1993.

72. Horrobin, D.F. Gamma-linolenic acid: an intermediate in essential fatty acid metabolism with potential as an ethical pharmaceutical and as a food. In: *Reviews in Contempoary Pharmacotherapy.* Johnson, S. and Johnson, F. N. (Eds.), vol. 1, No. 1, Marius Press, 1990, 1.

73. Swank, R.L. Multiple sclerosis: fat-oil relationship. *Nutr.*, 7, 368, 1991.

74. Hubbard, R.W., Westngard, J., Sanchez, A., and Barth, J. Chronic gluconeogenesis lowers urinary amino acids. *FASEB J.*, 13(Abstr 688.20) A935, 1999.

75. Asp, N-G. Nutritional classification and analysis of food carbohydrates. *Am. J. Clin. Nutr.*, 59 (suppl), 679S, 1994.

76. Bjorck, I., Granfeldt, Y., Liljeberg, H., Tovar, J., and Asp, N-G. Food properties affecting the digestion and absorption of carbohydrates. *Am. J. Clin. Nutr.*, 59 (suppl), 699S, 1994.

77. Mahan, L.K. and Escott-Stump, S. Carbohydrates. In: *Krause's Food, Nutrition, and Diet Therapy.* Mahan, L.K. and Escott-Stump, S., (Eds.), W. B. Saunders, Philadelphia, 1996, chap. 3, 31.

78. Raiten, D.J. and Talbot, J.M. (Eds.) Clinical trials for the treatment of secondary wasting and cachexia: selection of appropriate endpoints. *J. Nutr.*, 129, (1S), 223, 1999.

79. Mitch, W.W. and Goldberg, A.L. Mechanisms of muscle wasting (Review). In: Mechanisms of Disease. Epstein, H. (Ed.), *N. Eng. J. Med.*, 335, 25, 1897 1996.

80. Blaylock, R.L. *Excitotoxins: The Taste that Kills.* Health Press, Santa Fe, 1997.

81. Mahan, L.K., and Escott-Stump, S. Vitamins. In: *Krause's Food, Nutrition, and Diet Therapy.* Mahan, L.K., Escott-Stump, S. (Eds.), W. B. Saunders, Philadelphia, 77, 1996, chap. 6.

82. Herbert, V. Everyone should be tested for iron disorders. *J. Am. Diet. Assoc.*, 92, 1502, 1992.

83. Simopoulos, A., Herbert, V., and Jacobson, B. *Genetic Nutrition: Designing a Diet Based on Your Family Medical History.* Macmillan, New York, 1993.

84. Herbert, V. Staging vitamin B-12 (cobalamin) status in vegetarians. *Am. J. Clin. Nutr.*, 59 (suppl), 1213S, 1994.

85. Shaw, S., Herbert, V., Colman, N., and Jayatilleke, E. Effect of ethanol generated free radicals on gastric intrinsic factor and glutathione. *Alcohol*, 7, 153, 1990.

86. Norman, A.W. The vitamin D endocrine system: Identification of another piece of the puzzle. *Endocrinology*, 134, 1601A, 1994.

87. Norman, A.W. Sunlight, season, skin pigmentation, vitamin D, and 25-hydrdoxy vitamin D: Integral components of the vitamin D endocrine system. *Am J. Clin. Nutr.*, 67, 6, 1108, 1998.
88. MacLaughlin, J. and Hollick, M.F. Aging decreases the capacity of human skin to produce vitamin D-3. *J. Clin. Invest.*, 76, 1536, 1985.
89. Keane, E.M., Healy, M., O'Morre, R., Coakley, D., and Walsh, J.B. Vitamin D-fortified liquid milk a highly effective method of vitamin D administration for home-bound and institutionalized elderly. *Gerontology*, 38, 280, 1992.
90. Sterkel, B.B. Bone density and vitamin D intoxication. *Ann. Intern Med.*, 128, 6, 506, 1998.
91. Puig, J., Corocoy, R., and Rodriquez-Espinosa, J. Anemia secondary to vitamin D intoxication. *Ann. Intern. Med.*, 128, 7, 602, 1998.
92. Utiger, R.D. The need for more vitamin D. *N. Engl, J. Med.*, 338, 12, 828 1998.
93. Zineb, R., Zhor, B., Odile, W., and Marthe, R.R. Distinct, tissue-specific regulation of vitamin D receptor in the intestine, kidney, and skin by dietary calcium and vitamin D. *Endocrinology*, 139, 4, 1844, 1998.
94 Alisio, A., Canas, F., De Bronia, D.N., Pereira, E., and De Talamoni, N.T. Effect of vitamin D deficiency on lipid composition and calcium transport in basolateral membrane vesicles from chick intestine. *Biochem. Mol. Biol. Int.*, 42, 2, 339, 1997.
95. Carling, T., Ridefelt, P., Hellman, P., Rastad, J., Akerstrom, G. Vitamin D receptor polymorphisms correlate to parathyroid cell function in primary hyperparathyrodism. *J. Clin. Endocrinol. Metab.*, 82, 6, 1772, 1997.
96. Reid, I.R. The investigation of hypercalcaemia. *Clin. Endodrinology*, 41, 405, 1994.
97. Czajka-Narins, D. Minerals. In: *Krause's Food Nutrition and Diet Therapy*. Mahan, L.K. and Escott-Stump, S. (Eds.), W.B. Saunders, Philadelphia, 1996, chap 7.
98. Greger, J.L. Potential for trace mineral deficiencies and toxicities in the elderly. In: *Mineral Homeostasis in the Elderly*. Bales, C.W. (Ed.), Alan R. Liss, New York, 1989, 171.
99. Hardwick, L.L., Jones, M.R., Brauatbar, N., and Lee, D.B.N. Magnesium absorption: mechanisms and the influence of vitamin D, calcium and phosphate. *J. Nutr.*, 121, 13, 1991.
100. Chel, V.G.M., Ooms, M.E., Popp-Snijders, C., Pavel, S., Schothorst, A.A., Melemans, C.C.E., and Lips, P. Ultraviolet irradiation corrects vitamin D deficiency and suppresses secondary hyperparathyroidism in the elderly. *J. Bone and Min. Res.*, 13, 8, 1238, 1998.
101. Rude, R.K., Oldham, S.B., Sharp, C.F. Jr., and Singer, F.R. Parathyroid hormone secretion in magnesium deficiency. *J. Clin. Endocrinol. Metab.*, 47, 800, 1978.
102. Rude, R.K., Oldham, S.B., and Singer, F.R. Functional hypoparathyroidism and parathyroid hormone end-organ resistance in human magnesium deficiency. *Clin. Endocrinol.*, 5, 209, 1976.
103. Rude, R.K. Magnesium deficiency: a case of heterogeneous disease in humans. (Review) *J. Bone and Min. Res.*, 13, 4, 749, 1998.
104. Durlach, J. Bac., P, Durlach, V., Durlach, A., Bars, M., and Guiet-Bara, A. Are age-related neurodegenerative diseases linked with various types of magnesium depletion? *Magnesium Res.*, 10, 4, 339, 1997.

105. De Lourdes Lima, M., Cruz, T.P., Pousada, J.C., Rodrigues, L.E., Barbosa, K., and Canguqu, V. The effect of magnesium supplementation in increasing doses on the control of type 2 diabetes. *Diabetes Care*, 21, 5, 682, 1998.

106. Heath, D.L. and Vink, R. Neuroprotective effects of Mg SO_4 and $MgCl_2$ in closed head injury: a comparative phosphorus NMR study. *J. Neurotrauma.*, 15, 3, 183, 1998.

107. Mordes, J.P. and Wacker, W.E.C. Excessive magnesium. *Pharmacol. Rev.*, 29, 273, 1978.

108. Yoshizawa, K., Willett, W.C., Morris, S.J., Stampfer, M.J., Spiegelman, D., Rimm,, E.B., and Giovannucci, E. Study of prediagnostic selenium Level in toenails and the risk of advanced prostate cancer. *J. Nat. Can. Inst.*, 90, 16, 1219, 1998.

109. Clark, L.C., Combs, G.F.Jr., Turnbull, B.W., Slate, E.H., Chalker, D.K., Chow, J., Davis, L.S., Glover, R.A., Graham, G.F., Gross, E.G., Krongrad, A., Lesher, J.L., Jr., Park, H.K., Sanders, B.B., Jr., Smith, C.L., and Taylor, J.R. Effects of selenium supplementation for cancer prevention in patients with carcinoma of the skin. A randomized controlled trial. Nutritional Prevention of Cancer Study Group. *JAMA*, 276, 1957, 1996.

110. Taylor, P.R. and Albanes, D. Selenium, vitamin E, and prostate cancer — Ready for Prime Time? *J. Nat. Can. Inst.*, 90, 16, 184, 1998.

111. McKenzie, R.C., Rafferty, T.S., and Beckett, G.J. Selenium: an essential element for immune function. *Immunology Today*, 19, 8, 3432, 1998.

112. Schonberg, S.A., Rudra, P.K., Noding, R., Skorpen, F., Bjerve, K.S., and Krokan, H.E. Evidence that changes in Se-glutathionine peroxidase levels affect the sensitivity of human tumour cell lines to n-3 fatty acids. *Carcinogenesis*, 18, 10, 1897, 1997.

113. Rafferty, T.S., McKenzie, R.C., Hunter, J.A.A., Howie, A.F., Arthur, J.R., Nicol, F., and Beckett, G.J. Differential expression of selenoproteins by human skin cells and protection by selenium from UVB-radiation-induced cell death. *Biochem. J.*, 332, 231, 1998.

114. Stewart, M.S., Spallholz, J.E., Neldner, K.H., and Pence, B.C. Selenium compounds have disparate abilities to impose oxidative stress and induce apoptosis. *Free Rad. Biology Med.*, 25, 1/2, 42, 1999.

115. Hannigan, B.M. Diet and immune function. *Brit. J. Biomed. Sci.*, 51, 252, 1994.

116. Blumberg, J. Nutritional needs of seniors. *J. Amer. College Nutr.*, 16, 6, 517, 1997.

117. Gill, J.M.R., Murphy, M.H., and Hardman, A.E. Postprandial lipemia: effects of intermittent vs. continuous exercise. *Med. Sci. Sports and Exer.*, 30, 10, 1515, 1998.

118. Kostka, T., Drai, J., Berthouze, S.E., Lacour, J.R., and Bonnefoy, M. Physical activity, fitness and integrated antioxidant system in healthy active elderly women. *Int. J. Sports Med.*, 19, 461, 1998.

119. Yamada, K., Araki, S., Tamura, M., Sakai, I., Takahashi, Y., Kashihara, H., and Kono, S. Relation of serum total cholesterol, serum triglycerides and fasting plasma glucose to colorectal carcinoma in situ. *Int. J. Epid.*, 27, 794, 1998.

120. Subramaniam, R., Koppal, T., Green, M., Yatin, S., Jordan, B., Drake, J., and Butterfield, D.A. The free radical antioxidant vitamin E protects cortical synaptosomal membranes from amyloid beta-peptides (25–35) toxicity but not from hydroxynonenal toxicity: relevance to the free radical hypothesis of Alzheimer's disease. *Neurochemical Res.*, 23, 11, 1403, 1998.

12

IMPLICATIONS OF THE
VEGETARIAN DIET FOR
ATHLETES

David C. Nieman

CONTENTS

I. INTRODUCTION

Since the time of the ancient Greeks, athletes and their coaches have practiced special dietary regimens to improve performance and gain a competitive edge over their competitors.[1-4] Milo of Crotona, a legendary Greek wrestler who consumed gargantuan amounts of meat, was never once brought to his knees over five Olympiads (532–516 B.C.). Roman gladiators believed that meat made them better warriors, a belief that persists to this day among many football, basketball, and baseball athletes.

0-8493-8508-3/01/$0.00+$.50
© 2001 by CRC Press LLC

During the mid- to late-1800s, vegetarian athletes sought to prove, through excellence in endurance exercise, the superiority of the plant-based diet in opposition to the prevalent belief of that day that energy for muscular movement was produced by protein oxidation.[3] Vegetarian societies formed athletic and cycling clubs, and members often outperformed their carnivorous competitors in long endurance-race events.[3] Today, elite athletes such as triathlete Dave Scott, body builder Bill Pearl, long distance runner Paavo Numi, tennis players Martina Navratilova and Billy Jean King, Olympic wrestler Chris Campbell, and Olympic figure skater Surya Bonaly continue to demonstrate that the vegetarian diet is compatible with successful athletic endeavors.

Research during since the 1960s has emphasized that carbohydrate is the primary fuel of the working muscle for all athletic ventures, including weight lifting, team sports, and endurance activity (e.g., running, swimming, and cycling).[1] Since the plant-based diet is naturally high in carbohydrates, a growing number of athletes have become vegetarians (or near-vegetarians).[1-4] This has concerned some dietitians and sports nutritionists who believe that the vegetarian diet is associated with potential health and nutrient intake problems. In this chapter, these concerns will be addressed, with an emphasis on the following issues and conclusions:

1. **Performance:** Is the vegetarian diet associated with a decrement or improvement in athletic endeavor? Most research has indicated that the vegetarian diet, per se, is not associated with improved aerobic endurance performance; however, other benefits make this dietary regimen worthy of consideration by serious athletes.

2. **Carbohydrate intake:** A plant-based dietary facilitates a high intake of carbohydrates, which is essential for prolonged exercise.

3. **Potential for suboptimal intake of iron, zinc, and other minerals:** A well-planned vegetarian diet provides the athlete with adequate levels of all known nutrients, although the potential for suboptimal intake of iron, zinc, and trace elements exists if the diet is too restrictive. However, this concern exists for all athletes, vegetarian or non-vegetarian, who have poor dietary habits.

4. **Protein intake:** Although there has been some concern about protein intake for vegetarian athletes, data indicate that all essential and nonessential amino acids can be supplied by plant food sources alone, as long as a variety of foods is consumed and the energy intake is adequate to meet needs.

5. **Antioxidant nutrients:** Athletes consuming a diet rich in fruits, vegetables, and whole grains receive a high intake of antioxidant nutrients, which helps reduce the oxidative stress associated with heavy exertion.

6. **Menstrual irregularity:** There has been some concern that vegetarian female athletes are at increased risk for oligo-amenorrhea, but evidence suggests that low energy intake, not dietary quality, is a major cause.

7. **Health benefits:** While the athlete is most often concerned with performance, long-term health benefits and a reduction in risk of chronic disease have been associated with the vegetarian diet. Studies suggest that a combination of regular physical activity and vegetarian dietary practices provide lower mortality rates than the vegetarian diet or exercise alone.

II. THE EFFECT OF A VEGETARIAN DIET ON PERFORMANCE

Vegetarian dietary practices have been associated with many health benefits, including reduced death rates from ischemic heart disease, diabetes, and certain forms of cancer,[2,5-8] and decreased risk of obesity, dyslipidemia and hypertension.[2,9-11] Vegetarians, compared with non-vegetarians, typically have a higher intake of fruit and vegetables, dietary fiber, antioxidant nutrients, phytochemicals, and folic acid, with a lower intake of saturated fat and cholesterol,[12-15] each of which has been related to decreased risk of chronic disease.[16-21]

The question of whether the multiple benefits of vegetarian dietary practices extend to enhanced physical fitness and performance has been explored since early in the 20th century.[2-4] A few simple studies conducted prior to 1910 reported augmented muscular endurance (e.g., holding arms out horizontally, deep knee bends, and leg raises) in vegetarian vs. non-vegetarian subjects, but these results have not been confirmed in subsequent research.[2-4]

Modern-day research comparing physical fitness performance in vegetarians and non-vegetarians began in the 1970s. Cotes et al.[22] compared thigh muscle width, pulmonary function measures, and the cardiorespiratory response to submaximal cycle ergometry exercise in 14 vegan and 86 non-vegetarian women. Ventilation responses during rest or exercise did not differ between the groups, and thigh muscle width was similar. The authors concluded that the lack of animal protein did not impair the physiological response to submaximal exercise.

Meyer et al.[23] studied the effect of a vegetarian diet on running performance (5- to 8-kilometer test runs). The subjects completed the runs before and after being on the diet for 2 weeks, and then again 2 weeks after returning to a non-vegetarian diet. No significant differences were found between the trials, suggesting that the vegetarian diet had neither a beneficial nor detrimental effect on aerobic endurance.

Physical fitness, anthropometric, and metabolic parameters were compared by Hanne et al.[24] in 49 vegetarian and 49 non-vegetarian male and female Israeli athletes who were matched for age, sex, body size, and athletic activities. No significant differences were found between groups for pulmonary function, aerobic and anaerobic capacity, arm and leg circumferences, hand grip and back strength, hemoglobin, and total serum protein. The authors concluded that the specific influence of the vegetarian diet on physical performance is confounded by several factors, including the type of vegetarian diet ingested, the training regimen, and other lifestyle practices.

Twenty-one overweight females were fed a lacto-ovo-vegetarian diet for 5 weeks, with all meals prepared, weighed and served in a research kitchen.[25] Half of the subjects were randomized to a walk/jog exercise program (five 45-minute sessions each week at an intensity of 60% VO_{2max}), while the other half remained sedentary. Submaximal and maximal cardiorespiratory measures improved significantly in those who exercised, but no improvement was seen in the women who consumed the vegetarian diet without exercise. In other words, the vegetarian diet alone is an insufficient stimulus to improve physical performance unless accompanied by a regular exercise training program.

Snyder et al.[26] studied two groups of female runners who were matched for age, weight, and distance run per week. One group regularly consumed a semi-vegetarian diet (< 100 grams red meat per week), while the other group ingested a diet that included red meat. No significant difference in maximal aerobic capacity was found between the two groups.

A series of papers has been published on 110 runners who competed in a 1000-km race conducted over a 20-day period in West Germany.[27-29] Before and during the race, 60 of the runners consumed a conventional Western diet, and 50 consumed a lacto-ovo-vegetarian diet. During the race, diets for both groups were formulated to ensure a similar intake of carbohydrate for both groups (~ 60% total energy). Diet had no effect on the performance of the runners. Half of each group finished the 20-day race, the order of finishers was not influenced by the diet, and the average running time for the vegetarian runners was not significantly different from the non-vegetarians. (See Figure 12.1).

Nineteen long-term (mean of 46 years) vegetarian and 12 non-vegetarian, healthy, physically active elderly women (mean age of 71 years) were compared on a variety of hematological, anthropometric, and metabolic factors.[30] Although the vegetarian subjects had significantly lower blood glucose and cholesterol levels, no differences between groups were found for submaximal and maximal cardiorespiratory and electrocardiographic parameters measured during graded treadmill testing. The authors

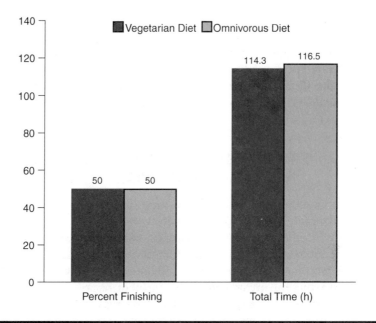

Figure 12.1 With a similar intake of carbohydrate (~ 60% total energy), the proportion of finishers and performance time following a 1000-km, 20-day race were not significantly different between vegetarian and non-vegetarian runners.[27-29].

concluded that a long-term vegetarian diet may be associated with several benefits, but these do not include greater cardiorespiratory fitness.

Two papers have been published on a study of eight well-trained male athletes in Denmark who consumed either a lacto-ovo-vegetarian or non-vegetarian diet for 6 weeks (cross-over design).[31,32] Both diets consisted of 57% total energy as carbohydrates, 14% protein, and 29% fat. Maximal aerobic capacity, aerobic endurance time to exhaustion, muscle glycogen levels, and isometric strength were unaffected by changes in the diet. This study demonstrated that when macronutrient intake is held constant, switching between a vegetarian and non-vegetarian diet should not be expected to have an influence on exercise performance.

Animal product intake was measured and related to VO_{2max} in a group of 80 women who varied widely in age, body mass, maximal aerobic power, and meat intake (1.1 to 31.6 meat exchanges per day).[33] Maximal aerobic power was not related to meat intake, an animal product index, or dietary cholesterol. Multiple regression analysis, using models to control for age and body composition, failed to alter these findings.

Together, these studies indicate that the vegetarian diet, even when practiced for several decades, is neither beneficial nor detrimental to cardiorespiratory endurance, especially when carbohydrate intake, age, training status, body weight, and other confounders are controlled for. Endurance exercise performance is strongly related to genetic factors, training regimens, and carbohydrate intake.[1] The inclusion or avoidance of meat in the dietary patterns of endurance athletes is not an important issue, especially when contrasted to the dominating influence of these three factors.

III. SPECIAL CONCERNS FOR ATHLETES ON VEGETARIAN DIETS

Scandinavian researchers in the 1960s were the first to demonstrate that the ability to exercise at a high intensity was related to the pre-exercise level of muscle glycogen.[1] Body glycogen stores play an important role in intense exercise (70–85% of peak aerobic power) that is either prolonged and continuous (e.g., running, swimming, and cycling), or of an extended intermittent, mixed anaerobic-aerobic nature (e.g., soccer, basketball, ice hockey, or repeated exercise intervals). Endurance athletes have been urged to ingest plant sources of carbohydrates to optimize muscle and liver glycogen stores.[1,34,35] At the high intensities necessary for athletic training and competition, the metabolism of body carbohydrate stores provides the major fuel for muscle contraction, and, when these reach low levels, fatigue occurs.[34,35] About 500–800 grams of carbohydrate per day (or 8–10 g/kg body weight or 60–70% of energy intake) have been recommended for athletes training intensively for more than 60–90 minutes per day.[1,34-36]

A near-vegetarian diet is often needed to take advantage of high carbohydrate plant foods such as cereals, pasta, grains, dried fruits, and legumes. In one study of 347 marathon runners, more than 75% reported higher intake of fruits, vegetables, and whole grains, and lower intake of red meat and eggs when compared with pre-running dietary habits.[37] (See Figure 12.2.) Nonetheless, in most studies, intake of carbohydrate by endurance athletes falls below recommended levels, although there are some noteworthy exceptions (e.g., Tarahumara Indian ultramarathon runners, and triathletes).[1,37-41] The Tarahumara Indians, a Ute-Aztecan tribe inhabiting the rugged Sierra Madre Occidental Mountains in the north-central state of Chihuahua, Mexico, are extraordinary endurance runners who consume a simple, near-vegetarian diet composed primarily of corn and beans (75–80% of total energy intake is carbohydrate).[38]

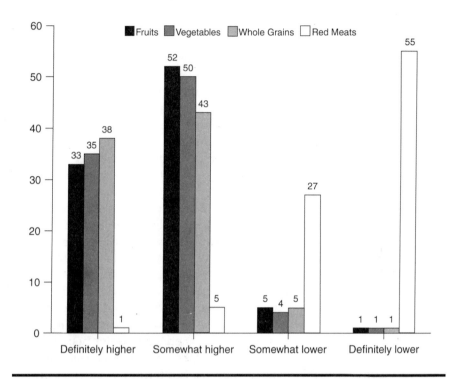

Figure 12.2 **In this study of 347 marathon runners, more than 75% reported higher intake of fruits, vegetables, and whole grains, and lower intake of red meat and eggs when compared with pre-running dietary habits.**[37]

A. Iron, Zinc, and Trace Minerals

Some athletes, especially elite male and female endurance athletes, test positive for mild iron deficiency.[1] Using serum ferritin as a criterion (less than 12 μg/l), between 10% and 80% of female athletes, depending on the study, have been described as having mild iron deficiency (in contrast to 5–11% of non-athletic females).[1] Concerns have been raised that an emphasis on plant foods to enhance carbohydrate intake by athletes may increase polyphenol (in certain vegetables), phytate (in bran), dietary fiber, and tannin (tea) intake to levels that reduce the bioavailability of several nutrients, including zinc, iron, and some trace minerals.[1,39-43] Furthermore, heme iron from meat is two to three times more absorbable than non-heme iron from plant-based foods and iron-fortified foods, increasing the risk of sports anemia in vegetarian athletes who are already at high risk for iron deficiency due to exercise-induced iron losses (via increased hemolysis, gastrointestinal bleeding, and high sweat rates).[1,40] These concerns may be especially apparent in certain subgroups such as female adolescent athletes.[41]

Most studies of long-term vegetarians (non-athletes) who have avoided dietary extremes indicate that, despite the apparent lower bioavailability of some minerals, the iron, zinc, and trace element status (as measured in the serum, hair, and urine) appears adequate.[42,43] Dietary intake of iron is typically above recommended levels in vegetarians, but serum ferritin levels and other iron status indicators are often lower than in non-vegetarians, although anemia is rare.[11,44-49] It appears that the gastrointestinal tracts of vegetarians can adapt by increasing the absorption of iron and trace elements, although concerns have been raised that adolescents on a vegetarian diet may have suboptimal zinc status because of their high zinc requirements for growth.[42,48]

Although inhibitors of dietary iron absorption are present in plant-based foods, plant foods also contain enhancers of dietary iron absorption, such as vitamin C and citric acid found in fruits and vegetables.[14,43] Although considered controversial, there is some evidence that a reduction in body iron stores may be associated with a reduced risk for both coronary artery disease and cancer.[50-52] Thus, the lower ferritin levels found in vegetarians may actually be advantageous, but further research is needed before this hypothesis can be accepted.

Although some athletes have been reported to be at risk for iron deficiency, iron deficient anemia is rare (about 2–5%, the same as measured in the general population).[1,53,54] There is a growing consensus, however, that mild iron deficiency has little or no meaningful impact on the health or performance capabilities of athletes.[1,53,54] Low intake of dietary iron, increased hemolysis, decreased iron absorption, and increased iron loss in sweat, feces, and urine have all been implicated as factors that may reduce body iron stores in some athletes, especially females.[1,53] In one large study of 1743 eastern Finnish men, the duration and frequency of physical activity were associated inversely with serum ferritin.[51] (Figure 12.3). The authors speculated that a reduction in stored iron levels could be one mechanism through which exercise training decreases the risk of coronary artery disease.[50,51]

There has been some concern that vegetarian female endurance athletes may be at special risk for iron deficiency.[39,40] A significant proportion (30–50%) of endurance athletes, especially women, have been reported to be semi-vegetarians, with a low intake of meat products.[26,39] Snyder et al.[26] compared iron status in nine non-vegetarian and nine semi-vegetarian female runners, and reported lower serum ferritin and higher total iron binding capacity in the semi-vegetarians. Serum iron, percent transferrin

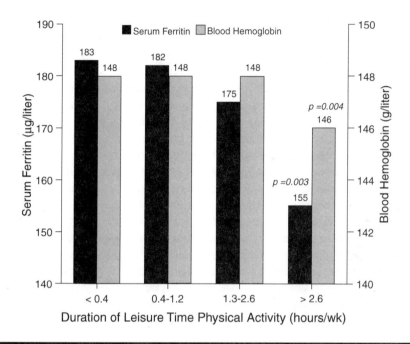

Figure 12.3 In this study of 1743 eastern Finnish men, the duration and frequency of physical activity were associated inversely with serum ferritin. There is some evidence that reduced body iron stores are inversely related to coronary heart disease risk.[51]

saturation, and hemoglobin levels, however, were not different between the groups.

Seiler et al.[28] has also reported lower ferritin levels in vegetarian vs. non-vegetarian runners (both male and female). However, no impairment in ability to compete in a 20-day, 1000-km race was measured in the vegetarian runners. During the 1000-km race, dietary iron intake was higher in the vegetarian group, but was of the non-heme variety from legumes, dried fruits, nuts, vegetables, and grain products. The high intake of vitamin C, together with the avoidance of tea, appeared to enhance iron absorption in that blood indicators of iron status were similar between the vegetarian and non-vegetarian runners.[29] The Tarahumara Indians have been found to have normal blood hemoglobin levels, despite diets that are 90% corn and pinto beans.[38,55] In the study of eight athletes who consumed a vegetarian or non-vegetarian diet for 6 weeks (cross-over design), despite an extremely high fiber intake while on the vegetarian diet (98 vs. 47 grams/day), blood hemoglobin, serum iron, and serum transferrin concentrations did not differ significantly between dietary regimens.[31,32]

Several studies have shown that acute exercise alters blood levels of trace elements, suggesting that exercise leads to a redistribution between body tissues.[56,57] There is some evidence that an acute bout of exercise increases urinary excretion of zinc.[56] However, most studies have failed to find that indicators of trace element status are different between athletes and non-athletes.[57] Concerns have been raised that athletes, especially adolescents, who avoid meat may have difficulty in maintaining appropriate levels of zinc in their bodies.[40] Insufficient data exist to determine whether these concerns are warranted. Beef, pork and poultry are major sources of zinc in the United States.[58] Milk products, cereal products, legumes and nuts are also good sources of zinc, but zinc from these sources is less bioavailable than from meat.[40,56,58]

Vegetarian athletes are urged to increase good sources of iron and zinc in their diets (e.g., fortified breakfast cereals, legumes, nuts and seeds), include vitamin C sources with each meal and avoid heavy tea intake.[40] Iron, zinc and trace element supplementation may be necessary for some vegetarian athletes with poor diets, but the supplements should be at a level no higher than 100% of the Recommended Dietary Allowance to avoid negative interactions with the absorption or function of other nutrients.[56,59]

B. Antioxidant Status

While there have been some concerns about the trace mineral status of vegetarian athletes, their dietary practices may be of benefit in another area of current interest in sports nutrition. Research has been directed toward the interaction of exercise, generation of reactive oxygen species or free radicals, and antioxidant nutrients (primarily vitamins E, C, and A, and the mineral selenium).[60-63] During exercise, oxygen consumption can increase 10- to 20-fold over rest to meet energy demands. Due to various means that are still being researched (e.g., increases in catecholamines, lactic acid, hyperthermia, and transient hypoxia), the rise in oxygen consumption results in an "oxidative stress" that leads to the generation of reactive oxygen species, such as the superoxide radical, hydrogen peroxide, and the hydroxyl radical.[60-63] These reactive oxygen species are defined as molecules or ions containing an unpaired electron that cause cell and tissue injury. Reactive oxygen species have been implicated in certain diseases and the aging process.

The body is equipped with a sophisticated defense system to scavenge oxygen reactive species.[1,60-63] Antioxidant enzymes (e.g., glutathione peroxidase, superoxide dismutase, catalase) provide the first line of defense, with antioxidant nutrients providing a second line. Because strenuous and prolonged exercise promotes reactive oxygen species production, considerable concerns have been raised among experts regarding the ability of the body to cope with the increased oxidative stress.

Most studies have shown that chronic physical training augments the physiological antioxidant defenses in several tissues of the body.[60-63] The activity of the various antioxidant enzymes is enhanced by physical training, helping to counter the exercise-induced increase in reactive oxygen species. In general, antioxidant supplementation does not appear necessary, and has not been consistently shown to improve performance, minimize exercise-induced muscle cell damage, or maximize recovery. However, until more is known, people who exercise regularly and intensely are urged to ingest foods rich in antioxidants (fruits, vegetables, nuts, seeds, and whole grains) to augment the body's defense system against reactive oxygen species.

C. Protein and Creatine

All essential and nonessential amino acids can be supplied by plant food sources alone, as long as a variety of foods is consumed and the energy intake is adequate to meet needs.[14,64] The American Dietetic Association has advised that conscious combining of various plant foods within a given meal is unnecessary.[14]

Interest in the influence of dietary protein intake on athletic performance has been evident since the days of the ancient Greeks and Romans.[1] Athletes consumed meat-rich diets in the belief that they would achieve the strength of the consumed animal. In 1842, the great German chemist and physiologist, Justus von Liebig, reported that the primary fuel for muscular contraction was derived from muscle protein, and he suggested that large quantities of meat be eaten to replenish the supply. However, a number of studies during the late 1800s, which measured urinary urea excretion, failed to confirm his results and the concept became established that changes in protein metabolism during exercise are nonexistent or minimal at best.[1-4] Studies since 1970 using modern technology and improved techniques, however, have concluded that protein is a much more important fuel source during exercise than previously thought.[65] Research based on nitrogen balance and protein kinetic methodology have clearly shown that athletes benefit from diets containing more protein than the current RDA of 0.8 grams per kilogram of body weight per day. Strength athletes probably need about 1.6–1.7 g/kg, and endurance athletes about 1.2–1.4 g/kg.[65]

Although most vegetarian diets meet or exceed dietary recommendations for protein, they often provide less protein than non-vegetarian diets[12,26,44,49] and concerns have been raised that vegetarian athletes may have intakes that fall below the added demands created by heavy exertion.[39,65] Most athletes are able to meet these extra demands without protein supplementation by keeping dietary protein intake near 15% of total energy intake.[65] The vegan athlete can achieve optimal protein intake by careful planning, with an emphasis on protein-rich plant foods such as legumes, nuts and seeds, and whole grain products.

Creatine supplementation has been urged as an ergogenic aid for athletes who engage in repeated bouts of short-term, high-intensity exercise.[66,67] Creatine is found in large quantities in skeletal muscle and binds a significant amount of phosphate, providing an immediate source of energy in muscle cells (adenosine triphosphate or ATP). The intent of consuming supplemental creatine is to increase the skeletal muscle's creatine content, in the hope that some of the extra creatine binds phosphate, increasing muscle phosphocreatine content. During repeated bouts of high intensity exercise (for example, five 30-second bouts of sprinting or cycling exercise separated by 1–4 minutes of rest), the increased availability of phosphocreatine may improve resynthesis and degradation rates, leading to greater anaerobic ATP turnover and high-power exercise performance.[66]

The estimated daily requirement for creatine is about 2 grams. Non-vegetarians typically get about 1 gram of creatine a day from the various meats they ingest, and the body synthesizes another gram in the liver, kidney, and pancreas using the amino acids arginine and glycine as precursors. Vegetarians have a reduced body creatine pool, suggesting that lack of dietary creatine from avoidance of meat is not adequately compensated by an increase in endogenous creatine production.[67]

Various studies have shown that consuming about 20–25 grams of creatine per day for 5 to 6 days in a row significantly increases muscle creatine in most people, especially those with low levels to begin with, such as vegetarians.[66-68] Four to five daily doses of 5 grams each are usually consumed by dissolving creatine in about 250 ml of a beverage throughout the day. Each 5-gram dose of creatine is the equivalent of 1.1 kg of fresh, uncooked steak. Creatine supplementation up to 8 weeks has not been associated with major health risks, but the safety of more prolonged creatine supplementation has not been established.[66-71]

Some, but not all studies have shown that supplemental creatine improves power performance during repeated bouts of short-term sprinting, cycling, or swimming.[66-71] A recent randomized, double-blind study with vegetarian subjects failed to demonstrate any effect of creatine on power performance.[69] Only about one-half of studies have shown a significant effect of creatine on power performance, and when a positive effect is reported, it is only 5–8% above placebo effects.[1,67,71] Additional laboratory and field research is needed to help resolve the conflicting findings regarding the ergogenic efficacy of creatine supplementation.[71] Creatine supplementation has no effect on aerobic exercise metabolism and performance.[66,67] At this point, there is no justification for creatine supplementation by vegetarian athletes involved in power sports.

D. Hormonal Alterations

High fiber, low fat vegetarian diets have been associated with reduced blood estrogen levels and increased menstrual irregularity.[72-75] Large volumes of exercise have also been related to menstrual irregularity.[1,76-78] Approximately 5–20% of women who exercise regularly and vigorously, and up to 50–65% of competitive athletes may develop oligo-amenorrhea.[76,77] The causes are hotly debated, but may include the effect of exercise itself on the hypothalamic-pituitary-ovarian axis, low energy intake, and depleted fat stores in the female athlete.[1,76-78] Amenorrheic athletes typically display reduced levels of estradiol and progesterone and have hormonal profiles more similar to those of postmenopausal women. The reduced levels of endogenous estrogen associated with athletic amenorrhea may prevent the formation of adequate bone density.[1,76,77] The syndrome of amenorrhea, disordered eating (and often excessive exercise), and osteoporosis is called the "female athlete triad."[76]

Although all physically active girls and women could be at risk for developing one or more components of the athlete triad, participation in the following sports is a major risk factor:[1,76]

- Sports in which performance is subjectively scored (dance, figure skating, diving, gymnastics, aerobics)
- Endurance sports emphasizing a low body weight (distance running, cycling, cross-country skiing)
- Sports requiring body-contour-revealing clothing for competition (volleyball, swimming, diving, cross-country running, cross-country skiing, track, cheerleading)
- Sports using weight categories for participation (horse racing, some martial arts, wrestling, rowing)
- Sports emphasizing a prepubertal body habitus for performance success (figure skating, gymnastics, diving)

Two reports (published as letters) suggested that a significant proportion of female athletes with amenorrhea were vegetarians.[79,80] However, these were descriptive studies that were not able to determine whether the cause was the vegetarian diet, heavy exercise training, lower energy intake or other factors. There is increasing evidence that low energy intake, not diet quality, is a major cause of oligo-amenorrhea in female athletes, and that when brought into positive energy balance, hormonal profiles return to normal and menstruation resumes.[81] There are many parallels between the amenorrhea induced by anorexia nervosa and by strenuous athletic training, with both causing an increased secretion of antirepro-ductive hormones, which inhibit the normal pulsatile secretion pattern of gonadotropins. Hanne et al.[24] have observed that when vegetarian female athletes are properly nourished, menstrual cycle function is normal, when compared with matched non-vegetarian controls.

IV. CONCLUSION

The available evidence does not support either a beneficial or detrimental effect of a vegetarian diet upon physical performance capacity, especially when carbohydrate intake is controlled. Concerns have been raised that an emphasis on plant foods to enhance carbohydrate intake to optimize body glycogen stores may increase dietary fiber and phytic acid intake to levels that reduce the bioavailability of several nutrients, including zinc, iron, and some other trace minerals. There are no convincing data, however, that vegetarian athletes suffer impaired nutrient status from the interactive effect of their heavy exertion and plant-food-based dietary practices, at least enough to impair performance or health. Although there has been some concern about protein intake for vegetarian athletes, data indicate that all essential and nonessential amino acids can be supplied by plant food sources alone, as long as a variety of foods is consumed and the energy intake is adequate to meet needs. Creatine, found in uncooked meat, has been urged as an ergogenic aid to athletes who perform repeated bouts of short-term high intensity exercise. However, further laboratory and field research is needed to help resolve the con-flicting findings regarding the ergogenic efficacy of creatine. At this point, there is no justification for creatine supplementation by vegetarian athletes involved in power sports. There has been some concern that vegetarian female athletes are at increased risk for oligo-amenorrhea, but evidence suggests that low energy intake, not dietary quality, is a major cause.

Although some concerns have been raised about the nutrient status of vegetarian athletes, a varied and well-planned vegetarian diet is compatible with successful athletic endeavor. Various benefits make this dietary reg-imen worthy of consideration by serious athletes. A plant-based dietary facilitates a high intake of carbohydrate, which is essential for prolonged exercise. A well-planned vegetarian diet provides the athlete with adequate levels of all known nutrients, although the potential for suboptimal iron, zinc, trace element, and protein intake exists if the diet is too restrictive. However, this concern exists for all athletes, vegetarian or non-vegetarian, who have poor dietary habits. Athletes consuming a diet rich in fruits, vegetables, and whole grains receive a high intake of antioxidant nutrients, which help reduce the oxidative stress associated with heavy exertion.

While the athlete is most often concerned with performance, long-term health benefits and a reduction in risk of chronic disease have been associated with the vegetarian diet. In two studies, a combination of regular physical activity and vegetarian dietary practices provided lower mortality rates than the vegetarian diet or exercise alone.[6,82] There are interesting health parallels between vegetarian and endurance athlete populations. Both have been associated with the following health benefits:[1-21]

- Decreased prevalence of hypertension, dyslipidemia, and other risk factors
- Decreased body fat
- Decreased death rates for coronary heart disease and some types of cancer
- Decreased iron stores (but rare anemia) (with potential to reduce heart disease risk)
- Decreased levels of estrogen (with potential to reduce breast cancer risk)

As summarized in Figure 12.4, a plant-based diet is associated with a macro- and micro-nutrient profile that is conducive to both health and endurance performance.

Diet-Performance Continuum

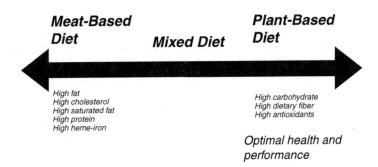

Meat-Based Diet   **Mixed Diet**   **Plant-Based Diet**

High fat
High cholesterol
High saturated fat
High protein
High heme-iron

High carbohydrate
High dietary fiber
High antioxidants

Optimal health and performance

Figure 12.4   A plant-based diet is associated with a macro- and micro-nutrient profile that is conducive to both health and endurance performance.

REFERENCES

1. Nieman, D.C. *Exercise Testing and Prescription, A Health-Related Approach.* Mayfield Publishing Company, Mountain View, CA, 1999.
2. Messina, M. and Messina, V. *The Dietitian's Guide to Vegetarian Diets: Issues and Applications.* Aspen Publishers, Inc., Gaithersburg, MD, 1996.
3. Nieman, D.C. Vegetarian dietary practices and endurance performance. *Am. J. Clin. Nutr.,* 48:754, 1988.
4. Nieman, D.C. Physical fitness and vegetarian diets: is there a relationship. *Am. J. Clin. Nutr.,* 48:754, 1999.
5. Thorogood, M., Mann, J., Appleby, P., and PcPherson, K. Risk of death from cancer and ischemic heart disease in meat and non-meat eaters. *BMJ,* 308:1667, 1994.
6. Fraser, G.E., Lindsted, K.D., and Beeson, W.L. Effect of risk factor values on lifetime risk of and age at first coronary event. The Adventist Health Study. *Am. J. Epidemiol.,* 142:746, 1995.
7. Burr, M.L. and Sweetnam, P.M. Vegetarianism, dietary fiber, and mortality. *Am. J. Clin. Nutr.,* 36:873, 1982.
8. Snowdon, D.A., Phillips, R.L., and Fraser, G.E. Meat consumption and fatal ischemic heart disease. *Prev. Med.,* 13:490, 1984.
9. Toohey, M.L., Harris, M.A., DeWitt, W., Foster, G., Schmidt, W.D., and Melby, C.L. Cardiovascular disease risk factors are lower in African-American vegans compared to lacto-ovo-vegetarians. *J. Am. Coll. Nutr.,* 17:425, 1998.
10. Thorogood, M., Carter, R., Benfield, L., McPherson, K., and Mann, J.I. Plasma lipids and lipoprotein cholesterol concentrations in people with different diets in Britain. *BMJ,* 295:351, 1987.
11. Appleby, P.N., Thorogood, M., Mann, J.I., and Key, T.J. Low body mass index in non-meat eaters: the possible roles of animal fat, dietary fiber and alcohol. *Int. J. Obes. Relat. Metab. Disord.,* 22:454, 1998.
12. Nieman, D.C., Underwood, B.C., Sherman, K.M., Barbosa, J.C., Johnson, M., and Shultz, T.D. Dietary status of Seventh-Day Adventist vegetarian and non-vegetarian elderly women. *J. Am. Diet. Assoc.,* 89:1763, 1989.
13. Neumark-Sztainer, D., Story, M., Resnick, M.D., and Blum, R.W. A behavioral profile of a school-based population in Minnesota. *Arch. Pediatr. Adolesc. Med.,* 151:833, 1997.
14. Krajcovicova-Kudlackova, M., Simoncic, R., Babinska, K., Bederova, A., Brtkova, A., Magalova, T., and Grancicova, E. Selected vitamins and trace elements in blood of vegetarians. *Ann. Nutr. Metab.,* 39:334, 1995.
15. American Dietetic Association. Position of the American Dietetic Association: Vegetarian diets, *J. Am. Diet. Assoc.,* 97:1317, 1997.
16. Key, T.J.A., Thorogood, M., Appleby, P.N., and Burr, M.L. Dietary habits and mortality in 11000 vegetarians and health conscious people: results of a 17 year follow up. *BMJ,* 313:775, 1996.
17. Pietinen, P., Rimm, E.B., Korhonen, P., Hartman, A.M., Willett, W.C., Albanes, D., and Virtamo, J. Intake of dietary fiber and risk of coronary heart disease in a cohort of Finnish men. The Alpha-Tocopherol, Beta-Carotene Cancer Prevention Study. *Circulation,* 94:2720, 1996.

18. Rimm, E.B., Ascherio, A., Giovannucci, E., Spiegelman, D., Stampfer, M.J., and Willett, W.C. Vegetable, fruit, and cereal fiber intake and risk of coronary heart disease among men. *JAMA*, 275:447, 1996.

19. American Dietetic Association. Position of the American Dietetic Association: Phytochemicals and functional foods. *J. Am. Diet. Assoc.*, 95:493, 1995.

20. Steinmetz, K.A. and Potter, J.D. Vegetables, fruit, and cancer prevention: a review. *J. Am. Diet. Assoc.*, 96:1027, 1996.

21. Jacobs, D.R., Meyer, K.A., Kushi, L.H., and Folsom, A.R. Whole-grain intake may reduce the risk of ischemic heart disease death in postmenopausal women: the Iowa Women's Health Study. *Am. J. Clin. Nutr.*, 68:248-257, 1998.

22. Cotes, J.E., Dabbs, J.M., Hall, A.M., McDonald, A., Miller, D.S., Mumford, P., and Saunders, M.J. Possible effect of a vegan diet upon lung function and the cardiorespiratory response to submaximal exercise in healthy women. *J. Physiol. (Lond.)*, 209 (suppl):30P, 1970.

23. Williams, M.H. *Nutritional Aspects of Human Physical and Athletic Performance*. Charles C. Thomas Publisher, Springfield, IL, 1985, pp. 415.

24. Hanne, N., Dlin, R., and Rotstein, A. Physical fitness, anthropometric and metabolic parameters in vegetarian athletes. *J. Sports Med.*, 26:180, 1986.

25. Nieman, D.C., Haig, J.L., De Guia, E.D., Dizon, G.P., and Register, U.D. Reducing diet and exercise training effects on resting metabolic rates in mildly obese women. *J. Sports Med.*, 28:79, 1988.

26. Snyder, A.C., Dvorak, L.L., and Roepke, J.B. Influence of dietary iron source on measures of iron status among female runners. *Med. Sci. Sports Exerc.*, 21:7, 1989.

27. Nagel, D., Seller, D., Franz, H., Leitzmann, C., and Jung, K. Effects of an ultra-long (1000 km) race on lipid metabolism. *Eur. J. Appl. Physiol.*, 59:16, 1989.

28. Seiler, D., Nagel, D., Franz, H., Hellstern, P., Leitzmann, C., and Jung, K. Effects of long-distance running on iron metabolism and hematological parameters. *Int J. Sports Med.*, 10:357, 1989.

29. Eisinger, M. Nutrient intake of endurance runners with lacto-ovo vetetarian diet and regular Western diet. *Z. Ernahrungswiss*, 33:217, 1994.

30. Nieman, D.C., Sherman, K.M., Arabatzis, K., Underwood, B.C., Barbosa, J.C., Johnson, M., Shultz, T.D., and Lee, J.W. Hematological, anthropometric, and metabolic comparisons between vegetarian and non-vegetarian elderly women. *Int J. Sports Med.*, 10:243, 1989.

31. Richter, E.A., Kiens, B., Raben, A., Tvede, N., and Pedersen, B.K. Immune parameters in male athletes after a lacto-ovo-vegetarian diet and a mixed Western diet. *Med. Sci. Sports Exerc.*, 23:517, 1991.

32. Raben, A., Kiens, B., Richter, E.A., Rasmussen, L.B., Svenstrup, B., Micic, S., and Bennett, P. Serum sex hormones and endurance performance after a lacto-ovo-vegetarian and a mixed diet. *Med. Sci. Sports Exerc.*, 24:1290, 1992.

33. Nieman, D.C., Butterworth, D.E., Nehlsen-Cannarella, S.L., Henson, D.A., and Fagoaga, O.R. Animal product intake and immune function. *Veg. Nutr. Int. J.*, 1:5, 1997.

34. Hargreaves, M. Interactions between muscle glycogen and blood glucose during exercise. *Exerc. Sport Sci. Rev.*, 25:21, 1997.

35. Coyle, E.F. Substrate utilization during exercise in active people. *Am. J. Clin. Nutr.*, 61(suppl):968S, 1995.

36. Coggan, A.R., Plasma glucose metabolism during exercise: effects of endurance training in humans. *Med. Sci. Sports Exerc.*, 29:620, 1997.
37. Nieman, D.C., Butler, J.V., Pollett, L.M., Dietrich, S.J., and Lutz, R.D. Nutrient intake of marathon runners. *J. Am. Diet. Assoc.*, 89:1273, 1989.
38. Cerqueira, M.T., Fry, M.M., and Conner, W.E. The food and nutrient intakes of the Tarahumara Indians of Mexico. *Am. J. Clin. Nutr.*, 32:905, 1979.
39. Kleiner, S.M. The role of meat in an athlete's diet: its effect on key macro- and micronutrients. *Sports Sci. Exch.*, 8(5):1, 1995.
40. Centers for Disease Control and Prevention. Recommendations to prevent and control iron deficiency in the United States. *MMWR*, 47(No. RR-3):1-30.
41. American Dietetic Association. Timely statement of the American Dietetic Association: Nutrition guidance for adolescent athletes in organized sports. *J. Am. Diet. Assoc.*, 96:611, 1996.
42. Gibson, R.S. Content and bioavailability of trace elements in vegetarian diets. *Am. J. Clin. Nutr.*, 59(suppl):1223S, 1994.
43. Craig, W.J. Iron status of vegetarians. *Am. J. Clin. Nutr.*, 59 (suppl):1233S, 1994.
44. Alexander, D., Ball, M.J., and Mann, J. Nutrient intake and hematological status of vegetarians and age-sex matched omnivores. *Eur. J. Clin. Nutr.*, 48:538, 1994.
45. Nathan, I., Hackett, A.F., and Kirby, S. The dietary intake of a group of vegetarian children aged 7-11 years compared with matched omnivores. *Br. J. Nutr.*, 75:533, 1996.
46. Lowik, M.R., Schrijver, J., Odink, J., Van Den Berg, H., and Wedel. M. Long-term effects of a vegetarian diet on the nutritional status of elderly people (Dutch Nutrition Surveillance System). *J. Am. Coll. Nutr.*, 9:600, 1900.
47. Brants, H.A., Lowik, M.R., Westenbrink, S., Hulshof, K.F., and Kistemaker, C. Adequacy of a vegetarian diet at old age (Dutch Nutrition Surveillance System). *J. Am. Coll. Nutr.*, 9:292, 1990.
48. Donovan, U.M. and Gibson, R.S. Iron and zinc status of young women aged 14 to 19 years consuming vegetarian and omnivorous diets. *J. Am. Coll. Nutr.*, 14:463, 1995.
49. Janelle, K.C. and Barr, S.I. Nutrient intakes and eating behavior scores of vegetarian and non-vegetarian women. *J. Am. Diet. Assoc.*, 95:180, 1995.
50. Salonen, J.T., Nyyssönen, K., Korpella, H., Tuomilehto, J., Seppanen, R., and Salonen, R. High stored iron levels are associated with excess risk of myocardial infarction in eastern Finnish men. *Circulation*, 86:803, 1992.
51. Lakka, T.A., Nyyssönen, K., and Salonen, J.T. Higher levels of conditioning leisure time physical activity are associated with reduced levels of stored iron in Finnish men. *Am. J. Epidemiol.*, 140:148, 1994.
52. Stevens, R.G., Jones, Y., Micozzi, M.S., and Taylor, P.R. Body iron stores and the risk of cancer. *N. Engl. J. Med.*, 319:1047, 1988.
53. Selby, G.B. and Eichner, E.R. Hematocrit and performance: the effect of endurance training on blood volume. *Sem. Hematol.*, 31:122, 1994.
54. Nielsen, P. and Nachtigall, D. Iron supplementation in athletes: current recommendations. *Sports Med.*, 26:207, 1998.
55. Balke, B. and Snow, C. Anthropological and physiological observations on Tarahumara endurance runners. *Am. J. Phys. Anthropol.*, 23:293, 1965.
56. Clarkson, P.M. and Haymes, E.M. Trace mineral requirements for athletes. *Int. J. Sports Nutr.*, 4:104, 1994.

57. Fogelholm, M. Indicators of vitamin and mineral status in athletes' blood: a review. *Int. J. Sports Nutr.*, 5:267, 1995.
58. Mares-Perlman, J.A., Subar, A.F., Block, G., Greger, J.L., and Luby, M.H. Zinc intake and sources in the U.S. adult population: 1976-1980. *J. Am. Coll. Nutr.*, 14:349, 1995.
59. American Dietetic Association. Position of the American Dietetic Association: Vitamin and mineral supplementation. *J. Am. Diet. Assoc.*, 96:73, 1996.
60. Vasankari, T.J., Kujala, U.M., Vasankari, T.M., Vuorimaa, T., and Ahotupa, M. Increased serum and low-density-lipoprotein antioxidant potential after antioxidant supplementation in endurance athletes. *Am. J. Clin. Nutr.*, 65:1052, 1997.
61. Sen, C. K. Oxidants and antioxidants in exercise. *J. Appl. Physiol.*, 79:675, 1995.
62. Ji, L.L. Exercise and oxidative stress: role of the cellular antioxidant systems. *Ex. Sport Sci. Rev.*, 23:135, 1995.
63. Kanter, M. Free radicals and exercise: effects of nutritional antioxidant supplementation. *Ex. Sport Sci. Rev.*, 23:375, 1995.
64. Young, V.R. and Pellett, P.L. Plant proteins in relation to human protein and amino acid nutrition. *Am. J. Clin. Nutr.*, 59(suppl):1203S, 1994.
65. Lemon, P.W.R. Effects of exercise on dietary protein requirements. *Int. J. Sport Nutr.*, 8:426, 1998.
66. Greenhaff, P.L. Creatine and its application as an ergogenic aid. *Int. J. Sport Nutr.*, 5:S100, 1995.
67. Mujika, I. and Padilla, S. Creatine supplementation as an ergogenic aid for sports performance in highly trained athletes: a critical review. *Int J. Sports Med.*, 18:491, 1997.
68. Hultman, E., Söderlund, K., Timmons, J.A., Cederblad, G., and Greenhaff, P.L. Muscle creatine loading in men. *J. Appl. Physiol.*, 81:232, 1996.
69. Clarys, P.M., Zinzen, E.M., Hebbelinck, M., and Verlinden, M. The effect of oral creatine supplementation on torque production in a vegetarian and a non-vegetarian population: a double blind study. *Veg. Nutr: Int. J.*, 1:100, 1997.
70. Burke, L.M., Pyne, D.B., and Telford, R.D. Effect of oral creatine supplementation on single-effort sprint performance in elite swimmers. *Int. J. Sport Nutr.*, 6:222, 1996.
71. Williams, M.H. and Branch, J.D. Creatine supplementation and exercise performance: an update. *J. Am. Coll. Nutr.*, 17:216, 1998.
72. Bagga, D. Effects of a very low-fat, high-fiber diet on serum hormones and menstrual function — implications for breast cancer prevention. *Cancer*, 76:2491, 1995.
73. Pedersen, A.B., Bartholomew, M.J., Dolence, L.A., Aljadir, L.P., Netteburg, K.L., and Lloyd, T. Menstrual differences due to vegetarian and non-vegetarian diets. *Am. J. Clin. Nutr.*, 53:879, 1991.
74. Barbosa, J.C., Shultz, T.D., Filley, S.J., and Nieman, D.C. The relationship among adiposity, diet, and hormone concentrations in vegetarian and non-vegetarian postmenopausal women. *Am. J. Clin. Nutr.*, 51:798, 1990.
75. Goldin, B.R., Adlercreutz, H., Gorbach, S.L., Warram, J.H., Dwyer, J.T., Swenson, L., and Woods, M.N. Estrogen excretion patterns and plasma levels in vegetarian and omnivorous women. *N. Engl. J. Med.*, 307:1542, 1982.
76. American College of Sports Medicine. ACSM Position Stand on the Female Athlete Triad. *Med. Sci. Sports Exerc.*, 29:i-ix, 1997.

77. Loucks, A.B., Vaitukaitis, J., Cameron, J.L., Rogol, A.D., Skrinar, G., Warren, M.P., Kendrick, J., and Limacher, M.C. The reproductive system and exercise in women. *Med. Sci. Sports Exerc.*, 24(suppl):S288, 1992.
78. West, RV. The female athlete: The triad of disordered eating, amenorrhea and osteoporosis. *Sports Med.*, 26:63-71.
79. Brooks, S.M., Sanborn, C.F., Albrecht, B.H., and Wagner, W.W. Diet in athletic amenorrhea. *Lancet*, 1:559, 1984 (letter).
80. Slavin, J., Lutter, J., and Cushman, S. Amenorrhea in vegetarian athletes. *Lancet*, 1:1474, 1984 (letter).
81. Dueck, C.A., Matt, K.S., Manore, M.M., and Skinner, J.S. Treatment of athletic amenorrhea with a diet and training intervention program. *Int. J. Sport Nutr.*, 6:24, 1996.
82. Chang-Claude, J. and Frentzel-Beyme, R. Dietary and lifestyle determinants of mortality among German vegetarians. *Int. J. Epidemiol.*, 22:228, 1993.

IV

RECOMMENDATIONS FOR HEALTHY VEGETARIAN DIETS

13

NUTRIENTS OF CONCERN IN VEGETARIAN DIETS

Winston J. Craig and Laura Pinyan

CONTENTS

0-8493-8508-3/01/$0.00+$.50
© 2001 by CRC Press LLC

I. INTRODUCTION

Well-balanced vegetarian diets offer many health benefits including decreased risk of cardiovascular disease, cancer, and possibly type II diabetes.[1] Vegetarian diets more closely approximate the recommendations for a reduced saturated fat and cholesterol intake, and an increased fruit and vegetable consumption. Since vegetarian diets vary widely, they are quite diverse in their nutrient profile. When appropriately planned, the majority of traditional vegetarian diets are nutritionally adequate. Some types of vegetarian diets, such as strict macrobiotic diets, raise concerns about multiple nutrient deficiencies.

Vegetarians in Western countries typically fall into three main categories: lacto-ovo-vegetarians (LOVs), vegans, or other vegetarians. LOVs use dairy products and eggs, but do not use meat, fish, or poultry. Many individuals, such as Seventh-Day Adventists, have been following LOV diets since the mid-1800s. They are less likely to have low intakes of vitamin B_{12} and calcium than other vegetarians.

Those who follow traditional Western vegan diets use a wide variety of fruits, grains, nuts, legumes, and vegetables, but do not use meat, fish, poultry, eggs, or dairy products. This usually corresponds to a lower intake of saturated fat and cholesterol than for omnivores or LOVs. Consequently, vegans have a decreased risk of cardiovascular disease.[2] Vegan diets are generally adequate except for the need for vitamin B_{12} supplementation. Some evidence suggests that female vegans may need to carefully plan their calcium intake to ensure optimal bone mass. This may necessitate the use of calcium-fortified foods or supplements.[3]

While most vegetarians do not follow unhealthful fad diets, there is a sizable minority that do. Vegetarians who follow trendy new diets may be at risk for nutrient deficiencies and attendant health problems. Such diets need to be modified to more nearly resemble those of traditional vegetarian diets.

The most liberal of macrobiotic diets may provide a fair variety of foods but still be inadequate in nutrients such as calcium.[4] The more restrictive macrobiotic diets, which are considered superior by their followers, are actually inadequate. They use little fruit and hardly any grains except rice. The diets may be low in protein, calories, and other nutrients. There have been serious medical complications, including death, in children on macrobiotic diets.[5] These diets should be liberalized to include more kinds of fruits, a variety of grains, and ample amounts of vegetable protein.

The generous use of raw foods can be healthful for most individuals. However, diets that are largely composed of raw foods may be difficult to plan to ensure nutritional adequacy. An entirely raw diet has been shown to cause 9% weight loss within 3 months despite adequate caloric intake, due to poor macronutrient absorption.[6] The use of cooked grains rather than raw, and the inclusion of legumes, along with other dietary planning can improve nutritional adequacy.

II. PROTEIN

It is recommended that American adults receive about 45–65 grams of protein. While vegetarians typically consume lower amounts of protein than omnivores, they generally have an adequate protein intake,[7] provided they receive adequate calories and eat a variety of foods such as soy beans and soy products (soy burgers, tofu, soy beverages, soy nuts, etc.), other legumes, nuts and seeds, and grains. Those with greater protein needs should increase the number of servings of legumes they consume. Soy products are considered complete proteins,[8] since they provide a balanced amount of all nine essential amino acids. Combining plant foods such as whole grains and legumes also provides a dietary protein combination that has an adequate biological value.

The amino acid pool available for absorption derives from a combination of exogenous and endogenous proteins. Endogenous protein, which contains essential amino acids, enters the digestive tract every day from two different sources, the digestive enzymes and the intestinal cells sloughed off into the intestinal tract. Clearly, the quality of protein eaten at each meal is important but not critical since the endogenous protein supplies a significant amount of essential amino acids. For the different types of plant proteins to complement each other, they should be eaten during the same day, but not necessarily within the same meal. This allows for flexibility in food preferences and removes the concern about whether each meal contains properly balanced protein sources.[9]

Protein is used for growth and tissue repair, and for the synthesis of enzymes and hormones. Hence, children will require a greater proportion of their proteins to be of high biological value than adults. Vegan children, especially, should receive ample quantities of legumes or soy products on a regular basis. The National Academy of Sciences recommends that children over the age of 1 receive 23–34 grams of protein, depending on their age. The typical American adult usually gets far more protein than required, and because protein consumption at or above the recommended level causes an increased excretion of calcium, the high protein diet typically eaten by Americans may also be a contributing factor in the decline of kidney function seen in certain diseases and in aging.

III. IRON

Iron provides a diversity of vital functions. While two thirds of body iron is present in hemoglobin, 10% of total body iron is found in myoglobin. The important iron-containing cytochromes located in the mitochondria facilitate energy production. The human body typically contains less than 5 grams of iron, and carefully guards against iron losses and conserves iron wherever possible. Iron can be stored in bone marrow and liver mostly as ferritin. The amount of iron stored in the body can vary over a wide range without any apparent impairment in body function.[10] Male adults typically have iron stores of about 1 gram, while female stores are usually less than one-half gram of iron.

Iron stores tend to be lower in premenopausal women, adolescents, and young children. Such groups are at highest risk of iron deficiency. In such individuals, iron absorption may be enhanced by the body's need for iron. In pregnant women, additional iron above the woman's normal needs is required for fetal growth. In growing children and adolescents, there is a rapidly expanding blood volume and muscle mass that requires iron. Women of childbearing years have higher iron needs due to additional menstrual losses of iron.

A. Iron Deficiency

Over 500 million people worldwide may have iron-deficiency anemia.[11] A major reason for this situation is that the common forms of iron in food are poorly absorbed. Furthermore, in Third World countries, there is a substantial drain on iron caused by malaria, hookworm, and other parasitic infections, in addition to the heavy burden on the iron stores of women caused by repeated pregnancies.

Iron deficiency results when absorption from the gastrointestinal tract is not sufficient to meet the needs of the body. Iron deficiency initially begins when iron stores decrease, followed by a drop in serum ferritin levels. However, low serum ferritin levels have not been associated with any known adverse physical effects. Iron is delivered to the tissues by the transport protein transferrin. Specific receptors bind transferrin, facilitating the uptake of iron by the cell. In iron deficiency the number of transferrin receptors increase. Iron-deficiency anemia results when hemoglobin levels drop and hematocrit values decrease below normal.[12] The use of iron supplements when needed (such as during pregnancy), and an adequate iron intake during times of rapid growth are important steps in the prevention of iron-deficiency anemia.

Iron deficiency is commonly caused by a poor absorption of iron from the diet due to a low intake of iron-rich foods or the consumption of a diet high in substances that block iron absorption. Anemia can result not only from a dietary deficiency of iron but also from infections, inflammatory conditions, achlorhydria, and hemorrhaging. There are a number of consequences of iron deficiency, some of which may be quite serious. The more common effects include a decreased capacity for work, impaired intellectual performance, a decrease in attentiveness, a tendency to fatigue, a greater risk of premature delivery, a low-birth-weight child, complications of pregnancy, and an impaired immune function with a decreased resistance to infection.[13-16]

B. Iron Absorption

The body regulates iron balance primarily by absorption. Iron absorption can vary greatly from as little as 1% to as much as 40%,[17] depending on the iron content of the meal, the chemical form of the iron, the composition of the ingested food, and the iron status and need of the individual.[13] Late in pregnancy, when the fetus is rapidly growing and developing significant liver stores of iron, iron absorption may increase to about 35–40%. Normally, iron absorption is only about 10–15%. With low iron stores, iron absorption increases, while absorption decreases as body iron stores increase. This is a regulatory mechanism to help the body fight iron deficiency and iron overload.[18]

Two types of iron exist in food — heme and non-heme iron. Almost one-half of the iron present in meat, poultry and fish is heme iron, which is generally better absorbed (15–35%) than non-heme iron (typically 5–10%) and its absorption tends to be unaffected by other dietary components.[19] Heme iron is more efficiently absorbed since there are specific heme-binding sites in the intestinal tract that facilitate its absorption.[13] The vegetarian diet, which contains plant foods with or without dairy products and eggs, contains only non-heme iron. The absorption of non-heme iron depends upon iron stores as well as its solubility in the small intestine. Phytates and polyphenolics in whole grain cereals, legumes, and nuts tend to bind non-heme iron and greatly reduce its absorption.[20] On the other hand, vitamin C enhances absorption. About 75 mg of vitamin C increases non-heme iron absorption 3- to 4-fold.[19,21] The polyphenolics in tea and coffee can reduce non-heme iron absorption from a meal by about 60% and 40% respectively, while the polyphenolics in herbal teas may also adversely effect iron uptake.[22-25] Diets high in phytates and tannins inhibit iron absorption and may produce iron deficiency. Such is the case where large quantities of unleavened chapatis and Indian tea are consumed.[22,26]

Vitamin C facilitates iron absorption by converting iron to ferrous iron, a form that is better absorbed than ferric iron.[20] Vitamin C can also chelate ferric iron, thus enhancing its solubility and improving its absorption. In addition, small amounts of citric, malic, and tartaric acids, as found in fruits and vegetables, and lactic acid in sauerkraut can enhance iron absorption 2- to 3-fold.[13,23] Iron absorption from fermented soy products such as miso and tempeh appears to be superior to that of the whole soybean.[27] Moderate amounts of vitamin C in the diet may negate the inhibitory effect on iron absorption of the phytates in cereals and nuts.[28,29]

Whole grain and fortified cereals, dark green leafy vegetables, fruits and dried fruits, nuts, and legumes provide a vegetarian diet with substantial amounts of iron (see Table 13.1). While the percentage of iron absorbed from refined cereal products is twice to three times greater than from whole grain products, the net absorption of iron from whole grain and refined products is about the same, since whole wheat bread and brown rice contain about twice to three times the amount of iron found in white bread and white rice. The same applies to soy beans. While the percentage of iron absorbed from soy may be low, the total amount of iron absorbed is adequate, because soy beans naturally contain relatively large amounts of iron.[30,31] Factors that influence the absorption of non-heme iron are summarized in Table 13.2.

C. Iron Status of Vegetarians

What then is the iron status of someone following a balanced vegetarian diet? While vegetarians tend to have reduced iron stores and lower serum ferritin levels, a number of studies have shown that serum iron and hemoglobin levels of vegetarians are similar to those of non-vegetarians.[32-36] This is also true for vegans who follow a well-planned diet. Since milk is not a good source of iron, and the iron in egg has a low bioavailability,[13,20] an LOV would have no advantage over a vegan as far as iron status is concerned. In a British study, adult vegans who consumed a total vegetarian diet for 6 or more years had hemoglobin levels similar to those of omnivorous subjects, and no subject had a hemoglobin level below the normal lower limit.[37] Children consuming a balanced LOV or vegan

Table 13.1 Iron Content of Plant Foods

	Iron (mg)
Legumes	
1/2 cup soybeans	2.7
1/2 cup red kidney beans	1.8
1/2 cup lentils	1.6
1/2 cup peas	1.5
Grains and pasta	
1 cup oatmeal	1.7
1 cup spaghetti, enriched	1.4
1 cup brown rice	0.8
1 slice whole-wheat bread	0.8
Vegetables	
1/2 cup collards, cooked	1.0
1 tomato, medium	0.8
1/2 cup broccoli	0.7
1 potato, medium	0.7
Nuts and seeds	
1 oz almonds	1.3
1 oz peanuts	1.0
Fruits and dried fruits	
5 prunes, large	1.7
5 dates, medium	1.5
1 slice watermelon (15 cm dm x 2 cm)	1.5
10 strawberries, large	1.0
1 oz raisins	1.0
1 cup orange juice	1.0
3 figs, medium	0.9
1 orange, medium	0.6

diet were also shown to have an iron status similar to children following a non-vegetarian diet.[38] However, children consuming a restricted macrobiotic diet consisting of rice, sea vegetables, and some fruit commonly manifest iron deficiencies.[39]

In summary, while the iron stores of some vegetarians may be marginal, the risk of iron-deficiency anemia resulting from the consumption of a well-balanced Western vegetarian diet appears to be no different from that of following a non-vegetarian diet. Some have suggested that high intakes of iron may actually be associated with greater risk of heart disease.[40] Iron is a strong pro-oxidant and may assist with the formation of free radicals, which promote the formation of atherogenic oxidized LDL particles. Non-

Table 13.2   Factors that Influence the Absorption of Non-Heme Iron

Plant Substances that Enhance Non-heme-Iron Absorption
    Ascorbic acid
    Citric, malic, lactic, tartaric, and other organic acids
    Fermented soy products
    Other factors include:
        Low iron stores of individuals
        Low iron content of meals
        Iron in ferrous form
Substances that Inhibit Non-heme-Iron Absorption
    Phytates
    Plant polyphenolics
    High intake of zinc supplements
    Soy protein
    Bran
    Milk and egg
    Tea and coffee
    Calcium phosphates

vegetarians are more likely to absorb excessive amounts of iron since the heme iron in meat products allows for a greater availability.

IV. ZINC

While overt zinc deficiency is rare in the U.S., it has been commonly seen in the Middle East.[41] The U.S. RDAs for zinc are 15 mg/day for adult males and 12 mg for adult females, 15 mg for pregnant women and 19 mg for lactating women. The precise zinc requirements are still a matter of debate — Canadian recommendations for zinc are about 35% lower than the U.S. recommendations. The absorption of zinc is quite variable (normally about 20–30%), and the absorption of zinc does increase with a lower intake or an increased need. Zinc is required for normal growth and development, a healthy immune system, taste acuity, and healthy epithelial tissue.

The zinc intake of children may not be adequate on some vegetarian diets. Whole grains, legumes, and nuts are high in phytates, which are known to bind zinc. Phytates may therefore limit zinc absorption and impair growth and reproductive development in children consuming a vegetarian diet.[42] Since zinc is less effectively absorbed from a vegetarian diet than from an omnivorous diet, it is important that vegetarians select zinc-rich foods.[43] A vegetarian diet can be satisfactorily devised whereby adequate levels of zinc are provided.[44] For example, zinc bioavailability from leavened bread is greater than from unleavened products, as the leavening process in breadmaking activates phytase, which breaks down phytic acid. The result is an improved bioavailability of zinc.

Even though adult vegetarians often have a mean zinc intake lower than omnivores, they generally appear to have adequate zinc status, as reflected by serum zinc levels[35] and zinc balance studies.[45] Over time, people appear to adapt to a vegetarian diet, which results in an improved zinc utilization.[46] Female vegetarians may be more likely to be at risk of low serum zinc levels than males, due to their lower zinc intake. An Australian study found that vegetarian and non-vegetarian men had a similar mean intake of zinc,[47] while vegetarian women had a significantly lower mean daily zinc intake than omnivorous women (6.8 mg vs. 8.4 mg). Even though vegetarian women had a lower zinc intake, the mean serum zinc levels were similar in female omnivores and vegetarians. A similar disparity in zinc intakes was observed for adolescent females following a vegetarian diet (6.7 mg) compared with those following an omnivorous diet (7.8 mg).[48]

The elderly, both vegetarians and omnivores, have an increased risk of zinc deficiency, which may be associated with altered taste acuity and a decreased immune function. In a study of elderly women, mean zinc intakes were low for both vegetarians and omnivores (6.3 mg).[33] By contrast, a study of elderly Dutch persons found serum zinc levels in vegetarians lower than in omnivores.[49]

In summary, while clinical zinc deficiency is not common in the West, relatively few individuals meet the U.S. RDAs. Adult male vegetarians appear to approximate the RDAs more closely than do female vegetarians. Generally, female vegetarians tend to have lower zinc intakes than female omnivores. Elderly people, both vegetarian and omnivores, are at increased risk for zinc deficiency. Vegan children and adolescents, and pregnant and lactating women may need to increase their zinc intake. Those on macrobiotic diets may have particularly low zinc intakes. Adults who follow an LOV diet do not appear to be at any greater risk of low zinc status than omnivores.[47]

V.   CALCIUM

Daily requirements for calcium were recently increased due to concerns about bone health of the elderly. Current U.S. DRIs for calcium vary depending on age. Adolescents are recommended to have 1300 mg of calcium/day; adults and pregnant and lactating women, 1000 mg/day; and persons over 50, 1200 mg/day. About 10 million Americans currently have osteoporosis and 18 million more are at risk due to low bone mineral density (BMD). In the U.S., the prevalence of osteoporosis among postmenopausal women is reported to be 21% in Caucasian and Asian, 16% in Hispanic, and 10% in African-American women.[50] Those who do not attain an appropriate peak BMD early in life are at risk for osteoporosis even if their rate of bone loss is not excessive.[51] Optimization of bone health at all stages of the life cycle is the most effective means of preventing osteoporosis. In order to optimize bone mass, adequate intakes of calcium throughout the life cycle is essential. However, maintaining desirable BMD involves many factors besides calcium intake (see Table 13.3).[52]

Table 13.3   Factors Negatively Affecting Calcium Balance

Not modifiable
  Female
  Premature menopause
  Caucasian (non Hispanic) or Asian ethnicity
  Elderly
  Small frame
  Family history
Modifiable
  Lack of vitamin D (sunlight or oral intake) especially in elderly shut-ins
  Amenorrhea
  Lack of estrogen
  Underweight
  Sedentary lifestyle
  Lack of adequate calcium
  High sodium intake
  Low isoflavone intake
  Alcohol
  Tobacco
  Caffeine
  Excessive or insufficient protein intake
  High phosphorus intake
  High consumption of phytate
  Insufficient magnesium
  Insufficient boron

A. Dietary Effects on Calcium Balance

The average American diet, high in protein and low in fruits and vegetables, can generate over 100 meq of acid a day, mainly as sulfate and phosphate.[53] Fruits and vegetables produce a high renal alkaline load whereas fish, meat, grains, and cheeses produce a high renal acid load.

Active bone resorption helps to buffer this acid. The kidneys also respond to the acid challenge with net acid excretion. Hence, a diet high in acid-ash proteins will cause hypercalciuria, whereas adding fruit and vegetables to the diet will slow or halt bone resorption and decrease calcium losses in the urine.[53] Aging kidneys cannot excrete hydrogen ions as well as young kidneys, so the elderly require more buffering action. This means that high protein diets are more detrimental to the bones of the elderly.

Studies reveal that a high protein intake increases glomerular filtration rate and decreases the fraction of calcium reabsorbed by the kidney.[54] The result is an increased urinary excretion of calcium. Calcium balance was reported to be positive on a low protein diet (48 g/day), but negative on a moderate or high protein diet (95 and 142 g/day).[55] Urinary calcium increased from 90 mg/day to 171 mg/day when elderly persons switched from a low protein diet (0.8 g /kg body weight) to a high protein diet (2.0 g/kg).[56] A dietary calcium (mg) to protein (g) ratio of at least 20 to 1[54] or at least 16 to 1[57] has been suggested as desirable to provide adequate protection for the skeleton. Using the more conservative number of 16 to 1, a person consuming 85 g protein/day would need to consume at least 1360 mg calcium/day.

Calcium excretion is a more important determinant of the calcium status than calcium absorption. Hence, dietary factors such as protein and sodium intake that increase urinary calcium losses have a negative effect on bone health. On average, for every 10 g of protein consumed, urinary calcium increases about 10 mg. On the other hand, for every gram of sodium ingested, there is an additional 25 mg of urinary calcium.[58] At the present level of intake in North America, dietary sodium intake would appear to have a greater effect on calcium balance than dietary protein. The long-term consequence of a small change in calcium balance can be quite substantial. A 30-mg increase in urinary calcium loss/day will result in a 11 g loss/year, or 220 g loss over 20 years. This corresponds to about 22% and 30% of typical male and female skeletal stores, respectively.[53]

One might think that increased milk consumption would guarantee a positive calcium balance and strong healthy bones, but this is not necessarily the case. Hegsted has reported that hip fractures worldwide actually occur more frequently in populations that consume higher levels of calcium, derived mainly from dairy products, and higher intakes of protein.[59] In the Nurses' Health Study, there was no evidence that a higher consumption of milk or calcium-rich foods provided any protective effect against hip or forearm fractures in middle-aged women.[60] Women who drank two or more glasses of milk/day had relative risks of 1.45 for hip fracture and 1.05 for forearm fracture when compared with women consuming one glass or less/week.

B. The Vegetarian Advantage

In addition to a diet rich in calcium, low in sodium, modest in protein, and adequate in vitamin D, an adequate intake of boron may also help to maintain a positive calcium balance and reduce the risk of osteoporosis. Postmenopausal women consuming diets supplemented with 3 mg of boron excreted about 20% less urinary calcium than unsupplemented women. In addition, blood estrogen levels of the women receiving boron more than doubled, giving a blood level similar to those women who were on estrogen replacement therapy.[61] Vegetarians would be more likely to consume adequate amounts of boron because meats and fish are poor sources of boron while fruits, dried fruits, and nuts are rich sources. Soy, almonds, peanuts, raisins, prunes, and hazel nuts are reported as having high levels of boron.[62]

In contrast to diets containing animal protein, vegetarian diets produce metabolizable anions such as acetate and bicarbonate that help reduce calcium excretion.[63,64] Furthermore, vegetarians generally consume more leafy vegetables than the general population. Green, leafy vegetables such as broccoli, cabbage, and lettuce supply sizeable quantities of vitamin K, which is essential for bone metabolism. Low intakes of vitamin K are associated with increased risk of hip fracture. One or more servings/day of lettuce has been associated with a 45% reduced risk of hip fracture.[65]

Animal-protein diets, with their high levels of sulfur-containing amino acids, produce excess sulfate ions that lead to a reduced renal reabsorption of calcium and an increased level of urinary calcium. Daily urinary net acid excretion was 27 meq higher and daily urinary calcium was 47 mg higher in young adults consuming an animal-protein diet vs. a vegetarian diet.[66] Since legumes are low in the sulfur-containing amino acids, we might expect that calcium losses would be less in vegetarians. A significantly greater titratable acid output was observed with omnivorous women (48.9 meq/24h) compared with vegetarian women (35.3 meq/24h). Although the dietary intake of calcium was not different between the two groups, urinary calcium excretion of the omnivores was 20% higher (3.87 vs. 3.22 mmol/24 h) than that of the vegetarians.[67]

In the Nurses' Health Study, consumption of meat had an adverse effect on bone health. The total protein intake was associated with a 22% increased risk of forearm fracture for women who consumed more than 95 g protein per day compared with those who consumed less than 68 g per day. A similar increase in risk was observed for animal protein, but no association was found for consumption of vegetable protein. Women who consumed at least five servings of red meat/week had a 23% increased risk of forearm fracture compared with women who ate red meat less than once per week.[68] No association was observed between protein intake and the incidence of hip fractures.

BMD has been compared in several cross-sectional studies of vegetarians and omnivores. Postmenopausal LOV women over 50 years of age are reported to have substantially higher cortical bone mass than non-vegetarian women who consumed similar levels of calcium.[69] In this study, no difference in BMD was seen between the two dietary groups for women aged 20 to 49 years. Other researchers have found an LOV diet associated with a higher cortical bone mass in post-menopausal women.[70]

Not all studies have found that a vegetarian diet has a protective effect on bone health. In a 5-year prospective study in North Carolina, post-menopausal LOV and omnivorous women (mean age, 81 years) lost radius BMD at a similar annual rate of about 1%.[71] The LOVs consumed about 150 mg/d less calcium than the omnivores. However, bone loss was independent of calcium intake perhaps due to the modestly high calcium intake of the women. The single most critical factor for BMD retention in these older women was maintenance of their lean body mass.[71] In another study of Caucasian postmenopausal women in Florida, no differences were observed in trabecular and cortical bone density between the LOVs and omnivores, despite a slightly lower calcium intake in vegetarians.[72] Lloyd, et al. also found that, for premenopausal women, spinal BMD did not differ significantly between vegetarians and omnivores.[73]

In a study of young Canadian women, vegetarians tended to have lower spinal BMD than the omnivores (5.6% lower, $p = 0.06$) although the difference appeared to result from a lower body weight in the vegetarians.[74] After 1 year of follow-up, the spinal BMD of the omnivores had increased 1.7%, while that of the vegetarians experienced only a non-significant 0.5% increase.[74] In at least one study of elderly women, vegetarians were seen to be at greater risk of osteoporosis. In the study by Lau et al.,[75] BMD at the hip, but not the spine, was observed to be significantly lower in elderly vegetarian women compared with matched omnivores.

C. Vegan Studies

While the dietary calcium intake of LOVs compares favorably with that of omnivores, the calcium intake of vegans is generally lower than the general population.[76-78] For example, Canadian vegan women were found to consume 578 mg of calcium per day, compared with 950 mg for omnivores and 875 mg for LOV.[77] Female vegans are more likely to have lower calcium intakes, while male vegans have substantially higher calcium intakes, probably due to their higher caloric intake.[78] Vegan women are also reported to have a calcium to protein ratio of only 10 or 11, substantially lower than that of LOVs and omnivores.[77,78] The low calcium intake of vegans would place them at higher risk of low BMD. In the unpublished work of Dr. Marsh, vegans were observed to have substantially lower BMD than LOVs. On the other hand, in a study of elderly Chinese women, there was no significant difference in BMD between vegans and lacto-vegetarians.[75] Furthermore, Barr et al. found that vegan women did not have lower spinal BMD than LOVs, despite daily calcium intakes averaging almost 300 mg lower.[74]

A study in Taiwan found that long-term vegans may have a lower BMD than other vegetarians.[79] The mean calcium intakes for both the vegans and LOVs was less than 400 mg/day. Lumbar spine and femoral neck BMD were measured in postmenopausal vegetarian women. The long-term vegans were found to be at a higher risk of lumbar spine fracture (odds ratio, 2.48) and of being classified as having osteopenia of the femoral neck (OR = 3.94). In multiple regression analysis, long term vegan status was found to be strongly associated with lower femoral neck BMD. With a very low calcium intake in these women, a higher protein intake was associated with a modest increase in BMD. Apparently, an adequate intake of both calcium and protein is important. The authors suggested that calcium supplements may be necessary to improve BMD and to reduce the risk of osteoporosis among long-term elderly female vegetarians.

For optimal bone density, calcium intake should be adequate all through childhood and adulthood. Vegans, especially, should ensure an adequate calcium intake by consuming high-calcium foods and calcium-fortified foods. When sufficient servings of calcium-rich foods are not consumed, supplemental calcium may be needed to maintain optimal bone health, especially for Caucasian and Asian females.

D. Phytoestrogens

Estrogen down-regulates the activity of osteoclasts, and thereby limits bone resorption.[80] The isoflavones in soy protein, such as genistein and daidzein, act as phytoestrogens by binding to the estrogen receptors in bone tissue,[81] and inhibit bone resorption.[82,83] Ipriflavone, a synthetic isoflavone, is successfully used as an estrogen replacement for menopausal women, as it increases bone mass in women with low bone density.[82] Ipriflavone has been shown to be effective against osteoporosis of the spine, wrist, and femur and may be administered along with 1000 mg calcium per day.

Recently, postmenopausal women who were consuming isoflavone-rich soy protein were observed to be protected against spinal bone loss.[84] The protection against vertebral bone loss was observed with a daily dose of 90 mg of isoflavones over a period of 6 months. The effect was not observed with 40 mg of isoflavones, nor was it observed at other skeletal sites. It is possible that larger amounts of isoflavones, or a greater time period, might have a greater effect on BMD, but, to date, no human studies have explored this possibility. Ninety milligrams is obtainable from food sources (see Table 13.4), but larger amounts of isoflavones would be difficult to achieve without supplements. Very high doses of genistein have been shown to decrease bone loss in ovariectomized rats with equal or greater efficacy than Premarin.[85,86] Genistein, diadzen, and ipriflavone all appear to selectively modulate estrogen receptors in bone but not the uterus or breast. Such agents apparently do not increase the risk of breast or uterine cancer even with long-term use.[87] In fact, genistein has been shown to strongly inhibit the growth of human breast cancer cells, whether estrogen positive or negative.[88,89] Further studies would be helpful on the possible efficacy of long-term use of phytoestrogen-rich foods, chiefly soy products, in slowing bone loss during menopause.

Table 13.4　Isoflavone Content (Genistein plus Diadzen) in Selected Foods[140]

Food, 100 g	Isoflavones (mg)
Soybeans, dry roasted	128
Defatted soy flakes	126
Powdered soy drink, dry*	109
Soy protein concentrate, aqueous washed **	102
Soy protein isolate	97
Soybeans, cooked	55
Tofu	28–33
Soy meat substitutes	6–14***
Soy cheese	7

*　Reconstituted. liquid soy milk has about 25–40 mg of isoflavones/cup

**　Alcohol-extracted soy protein is reduced to 13 isoflavone/cup

*** Per serving

E. Macrobiotic Diets

Data suggest that those who follow low-calcium diets during their childhood may carry the consequences for years to come. A Dutch study of adolescents who had followed a macrobiotic diet as children found that their hip bone mineral density was 8% lower than omnivores,[4] despite higher calcium intakes during adolescence. In another Dutch study, 28% of macrobiotic infants studied had clinical symptoms of rickets related to low calcium intake.[90] Other studies also indicate low calcium and vitamin D intake, with an increased risk of rickets among macrobiotic children, especially in regions where the weather does not permit regular exposure to the sun.[91,92] A low calcium intake in childhood could result in earlier osteoporosis in adult life. Since the volume of food that a child can eat is lower than that of an adult, their food may need to be calcium fortified. Macrobiotic diets consumed by adults may also be low in calcium. Lactating women consuming a macrobiotic diet had a mean daily calcium intake of only 486 mg, less than one half that consumed by omnivores.[93]

F. Postmenopausal Women

It is important that both omnivorous and vegetarian women maximize their calcium stores before menopause, since decreased estrogen production at menopause is associated with accelerated bone loss for about 5 years.[94] During this 5-year period, women can lose an average of about 3% of their skeletal mass per year. The decrease in BMD experienced by postmenopausal women may be attenuated by regular weight-bearing exercise, hormone replacement, or high-dose calcium supplementation. However, calcium supplementation does not appear to prevent the rapid trabecular bone loss that occurs in the first 5 years after menopause although it can significantly reduce bone loss in women more than 5 years beyond menopause.[95,96]

For late postmenopausal women, supplementation may be more effective. Elderly women aged 62 to 92 years who had a calcium intake of less than 300 mg/day were given a calcium supplement of 800 mg (as calcium lactate gluconate) or a placebo tablet daily. After 10 months, the BMD at Ward's triangle and the intertrochanteric area significantly increased in the women on the calcium supplement, although there was no significant change in BMD at the spine and femoral neck.[97] The parathyroid hormone levels also fell significantly in those subjects on calcium supplements. The calcium supplements were considered effective in the reducing hip bone loss in elderly women.[97]

G. Plant Sources of Calcium

Dairy products are known to be a rich source of readily available calcium for both the LOV and omnivore. The low-fat dairy products are the preferred choice, because regular dairy products supply substantial amounts of saturated fat and cholesterol. Additionally, a good supply of calcium is obtained by consuming moderate amounts of greens such as collard greens and kale, calcium-fortified breakfast cereals, calcium-forti-fied soy beverages, calcium-fortified orange juice, tofu, and other calcium-rich foods (see Table 13.5). The calcium content of tofu can vary by a factor of 20, depending on its preparation. The calcium content is much higher if the tofu has been precipitated with calcium sulfate. Unfortified soy milk, sunflower seeds, and alfalfa sprouts are not rich sources of calcium, even though many vegans commonly believe them to be excellent sources.[98] Tahini and almonds have also been considered good calcium sources by vegans, but they are only fair sources of calcium.

Table 13.5   Plant Sources of Calcium[98]

Food	Calcium (mg)
Blackstrap molasses, 1.5 Tbsp.	258
Beverages, 1 cup	
Soy Milk, calcium-fortified	160–300
Orange Juice, calcium- fortified	350
Greens, 1 cup	
Collard greens, cooked*	357
Turnip greens, cooked*	249
Kale, cooked*	180
Chinese cabbage, cooked	158
Okra, cooked*	154
Mustard greens, cooked*	151
Legumes, 1 cup	
Soybeans, green, boiled	261
Black-eyed peas, cooked	211
Tofu, 100 gm	
Tofu, firm, prepared with calcium sulfate	683
Tofu, regular, prepared with calcium sulfate	350
Tofu, firm, prepared with nigari**	162
Tofu, soft, prepared with nigari**	111
Tofu, Mori Nu type, silken, firm	31

* Nutrient content for cooked vegetables varies depending on process-ing. These calculations are for frozen, cooked vegetables, which are higher in calcium than fresh vegetables, probably due to inclusion of a higher proportion of the stem. Mineral content per cup, including calcium, of frozen, cooked green vegetables is often higher because the cooking method renders them more compact. Broccoli stems are higher in calcium than broccoli flowers.

** Calcium sulfate and magnesium chloride

The bioavailability of calcium is also an important matter to consider. The calcium in most greens is well absorbed. In the case of kale, its calcium is absorbed substantially better than that of milk.[99] By contrast, the calcium in spinach, which contains oxalic acid, has a low bioavailability.[100] Wheat bran may also substantially reduce the bioavailability of calcium.[101] Both low- and high-phytate soybeans contain calcium that is well absorbed. Heaney reported that high-phytate soybeans had a calcium absorption that is 82% that of milk, while the calcium absorption in low-phytate soybeans was 10% greater than that of milk.[102]

H. Calcium Supplements

The most readily absorbed supplements suitable for vegetarians include calcium citrate malate (often found in calcium-fortified fruit juices), calcium lactate gluconate, calcium citrate, and calcium carbonate. Calcium obtained from oyster shell is not acceptable to vegetarians because of its animal origin. Calcium hydroxyapatite, derived from bone, and bone meal are both unacceptable to those wishing to avoid animal products. Dolomite and bone meal are also unacceptable due to their lead content.[103]

When taken on an empty stomach, calcium carbonate is not as well absorbed as calcium citrate.[104] There is evidence that ultradense calcium citrate may be much better absorbed than calcium carbonate by postmenopausal women when it is taken with food.[105] The capacity to absorb supplemental calcium in the form of calcium carbonate varies widely after menopause.[106]

I. Summary

Lacto-ovo-vegetarians have dietary calcium intakes similar to omnivores' and do not appear to be at increased risk for calcium deficiency. Adequate calcium is generally obtained by consuming two to three servings of calcium-rich foods daily. On the other hand, it may be difficult for vegans, especially females and children, to get enough calcium on a vegan diet without using calcium-fortified foods or calcium supplements. Postmenopausal women need to pay special attention to their calcium intake since they are at increased risk of osteoporosis.

VI. VITAMIN D

Vitamin D is essential for calcium absorption and optimal bone health. The current U.S. DRIs for vitamin D are 5 to 15 mcg. (200 to 600 IU) depending on age. Those under 50 years. of age require 5 mcg, those 51–70 require 10 mcg, and those over 70 require 15 mcg. Most individuals can manufacture sufficient vitamin D with adequate sunlight exposure. In addition, there are some readily obtainable vitamin D-fortified foods. These include cow's milk, some cereals, and some soy beverages. Because of the less efficient vitamin D metabolism, elderly individuals may require vitamin D supplementation, especially if they are institutionalized and have limited sunlight exposure. Others who may be at risk of becoming vitamin D deficient include those who live in northern latitudes and some temperate latitudes where there is not enough exposure to sunlight during the late fall, winter, and early spring months to ensure optimal vitamin D levels.[107]

Geographical latitude was a significant factor in the 15-country population study on bone fractures.[108] Countries with the lowest fracture rates typically occurred in regions of high sunlight exposure while the three countries with the highest fracture rates were all Scandinavian. While Finland has lower fracture rates than its neighboring countries, the Finnish do fortify foods with vitamin D, as well as having higher calcium intakes than their Scandinavian neighbors. Countries with similar protein intakes may have hip fracture rates that vary two- to threefold, depending largely on latitude, suggesting that obtaining adequate vitamin D is important for bone health. Results from a meta-analysis suggest a need for vitamin D fortification in foods, since hypovitaminosis D was more frequently seen in those countries in which vitamin D supplementation was less common.[109]

A Boston study of postmenopausal omnivorous women showed that a vitamin D intake of 200 IU per day was less efficient at preventing femur bone mineral loss than an intake of 800 IU per day.[110] Both regimens included modest calcium supplementation. Those who received the higher vitamin D supplementation lost less than 1.1% of BMD at the hip, compared with a loss of 2.5% for the low-dosage group. Seventy percent of bone loss occurred during the winter and spring, when vitamin D levels were the lowest. Both levels of supplementation had similar results in preventing whole-body and spinal bone mineral loss.

A. Vegetarian Studies

Vegetarians have been shown to have a lower mean intake of vitamin D and a lower mean serum vitamin D level. In a study of Finnish women, the dietary intake of vitamin D in vegans was found to be insufficient to maintain blood levels of 25-hydroxyvitamin D and parathyroid hormone within normal ranges during the winter.[111] Both LOV and vegan premenopausal women had vitamin D intakes significantly lower than the omnivores. The vegans had significantly lower (12%) bone mineral density (BMD) in the lumbar region of the spine than the omnivores, and the vegans' spinal BMD tended to be lower than the LOVs. In addition, BMD in the neck of the femur tended to be lower in the vegans. The higher levels of parathyroid hormone found in the vegans would indicate that low vitamin D levels had a negative effect on their BMD. The serum vitamin D levels of the vegans were lower, and their parathyroid hormones higher, throughout the year. The researchers concluded that vitamin D supplementation or fortification should routinely be recommended to vegans living in northern latitudes, at least during winter months. In an earlier Finnish study, male and female vegans were reported to have serum 25-hydroxyvitamin D levels 43% lower and serum parathyroid hormone 104% higher than omnivores.[112] Six of the 10 vegans had serum vitamin D levels that indicated vitamin D deficiency. The dietary vitamin D intake for the vegans averaged only 0.3 mcg/d.[112]

A New Zealand study also found that both LOVs and vegans had significantly lower vitamin D intakes than did omnivores.[113] Daily vitamin D intake for the vegans was 1.9 mcg. (76 IU) while the omnivores had a mean daily vitamin D intake of 3.4 mcg. (132 IU). Among elderly Seventh-Day Adventist women in California, vitamin D intake of vegetarians was 16% lower than that of the omnivores.[33] Serum vitamin D levels in elderly Dutch vegetarians (not vegans) were also lower than those of omnivores.[49] American women on macrobiotic diets had up to 50% lower serum 25-hydroxyvitamin D levels than did omnivores.[93] Children under 6 years of age consuming macrobiotic diets show evidence of vitamin D deficiency due to very low vitamin D intakes.[91]

B. Summary

Vegetarians generally have lower levels of vitamin D than omnivores. Lower levels of vitamin D are associated with a decreased ability to absorb calcium. In vegans, the levels have been shown to be far lower than the DRIs. In most climates, a 5- to 10-mcg supplement of vitamin D during the winter and early spring would be a safe, reasonable, and appropriate step for vegans. Lacto-ovo-vegetarians may also benefit from supplemental vitamin D during the winter months. The institutionalized elderly, and those who are unable to obtain or tolerate sun exposure, would likely benefit from vitamin D supplementation year round — irrespective of diet.

VII. VITAMIN B$_{12}$

Vitamin B$_{12}$ is required for the normal maturation of red blood cells and for the synthesis of sphingomyelins, which occur in large amounts in the myelin sheath of nerve tissue. Without sufficient B$_{12}$, changes will occur in nerve function, and red blood cells remain as large immature megaloblasts, producing macrocytic anemia. Because vitamin B$_{12}$ is not naturally found in any significant amounts in plant foods, some vegetarians, especially vegans, may be at risk of vitamin B_{12} deficiency. Lacto-ovo-vegetarians, however, could obtain sufficient vitamin B_{12} from eggs and dairy products, provided these products are consumed in significant amounts.

A. Absorption of Vitamin B_{12}

The average absorption of vitamin B_{12} is about 70%, but may drop to below 20% when large supplements are ingested.[114] Less than 5% of the total B_{12} absorption is absorbed by passive diffusion across the intestinal wall without the intrinsic factor. From 1 to 10 µg of vitamin B_{12} per day is excreted via bile, and most of this is reabsorbed via the enterohepatic circulation. A deficiency of B_{12} may not readily develop as long as there is effective vitamin B_{12} absorption. However, it may take only about 3 years to become B_{12} deficient if one stops absorbing the vitamin.[115] The major reason for vitamin B_{12} deficiency is a lack of adequate B_{12} absorption. This may result from a lack of B_{12} in the diet because of food selection; a lack of intrinsic factor secretion due to aging, gastritis or a gastrectomy; ileal resection; ileitis; or achlorhydria.

By age 60, about 1% of adults develop gastric atrophy. With aging, there is also a decrease in the level of proteases, as well as a drop in the level of acid in the stomach. The result is that B_{12} is not effectively removed from the food proteins to which it is attached, and B_{12} absorption is diminished. A decreased absorption of B_{12} also results when the intrinsic factor production decreases.

B. Symptoms of B_{12} Deficiency

In vitamin B_{12} deficiency, the blood levels of B_{12} normally drop to subnormal levels, that is, below 200 pg/ml. Blood and urinary levels of methylmalonate and homocysteine are elevated in true B_{12} deficiency because the metabolism of both these substances requires B_{12} as a coenzyme. Normal serum levels of methylmalonic acid and homocysteine are 73-271 nmol/L and 5.1–13.9 µmol/L, respectively.[116]

Other characteristic features seen with B_{12} deficiency include paresthesia in the limbs, inability to maintain balance when walking, weakness and excessive fatigue, loss of vibration and position sense, and a range of psychiatric disorders including disorientation, depression, mood disturbances, irritability, memory loss, and dementia. The lesions result from the patchy and progressive demyelination in peripheral nerves, the spinal cord, and the brain. Vitamin B_{12} deficiency is fairly common in the elderly and is associated with impairment in cognitive function or the exacerbation of coexisting dementia in the geriatric population.[117]

Studies have shown the presence of neurological damage in B_{12}-deficient elderly subjects, without showing any blood cell abnormalities. Researchers found that, in almost one third of their patients who had a range of neuropsychiatric disorders caused by vitamin B_{12} deficiency, there was an absence of anemia and red blood cell changes expected in B_{12}-deficient patients.[118] The neurologic abnormalities due to B_{12} deficiency were responsive to cobalamin therapy. Early diagnosis and treatment of the disorders is considered important to prevent permanent damage. Some now propose 350 pg/ml (258 pmol/L) to be the cut-off for normal serum cobalamin levels, rather than 200 pg/ml (147 pmol/L), due to the need to better identify B_{12} deficiency in the elderly.[119]

A report from Israel further documents B_{12} deficiency with neurologic disorders without hematologic abnormalities. About one half of a group of persons who were strict vegans for 5–35 years had below normal blood levels of B_{12}. The four vegans with the lowest B_{12} levels all had histories of neurologic complaints, including muscle pain, paraesthesia in the legs, and difficulty in mental concentration.[120] All showed improvement with intramuscular B_{12} treatment.

Since folic acid may partly substitute for B_{12} in bone marrow activity, an adequate folic acid intake can prevent or delay the development of macrocytic anemia in B_{12} deficiency. However, folate cannot prevent nerve damage. If the macrocytic anemia of B_{12}-deficient patients is treated with folic acid, it might allow neurological problems to develop or worsen while normalizing the red blood cell picture. Neurological damage could require weeks and months for recovery, if it occurs at all.

C. Are Vegetarians at Risk?

Many long-term vegans are reported to have low serum B_{12} levels.[121] While oral B_{12} supplements can restore serum levels of B_{12} and eliminate macrocytic anemia, in some cases, the damage done to the nervous system is not reversible and the neurological disorders may persist even months after treatment.[122,123] The use of a macrobiotic diet is also associated with a marginal vitamin B_{12} status. Serum B_{12} levels are observed to decrease with increasing time on the macrobiotic diet as B_{12} stores are depleted.[124] Occasionally, an LOV may also have a low serum B_{12} level.[125,126] Most of those with low serum B_{12} levels can have the megaloblastic anemia corrected by oral B_{12} supplements or an injection of B_{12}. In one study, the serum B_{12} levels of adult LOVs dropped 35% 2 months after they switched to a vegan diet.[127]

D. How Much Vitamin B$_{12}$ Do We Need?

Fortunately, vitamin B$_{12}$ is required only in very small amounts, probably no more than 1 µg/day.[115] The present RDA is set at 2 µg/day for adults and teenagers, about 2.5 µg for pregnant and breast-feeding women, and one microgram or less for children. Minimum needs are actually less than those amounts. In fact, 1 µg/day can effectively treat anemic vegans[128,129] and return people without B$_{12}$ stores to normal. Human vitamin B$_{12}$ deficiency may be slow to develop because of large liver stores. It is estimated that about 3000 µg are stored in an adult, and 30–50 µg are stored in an infant or child.[130] Persons who completely give up animal products may go for years before any nervous system disorders or other signs and symptoms of a B$_{12}$ deficiency are manifested.

It is essential that pregnant and breast-feeding women have adequate B$_{12}$ intakes, especially when following a vegan diet. During the latter half of pregnancy, the fetus removes about one fifth of a microgram of B$_{12}$ per day from the mother's stores, while a nursing mother may give up one third of a microgram of B$_{12}$ per day in her breast milk. Without a proper B$_{12}$ intake, fetal stores and breast milk levels of B$_{12}$ may fall to very low levels, especially in a vegan consuming a diet without any B$_{12}$ supplement.[131] The infant born to a mother who has been a vegetarian for many years is clearly at high risk of vitamin B$_{12}$ deficiency. Even though the mother may not show signs of deficiency, her child may not receive adequate stores of the vitamin from the mother. Vitamin B$_{12}$ deficiency may develop in the breast-fed infant within 3–6 months of age.[132-134] The B$_{12}$-deficient child may have seizures, become apathetic, lethargic, anemic, and show signs of developmental delay or regression and failure to thrive.

E. Vitamin B$_{12}$ Levels in Foods

Vitamin B$_{12}$ is found in milk, eggs, and meat due to the action of bacteria in the gastrointestinal tract of the animal. The bacteria in the large bowel of humans can also manufacture vitamin B$_{12}$. However, the vitamin B$_{12}$ cannot be absorbed because its synthesis occurs past the ileum, the site of B$_{12}$ absorption. Some vegetarians have the notion that vitamin B$_{12}$ is present in a variety of plant foods such as fermented soy products (miso and tempeh), shiitake mushrooms, and algae (spirulina and nori). While these products are often sold in health food stores as excellent sources of B$_{12}$ and are widely used by the macrobiotic community, they actually contain little, if any, vitamin B$_{12}$.[115,135] Instead, they contain analogs of B$_{12}$ that are not active and may actually block the absorption of true vitamin B$_{12}$ when its intake is low.

The standard method for determining vitamin B_{12} levels in foods involves an old microbiological assay using the bacterium *Lactobacillus leichmannii*. Food levels of B_{12} are greatly overestimated by this method because the bacterium measures not only the active vitamin B_{12} (cobalamin) levels, but also the whole family of related corrinoids that are inactive in humans. As much as 80% of the vitamin B_{12} activity determined by this method is due to the inactive corrinoid analogs of B_{12}.[115] A new radioimmunoassay method specifically measures only cobalamin.

For the LOV, dairy products and eggs can supply substantial amounts of B_{12} (see Table 13.6). However, since the vitamin B_{12} in an egg resides almost totally within the cholesterol-laden yolk, it would be better for the LOV to rely on low-fat dairy products for their source of B_{12}. Foods that are high in B_{12} should be included in the diet of a total vegetarian. This is especially true if one is pregnant or nursing a child. Vegans should obtain their dietary needs either from foods fortified with B_{12}, such as some ready-to eat cereals, a fortified yeast (Nutritional Support Formula), fortified soy beverages, fortified meat analogs, or from the regular use of a vitamin B_{12} supplement.

Table 13.6　Vitamin B_{12} Levels in Dairy and Egg Products (in micrograms)

6 ozs. yogurt	1.1
8 ozs. milk	0.9*
1/2 c. cottage cheese	0.7
1 oz. aged cheese	0.07–0.47
1 egg	0.8
1 egg white	0.02

*skim, 2% or whole milk

With normal absorption, a vitamin B_{12} supplement of 5 µg/day would daily provide 1–2 µg B_{12}. For an oral B_{12} supplement to have any beneficial effect, the tablet should be thoroughly chewed, rather than swallowed whole. A new painless delivery of cobalamin using intranasal or sublingual application provides fast absorption without any side effects. Substantial increases in plasma vitamin B_{12} levels have resulted after the intranasal application of hydroxocobalamin.[136]

VIII.　RIBOFLAVIN

Riboflavin deficiency among vegetarians should not be a major concern in the West since there are good riboflavin sources available for the vegetarian. These include dairy products, whole grains, leafy green vegetables, legumes, and sea vegetables. While vegetarian adults in Western nations generally have somewhat lower riboflavin intakes than do omnivores,[77] they still have intakes of riboflavin above the U.S. RDAs (1.3 mg for males; 1.1 mg for females). Vegans often report a lower riboflavin intake than omnivores or LOVs, but their intakes are still generally adequate.[78] In a study of elderly women in California, the lacto-vegetarians reported slightly higher riboflavin intakes (1.46 mg/d) than the omnivores (1.36 mg/d).[33] Many teenagers have a marginal riboflavin intake, possibly due to poor dietary choices. Among Canadian teenagers, slightly more lacto-vegetarians and semi-vegetarians had inadequate riboflavin intakes than did omnivores.[48]

IX. IODINE

Iodine deficiency disorders are very rare in the U.S. today. However, national nutrition surveys reveal that the dietary intake of iodine has substantially declined over the past 2 decades. The U.S. RDA for iodine is 150 mcg. per day, an amount supplied by only 2 grams of iodized salt or one kelp tablet. In addition to iodized salt and sea vegetables, foods that provide significant amounts of iodine include dairy foods and bakery products. The dairy industry uses iodine-containing disinfectants to clean milk processing equipment, while the baking industry uses iodine-containing dough stabilizers.

There is no evidence that LOVs have a higher risk of iodine deficiency than the population at large. Some studies suggest that vegans have a low iodine intake,[137] although there is no evidence of iodine deficiency among vegans. In two European studies, the mean iodine intake of vegans was substantially below recommended levels.[138,139] In addition to low iodine intakes, certain foods can alter iodine bioavailability. Goitrogenic compounds, which decrease iodine utilization, occur in nuts, cruciferous vegetables, millet, lima beans, sweet potatoes, and soy products, foods which are commonly eaten by many vegetarians. While LOVs are unlikely to have low intakes of iodine, it seems prudent for vegans to use iodized salt or sea vegetables on a regular basis to avoid an inadequate iodine status.

X. THE ELDERLY

In a study of 37 elderly women, vegetarians were observed to consume higher levels of many vitamins and minerals.[33] However, both non-vegetarians and vegetarians had some risk of deficiency of key nutrients such as calcium, zinc, vitamin B_6, and vitamin E. Vegetarians were significantly more likely to be deficient in vitamins D and B_{12}. The nutritional status of all elderly, both vegetarians and non-vegetarians, should be individually evaluated, paying special attention to vitamin D, B_{12}, calcium, zinc, and folate. Evaluation of vitamin B_{12} status is particularly important in geriatric patients due to the increased risk of anemia and dementia from atrophy of the small bowel, lack of intrinsic factor, and achlorhydria. A significant number of elderly persons with dementia have been found to be vitamin B_{12} deficient.[117]

XI. CONCLUSIONS

Vegetarian diets normally contain substantial amounts of potassium, folic acid, magnesium, manganese, copper, fiber, vitamins C, E, and K, and vitamin A (carotenoids). Since the different types of vegetarian diets are quite varied in their composition, nutrient concerns will vary from one to another. Appropriately planned vegan or LOV diets can be nutritionally adequate. However, there are significant nutritional concerns regarding vegetarian diets such as a strict macrobiotic diet.

Lacto-ovo-vegetarians and vegans tend to consume sufficient protein in their diets. Even though vegetarians consume iron in a less bioavailable form (non-heme iron), the consumption of a well-balanced vegetarian diet is not associated with any greater risk of iron deficiency. Vegetarian females, especially vegans, tend to have a lower zinc intake and possibly a lower zinc status than omnivores. However, the zinc intake of vegetarian males, both LOV and vegan, appears to be adequate. Female vegans should be encouraged to consume greater levels of zinc-rich foods.

In Western countries, there is a heightened interest to provide adequate calcium to support the attainment of optimal bone mineral density. Lacto-ovo-vegetarian diets are not likely to be deficient in calcium when low-fat dairy foods are regularly eaten. Vegan diets need to be appropriately planned to contain adequate calcium. Some vegans, particularly Caucasian and Asian females, may need to consume calcium-fortified foods or supplemental calcium to ensure nutritional adequacy.

Vegetarians can obtain vitamin D from exposure to sunlight or from consuming vitamin D-fortified foods such as cow's milk, many soy beverages, and some breakfast cereals. Vegetarians who live in northern climates may need to take supplemental vitamin D during the winter months, particularly if their exposure to sunlight is limited. Vegetarians who regularly use dairy products or eat vitamin B_{12}-fortified foods generally have an adequate B_{12} status. Vegans may need a daily supplement of vitamin B_{12}, unless they are consuming vitamin B_{12}-fortified foods. Preliminary data indicates that many vegans may have low iodine intakes, which can be easily remedied by the regular use of iodized salt. For optimal health, elderly vegetarians need to pay special attention to getting adequate vitamin D and B_{12} intakes.

REFERENCES

1. Messina, V.K. and Burke, K.I. Position of the American Dietetic Association: vegetarian diets. *J. Am. Diet. Assoc.*, 97, 1317, 1997.
2. Thorogood, M., Carter, R., Benfield, L., McPherson, K., and Mann, J.I. Plasma lipids and lipoprotein cholesterol concentrations in people with different diets in Britain. *Br. Med. J. (Clin. Res. ed.)*, 295, 351, 1987.
3. Weaver, C.M. and Plawecki, K.L. Dietary calcium: adequacy of a vegetarian diet. *Am. J. Clin. Nutr.*, 59, 1238S, 1994.
4. Parsons, T.J., van Dusseldorp, M., van der Vliet, M., van de Werken, K., Schaafsma, G., and van Staveren, W.A. Reduced bone mass in Dutch adolescents fed a macrobiotic diet in early life. *J. Bone Miner. Res.*, 12, 1486, 1997.
5. Zmora, E., Gorodischer, R., and Bar-Ziv, J. Multiple nutritional deficiencies in infants from a strict vegetarian community. *Am. J. Dis. Child.*, 133, 141, 1979.
6. Rauma, A.L., Nenonen, M., Helve, T., and Hanninen, O. Effect of a strict vegan diet on energy and nutrient intakes by Finnish rheumatoid patients. *Eur. J. Clin. Nutr.*, 47, 747, 1993.
7. Hardinge, M. Nutritional studies of vegetarians. *Am. J. Clin. Nutr.*, 2, 73, 1943.
8. Young, V.R. and Pellett, P.L. Plant proteins in relation to human protein and amino acid nutrition. *Am. J. Clin. Nutr.*, 59, 1203S, 1994.
9. Messina, M. and Messina, V. *The Dietitian's Guide to Vegetarian Diets. Issues and Applications.* Aspen, Gaithersburg, 1996.
10. Dallman, P. Biochemical basis for the manifestations of iron deficiency. *Am. Rev. Nutr.*, 6, 13, 1986.
11. DeMaeyer. The prevalence of anemia in the world. *World Health Stat. Q.*, 38, 302, 1985.
12. Herbert, V. Recommended dietary intakes (RDI) of iron in humans. *Am. J. Clin. Nutr.*, 45, 679, 1987.
13. Baynes, R.D. and Bothwell, T.H. Iron deficiency. *Annu. Rev. Nutr.*, 10, 133, 1990.
14. Cook, J.D. and Lynch, S.R. The liabilities of iron deficiency. *Blood*, 68, 803, 1986.
15. Dallman, P. Iron deficiency: does it matter? *J. Int. Med.*, 226, 367, 1989.
16. Dallman, P. Present knowledge in nutrition. In: *Iron*. Brown, M. (Ed.), ILSI-Nutrition Foundation, Washington, D.C., 1990.
17. Charlton, R.W. and Bothwell, T.H. Iron absorption. *Annu. Rev.Med.*, 34, 55, 1983.
18. Finch, C.A. and Cook, J.D. Iron deficiency. *Am. J. Clin. Nutr.*, 39, 471, 1984.
19. Monsen, E.R. Iron nutrition and absorption: dietary factors which impact iron bioavailability. *J. Am. Diet. Assoc.*, 88, 786, 1988.
20. Hallberg, L. Bioavailability of dietary iron in man. *Annu. Rev. Nutr.*, 1, 123, 1981.
21. Cook, J.D. and Monsen, E.R. Vitamin C, the common cold, and iron absorption. *Am. J. Clin. Nutr.*, 30, 235, 1977.
22. Disler, P.B., Lynch, S.R., Charlton, R.W., Torrance, J.D., Bothwell, T.H., Walker, R.B., and Mayet, F. The effect of tea on iron absorption. *Gut*, 16, 193, 1975.

23. Gillooly, M., Bothwell, T.H., Torrance, J.D., MacPhail, A.P., Derman, D.P., Bezwoda, W.R., Mills, W., Charlton, R.W., and Mayet, F. The effects of organic acids, phytates and polyphenols on the absorption of iron from vegetables. *Br. J. Nutr.*, 49, 331, 1983.

24. Morck, T.A., Lynch, S.R., and Cook, J.D. Inhibition of food iron absorption by coffee. *Am. J. Clin. Nutr.*, 37, 416, 1983.

25. Brune, M., Rossander, L., and Hallberg, L. Iron absorption and phenolic compounds: importance of different phenolic structures. *Eur. J. Clin. Nutr.*, 43, 547, 1989.

26. El-Guindi, M., Lynch, S., and Cook, J. Iron absorption from fortified flat breads. *Br. J. Nutr.*, 59, 205, 1988.

27. Macfarlane, B.J., van der Riet, W.B., Bothwell, T.H., Baynes, R.D., Siegenberg, D., Schmidt, U., Tal, A., Taylor, J.R., and Mayet, F. Effect of traditional oriental soy products on iron absorption. *Am. J. Clin. Nutr.*, 51, 873, 1990.

28. Hallberg, L., Brune, M., and Rossander, L. Iron absorption in man: ascorbic acid and dose-dependent inhibition by phytate. *Am. J. Clin. Nutr.*, 49, 140, 1989.

29. Macfarlane, B.J., Bezwoda, W.R., Bothwell, T.H., Baynes, R.D., Bothwell, J.E., MacPhail, A.P., Lamparelli, R.D., and Mayet, F. Inhibitory effect of nuts on iron absorption. *Am. J. Clin. Nutr.*, 47, 270, 1988.

30. Hallberg, L. and Rossander, L. Effect of soy protein on non-heme iron absorption in man. *Am. J. Clin. Nutr.*, 36, 514, 1982.

31. Hallberg, L. and Rossander, L. Improvement of iron nutrition in developing countries: comparison of adding meat, soy protein, ascorbic acid, citric acid, and ferrous sulphate on iron absorption from a simple Latin American-type of meal. *Am. J. Clin. Nutr.*, 39, 577, 1984.

32. Reddy, S. and Sanders, T.A. Haematological studies on premenopausal Indian and Caucasian vegetarians compared with Caucasian omnivores. *Br. J. Nutr.*, 64, 331, 1990.

33. Nieman, D.C., Underwood, B.C., Sherman, K.M., Arabatzis, K., Barbosa, J.C., Johnson, M., and Shultz, T.D. Dietary status of Seventh-Day Adventist vegetarian and non-vegetarian elderly women. *J. Am. Diet. Assoc.*, 89, 1763, 1989.

34. Latta, D. Iron and zinc status of vegetarian and non-vegetarian males. *Nutr. Rep. Int.*, 141, 1984.

35. Anderson, B.M., Gibson, R.S., and Sabry, J.H. The iron and zinc status of long-term vegetarian women. *Am. J. Clin. Nutr.*, 34, 1042, 1981.

36. Armstrong, B.K., Davis, R.E., Nicol, D.J., van Merwyk, A.J., and Larwood, C.J. Hematological, vitamin B 12, and folate studies on Seventh-Day Adventist vegetarians. *Am. J. Clin. Nutr.*, 27, 712, 1974.

37. Sanders, T.A., Ellis, F.R., and Dickerson, J.W. Haematological studies on vegans. *Br. J. Nutr.*, 40, 9, 1978.

38. Kim, Y. M.S. University of Massachusetts (1988).

39. Dwyer, J.T., Dietz, W.H., Jr., Andrews, E.M., and Suskind, R.M. Nutritional status of vegetarian children. *Am. J. Clin. Nutr.*, 35, 204, 1982.

40. Salonen, J.T., Nyyssonen, K., Korpela, H., Tuomilehto, J., Seppanen, R., and Salonen, R. High stored iron levels are associated with excess risk of myocardial infarction in eastern Finnish men. *Circulation*, 86, 803, 1992.

41. Prasad, A. Nutritional zinc today. *Nutr. Today*, 16, 4, 1981.

42. North, K. and Golding, J. A maternal vegetarian diet in pregnancy is associated with hypospadias. The ALSPAC Study Team. Avon Longitudinal Study of Pregnancy and Childhood. *BJ.U Int.*, 85, 107, 2000.

43. Gibson, R.S. Content and bioavailability of trace elements in vegetarian diets. *Am. J. Clin. Nutr.*, 59, 1223S, 1994.

44. Gibson, R.S., Donovan, U.M., and Heath, A.L. Dietary strategies to improve the iron and zinc nutriture of young women following a vegetarian diet. *Plant Foods Hum. Nutr.*, 51, 1, 1997.

45. Hunt, J.R., Matthys, L.A., and Johnson, L.K. Zinc absorption, mineral balance, and blood lipids in women consuming controlled lacto-ovo-vegetarian and omnivorous diets for 8 wk. *Am. J. Clin. Nutr.*, 67, 421, 1998.

46. Kies, C., Young, E., and McEndree, L. Zinc bioavailability from vegetarian diets. In: *Nutritional Bioavailability of Zinc*, Vol. 210. Inglett, G.E. (Ed.), American Chemical Society, Washington, D.C., 1983.

47. Ball, M.J. and Ackland, M.L. Zinc intake and status in Australian vegetarians. *Br. J. Nutr.*, 83, 27, 2000.

48. Donovan, U.M. and Gibson, R.S. Dietary intakes of adolescent females consuming vegetarian, semi-vegetarian, and omnivorous diets. *J. Adolesc. Hlth.*, 18, 292, 1996.

49. Lowik, M.R., Schrijver, J., Odink, J., van den Berg, H., and Wedel, M. Long-term effects of a vegetarian diet on the nutritional status of elderly people (Dutch Nutrition Surveillance System). *J. Am. Coll. Nutr.*, 9, 600, 1990.

50. Looker, A.C., Johnston, C.C., Jr., Wahner, H.W., Dunn, W.L., Calvo, M.S., Harris, T.B., Heyse, S.P., and Lindsay, R.L. Prevalence of low femoral bone density in older U.S. women from NHANES III. *J. Bone Miner. Res.*, 10, 796, 1995.

51. NIH. Osteoporosis Prevention, Diagnosis, and Therapy. Vol. 2000 (NIH Consensus Statement 2000, 2000).

52. Craig, W.J. *Nutrition and Wellness. A Vegetarian Way to Better Health.* Golden Harvest Books, Berrien Springs, Michigan, 1999.

53. Barzel, U.S. and Massey, L.K. Excess dietary protein can adversely affect bone. *J. Nutr.*, 128, 1051, 1998.

54. Massey, L.K. Does excess dietary protein adversely affect bone? Symposium overview. *J. Nutr.*, 128, 1048, 1998.

55. Linkswiler, H.M., Zemel, M.B., Hegsted, M., and Schuette, S. Protein-induced hypercalciuria. *Fed. Proc.*, 40, 2429, 1981.

56. Licata, A.A., Bou, E., Bartter, F.C., and West, F. Acute effects of dietary protein on calcium metabolism in patients with osteoporosis. *J. Gerontol.*, 36, 14, 1981.

57. Heaney, R.P. Protein intake and the calcium economy. *J. Am. Diet. Assoc.*, 93, 1259, 1993.

58. McBean, L.D., Forgac, T., and Finn, S.C. Osteoporosis: visions for care and prevention — a conference report. *J. Am. Diet. Assoc.*, 94, 668, 1994.

59. Hegsted, D.M. Calcium and osteoporosis. *J. Nutr.*, 116, 2316, 1986.

60. Feskanich, D., Willett, W.C., Stampfer, M.J., and Colditz, G.A. Milk, dietary calcium, and bone fractures in women: a 12-year prospective study. Am. J. Public Health., 87, 992, 1997.

61. Nielsen, F., Mullen, L., and Gallagher, S. Effect of boron depletion and repletion on blood indicators of calcium status in humans fed a magnesium-low diet. *J. Trace Elem. Exp. Med.*, 3, 45, 1990.

62. Nielsen, F. Boron — An overlooked element of potential nutritional importance. *Nutr. Today,* 23, 4, 1988.
63. Berkelhammer, C.H., Wood, R.J., and Sitrin, M.D. Acetate and hypercalciuria during total parenteral nutrition. *Am. J. Clin. Nutr.,* 48, 1482, 1988.
64. Sebastian, A., Harris, S.T., Ottaway, J.H., Todd, K.M., and Morris, R.C., Jr. Improved mineral balance and skeletal metabolism in postmenopausal women treated with potassium bicarbonate [see comments]. *N. Engl. J. Med.,* 330, 1776, 1994.
65. Feskanich, D., Weber, P., Willett, W.C., Rockett, H., Booth, S.L., and Colditz, G.A. Vitamin K intake and hip fractures in women: a prospective study. *Am. J. Clin. Nutr.,* 69, 74, 1999.
66. Breslau, N.A., Brinkley, L., Hill, K.D., and Pak, C.Y. Relationship of animal-protein-rich diet to kidney stone formation and calcium metabolism. *J. Clin. Endocrinol. Metab.,* 66, 140, 1988.
67. Ball, D. and Maughan, R.J. Blood and urine acid-base status of premenopausal omnivorous and vegetarian women. *Br. J. Nutr.,* 78, 683, 1997.
68. Feskanich, D., Willett, W.C., Stampfer, M.J., and Colditz, G.A. Protein consumption and bone fractures in women. *Am. J. Epidemiol.,* 143, 472, 1996.
69. Marsh, A.G., Sanchez, T.V., Midkelsen, O., Keiser, J., and Mayor, G. Cortical bone density of adult LOV and omnivorous women. *J. Am. Diet. Assoc.,* 76, 148, 1980.
70. Tylavs.ky, F.A., and Anderson, J.J. Dietary factors in bone health of elderly lacto-ovo-vegetarian and omnivorous women. *Am. J. Clin. Nutr.,* 48, 842, 1988.
71. Reed, J.A., Anderson, J.J., Tylavsky, F.A., and Gallagher, P.N., Jr. Comparative changes in radial-bone density of elderly female lacto-ovo-vegetarians and omnivores [published erratum appears in *Am. J. Clin. Nutr.,* 1994 Dec; 60(6):981]. *Am. J. Clin. Nutr.,* 59, 1197S, 1994.
72. Tesar, R., Notelovitz, M., Shim, E., Kauwell, G., and Brown, J. Axial and peripheral bone density and nutrient intakes of postmenopausal vegetarian and omnivorous women. *Am. J. Clin. Nutr.,* 56, 699, 1992.
73. Lloyd, T., Schaeffer, J.M., Walker, M.A., and Demers, L.M. Urinary hormonal concentrations and spinal bone densities of premenopausal vegetarian and non-vegetarian women [published erratum appears in *Am. J. Clin. Nutr.,* 1992 Nov; 56(5):954]. *Am. J. Clin. Nutr.,* 54, 1005, 1991.
74. Barr, S.I., Prior, J.C., Janelle, K.C., and Lentle, B.C. Spinal bone mineral density in premenopausal vegetarian and non-vegetarian women: cross-sectional and prospective comparisons. *J. Am. Diet. Assoc.,* 98, 760, 1998.
75. Lau, E.M., Kwok, T., Woo, J., and Ho, S.C. Bone mineral density in Chinese elderly female vegetarians, vegans, lacto-vegetarians, and omnivores. *Eur. J. Clin. Nutr.,* 52, 60, 1998.
76. Calkins, B.M., Whittaker, D.J., Nair, P.P., Rider, A.A., and Turjman, N. Diet, nutrition intake, and metabolism in populations at high and low risk for colon cancer. Nutrient intake. *Am. J. Clin. Nutr.,* 40, 896, 1984.
77. Janelle, K.C. and Barr, S.I. Nutrient intakes and eating behavior scores of vegetarian and non-vegetarian women. *J. Am. Diet. Assoc.,* 95, 180, 1995.
78. Mejia, A. M.S. Thesis, Loma Linda University, CA, 1994.
79. Chiu, J.F., Lan, S.J., Yang, C.Y., Wang, P.W., Yao, W.J., Su, L.H., and Hsieh, C.C. Long-term vegetarian diet and bone mineral density in postmenopausal Taiwanese women. *Calcif. Tissue Int.,* 60, 245, 1997.

80. Eriksen, E.F., Colvard, D.S., Berg, N.J., Graham, M.L., Mann, K.G., Spelsberg, T.C., and Riggs, B.L. Evidence of estrogen receptors in normal human osteoblast-like cells. *Science*, 241, 84, 1988.

81. Setchell, K.D. Phytoestrogens: the biochemistry, physiology, and implications for human health of soy isoflavones. Am. J. Clin. Nutr., 68, 1333S, 1998.

82. Setchell, K.D. and Cassidy, A. Dietary isoflavones: biological effects and relevance to human health. *J. Nutr.*, 129, 758S, 1999.

83. Arjmandi, B.H., Birnbaum, R., Goyal, N.V., Getlinger, M.J., Juma, S., Alekel, L., Hasler, C.M., Drum, M.L., Hollis, B.W., and Kukreja, S.C. Bone-sparing effect of soy protein in ovarian hormone-deficient rats is related to its isoflavone content. *Am. J. Clin. Nutr.*, 68, 1364S, 1998.

84. Potter, S.M., Baum, J.A., Teng, H., Stillman, R.J., Shay, N.F., and Erdman, J.W., Jr. Soy protein and isoflavones: their effects on blood lipids and bone density in postmenopausal women. *Am. J. Clin. Nutr.*, 68, 1375S, 1998.

85. Ishimi, Y., Miyaura, C., Ohmura, M., Onoe, Y., Sato, T., Uchiyama, Y., Ito, M., Wang, X., Suda, T., and Ikegami, S. Selective effects of genistein, a soybean isoflavone, on B-lymphopoiesis and bone loss caused by estrogen deficiency. *Endocrinology*, 140, 1893, 1999.

86. Anderson, J.J., Ambrose, W.W., and Garner, S.C. Biphasic effects of genistein on bone tissue in the ovariectomized, lactating rat model. *Proc. Soc. Exp. Biol. Med.*, 217, 345, 1998.

87. Guzzo, J.A. Selective estrogen receptor modulators — a new age of estrogens in cardiovascular disease? *Clin. Cardiol.*, 23, 15, 2000.

88. Shen, F., Xue, X., and Weber, G. Tamoxifen and genistein synergistically downregulate signal transduction and proliferation in estrogen receptor-negative human breast carcinoma MDA-MB-435 cells. *Anticancer Res.*, 19, 1657, 1999.

89. Zava, D.T. and Duwe, G. Estrogenic and antiproliferative properties of genistein and other flavonoids in human breast cancer cells in vitro. *Nutr. Cancer.*, 27, 31, 1997.

90. Dagnelie, P.C., Vergote, F.J., van Staveren, W.A., van den Berg, H., Dingjan, P.G., and Hautvast, J.G. High prevalence of rickets in infants on macrobiotic diets. *Am. J. Clin. Nutr.*, 51, 202, 1990.

91. Dwyer, J.T., Dietz, W.H., Jr., Hass, G., and Suskind, R. Risk of nutritional rickets among vegetarian children. *Am. J. Dis Child.*, 133, 134, 1979.

92. van Staveren, W.A., Dhuyvetter, J.H., Bons, A., Zeelen, M., and Hautvast, J.G. Food consumption and height/weight status of Dutch preschool children on alternative diets. *J. Am. Diet. Assoc.*, 85, 1579, 1985.

93. Specker, B.L. Nutritional concerns of lactating women consuming vegetarian diets. *Am. J. Clin. Nutr.*, 59, 1182S, 1994.

94. Gallagher, J.C., Goldgar, D., and Moy, A. Total bone calcium in normal women: effect of age and menopause status. *J. Bone Miner. Res.*, 2, 491, 1987.

95. Hosking, D.J., Ross, P.D., Thompson, D.E., Wasnich, R.D., McClung, M., Bjarnason, N.H., Ravn, P., Cizza, G., Daley, M., and Yates, A.J. Evidence that increased calcium intake does not prevent early postmenopausal bone loss. *Clin. Ther.*, 20, 933, 1998.

96. Dawson-Hughes, B., Dallal, G.E., Krall, E.A., Sadowski, L., Sahyoun, N., and Tannenbaum, S. A controlled trial of the effect of calcium supplementation on bone density in postmenopausal women. *N. Engl. J. Med.*, 323, 878, 1990.

97. Lau, E.M., Woo, J., Leung, P.C., Swaminathan, R., and Leung, D. The effects of calcium supplementation and exercise on bone density in elderly Chinese women. *Osteopor. Int.*, 2, 168, 1992.

98. USDA. USDA nutrient database for standard reference, release 13. *Nutrient data laboratory home page* 1999.

99. Heaney, R.P. and Weaver, C.M. Calcium absorption from kale. *Am. J. Clin. Nutr.*, 51, 656, 1990.

100. Heaney, R.P., Weaver, C.M., and Recker, R.R. Calcium absorbability from spinach. *Am. J. Clin. Nutr.*, 47, 707, 1988.

101. Weaver, C.M., Heaney, R.P., Teegarden, D., and Hinders, S.M. Wheat bran abolishes the inverse relationship between calcium load size and absorption fraction in women. *J. Nutr.*, 126, 303, 1996.

102. Heaney, R.P., Weaver, C.M., and Fitzsimmons, M.L. Soybean phytate content: effect on calcium absorption. *Am. J. Clin. Nutr.*, 53, 745, 1991.

103. Bourgoin, B.P., Evans, D.R., Cornett, J.R., Lingard, S.M., and Quattrone, A.J. Lead content in 70 brands of dietary calcium supplements. *Am. J. Public Health*, 83, 1155, 1993.

104. Harvey, J. Superior calcium absorption from calcium citrate than calcium carbonate using external forearm counting. *J. Am. Coll. Nutr.*, 9, 583, 1990.

105. Heller, H.J., Stewart, A., Haynes, S., and Pak, C.Y. Pharmacokinetics of calcium absorption from two commercial calcium supplements. *J. Clin. Pharmacol.*, 39, 1151, 1999.

106. Recker, R.R., Bammi, A., Barger-Lux, M.J., and Heaney, R.P. Calcium absorbability from milk products, an imitation milk, and calcium carbonate. *Am. J. Clin. Nutr.*, 47, 93, 1988.

107. Webb, A.R., Kline, L., and Holick, M.F. Influence of season and latitude on the cutaneous synthesis of vitamin D3: exposure to winter sunlight in Boston and Edmonton will not promote vitamin D3 synthesis in human skin. *J. Clin. Endocrinol. Metab.*, 67, 373, 1988.

108. Abelow, B.J., Holford, T.R., and Insogna, K.L. Cross-cultural association between dietary animal protein and hip fracture: a hypothesis. *Calcif. Tissue Int.*, 50, 14, 1992.

109. McKenna, M.J. Differences in vitamin D status between countries in young adults and the elderly. *Am. J. Med.*, 93, 69, 1992.

110. Dawson-Hughes, B., Harris, S.S., Krall, E.A., Dallal, G.E., Falconer, G., and Green, C.L. Rates of bone loss in postmenopausal women randomly assigned to one of two dosages of vitamin D. *Am. J. Clin. Nutr.*, 61, 1140, 1995.

111. Outila, T.A., Karkkainen, M.U., Seppanen, R.H., and Lamberg-Allardt, C.J. Dietary intake of vitamin D in premenopausal, healthy vegans was insufficient to maintain concentrations of serum 25-hydroxyvitamin D and intact parathyroid hormone within normal ranges during the winter in Finland. *J. Am. Diet. Assoc.*, 100, 434, 2000.

112. Lamberg-Allardt, C., Karkkainen, M., Seppanen, R., and Bistrom, H. Low serum 25-hydroxyvitamin D concentrations and secondary hyperparathyroidism in middle-aged white strict vegetarians. *Am. J. Clin. Nutr.*, 58, 684, 1993.

113. Alexander, D., Ball, M.J., and Mann, J. Nutrient intake and haematological status of vegetarians and age–sex-matched omnivores. *Eur. J. Clin. Nutr.*, 48, 538, 1994.

114. Herbert, V. Recommended dietary intakes (RDI) of vitamin B-12 in humans. *Am. J. Clin. Nutr.*, 45, 671, 1987.

115. Herbert, V. Vitamin B-12: plant sources, requirements, and assay. *Am. J. Clin. Nutr.*, 48, 852, 1988.

116. Kuzminski, A.M., Del Giacco, E.J., Allen, R.H., Stabler, S.P., and Lindenbaum, J. Effective treatment of cobalamin deficiency with oral cobalamin. *Blood*, 92, 1191, 1998.

117. Kwok, T., Tang, C., Woo, J., Lai, W.K., Law, L.K., and Pang, C.P. Randomized trial of the effect of supplementation on the cognitive function of older people with subnormal cobalamin levels. *Int J. Geriatr Psychiatry*, 13, 611, 1998.

118. Lindenbaum, J., Healton, E.B., Savage, D.G., Brust, J.C., Garrett, T.J., Podell, E.R., Marcell, P.D., Stabler, S.P., and Allen, R.H. Neuropsychiatric disorders caused by cobalamin deficiency in the absence of anemia or macrocytosis. *N. Engl. J. Med.*, 318, 1720, 1988.

119. Lindenbaum, J., Rosenberg, I.H., Wilson, P.W., Stabler, S.P., and Allen, R.H. Prevalence of cobalamin deficiency in the Framingham elderly population [see comments]. *Am. J. Clin. Nutr.*, 60, 2, 1994.

120. Bar-Sella, P., Rakover, Y., and Ratner, D. Vitamin B-12 and folate levels in long-term vegans. *Isr. J. Med Sci.*, 26, 309, 1990.

121. Immerman, A. Vitamin B-12 status on a vegetarian diet. A critical review. *World Rev. Nutr. Diet.*, 37, 38, 1981.

122. Campbell, M., Lofters, W.S., and Gibbs, W.N. Rastafarianism and the vegans syndrome. *Br. Med. J. (Clin. Res. ed.)*, 285, 1617, 1982.

123. Jones, S.J., Yu, Y.L., Rudge, P., Kriss, A., Gilois, C., Hirani, N., Nijhawan, R., Norman, P., and Will, R. Central and peripheral SEP defects in neurologically symptomatic and asymptomatic subjects with low vitamin B-12 levels. *J. Neurol. Sci.*, 82, 55, 1987.

124. Miller, D.R., Specker, B.L., Ho, M.L., and Norman, E.J. Vitamin B-12 status in a macrobiotic community. *Am. J. Clin. Nutr.*, 53, 524, 1991.

125. Ellis, F. The treatment of dietary deficiency of B-12 with vegetable protein food. *Nutrition et Dieta*, 9, 81, 1967.

126. Dong, A. Serum vitamin B-12 and blood cell values in vegetarians. *Am. Nutr. Metab.*, 26, 209, 1982.

127. Crane, M. Vitamin B-12 in a group of vegans. *Am. J. Clin. Nutr.*, 48, 927, 1988.

128. Baker, S. Evidence regarding the minimal daily requirements of dietary vitamin B-12. *Am. J. Clin. Nutr.*, 34, 2423, 1981.

129. Stewart, J. Response of dietary vitamin B-12 deficiency to physiological oral doses of cyanocobalamin. *Lancet*, 2, 1970.

130. Roberts, P.D., James, H., Petrie, A., Morgan, J.O., and Hoffbrand, A.V. Vitamin B-12 status in pregnancy among immigrants to Britain. *Br. Med. J.*, 3, 67, 1973.

131. Sanders, T. Growth and development of British vegan children. *Am. J. Clin. Nutr.*, 48, 822, 1988.

132. Davis, J. Nutritional B-12 deficiency in infants. *Am. J. Dis Child.*, 135, 566, 1981.

133. Doyle, J., Langerin, A., and Zipursky, A. Nutritional vitamin B-12 deficiency in infancy: three case reports and a review of the literature. *Pediatr. Hematol. Oncol.*, 6, 161, 1989.

134. Specker, B., and Miller, D. Increase urinary methylmalonic acid excretion in breast fed infants of vegetarian mothers and identification of an acceptable dietary source of vitamin B-12. 1988.

135. Dagnelie, P., van Staveren, W., and van den Berg, H. Vitamin B-12 from algae appears not to be available. *Am. J. Clin. Nutr.*, 53, 695, 1991.

136. Slot, W., Merkus, F., and Van Deventer, S. Normalization of plasma vitamin B-12 concentration by intranasal hydrozocobalamin in vitamin B-12 deficient patients. *Gastroenterology*, 113, 430, 1997.

137. Lightowler, H.J. and Davies, G.J. Iodine intake and iodine deficiency in vegans as assessed by the duplicate-portion technique and urinary iodine excretion. *Br. J. Nutr.*, 80, 529, 1998.

138. Draper, A., Lewis, J., Malhotra, N., and Wheeler, E. The energy and nutrient intakes of different types of vegetarian: a case for supplements? [published erratum appears in Br. J. Nutr., 1993 Nov;70(3):812]. *Br. J. Nutr.*, 69, 3, 1993.

139. Abdulla, M., Andersson, I., Asp, N.G., Berthelsen, K., Birkhed, D., Dencker, I., Johansson, C.G., Jagerstad, M., Kolar, K., Nair, B.M., Nilsson-Ehle, P., Norden, A., Rassner, S., Akesson, B., and Ockerman, P.A. Nutrient intake and health status of vegans. Chemical analyses of diets using the duplicate portion sampling technique. *Am. J. Clin. Nutr.*, 34, 2464, 1981.

140. USDA-Iowa State University Database on Isoflavone Content of Foods, Release 1.1–1999. (1999).

14

HEALTH-PROMOTING PHYTOCHEMICALS: BEYOND THE TRADITIONAL NUTRIENTS

Winston J. Craig

CONTENTS

0-8493-8508-3/01/$0.00+$.50
© 2001 by CRC Press LLC

I. INTRODUCTION

It is now recognized that foods contain a wide variety of physiologically active substances, in addition to the macronutrients, vitamins, minerals, and dietary fiber components.[1] These additional substances, called phytochemicals, are found almost exclusively in plant foods. Extensive research on the distribution and physiological activities of the phytochemicals has been fueled by the intense interest in their health-promoting properties and the protection they afford against chronic diseases, such as heart disease and cancer. Thousands of different phytochemicals have been identified in legumes, whole grains, fruits, vegetables, nuts and seeds — foods that are commonly eaten in a vegetarian diet. Many of the phytochemicals, such as the terpenoids, flavonoids, and carotenoids, add flavor and color to food and possess significant antioxidant activity, in some cases greater than that provided by vitamins C and E.[2]

II. FRUITS AND VEGETABLES

A. Population Studies

More than 200 epidemiological studies have investigated the relationship between vegetable and fruit consumption and the risk of cancer. When examining the studies of all cancer sites, more than three quarters of these studies show a significant reduction in risk for a higher intake of at least one vegetable or fruit category.[3] People who eat higher amounts of fruits and vegetables have about one half the risk of cancer and less mortality from cancer.[4,5] Pickled vegetables would not be included in the list of recommended vegetables, since these have been associated with an increased risk of esophageal cancer.[6] Fruits and vegetables are most effective against those cancers that involve epithelial cells, such as cancer of the lung, cervix, esophagus, stomach, colon, and pancreas. Results from a large-scale Italian study revealed that relative risk of common epithelial cancers ranged from 0.2 to 0.5, for the highest tertile, compared with the lowest tertile of vegetable intake.[7] High intakes of fruit provided reduced risk of many epithelial cancers although the protection was generally less than that seen with a high vegetable intake.

The protective effect of vegetables has also been observed for hormone-related cancers, such as breast cancer. A recently published case control study found a strong inverse association between total vegetable intake and breast cancer risk in premenopausal women.[8] A risk reduction of 54% was seen in women with the highest intake of vegetables compared with those with the lowest intake. The protective effect appeared to be due to the synergistic effect of a variety of substances in the vegetables. A Greek study also noted that vegetable and fruit consumption was independently associated with significant reductions in the incidence of breast cancer.[9] Women consuming four to five servings of vegetables per day had a 46% lower risk of breast cancer, compared with women consuming less than two servings a day. Furthermore, women consuming six servings of fruit a day had a 35% lower risk of breast cancer than women consuming less than two servings a day.

Different fruits and vegetables have been investigated separately and appear to provide protection against cancer at certain locations. For example, the use of carrots and green, leafy vegetables provides substantial protection against lung and stomach cancers, while the cruciferous vegetables (cabbage, broccoli, cauliflower, etc.) provide useful protection against colorectal and thyroid cancers. In addition, the regular use of onions or garlic can decrease the risk of stomach and colon cancer by 50–60%,[3,10,11] while the regular consumption of tomatoes and strawberries was recently found to substantially protect against prostate cancer.[12]

A regular fruit and vegetable consumption may also reduce the risk of ischemic heart disease.[13,14] A study of 11,000 health conscious people in the U.K. noted that a daily consumption of fresh fruit was associated with a 24% reduction in mortality from heart disease and a 32% reduction in death from cerebrovascular disease, compared with less frequent fruit consumption. Daily consumption of raw salad was associated with a 26% reduction in mortality from heart disease.[15]

Stroke kills over 150,000 Americans a year. Research at Harvard found that persons in the highest quintile of fruit and vegetable intake (men who consumed an average of 5.1 servings/day and women who consumed an average of 5.8 servings/day) experienced a 31% lower risk of stroke, than those in the lowest quintile (men and women consuming less than three servings a day). Cruciferous vegetables, green leafy vegetables, citrus fruits and citrus juices, but not potatoes or legumes, contributed the most to the protective effect of fruit and vegetables.[16]

The World Health Organization has recommended that, for good health, we consume at least 400 grams (14 ozs.) of fruits and vegetables a day.[17]

The National 5-A-Day for Better Health campaign was designed to increase the consumption of vegetables and fruit to at least five servings a day. When surveyed, only one in 11 Americans actually met this recommended guideline.[18] A lack of knowledge about the value of fruit and vegetables possibly explains the low intake. Two out of every three Americans surveyed said they thought that not more than two servings of fruit and vegetables a day were sufficient for good health.[19]

A high intake of fruit and vegetables is often associated with a lower meat intake and hence, a reduced saturated fat intake. Fruit and vegetables are known to be rich in dietary fiber, folic acid, potassium, magnesium, vitamin C, and other micronutrients that provide protection against cardiovascular disease and cancer. Beyond all these factors, there are additional protective substances: the phytochemicals.

B. Phytochemical Feast

A variety of foods have been reported to be cardio-protective and cancer-preventive. The foods and herbal seasonings that have been reported to exhibit anticancer activity include soybeans, the cruciferous vegetables, the umbelliferous vegetables (carrots, celery, cilantro, caraway, dill, fennel, parsley, and parsnips), flax, citrus, garlic, onions, ginger, turmeric, licorice root, solanaceous vegetables (tomatoes and peppers), brown rice, whole wheat, oats, cucumber, cantaloupe, berries, green tea, and the Labiatae herbs (mints, rosemary, thyme, oregano, sage, basil).[20]

A host of cancer-preventive and cardio-protective phytochemicals have been identified in these foods (see Table 14.1).[21] Some of these phytochemicals may reduce the risk of cardiovascular disease by improving blood flow, inhibiting LDL oxidation, inhibiting platelet aggregation, interfering with cholesterol absorption and modulating cholesterol metabolism. The phytochemicals effectively involved in these processes include the carotenoids, flavonoids, tocotrienols, terpenoids, isoflavones, phytosterols, and various sulfur compounds from the Allium herbs. Furthermore, many of these phytochemicals block various hormone actions and metabolic pathways that are associated with the development of cancer; stimulate the immune system; block the formation of adducts between DNA and a carcinogen; induce phase I enzymes (such as cytochrome P-450) and phase II enzymes (such as glutathione-S-transferase); and have antioxidant activity.[1,11,20,22-28]

For example, the indoles in cruciferous vegetables strongly induce estrogen 2-hydroxylase, which produces metabolites that decrease the risk of cancer.[22] Sulforaphane, the isothiocyanate in cruciferous vegetables,

Table 14.1   Health-Promoting Phytochemicals in Plants[21]

Phytochemical	Food Source
Carotenoids	Yellow-orange vegetables and fruits; green, leafy vegetables; red fruits
Coumarins	Celery, parsnips, figs, parsley
Curcumins	Turmeric, ginger
Dithiolthiones	Cruciferous vegetables
Ellagic acid	Grapes, strawberries, raspberries, nuts
Flavonoids	Most fruits and vegetables
Indoles, isothiocyanates	Broccoli, cabbage, cauliflower, Brussels sprouts, and radish
Isoflavones	Soybeans, tofu
Glucarates	Citrus, grains, tomatoes, bell peppers
Lignans	Soybeans, flax seed
Liminoids	Citrus
Phthalides, polyacetylenes	Caraway, celery, cumin, dill, fennel, parsley, carrots, coriander
Phenolic acids	Berries, grapes, nuts, whole grains
Phytates	Grains, legumes
Phytosterols	Seeds, legumes
Protease inhibitors	Grains, seeds, nuts, legumes
Saponins	Legumes, herbs
Sulfides	Onions, garlic, chives, leeks
Terpenes	Cherries, citrus, herbs
Tocotrienols	Nuts, seeds

and especially broccoli, induces phase II enzymes that detoxify carcinogens. Broccoli sprouts are reported to have 10–100 times the cancer-protective activity of mature broccoli plants.[29] The activity in the sprouts is largely due to glucoraphanin, a precursor of sulforaphane. The citrus flavonoids, tangeretin and nobiletin, are known to activate the detoxifying P-450 enzyme system and are potent inhibitors of tumor cell growth.[30] Limonin and nomilin, the principal limonoids in citrus, occur in high concentrations in grapefruit and orange juice, and partly provide the bitter taste in citrus. These limonoids possess the ability to inhibit tumor formation by stimulating the enzyme glutathione S-transferase.[31] The pulp and albedo of an orange and other citrus are rich in glucarates, which significantly reduce the incidence and multiplicity of mammary tumors, and increase tumor latency.[32] The oil in orange rind contains substantial amounts of limonene, a terpenoid that possesses anti-cancer activity.[33]

C. Carotenoids

Hundreds of carotenoids have been identified in plants. These pigments are responsible for the yellow-orange and red colors of many of the commonly eaten fruits (such as mango, citrus, peach, pineapple, tomato, strawberries, apricots, guava, watermelon, cantaloupe) and vegetables (such as carrots, pumpkin, sweet potato).[34] Dark-green leafy vegetables are also rich sources of carotenoids. In all cases, the deeper the color, the greater the amount of carotenoid pigment. Persons with a high carotenoid intake or who have high levels of serum carotenoids have a reduced risk of cancer.[35,36] The carotenoids have significant antioxidant activity and the ability to quench free radicals, thereby protecting DNA, cell membranes, and other cellular components from oxidative damage that might lead to the development of tumor cells. The consumption of tomato products substantially reduces the susceptibility of DNA to oxidative damage.[37]

High levels of lycopene are found in the prostate. The consumption of tomato products, rich in the red lycopene pigment, is associated with a reduced risk of prostate cancer. In the Adventist Health Study, men who consumed tomatoes more than five times a week had a 40% lower risk of prostate cancer than men consuming tomatoes less than once a week.[38] In the Health Professionals Study, lycopene intake was inversely related to risk of prostate cancer.[12] Risk of prostate cancer was 22% lower and 35% lower in those men consuming four to seven servings per week and more than 10 servings of tomato products per week, respectively, compared with those consuming less than 1.5 servings per week. Studies also suggest that lycopene may play a role in protection against cancer of the breast and cervix.[39,40] Tomato and tomato-based products account for over 85% of dietary lycopene in American diets. The rich sources of lycopene (given in μg lycopene per g wet weight) include fresh tomatoes (9–42), tomato paste (54–1500), tomato juice (50–116), pizza sauce (127), watermelon (23–72), pink guava (54), pink grapefruit (34) and papaya (20–53).[41] Many factors influence the absorption and bioavailability of lycopene, such as heat and food processing and the presence of dietary fat. The availability of lycopene from tomato paste was found to be greater than from fresh tomatoes. Lycopene concentrates in LDL and VLDL serum fractions.[41]

Carotenoids protect against cholesterol oxidation. Persons with high levels of serum carotenoids have a reduced risk of heart disease.[25,42] The recent EURAMIC study found that a high intake of lycopene (the red pigment in tomatoes, pink grapefruit, guava, and watermelon) in men was associated with a 48% lower risk of a myocardial infarction, compared with a low intake of lycopene.[43] Carotenoids act as modest hypocholesterolemic agents, secondary to their inhibitory effect on HMG-CoA reductase, the rate-limiting enzyme in cholesterol synthesis. Cholesterol synthesis is suppressed and LDL receptor activity is augmented by the carotenoids ß-carotene and lycopene, similar to that seen with the drug fluvastatin. When lycopene supplements (60 mg/day) were given to men for a 3-month period, a 14% reduction in their LDL cholesterol levels occurred.[44] Therefore, lycopene may be useful for decreasing the risk of coronary heart disease.

Citrus fruits contain a variety of carotenoids. Pink grapefruits have a high content of lycopene and ß-carotene, while other citrus (such as tangerines, oranges) contain high levels of different carotenoids (lutein, zeaxanthin, ß-cryptoxanthin)[34] that have significant antioxidant activity. These carotenoids are associated with a lower incidence of age-related macular degeneration,[45] the leading cause of vision loss in Americans after the age of 55. A diet rich in carotenoids (such as lutein, zeaxanthin or ß-carotene) enhances several aspects of immune function in the body, including those linked to tumor cell destruction.[46]

Carotenoids, along with other antioxidants, may play a role in preventing age-related cataracts. In the Nurses' Health Study, an increased intake of spinach and kale (foods rich in the carotenoid lutein) was associated with a moderate decrease (22%) in risk of cataract.[47] In the Health Professionals' Study, broccoli and spinach consumption were consistently associated with a lower risk of cataract. Men in the highest quintile of lutein and zeaxanthin intake (carotenoids found in green vegetables) had a 19% lower risk of cataract, relative to men in the lowest quintile.[48]

D. Flavonoids

Polyphenols constitute one of the most numerous groups of plant metabolites. They include molecules such as coumarins, the 13 classes of flavonoids (numbering over 5000 substances), as well as highly polymerized compounds such as lignans and tannins. In berries, the main polyphenols are anthocyanins; fruits and vegetables are rich in phenolic acids, citrus are rich in flavonoids, and vegetables are rich in flavonoids and coumarins.[49]

The many flavonoids in fruit and vegetables have extensive biological properties that reduce the risk of cardiovascular disease. Flavonoids are among the most potent antioxidants. They protect LDL cholesterol from oxidation; inhibit the formation of blood clots; and have vasopressive and hypolipidemic effects and anti-inflammatory action.[49,50] Some polyphenols have hypocholesterolemic effects mediated by reduced intestinal cholesterol absorption and increased bile acid excretion. European studies have found flavonoid intake to be inversely associated with heart disease mortality, and the incidence of heart attack and stroke over a 5-year period.[51-53] Those who had the highest consumption of flavonoids had 60% less mortality from heart disease and 70% lower risk of stroke than the low-flavonoid consumers. Among other things, flavonoids extend the activity of vitamin C, and have anti-tumor activity.[50] The citrus flavonoids, tangeretin and nobiletin, are known to be potent inhibitors of tumor cell growth and can activate the P-450 enzyme system.[30]

The flavonoid content of a food depends on the growing conditions, the part of the plant consumed, the degree of ripeness, and method of processing. The levels are greater in immature organs of the plant where there is active cell division, and in external tissues exposed to sunlight. Fruits have a relatively high level of flavonoids, especially when ripe. Peeling will eliminate a substantial amount of flavonoids, since the skin contains 8- to 10-fold more than the pulp. Flavonoid levels in processed foods (canned, in glass jars, or frozen) are significantly lower than in fresh products. Flavonoids are carried in the LDL particle along with other antioxidants such as vitamin E and carotenoids. The oxidation of LDL cholesterol can occur only when these endogenous antioxidants are exhausted.[50]

E. Pigments in Grapes and Cherries

Anthocyanin pigments, the water-soluble, reddish pigments found in fruits such as strawberries, cherries, cranberries, raspberries, blueberries, grapes, and black currants, are reported to be antioxidants and are very effective in scavenging free radicals, inhibiting LDL cholesterol oxidation and platelet aggregation, and protecting against cardiovascular disease.[54-56] A variety of anthocyanins and flavonoids have been identified in tart cherries, which possess very strong antioxidant and anti-inflammatory activity. These compounds could account for antiallergenic, antiviral, anticancer, and cardio-protective activities.[57] It has been suggested that the composition of tart cherries may protect against various chronic diseases and reduce arthritic- and gout-related pain.[57]

The regular use of red wine is suggested for lowering the risk of heart disease. Two possible mechanisms explain this effect. First, alcohol raises HDL cholesterol levels.[58] Second, wine inhibits the formation of blood clots. Since purple grape juice and dealcoholized red wine inhibit platelet aggregation, it is clearly not an effect of alcohol, but appears to be related to the flavonoid pigments in the grape juice or wine.[59,60] Dealcoholized red wines and red grape juice inhibit platelet aggregation by blocking thromboxane B_2 synthesis in the platelets. This inhibition was found to be in direct proportion to the content of a stillbene, trans-resveratrol, which is found in wine and grape juice.[59] Resveratrol is a phytochemical found mainly in the skins of grapes and is readily transferred to red wine by alcohol extraction. It is also recovered during the hot-press-extraction process in the manufacture of purple grape juice.

Dealcoholized red wine and red grapes are also rich in phenolic compounds such as anthocyanins, flavonols, flavan-3-ols, and hydroxycinnamates, which act as antioxidants. These compounds strongly inhibit LDL oxidation and diminish the development of atherosclerotic plaque formation.[61-64] The antioxidants in wine and grape juice may be even more potent than vitamins C and E.[63,64] In a new study from the University of Wisconsin, grape juice was shown to improve blood flow by 6.4% and protect LDL from oxidation by 35.4%. Wines also contain lignans, with the red wines having four to nine times more lignans than the white wines.[65] White wine, white grape juice, and green grapes generally have polyphenolic compounds similar to the red varieties, but occur in lesser amounts.[55]

In preliminary studies, the stilbene, resveratrol, has been shown to reduce the risk of breast, colon, and liver cancers. Dannenberg has shown that resveratrol inhibits cyclooxygenase-2, an enzyme linked to breast cancer.[66] Others have shown that compounds in grapes inhibit breast cancer by suppressing the estrogen-producing enzyme aromatase.[67]

F. Isoprenoids and Phenolics

Fruits, vegetables, and cereal grains contain a variety of isoprenoid compounds that exhibit anticancer activities. These compounds, which derive from mevalonate metabolism, include the tocotrienols and monoterpenes such as limonene, geraniol, menthol, carvone, and perillyl alcohol. The isoprenoids can suppress tumor growth by inhibiting HMG-CoA reductase, the rate-limiting step in cholesterol synthesis. Overall, the terpenoids and tocotrienols increase tumor latency and decrease tumor multiplicity.[68] In addition, many of the terpenoids such as limonene, geraniol, menthol, and carvone exhibit anti-tumor activity by stimulating the activity of the phase II enzyme, glutathione S-transferase. Finally, the terpenoids may also facilitate a reduction in blood cholesterol levels.[69,70]

A whole variety of phenolic compounds are widely distributed in fruits and vegetables. These phenolics act as antioxidants and influence the sensory quality and stability of foods. Many of these compounds (such as caffeic, ellagic and ferulic acids, sesamol and vanillin) exhibit anticarcinogenic activity and inhibit atherosclerosis.[24] Ellagic acid, in raspberries and strawberries, inhibits certain carcinogen-induced cancers and has other chemopreventive properties. Ellagic acid also has a role in cell cycle regulation of cancer cells.[71] A number of fruits and vegetables contain the phytoestrogenic lignans. Those with the highest level of lignans were found to be strawberries, pomegranates, cranberries, melons, asparagus, pumpkin, chives, guava, broccoli, black currant, and garlic.[65] The predominant lignan measured in these foods was secoisolariciresinol, with much lesser amounts of matairesinol.

G. Fructose Oligosaccharides

Fructose oligosaccharides (FOS) are widely distributed in plants, with the best sources being artichokes, onions, garlic, leeks, wheat, dandelion greens, asparagus, banana, and rye.[72] About 95% of FOS, or oligofructose, in the American diet comes from wheat and onions, with another 4% being derived from bananas and garlic.[72] The functional and nutritional properties of oligofructose have led many to see its significance and value in the human diet. Oligofructose can be considered a carbohydrate, similar to dietary fiber. It has been used to replace sugar in foods due to its sweet, pleasant flavor and high solubility. It causes a shift in the composition of colonic microflora by selectively stimulating the growth of bifidobacteria.[73] Other health-promoting properties reported for oligofructose include increasing intestinal motility, decreasing blood triglycerides and blood cholesterol levels, blunting of alimentary glycemia, decreasing the growth rate of tumors, increasing the absorption of calcium and magnesium, and enhancing the immune system.[73]

III. LEGUMES

A number of studies have shown that legumes, such as beans and lentils, lower blood cholesterol levels, improve blood sugar control, lower triglyceride levels, and lower the risk of heart disease.[74-76] While beans are good sources of polyunsaturated fat, folic acid, potassium, copper, and soluble fiber, they also contain a variety of important phytochemicals such as flavonoids, protease inhibitors, saponins, phytates, and phytosterols that have cardio-protective and cancer-preventive properties.[3,77,78] The anthocyanin pigments isolated from the bean seed coat of *Phaseolus vulgarus*, the common bean, exhibit strong antioxidative activity.[79] These pigments may provide protection against oxidative damage of cell membrane lipids and cell contents.

A. Soy Isoflavones

Intense research over the past decade has shown that soybean has health-promoting properties and may be useful in lowering the risk of heart disease, cancer, osteoporosis, menopausal symptoms, and other problems. Soy is now available in many different kinds of foods such as tofu, soy beverages, soy cheese, soy sauce, tempeh, soy-based meat substitutes, soy nuts, and soy-based frozen desserts.

Soy protein is unique in its rich content of isoflavones. The isoflavones in soybeans occur principally as glucosides of genistein, daidzein, and glycitein, with or without an acetyl or malonyl group attached to the glucose. Different soy products contain various amounts of these glucoside derivatives (see Table 14.2), and these compounds have different rates of absorption and possibly metabolism.[80] The isoflavone glucosides are hydrolyzed in the gut and the resulting aglycones may be further metabolized before absorption. For example, daidzein is partly metabolized to equol. The isoflavone metabolites are fat-soluble and are absorbed from the gut by diffusion via the fat-rich micelles. Clearly, a diet that is highly restricted in fat content will impede the absorption of soy isoflavones and their metabolites.

Table 14.2 Isoflavone Contents of Soyfoods

	(μg/g)		
	Genistein*	Daidzein*	Glycitein*
Soybeans	1696	1548	187
Soyflour, roasted	2860	3087	181
Soynuts, roasted	781	604	256
TVP	1222	825	332
Tofu	1556	1376	287
Tempeh	1690	907	164
Miso	1140	1398	265
Soy milk	2420	1140	203

* The values include the glucoside, malonyl and acetyl derivatives as well as the aglycones. Adapted from Reference 80.

During processing, the relative amounts of these isoflavones in soy may change (see Table 14.2). However, the total isoflavone concentration in soy foods is not altered under normal household cooking conditions. The total isoflavone content of the unprocessed soybean can itself vary by a factor of five, depending upon the source and variety of the bean,[80] and different analyses will reflect this variation. Ethyl alcohol extraction of soy flour to give a soy protein concentrate removes most of the isoflavones.[4] Low-fat choices of soy milk and tofu are markedly reduced in isoflavones.[81] Baking or frying of textured vegetable protein (TVP) and baking of soy flour in cookies does not alter the total isoflavone content. Fermentation of soy to produce miso and tempeh causes a breakdown of the glucosides to form the aglycones (the free forms of genistein and daidzein).[81]

Intestinal metabolism of the glucosides is essential for isoflavone absorption and bioavailability, as there is no evidence to support absorption of the conjugated forms of isoflavones. In addition, it is the aglycone forms that have an affinity for estrogen receptors. The use of antibiotics adversely affects the gut metabolism of isoflavone glycosides. The net result is that fewer aglycones are formed. This is reflected in lower serum isoflavone levels. Hence, the regular use of antibiotics may negate the positive health effects of dietary soy.

The isoflavones are well known for their estrogenic activity, which varies substantially from one compound to another. These nonsteroidal phytoestrogens have an array of potent biological activities, of both a hormonal and non-hormonal nature, which influence the development of chronic diseases. The isoflavones can undergo enterohepatic recycling and reach circulating levels that exceed, by several orders of magnitude, the amounts of natural endogenous estrogens.[82] The major tissues targeted by the phytoestrogens are the reproductive tissues (uterus, breast, and prostate), the cardiovascular tissues (arteries and blood lipids) and the skeletal tissues.[83] About 30–60 mg of isoflavones, per day appear to be the required threshold level needed to lower the risk of heart disease and cancer in humans. Higher levels are apparently needed for improving bone health.[82,84] These levels can be achieved from a modest intake of a variety of soy products in the diet (see Table 14.3).

B. Effects on Lipid Levels

Over the past 20 years, a number of human studies have shown that the consumption of 30–60 g of soy protein decreases total and LDL cholesterol levels by as much as 10–20% in persons with elevated blood cholesterol levels.[86-88] In some instances, persons with normal blood cholesterol levels have also benefited by lowered blood LDL cholesterol and raised HDL cholesterol levels after using soy.[89] The use of soy protein may also lower triglyceride levels, especially in subjects with elevated counts.[87] In addition to the soy protein, the fiber and polyunsaturated fat in soy will have a hypocholesterolemic effect.

A meta-analysis of 38 clinical studies revealed that persons with elevated blood cholesterol levels experienced, on average, a 9 and 13% drop in their serum total cholesterol and LDL cholesterol levels, respectively, while consuming an average of 47 g of soy protein a day for 4 weeks.[90] Furthermore, triglyceride levels decreased 10%, while HDL cholesterol levels typically showed no change, or were slightly increased. The reduc-

Table 14.3   Isoflavone Content of Soy Products

Soy Food	Isoflavone Content (mg)
1/2 c. soybeans, cooked	35
1/4 c. dry TVP	35
1/3 c. soy nuts, dry, roasted	35
4 ozs. tofu	33
2 ozs. soy flour	30
2 ozs. soy protein isolate	30
1 c. soymilk	25–40
1 oz. SoyBoy Breakfast Links	20
1 oz. soybean chips	15.3
1 oz. tempeh	12.3
1 oz. miso	12
1 oz. soy cheese	2–9
1/2 c. Ice bean	8
1 oz. Green Giant Harvest Burger	2.6
1 oz. soy noodles	2.4
1/2 c. Tofutti	2
1 Tbsp. soy sauce	0.3
1 Tbsp. soy oil	0

Data from references 21 and 85.

tions in blood lipids were normally greater in those subjects with initially high cholesterol levels.

Numerous mechanisms have been proposed to explain the effects of soy, such as an altered hepatic metabolism of cholesterol that includes an altered LDL receptor activity, altered thyroid hormone and altered estrogenic activity.[91] The phytosterols and the saponins in soy can block the absorption of cholesterol and bile acids or increase their excretion from the body, thus lowering blood cholesterol levels.[77,92] Recent research shows that the isoflavones in soy may also be involved. They are known to prevent the oxidation of LDL cholesterol, inhibit proliferation in the artery wall, lower blood cholesterol levels, and attenuate events leading to the formation of blood clots. Genistein is a well-known inhibitor of tyrosine kinase, an enzyme active in the cascade of events that occurs in the formation of clots, as well as in tissues actively producing plaque.[91,93] The isoflavones also alter the activity of cytokines and specific growth factors that influence lesion formation, have an antioxidative effect, promote enlargement of the artery lumen after arterial injury, maintain normal vascular reactivity, and diminish angina by improving vasodilation in atherosclerotic arteries.[82] Isoflavones have also improved arterial compliance in menopausal women.[94]

C. Protection against Cancer

Consumption of soybeans is suggested as a contributing factor in the low incidence of breast and prostate cancer in Japanese women and men, respectively. Asian women who consume large amounts of soy foods have only one fifth as much breast cancer as Western women, along with a reduced mortality from breast cancer. Chinese populations having a regular consumption of soybeans, fermented soy products or tofu, have only one half as much cancer of the stomach, colon, rectum, breast, prostate, and lung compared with those Chinese people who rarely consume soy products.[95] A high consumption of soy products and other legumes was associated with a 54% reduction in risk of endometrial cancer in Hawaiian women.[96] Decreased prostatic cancer was observed in Hawaiian men of Japanese descent who consumed substantial amounts of tofu,[97] while the use of soy milk more than once a day was associated with a 70% reduction in risk of prostate cancer in Adventist men in California.[98]

Studies on young women revealed that regular consumers of soy protein had their menstrual cycles lengthened 2–3 days due to the lengthening of the follicular phase.[99] In addition, the soy diet suppressed the normal midcycle surge in luteinizing hormone and follicle-stimulating hormone, which translates into a decreased risk of breast cancer. During the luteal phase of the cycle, when hormone levels are normally high, there is a stimulation of breast cell proliferation. A diet that lengthens the follicular phase may mean fewer luteal phases over a lifetime, which may translate into a reduced risk of breast cancer.[99] Soy has been suggested as an effective alternative to the drug tamoxifen for the prevention of breast cancer in high risk women.[82]

A large majority of the studies involving experimental animals reported that either soy or soy isoflavones had cancer-preventive effects. However, the protective effect of soy is lost when the isoflavones are removed. The isoflavones are reported to display antioxidant, antiproliferative, and antiangiogenic activities, inhibit the actions of cytokines and growth factors, inhibit nitric oxide formation, inhibit the enzyme aromatase, and stimulate the synthesis of sex-hormone-binding globulin.[82] Recent experiments suggest that genistein may inhibit cell growth by modulating and transforming growth factor ß1 signaling pathways.[100] The isoflavones in soy inhibit the growth of hormone-dependent and hormone-independent cancer cells in culture,[101] and have been shown to inhibit the growth of both breast and prostate cancer.[95] Genistein is also known to block carcinogens from forming adducts with DNA, and is a specific inhibitor of protein tyrosine kinases and DNA topoisomerases I and II.[82]

The growth of mammary tumors in experimental animals is stimulated by estrogen. Genistein functions as an estrogen antagonist, competitively binding to the estrogen receptors, reducing the activity of endogenous estrogen, and reducing the risk of growth of estrogen-sensitive tumors.[102] Genistein and daidzein have only about 1/1000th to 1/10,000th the activity of estradiol, with genistein having 6.5 and 1.4 times the estrogenic activity of daidzein and equol, respectively.[83] Soybeans are not the only legume that have isoflavonoid phytoestrogens. Kidney beans, garbanzos, pinto beans, and black-eyed beans were found to have small amounts of biochanin A (which is metabolized to genistein), lima beans and alfalfa sprouts reported significant levels of coumestrol, while green split peas had 73 µg/g of daidzein. On the other hand, lentils, green peas, and sesame seeds had no detectable phytoestrogens.[83] In another study, the best sources of genistein in legumes other than soy were pinto beans, navy beans, mung beans, and pigeon peas, while low levels were seen in split peas, lima beans, and lentils.[103]

In addition to the isoflavones, soybeans also contain fairly high levels of several other compounds with demonstrated anti-cancer activity, including phytates, protease inhibitors, phytosterols, and saponins.[78] These phytochemicals, which are commonly found in all legumes, are generally stable during soy processing, except for protease inhibitors, which are heat sensitive.

D. Help for Menopause and Bone Loss

Soy products are being studied for their potential use as hormone replacement therapy during menopause. Japanese women who regularly consume soy products report less frequent and fewer hot flushes and other menopausal symptoms than American and European women who do not eat soy products. A 3-month clinical trial observed a beneficial effect of soy protein on the frequency of hot flushes in postmenopausal women.[104] Italian researchers observed a significant decrease in the average number of hot flushes experienced by postmenopausal women taking 60 g of soy protein isolate daily for 12 weeks. In a double-blind, placebo-controlled study, the women taking soy experienced a 45% reduction in their daily hot flushes, compared with a 30% reduction in women taking a placebo.[105] The soy isoflavones are believed to bind at the estrogen receptors and act as mild agonists for estrogen in postmenopausal women, thus alleviating some menopausal symptoms experienced in estrogen deficiency.

The isoflavones in soy appear to inhibit bone resorption and benefit bone health in postmenopausal women. Estrogen is known to down-regulate the activity of osteoclasts, thereby limiting bone resorption. The isoflavones in soy protein, acting as phytoestrogens, can bind to the estrogen receptors in bone tissue.[82] Animal studies reveal that soy isoflavones have a positive effect on bone density and counteract the effects of estrogen deficiency on bone. Ovariectomized rats normally experience bone loss due to their estrogen deficiency. However, when given either estradiol- or soy protein-containing isoflavones, these rats do not experience a loss in bone density.[82] It is also known that ipriflavone, a synthetic isoflavone, is suc-cessfully used as an estrogen replacement in menopausal women, as it increases bone mass in women with low bone density.[106] Recently, post-menopausal women who were consuming isoflavone-rich soy protein for 6 months were found to be protected against spinal bone loss.[84]

IV. WHOLE GRAINS

A. Population Studies

Epidemiological studies support the notion that whole grains are protective against cardiovascular disease and cancers, especially gastrointestinal can-cers.[107,108] In a review of 40 case-control studies involving 20 cancers and colon polyps, 95% of the studies showed whole grains to be protective. Overall, the risk of most cancers was 20–50% lower (average risk was 34% lower) in those with a high vs. low consumption of whole grains.[109] The risks of breast and prostate cancer were only 14% and 10% lower, respectively. In a recent study from northern Italy, researchers found that those who had the highest consumption of refined cereals (pasta, breads, or rice) experienced a 30 to 60% higher incidence of cancer of the gastrointestinal tract (mouth, esophagus, stomach, colon, and rectum) than those who had the lowest intake of refined grains.[110] Americans are encouraged to consume at least three of their daily servings of grains and cereals in the form of whole grains.[107] At present, the average American consumes as little as one half of a serving of whole-grain products per day.

In the Iowa Women's Study, women in the highest quintile of whole-grain consumption (22 servings per week) had a risk of death from heart disease that was 30% lower than the women in the lowest quintile (1–2 servings per week).[109] In the Nurses' Health Study, involving over 75,000 women, those in the top quintile of whole-grain consumption (median of 2.7 servings/d) experienced a 33% lower risk of coronary heart disease than women in the lowest quintile (median of 0.13 servings/d). In this study, whole grain included dark bread, whole-grain breakfast cereal (at least 25% whole-grain or bran content by weight), popcorn, cooked oatmeal, wheat germ, brown rice, bran, bulgar, kasha, and couscous. The lower risk of coronary heart disease associated with whole-grain intake was not fully explained by the dietary fiber, folate, vitamin B[6], and vitamin E content of the whole grains.[111] Recent studies consistently demonstrate higher rates of cardiovascular disease and type II diabetes in individuals deriving a greater percentage of energy from refined grains and simple carbohydrates than from whole grains.[112,113]

B. Contents of the Grains

The active phytochemicals are located principally in the bran and the germ, which compose less than 20% of the kernel. Hence, the refining of wheat causes very substantial losses of phytochemicals.[114] The protective substances include those that affect the gut environment, such as dietary fiber, resistant starch, and oligosaccharides; compounds that function as antioxidants, such as selenium, tocopherols, tocotrienols, flavonoids, ellagic acid; and phenolic acids, such as ferulic, caffeic, vanillic and p-coumaric acids (these phenolic acids occur in high levels in whole grains); and lignans (phytoestrogens).[107,108] Rye and barley contain the highest level of lignans among the grains, while wheat and corn have the least.[65] Other important health-promoting phytochemicals in whole grains include phytosterols, phytates, and saponins.[107]

Brans have various effects on blood lipid levels. Rice bran and oat bran are both effective for lowering cholesterol levels while wheat bran has little, if any, effect. Rice bran oil effectively lowers blood cholesterol levels, due to its rich content of unsaturated fat, as well as γ-oryzanol, triterpene alcohols (cycloartenol and 24-methylene cycloartanol), plant sterols (β-sitosterol and campesterol) and β- and γ-tocotrienols, all of which interfere with cholesterol metabolism.[115] Wheat germ also lowers cholesterol and triglyceride levels in hypercholesterolemic subjects.[116]

V.   NUTS, SEEDS AND OILS

Nuts are typically classified as tree nuts (often encased in a hard shell) or peanuts (actually a legume). For most of the year, Americans eat nuts and seeds somewhat sparingly (less than one-half ounce per day) because of their high fat content. Nuts account for only 2 to 3% of the total fat intake in the American diet.[117] People in the Mediterranean countries, who are noted for their healthy diet, consume twice as many nuts per person as Americans do.

A. Nuts and Heart Disease

A number of epidemiological studies have consistently reported that frequent consumption of nuts is associated with a reduced risk of coronary heart disease (CHD). For example, in the Adventist Health Study, people who ate nuts (mostly almonds and walnuts with lesser amounts of peanuts) one to four times per week had a 25% reduced risk of CHD, while those who ate nuts five or more times a week experienced a 50% reduction in risk of CHD, compared with people who ate nuts less than once a week.[118] In a 9-year follow-up study of African-American Californians, the observed mortality rate for those who frequently consumed nuts was 44% lower than in those who consumed nuts very infrequently.[119] In the Women's Health Study in Iowa, those women with the highest nut intake had a 60% lower risk of CHD than the women who never ate nuts.[120] In the Nurses' Health Study, women who ate nuts five or more times per week had a 39% lower risk of fatal CHD and a 32% lower risk of nonfatal myocardial infarction than those eating nuts less than once a month.[121]

While 73 to 95% of the calories in nuts come from fat, they are low in saturated fat. On average, nuts contain about 60% of their calories from monounsaturated fat, which facilitates a reduction in blood total- and LDL cholesterol levels, without lowering the HDL cholesterol levels. A number of clinical trials have demonstrated the effectiveness of diets that contain either almonds, pecans, peanuts, hazelnuts, macadamia nuts, pistachios, or walnuts to significantly lower blood cholesterol levels.[122-129] Human feeding trials that incorporated these nuts into the diet produced significant reductions in LDL cholesterol levels ranging from an 8% decrease with macadamia nuts to a 16% decrease with walnuts. Except for the studies with almonds and pistachios, all of the clinical trials involved normocholesterolemic subjects. Only in the case of the pistachio study did HDL cholesterol levels increase (up 12%).[129] In an analysis of the nut-feeding studies, Kris-Etherton reports that the lipid-lowering effect of the test diets was 25% greater than that suggested by predictive equations that involve fat composition.[130] It was suggested that phytochemicals and other non-fatty-acid constituents in the nuts provided the additional cardio-protective effects.

B. The Content of Nuts and Seeds

Nuts are known to contain a number of vitamins (folic acid, vitamin E), minerals (potassium, copper, magnesium), dietary fiber, and other substances important for cardiovascular health.[118] Almonds and hazelnuts also have high levels of α-tocopherol, whereas pecans and walnuts are rich in γ-tocopherol. The tocopherols are known to prevent the oxidation of LDL cholesterol. Nuts and seeds are also a rich source of tocotrienols, which are inhibitors of HMG-CoA reductase in the biosynthesis of cholesterol. Hence, tocotrienols are effective hypocholesterolemic agents, as well as potent cancer-preventive substances.[68-70] Peanuts contain substantial levels of trans-resveratrol, the protective compound in red wine and grape juice shown to inhibit the formation of blood clots. As far as phytoestrogens are concerned, nuts and sunflower seeds have a substantial lignan content, while peanuts contain small amounts of isoflavones.[65,85]

Nuts and seeds are also a rich source of flavonoids,[117] and contain high levels of phytosterols.[131] Nuts typically contain 30–60 mg of phytosterols per ounce, with peanuts and pistachios having the highest levels. β-sitosterol is the major phytosterol, composing about three quarters of the total phytosterol content. Plant sterols can interfere with cholesterol absorption and lower blood cholesterol levels.[132,133] The esters of phytosterols from soybean oil (esters of β-sitosterol, campesterol, and stigmasterol) were shown to be as effective as their synthetic saturated derivatives (sitostanol esters) in lowering blood total cholesterol (7–8%) and LDL cholesterol levels (12–13%), without affecting HDL cholesterol levels, in healthy, nonobese subjects.[134] Two new cholesterol-lowering margarines have become popular spreads. One is fortified with the esters of sitostanols (from wood pulp) and the other with soy phytosterols. Various studies show that these margarines can lower elevated blood cholesterol levels by as much as 10%.[134] However, new research shows that persons using these sterol-fortified margarines experienced a 25–30% drop in their blood levels of beta-carotene, a change that might result in reduced protection against cancer and heart disease.

Nuts, especially peanuts, are a good source of saponins which are reported to have both anticarcinogenic activity and hypocholesterolemic activity.[135,136] Most nuts and oilseeds are a good source of phenolic acids (such as caffeic and ellagic acids). In particular, pecans and walnuts have high levels of the cancer-preventive ellagic acid,[71] the majority of which is lost when the nuts are blanched.[137] Typically, nuts also contain 300–500 mg of phytates per ounce.[138] Phytates are known to reduce the risk of various cancers and reduce cell proliferation.[139] Nuts are also rich in tannins, which are water-soluble polyphenolic compounds.[49] Tannins have antioxidant, mutagenic and antimicrobial activities. Some are reported to possess anticarcinogenic activity.[140] Tannins have also been reported to decrease blood lipid and blood pressure levels and modulate immunoresponses, depending on the amount and type of tannins consumed.[140] With such an array of cancer-preventive substances in nuts, it comes as no surprise that nuts have been reported to also be protective against prostate cancer.[141]

The use of flaxseed can lower both total- and LDL cholesterol levels, due, in part, to its very low saturated fat content and its rich content of polyphenolics.[142] Oilseeds, such as sesame seed and especially flax seed, are very rich sources of lignans.[65] Plant lignans are converted to mammalian lignans (enterolactone and enterodiol) by bacterial fermentation in the colon.[143] The lignan metabolites bear a structural similarity to estrogens and can bind to estrogen receptors and inhibit the growth of estrogen-stimulated breast cancer.[144]

C. Olive Oil

The increased life expectancy and low rates of chronic diseases such as heart disease, high blood pressure, diabetes, and cancer among the southern Europeans, may be, in part, due to their physically active, simple lifestyle and unique Mediterranean diet, which is especially rich in a variety of phytochemicals such as those found in olive oil, garlic and other herbs, beans, fresh fruit and vegetables.[145,146]

In the Lyon Diet Heart Study, it was observed that the Mediterranean diet reduced the risk of recurrence of heart disease after the first myocardial infarction, and that the protective effect persisted for at least 4 years. The advantage of a traditional Mediterranean diet over a prudent Western diet could not be explained by the typical risk factors, such as blood pressure levels; total, LDL or HDL blood cholesterol or triglyceride levels; smoking or alcohol use. It was suggested that the critical components in a Mediterranean diet rich in vegetables, legumes, and virgin olive oil may be the abundant flavonoids and other antioxidants that have antithrombotic activity and that quench free radicals.[147]

Many of the non-glyceride components of virgin olive oil are known to protect against heart disease and cancer. Because olive oil is obtained by a mild extraction method, it retains substantial amounts of bioactive phytochemicals such as phytosterols, polyphenolics, and many unique flavor compounds.[148] The polyphenolics, which include anthocyanins, flavonoids (luteolin, apigenin), tyrosol, 3-hydroxytyrosol, oleuropein and phenolic acids (caffeic, vanillic, p-coumaric, and ferulic acids), amount to 50–800 mg/kg depending on the cultivar, soil, ripeness of the olives and the way the oil is produced and stored.[149] Olive oil may contain as much as 2500 ppm of β-sitosterol, the major sterol in olive oil, which is believed to block cholesterol absorption. Another sterol, cycloartenol, aids in the excretion of cholesterol through increased bile acid secretion.[150]

A variety of water-soluble polyphenolics are found in olive pulp and are responsible for the bitter taste of olives. Measurable amounts of these compounds end up in the oil extract, with extra-virgin olive oil containing the highest levels. Tyrosol and 3-hydroxytyrosol, the major polyphenolics in olives, are found at levels of 120 to 150 ppm.[148] The antioxidant activities of oleuropein and 3-hydroxytyrosol are similar to those of vitamins C and

E. The polyphenolics in olive oil inhibit LDL oxidation by scavenging free radicals and chelating free metal ions.[149] The polyphenolics also enhance the synthesis of prostacyclin, PGI_2, and thus inhibit platelet aggregation. These phenolic compounds are antioxidants that reduce eicosanoid production by leukocytes, so as to modulate inflammation and protect the cell against cancer-forming substances. Olive oil also contains up to 150 ppm of the antioxidant vitamin E, which can also inhibit platelet aggregation. Polyphenolics have also been shown to lower blood glucose levels.[151]

VI. HERBS

Many of the commonly used herbs contain phytochemicals, such as the carotenoids, flavonoids, terpenoids, phytosterols, saponins, and phenolic acids, which are similar to those found in fruit, vegetables, and whole grains, and also those associated with disease prevention (see Table 14.4). The therapeutic value of many of these herbs owe their health-promoting properties to the phytochemicals they contain.[152]

Table 14.4   Phytochemicals in Common Herbs also Found in Vegetables, Fruit and Whole Grains

Phytochemical Class	Herbal Source[152,153]
Carotenoids	Rose hips
Coumarins	Alfalfa, chamomile, fenugreek, red clover
Flavonoids	Chamomile, ginkgo, hawthorn, licorice root, milk thistle
Lignans	Flax seed, milk thistle
Phthalides	Caraway, cilantro, cumin, dill, fennel, parsley
Phytosterols	Nettles, pumpkin seeds, saw palmetto
Phenolic acids	Echinacea, rosemary, sage, St John's Wort, thyme
Polyacetylenes	Caraway, cilantro, cumin, dill, fennel, parsley
Saponins	Alfalfa, black cohosh, ginseng, licorice root
Terpenes	Basil, eucalyptus, feverfew, ginkgo, oregano, rosemary, sage, thyme, valerian

A number of herbs, along with some fruits and vegetables, contain compounds that stimulate the activity of the protective phase II enzyme glutathione S-transferase (GST). The substances that stimulate GST activity include the phthalides in celery seed, the sulfides in garlic and onions, the courmarins in umbelliferous vegetables and herbs, catechins in green tea, dithiolthiones and isothiocyanates in broccoli and other cruciferous vegetables, limonene and the liminoids (such as limonin and nomilin) in citrus and the curcumins in ginger and turmeric.[11,31,154-156]

Rosemary, sage, oregano, thyme, and other flavoring herbs that belong to the *Labiatae* family are known to possess strong antioxidative activity.[157] Of the *Labiatae* herbs, rosemary has the most effective antioxidant activity. It contains substantial levels of carnosol and ursolic acid, potent antioxidants that possess anti-tumor activity.[158] Rosemary also contains a family of diterpenoids with powerful antioxidant activity, including rosmanol, epirosmanol, isorosmanol, and rosmarinic acid.[157] Ginger contains a dozen phenolic compounds known as gingerols and diarylhaptanoids, which have an antioxidant activity that is even greater than α-tocopherol.[159] The compounds responsible for the flavors of many common herbs and seasonings are terpenoids (see Table 14.5), reported to be cancer-chemopreventive agents.[152,160-163] Phase I clinical trial testing of the cancer preventive activity of limonene and perillyl alcohol is in progress.[160] Both terpenoids show activity against mammary tumors and perillyl alcohol is active against pancreatic tumors.

Table 14.5   Terpenoids Known to Inhibit Tumors

Terpenoid	Food/Herb Containing the Terpenoid[152,160]
carvocrol	dill, marjoram, mint, thyme
carvone	caraway, spearmint
farnesol	chamomile, lemongrass
geraniol	basil, coriander, lemongrass, rosemary
β-ionone	black and green tea, passionflower
limonene	caraway, citrus peel, cardamom, celery seed, coriander, dill, fennel
menthol	peppermint
perillyl alcohol	cherries, spearmint
thymol	thyme, oregano

A number of herbs are cardio-protective. Flaxseed, which is rich in soluble fiber and phytosterols, and fenugreek, which is rich in soluble fiber and saponins, are both reported to lower blood cholesterol levels.[142,164] Cholesterol levels can also be lowered by the regular use of lemon grass oil, a flavoring used in Oriental cooking that is rich in the terpenoids geraniol and farnesol.[165] The catechins, especially epigallocatechin gallate in green tea, and the theaflavins in black tea, are more potent than vitamin E in protecting LDL from oxidation, and hence have a role in ameliorating atherosclerosis.[166] Glabrin, an isoflavan in licorice root, and the proanthocyanidins in grape seed extract, also significantly protect

LDL against lipid oxidation.[167,168] The diterpene dialdehydes in ginger are known to exhibit a strong inhibitory effect on platelet aggregation.[169] The flavonoids and proanthocyanidins in hawthorn and the terpenoids and flavonoids in ginkgo are reported to improve blood flow in cases of impaired circulation.[170,171]

A. The Value of Onions and Garlic

Onion extracts are useful in the treatment of asthma and bronchitis because they produce a decrease in bronchial spasms.[172] Administration of an onion extract was found to decrease allergy-induced bronchial constriction in asthma patients.[173] Studies in India found low blood triglyceride levels associated with the regular consumption of onions and garlic.[174] Onions are natural anti-clotting agents, as they possess substances with fibrinolytic activity and can suppress platelet clumping.[175-177] Onion extracts provide protection against tumor growth.[178] Studies in Greece have shown a high consumption of onions, garlic, and other alliums to be protective against stomach cancer.[11] Elderly Dutch men and women with the highest onion consumption (at least one-half onion/day), had half the level of cancer in the noncardia section of the stomach, compared with those consuming no onions at all.[10] A Chinese study found chives had a strong protective effect against colorectal cancer.[179]

Garlic has broad-spectrum antibiotic activity inhibiting a variety of microorganisms, including bacteria (*Staphylococcus, Streptococcus, Salmonella, Vibrio cholerae*), molds and yeasts (*Candida albicans*), viruses (influenza and Herpes), and parasites. In China, cases of cryptococcal meningitis have been successfully treated with garlic extracts. Whole cloves of garlic (*Allium sativum*) contain 0.8% (by fresh weight) of an odorless sulfur compound called alliin (S-allyl-L-cysteine sulfoxide). When a clove is cut or crushed, the enzyme alliinase breaks alliin down to produce allicin (diallyl thiosulfinate), a substance with a strong odor that has powerful antimicrobial properties.[180] Allicin produces a variety of sulfides (such as diallyl trisulfide and diallyl disulfide) when heated in water or steam. When heated in vegetable oil, allicin produces 1,3- and 1,2-vinyldithiins and ajoenes.[180]

The *Allium* spp. are all characterized by a rich content of thiosulfinates, sulfides, polysulfides, mercaptans, and other odoriferous sulfur compounds. The sulfur content of garlic is 3.3 mg/g fresh weight, four times the level in onions.[180] The various *Allium* spp. are characterized by different types of alkyl groups in the thiosulfinate compounds. The *n*-propyl group is the major alkyl group in chives, scallions, shallots, and leeks, but is absent in garlic.[181] While all the *Allium* contain the 1-propenyl group, it is the dominant group only in onions. Garlic has mostly allyl groups and some methyl groups.

B. Protection against Heart Disease

Studies have shown the beneficial value of garlic in reducing the risk of heart attacks and strokes.[174,175,182] Regular use of garlic can lower total cholesterol, LDL cholesterol, and triglyceride levels and possibly raise HDL cholesterol levels.[176,183] A meta-analysis revealed that, on average, one-half to one clove of garlic per day reduced hypercholesterolemia by about 25 mg/dl (0.65 mmol/L), or 9% of the initial value.[183] Garlic also lowers blood pressure levels, due to its vasodilator properties. The results of a meta-analysis suggested that garlic might be useful for patients with mild hypertension.[184] In addition, garlic inhibits platelet clumping, along with decreasing fibrinogen levels.[175,185] A daily ingestion of 3 g of garlic (one clove) for 6 months resulted in an 80% decrease in serum thromboxane B_2, as well as a 20% decrease in coronary heart disease in middle-aged men.[186] Garlic also has mild hypoglycemic effects, especially in patients with diabetes.[175,182]

The antithrombotic properties are due to the presence of ajoenes, allyl methyl trisulfide and vinyldithiins, which are produced from the breakdown of allicin. Garlic and onions contain various sulfur compounds, such as the disulfides that may lower blood cholesterol and triglyceride levels and blood pressure levels.[173,175,176] In animal models, garlic causes both direct antiatherogenic effects and regression. Garlic's direct effect on atherosclerosis may be explained by its capacity to reduce the lipid content in arterial cells and to prevent intracellular lipid accumulation.[187] In a double-blind, placebo-controlled clinical study in the elderly, the intake of high-dose garlic powder significantly reduced the increase in atherosclerotic plaque volume by as much as 18% and even effected a slight regression over a 4-year period.[188]

However, not all garlic preparations are effective. Recently, a steam-distilled garlic oil preparation was found to be inactive when fed for 3 months to hypercholesterolemic patients.[189] Enteric-coated pills, which dissolve in the intestinal tract, cut down on odor problems and improve the absorption of allicin, the key ingredient. Garlic powders represent the composition of garlic cloves better than any other processed garlic. Aged garlic extract (Kyolic), which is prepared by storing sliced garlic in 15–20% alcohol for 20 months, has lower amounts of sulfur and lacks allicin. Its chief sulfur substance is S-allyl cysteine.[180] Clinical studies regarding cardiovascular effects of aged garlic extract have been less conclusive than those with fresh garlic and garlic powder products. Aged garlic extract requires 5–6 months to lower blood lipids in some studies, while garlic cloves and standardized garlic powder show significant decreases after 1–2 months.[180] Sulfur compounds, other than from the breakdown of allicin, also contribute to the various therapeutic effects of garlic.

C. Protection against Cancer

Various studies show that garlic can reduce the development of bladder, skin, stomach, prostate, and colon cancer.[190-193] Risk of prostate cancer is reduced 44% in those using garlic two or more times/week.[194] In China, persons in the highest quartile of intake of garlic, onions, and other *Allium* vegetables had a risk of stomach cancer that was 40% lower than those in the lowest quartile of intake.[195] In the Iowa Women's Health Study, the consumption of garlic was associated with a 32% reduced risk of colon cancer for the uppermost vs. lowermost quartile of intake.[196] The sensitivity of the bacterium *Helicobacter pylori* to low levels of garlic may be related to the low risk of stomach cancer in those people with a high *Allium* vegetable intake.[197]

The anti-tumor properties of garlic are reported to be due to its rich content of organic sulfides, disulfides (such as diallyl disulfide), and trisulfides.[190,198] Components of garlic inhibit the activity of cancer-causing substances during both the initiation and promotion phases of cancer.[191] Tumor inhibition by garlic seems to be most effective when the tumor size is small. Garlic is reported to stimulate the immune system, even in AIDS patients;[199] enhance the activity of the lymphocytes and macrophages to destroy cancer cells; and disrupt the metabolism of tumor cells.[192] Ajoene, a major compound in garlic, induces apoptosis in human leukemic cells in a dose- and time-dependent fashion, possibly via the stimulation of peroxide production and the activation of nuclear factor kappa-B.[200] More research is needed to actually determine the quantity of garlic needed to minimize cancer risk.

Garlic oil also contains terpenoids, such as p-cymene and limonene, which have cancer preventive properties.[173] Garlic contains 0.2 ppm of selenium. The selenium level of garlic can be increased 2,500-fold by growing the garlic in selenium-enriched soils.[180] Diallyl selenide, in the selenium-enriched garlic, is 300 times more active in tumor inhibition than diallyl sulfide.[201] The formation of nitrosamines, potent carcinogens, are also inhibited by garlic.[198] Both onion and garlic contain health promoting compounds such as fructo-oligosaccharides, flavonoids, phenolic acids, tannins, phytosterols, and saponins, which protect against chronic diseases.[173,180]

VII. CONCLUSION

To maintain good health, a regular intake of plant foods is essential. The health benefits associated with plant foods goes far beyond their vitamin, mineral, and fiber content. Vegetables, fruits, whole grains, nuts, legumes, and herbs all contain a variety of phytochemicals (such as carotenoids, polyphenolics, terpenoids, phytosterols, and sulfides) that decrease the risk of cancer, cardiovascular disease, and other diseases.[2] Research efforts continue in an attempt to discover and understand the different mechanisms by which phytochemicals exert their health-promoting properties. It is known that some of the phytochemicals act synergistically to exert health benefits.[202] Are the phytochemicals destroyed by cooking? Most of the compounds are heat stable and are not significantly lost in the cooking water. The availability of carotenoids and the level of indoles in broccoli may actually be increased during cooking.[203] Lycopene, for example, is more available from processed tomatoes than from raw.[41]

The regular consumption of antioxidant-rich plant foods is positively associated with a wide spectrum of health benefits. However, for the best protection against disease, whole foods should be consumed, rather than phytochemical supplements.[204] The safety and health benefits of consuming concentrated extracts of fruits and vegetables that contain very high levels of phytochemicals is unknown and unwarranted at this time.

REFERENCES

1. Beecher, G.R. Phytonutrients' role in metabolism: effects on resistance to degenerative processes. *Nutr. Rev.*, 57: S3, 1999.
2. Bloch, A. and Thomson, C.A. Position of The American Dietetic Association: phytochemicals and functional foods. *J. Am. Diet. Assoc.*, 95: 493, 1995.
3. *Food, Nutrition and the Prevention of Cancer: a Global Perspective*, World Cancer Research Fund/American Institute for Cancer Research, Washington D.C., 1997.
4. Steinmetz, K.A. and Potter, J.D. Vegetables, fruit, and cancer. I. Epidemiology. *Cancer Causes Control*, 2: 325, 1991.
5. Ziegler, R.G. Vegetables, fruits, and carotenoids and the risk of cancer. *Am. J. Clin. Nutr.*, 53: 251S, 1991.
6. Lu, S.H., Camus, A.M., Tomatis, L., and Bartsch, H. Mutagenicity of extracts of pickled vegetables collected in Linhsien County, a high-incidence area for esophageal cancer in Northern China. *J. Natl. Cancer Inst.*, 66: 33, 1981.
7. Tavani, A. and La Vecchia, C. Fruit and vegetable consumption and cancer risk in a Mediterranean population. *Am. J. Clin. Nutr.*, 61: 1374S, 1995.
8. Freudenheim, J.L., Marshall, J.R., Vena, J.E., Laughlin, R., Brasure, J.R., Swanson, M.K., Nemoto, T., and Graham, S. Premenopausal breast cancer risk and intake of vegetables, fruits, and related nutrients. *J. Natl. Cancer Inst.*, 88: 340, 1996.

9. Trichopoulou, A., Katsouyanni, K., Stuver, S., Tzala, L., Gnardellis, C., Rimm, E., and Trichopoulos, D. Consumption of olive oil and specific food groups in relation to breast cancer risk in Greece. *J. Natl. Cancer Inst.*, 87: 110, 1995.

10. Dorant, E., van den Brandt, P.A., Goldbohm, R.A., and Sturmans, F. Consumption of onions and a reduced risk of stomach carcinoma. *Gastroenterology*, 110: 12, 1996.

11. Steinmetz, K.A. and Potter, J.D. Vegetables, fruit, and cancer. II. Mechanisms. *Cancer Causes Control*, 2: 427, 1991.

12. Giovannucci, E., Ascherio, A., Rimm, E.B., Stampfer, M.J., Colditz, G.A., and Willett, W.C. Intake of carotenoids and retinol in relation to risk of prostate cancer. *J. Natl. Cancer Inst.*, 87: 1767, 1995.

13. Law, M.R. and Morris, J.K. By how much does fruit and vegetable consumption reduce the risk of ischaemic heart disease? *Eur. J. Clin. Nutr.*, 52: 549, 1998.

14. Ness, A.R. and Powles, J.W. Fruit and vegetables, and cardiovascular disease: a review. *Int. J. Epidemiol.*, 26: 1, 1997.

15. Key, T.J., Thorogood, M., Appleby, P.N., and Burr, M.L. Dietary habits and mortality in 11,000 vegetarians and health conscious people: results of a 17 year follow up. *BMJ*, 313: 775, 1996.

16. Joshipura, K.J., Acherio, A., Manson, J.E., Stampfer, M.J., Rimm, E.B., Speizer, F.E., Hennekens, C.H., Spiegelman, D., and Willett, W.C. Fruit and vegetable intake in relation to risk of ischemic stroke. *JAMA.*, 282: 1233, 1999.

17. Diet, nutrition and the prevention of chronic diseases. A report of the WHO study on diet, nutrition and prevention of noncommunicable diseases. *Nutr. Rev.*, 49: 291, 1991.

18. Patterson, B.H., Block, G., Rosenberger, W.F., Pee, D., and Kahle, L.L. Fruit and vegetables in the American diet: data from the NHANES II survey. *Am. J. Public Health*, 80: 1443, 1990.

19. Subar, A.S., Heimendinger, J., Krebs-Smith, S.M. 5 A Day for Better Health: a Baseline Study of Americans' Fruit and Vegetable Consumption. National Cancer Institute, NIH, Rockville, MD, 1991.

20. Caragay, A.B. Cancer-preventive foods and ingredients. *Food Tech.*, 46: 65, 1992.

21. Craig, W.J. *Nutrition and Wellness. A Vegetarian Way to Better Health*, Golden Harvest Books, Berrien Springs, MI, 1999.

22. Michnovicz, J.J. and Bradlow, H.L. Dietary cytochrome P-450 modifiers in the control of estrogen metabolism. In: *Food Phytochemicals for Cancer Prevention I. Fruits and Vegetables* (Eds. Huang, M.J., Osawa, T., Ho, C.T. & Rosen, R.T.), American Chemical Society, Washington, D.C., 1994, 282.

23. Smith, T.J. and Yang, C.S. Effects of food phytochemicals or xenobiotic metabolism. In: *Food Phytochemicals for Cancer Prevention I. Fruits and Vegetables* (Eds. Huang, M.J., Osawa, T., Ho, C.T. & Rosen, R.T.), American Chemical Society, Washington, D.C., 1994, 17.

24. Decker, E.A. The role of phenolics, conjugated linoleic acid, carnosine, and pyrroloquinoline quinone as nonessential dietary antioxidants. *Nutr. Rev.*, 53: 49, 1995.

25. Kohlmeier, L. and Hastings, S.B. Epidemiologic evidence of a role of carotenoids in cardiovascular disease prevention. *Am. J. Clin. Nutr.*, 62: 1370S, 1995.

26. Craig, W.J. Health-promoting properties of common herbs. *Am. J. Clin. Nutr.*, 70: 491S, 1999.

27. Hecht, S.S. Chemoprevention of cancer by isothiocyanates, modifiers of carcinogen metabolism. *J. Nutr.*, 129: 768S, 1999.

28. Lampe, J.W. Health effects of vegetables and fruit: assessing mechanisms of action in human experimental studies. *Am. J. Clin. Nutr.*, 70: 475S, 1999.

29. Nestle, M. Broccoli sprouts in cancer prevention. *Nutr. Rev.*, 56: 127, 1998.

30. Attaway, J.A. Citrus juice flavonoids with anticarcinogenic and antitumor properties. In: *Food Phytochemicals for Cancer Prevention I. Fruits and Vegetables* (Eds. Huang, M.-J., Osawa, T., Ho, C.-T. & Rosen, R.T.), American Chemical Society, Washington D.C., 1994, 240.

31. Lam, L.K.T., Zhang, J., Hasegawa, S., and Schut, H.A.J. Inhibition of chemically induced carcinogenesis by citrus liminoids. In: *Food Phytochemicals for Cancer Prevention I. Fruits and Vegetables* (Eds. Huang, M.-J., Osawa, T., Ho, C.-T. & Rosen, R.T.), American Chemical Society, Washington, D.C., 1994, 209.

32. Abou-Issa, H., Moeschberger, M., el-Masry, W., Tejwani, S., Curley, R.W., Jr., and Webb, T.E. Relative efficacy of glucarate on the initiation and promotion phases of rat mammary carcinogenesis. *Anticancer Res.*, 15: 805, 1995.

33. D-Limonene, an anticarcinogenic terpene. *Nutr. Rev.*, 46: 363, 1988.

34. Mangels, A.R., Holden, J.M., Beecher, G.R., Forman, M.R., and Lanza, E. Carotenoid content of fruits and vegetables: an evaluation of analytic data. *J. Am. Diet. Assoc.*, 93: 284, 1993.

35. Shekelle, R.B., Lepper, M., Liu, S., Maliza, C., Raynor, W.J., Jr., Rossof, A.H., Paul, O., Shryock, A.M., and Stamler, J. Dietary vitamin A and risk of cancer in the Western Electric study. *Lancet*, 2: 1185, 1981.

36. van Poppel, G. and Goldbohm, R.A. Epidemiologic evidence for beta-carotene and cancer prevention. *Am. J. Clin. Nutr.*, 62: 1393S, 1995.

37. Riso, P., Pinder, A., Santangelo, A., and Porrini, M. Does tomato consumption effectively increase the resistance of lymphocyte DNA to oxidative damage? *Am. J. Clin. Nutr.*, 69: 712, 1999.

38. Mills, P.K., Beeson, W.L., Phillips, R.L., and Fraser, G.E. Cohort study of diet, lifestyle, and prostate cancer in Adventist men. *Cancer*, 64: 598, 1989.

39. Dorgan, J.F., Sowell, A., Swanson, C.A., Potischman, N., Miller, R., Schussler, N., and Stephenson, H.E., Jr. Relationships of serum carotenoids, retinol, alpha-tocopherol, and selenium with breast cancer risk: results from a prospective study in Columbia, Missouri (United States). *Cancer Causes Control*, 9: 89, 1998.

40. Kantesky, P.A., Gammon, M.D., Mandelblatt, J., Zhang, Z.F., Ramsey, E., Dnistrian, A., Norkus, E.P., and Wright, T.C., Jr. Dietary intake and blood levels of lycopene: association with cervical dysplasia among non-Hispanic, black women. *Nutr. Cancer.*, 31: 31, 1998.

41. Role of lycopene as antioxidant carotenoid in the prevention of chronic disease: a review. *Nutr. Res.*, 19: 305, 1999.

42. Morris, D.L., Kritchevsky, S.B., and Davis, C.E. Serum carotenoids and coronary heart disease. The Lipid Research Clinics Coronary Primary Prevention Trial and Follow-up Study. *JAMA*, 272: 1439, 1994.

43. Clinton, S.K. Lycopene: chemistry, biology, and implications for human health and disease. *Nutr. Rev.*, 56: 35, 1998.

44. Fuhrman, B., Elis, A., and Aviram, M. Hypocholesterolemic effect of lycopene and beta-carotene is related to suppression of cholesterol synthesis and augmentation of LDL receptor activity in macrophages. *Biochem. Biophys. Res. Commun.*, 233: 658, 1997.

45. Seddon, J.M., Ajani, A.U., Sperduto, R.D., Hiller, R., Blair, N., Burton, T.C., Farber, M.D., Gragoudas, E.J., Haller, J., Miller, D.T., Yannuzzi, L.A., and Willett, W. Dietary carotenoids, vitamins A, C, and E, and advanced age-related macular degeneration. Eye disease case-control study group. *JAMA*, 272: 1413, 1994.

46. Bendich, A. A Role for carotenoids in immune function. *Clin. Nutr.*, 7: 113, 1988.

47. Chasan-Taber, L., Willett, W.C., Seddon, J.M., Stampfer, M.J., Rosner, B., Colditz, G.A., Speizer, F.E., and Hankinson, S.E. A prospective study of carotenoid and vitamin A intakes and risk of cataract extraction in U.S. women. *Am. J. Clin. Nutr.*, 70: 509, 1999.

48. Brown, L., Rimm, E.B., Seddon, J.M., Giovannucci, E.L., Chasan-Taber, L., Spiegelman, D., Willett, W.C., and Hankinson, S.E. A prospective study of carotenoid intake and risk of cataract extraction in U.S. men. *Am. J. Clin. Nutr.*, 70: 517, 1999.

49. Bravo, L. Polyphenols: chemistry, dietary sources, metabolism, and nutritional significance. *Nutr. Rev.*, 56: 317, 1998.

50. Manach, C. Bioavailability, metabolism and physiological impact of 4-oxo-flavonoids. *Nutr. Res.*, 16: 517, 1996.

51. Hertog, M.G., Kromhout, D., Aravanis, C., Blackburn, H., Buzina, R., Fidanza, F., Giampaoli, S., Jansen, A., Menotti, A., Nedeljkovic, S., Pekkarinen, M., Simic, B.S., Toshima, H., Feskens, E.J.M., Hollman, P.C.H., and Katan, M.B. Flavonoid intake and long-term risk of coronary heart disease and cancer in the Seven Countries Study. *Arch. Intern. Med.*, 155: 381, 1995.

52. Hertog, M.G.L., Feskens, E.J.M., Hollman, P.C.H., Katan, M.B., and Kromhout, D. Dietary antioxidant flavonoids and risk of coronary heart disease. *Lancet*, 342: 1007, 1993.

53. Keli, S.O., Hertog, M.G., Feskens, E.J., and Kromhout, D. Dietary flavonoids, antioxidant vitamins, and incidence of stroke: the Zutphen Study. *Arch. Intern. Med.*, 156: 637, 1996.

54. Folts, J.D. Antithrombic potential of grape juice and red wine for preventing heart attacks. *Pharmaceut. Biol.*, 36: 21, 1998.

55. Frankel, E.N. and Meyer, A.S. Antioxidants in grapes and grape juices and their potential health effects. *Pharmaceut. Biol.*, 36 (suppl): 14, 1998.

56. Ghiselli, A., Nardini, M., Baldi, A., and Scaccini, C. Antioxidant activity of different phenolic fractions separated from an Italian wine. *J. Agric. Food Chem.*, 46: 361, 1998.

57. Balentine, D.A., Albano, M.C., and Nair, M.G. Role of medicinal plants, herbs, and spices in protecting human health. *Nutr. Rev.*, 57: S41, 1999.

58. Linn, S., Carroll, M., Johnson, C., Fulwood, R., Kalsbeek, W., and Briefel, R. High-density lipoprotein cholesterol and alcohol consumption in U.S. white and black adults: data from NHANES II. *Am. J. Public Health*, 83: 811, 1993.

59. Pace-Asciak, C.R., Hahn, S., Diamandis, E.P., Soleas, G., and Goldberg, D.M. The red wine phenolics trans-resveratrol and quercetin block human platelet aggregation and eicosanoid synthesis: implications for protection against coronary heart disease. *Clin. Chim. Acta.*, 235: 207, 1995.

60. Demrow, H.S., Slane, P.R., and Folts, J.D. Administration of wine and grape juice inhibits in vivo platelet activity and thrombosis in stenosed canine coronary arteries. *Circulation*, 91: 1182, 1995.

61. Frankel, E.N., Kanner, J., German, J.B., Parks, E., and Kinsella, J.E. Inhibition of oxidation of human low-density lipoprotein by phenolic substances in red wine. *Lancet*, 341: 454, 1993.

62. Inhibition of LDL Oxidation by phenolic substances in red wine: a clue to the French paradox. *Nutr. Rev.*, 51: 185, 1993.

63. Vinson, J.A. and Hontz, B.A. Phenol antioxidant index: Comparative antioxidant effectiveness of red and white wines. *J. Agric. Food Chem.*, 43: 401, 1995.

64. Kanner, J., Frankel, E., Granit, R., German, B., and Kinsella, J.E. Natural antioxidants in grapes and wines. *J. Agric. Food Chem.*, 42: 64, 1994.

65. Mazur, W. Phytoestrogen content in foods. *Baillieres Clin. Endocrinol. Metab.*, 12: 729, 1998.

66. Subbaramaiah, K., Michaluart, P., Chung, W.J., and Dannenberg, A.J. Resveratrol inhibits the expression of cyclooxygenase-2 in human mammary and oral epithelial cells. *Pharmaceut. Biol.*, 36: 35, 1998.

67. Chen, S., Sun, X-Z., Kao, Y-C., Kwon A., Zhou, D., and Eng, E. Suppression of breast cancer cell growth with grape juice. *Pharmaceut. Biol.*, 36 (suppl): 53, 1998.

68. Elson, C.E. and Yu, S.G. The chemoprevention of cancer by mevalonate-derived constituents of fruits and vegetables. *J. Nutr.*, 124: 607, 1994.

69. Pearce, B.C., Parker, R.A., Deason, M.E., Qureshi, A.A., and Wright, J.J. Hypocholesterolemic activity of synthetic and natural tocotrienols. *J. Med. Chem.*, 35: 3595, 1992.

70. Yu, S.G., Abuirmeilah, N.M., Quershi, A.A., and Elson, C.E. Dietary beta-ionone suppresses hepatic 3-hydroxy-3-methylglutaryl coenzyme A reductase activity. *J. Agric. Food Chem.*, 42: 1493, 1994.

71. Narayanan, B.A., Geoffroy, O., Willingham, M.C., Re, G.G., and Nixon, D.W. p53/p21(WAF1/CIP1) expression and its possible role in G1 arrest and apoptosis in ellagic acid treated cancer cells. *Cancer Lett.*, 136: 215, 1999.

72. Moshfegh, A.J., Friday, J.E., Goldman, J.P., and Ahuja, J.K. Presence of inulin and oligofructose in the diets of Americans. *J. Nutr.*, 129: 1407S, 1999.

73. Niness, K.R. Inulin and oligofructose: what are they? *J. Nutr.*, 129: 1402S, 1999.

74. Simpson, H.C., Simpson, R.W., Lousley, S., Carter, R.D., Geekie, M., Hockaday, T.D., and Mann, J.I. A high carbohydrate leguminous fibre diet improves all aspects of diabetic control. *Lancet*, 1: 1, 1981.

75. Jenkins, D.J., Wong, G.S., Patten, R., Bird, J., Hall, M., Buckley, G.C., McGuire, V., Reichert, R., and Little, J.A. Leguminous seeds in the dietary management of hyperlipidemia. *Am. J. Clin. Nutr.*, 38: 567, 1983.

76. Anderson, J.W., Smith, B.M., and Washnock, C.S. Cardiovascular and renal benefits of dry bean and soybean intake. *Am. J. Clin. Nutr.*, 70: 464S, 1999.

77. Potter, S.M. Overview of proposed mechanisms for the hypocholesterolemic effect of soy. *J. Nutr.*, 125: 606S, 1995.

78. Kennedy, A.R. The evidence for soybean products as cancer preventive agents. *J. Nutr.*, 125: 733S, 1995.

79. Tsuda Kohshima, T., Kawakishi, S., and Osawa, T. Antioxidative pigments isolated from the seed of Phaseolus vulgaris L. *J. Agric. Food Chem.*, 42: 248, 1994.

80. Song, T., Barua, K., Buseman, G., and Murphy, P.A. Soy isoflavone analysis: quality control and a new internal standard. *Am. J. Clin. Nutr.*, 68: 1474S, 1998.

81. Coward, L., Smith, M., Kirk, M., and Barnes, S. Chemical modification of isoflavones in soyfoods during cooking and processing. *Am. J. Clin. Nutr.*, 68: 1486S, 1998.

82. Setchell, K.D.R. Phytoestrogens: Biochemistry, physiology, and implications for human health of soy isoflavones. *Am. J. Clin. Nutr.*, 68: 1333S, 1998.

83. Anderson, J.J.B. and Garner, S.C. Phytoestrogens and human function. *Nutr. Today*, 32: 232, 1998.

84. Potter, S.M., Baum, J.A., Teng, H., Stillman, R.J., Shay, N.F., and Erdman, J.W., Jr. Soy protein and isoflavones: their effects on blood lipids and bone density in postmenopausal women. *Am. J. Clin. Nutr.*, 68: 1375S, 1998.

85. USDA Nutrient Database for Standard Reference, Release 13. Nutrient Data Laboratory Home Page. (U.S. Department of Agriculture, Agricultural Research Service, 1999).

86. Potter, S.M., Bakhit, R.M., Essex-Sorlie, D.L., Weingartner, K.E., Chapman, K.M., Nelson, R.A., Prabhudesai, M., Savage, W.D., Nelson, A.I., Winter, L.W., and Erdman Jr., J.W. Depression of plasma cholesterol in men by consumption of baked products containing soy protein. *Am. J. Clin. Nutr.*, 58: 501, 1993.

87. Carroll, K.K. Review of clinical studies on cholesterol lowering response to soy protein. *J. Am. Diet. Assoc.*, 91: 820, 1991.

88. Crouse, J.R., Morgan, T., Terry, J.G., Ellis, J., Vitolins, M., and Burke, G.L. A randomized trial comparing the effect of casein with that of soy protein containing varying amounts of isoflavones on plasma concentrations of lipids and lipoproteins. *Arch. Intern. Med.*, 159: 2070, 1999.

89. Nilausen, K. and Meinertz, H. Variable lipemic response to dietary soy protein in healthy, normolipemic men. *Am. J. Clin. Nutr.*, 68: 1380S, 1998.

90. Anderson, J., Johnstone, B.M., and Cook-Newell, M.E. Meta-analysis of the effects of soy protein intake on serum lipids. *N. Engl. J. Med.*, 333: 276, 1995.

91. Potter, S.M. Soy protein and cardiovascular disease: the impact of bioactive components in soy. *Nutr. Rev.*, 56: 231, 1998.

92. Moghadasian, M.H. and Frohlich, J.J. Effects of dietary phytosterols on cholesterol metabolism and atherosclerosis: clinical and experimental evidence. *Am. J. Med.*, 107: 588, 1999.

93. Anthony, M.S., Clarkson, T.B., and Williams, J.K. Effects of soy isoflavones on atherosclerosis: potential mechanisms. *Am. J. Clin. Nutr.*, 68: 1390S, 1998.

94. Nestel, P.J., Yamashita, T., Sasahara, T., Pomeroy, S., Dart, A., Komesaroff, P., Owen, A., and Abbey, M. Soy isoflavones improve systemic arterial compliance but not plasma lipids in menopausal and perimenopausal women. *Arterioscler. Thromb. Vasc. Biol.*, 17: 3392, 1997.

95. Messina, M.J., Persky, V., Setchell, K.D., and Barnes, S. Soy intake and cancer risk: a review of the in vitro and in vivo data. *Nutr. Cancer.*, 21: 113, 1994.

96. Goodman, M.T., Wilkens, L.R., Hankin, J.H., Lyu, L.C., Wu, A.H., and Kolonel, L.N. Association of soy and fiber consumption with the risk of endometrial cancer. *Am. J. Epidemiol.*, 146: 294, 1997.

97. Severson, R.K., Nomura, A.M., Grove, J.S., and Stemmermann, G.N. A prospective study of demographics, diet, and prostate cancer among men of Japanese ancestry in Hawaii. *Cancer Res.*, 49: 1857, 1989.

98. Jacobsen, B.K., Knutsen, S.F., and Fraser, G.E. Does high soy milk intake reduce prostate cancer incidence? The Adventist Health Study (United States). *Cancer Causes Control,* 9: 553, 1998.

99. Cassidy, A., Bingham, S., and Setchell, K.D. Biological effects of a diet of soy protein rich in isoflavones on the menstrual cycle of premenopausal women. *Am. J. Clin. Nutr.*, 6: 333, 1994.

100. Kim, H., Peterson, T.G., and Barnes, S. Mechanisms of action of the soy isoflavone genistein: emerging role for its effects via transforming growth factor beta signaling pathways. *Am. J. Clin. Nutr.*, 68: 1418S, 1998.

101. Herman, C., Adlercreutz, T., Goldin, B.R., Gorbach, S.L., Hockerstedt, K.A.V., Watanabe, S., Hamalainen, E.K., Markkanen, M.H., Makela, T.H., Wahala, K.T., Hase, T.A., and Fotsis, T. Soybean phytoestrogen intake and cancer risk. *J. Nutr.*, 125: 757S, 1995.

102. Messina, M. and Messina, V. Increasing use of soyfoods and their potential role in cancer prevention. *J. Am. Diet. Assoc.*, 91: 836, 1991.

103. Mazur, W.M., Duke, J.A., Wahala, K., Rasku, S., and Adlercreutz, H. Isoflavonoids and lignans in legumes: nutritional and health aspects in humans. *J. Nutr. Biochem.*, 9: 193, 1998.

104. Murkies, A.L., Lombard, C., Strauss, B.J., Wilcox, G., Burger, H.G., and Morton, M.S. Dietary flour supplementation decreases post-menopausal hot flushes: effect of soy and wheat. *Maturitas,* 21: 189, 1995.

105. Albertazzi, P., Pansini, F., Bonaccorsi, G., Zanotti, L., Forini, E., and De Aloysio, D. The effect of dietary soy supplementation on hot flushes. *Obstet. Gynecol.*, 91: 6, 1998.

106. Brandi, M.L. New treatment strategies: ipriflavone, strontium, vitamin D metabolites and analogs. *Am. J. Med.*, 95: 69S, 1993.

107. Slavin, J., Jacobs, D., and Marquart, L. Whole-grain consumption and chronic disease: protective mechanisms. *Nutr. Cancer.*, 27: 14, 1997.

108. Slavin, J.L., Martini, M.C., Jacobs Jr, D.R., and Marquart, L. Plausible mechanisms for the protectiveness of whole grains. *Am. J. Clin. Nutr.*, 70(suppl): 459S, 1999.

109. Jacobs, D.R., Jr., Marquart, L., Slavin, J., and Kushi, L.H. Whole-grain intake and cancer: an expanded review and meta-analysis. *Nutr. Cancer.*, 30: 85, 1998.

110. Chatenoud, L., La Vecchia, C., Franceschi, S., Tavani, A., Jacobs Jr, D.R., Parpinel, M.T., Soler, M., and Negri, E. Refined-cereal intake and risk of selected cancers in Italy. *Am. J. Clin. Nutr.,* 70: 1107, 1999.

111. Liu, S., Stampfer, M.J., Hu, F.B., Giovannucci, E., Rimm, E., Manson, J.E., Hennekens, C.H., and Willett, W.C. Whole-grain consumption and risk of coronary heart disease: results from the Nurses' Health Study. *Am. J. Clin. Nutr.*, 70: 412, 1999.

112. Morris, K.L. and Zemel, M.B. Glycemic index, cardiovascular disease, and obesity. *Nutr. Rev.,* 57: 273, 1999.

113. Salmeron, J., Ascherio, A., Rimm, E.B., Colditz, G.A., Spiegelman, D., Jenkins, D.J., Stampfer, M.J., Wing, A.L., and Willett, W.C. Dietary fiber, glycemic load, and risk of NIDDM in men. *Diabetes Care.*, 20: 545, 1997.

114. Thompson, L.U. Antioxidants and hormone-mediated health benefits of whole grains. *Crit. Rev. Food Sci. Nutr.*, 34: 473, 1994.

115. Sugano, M. and Tsuji, E. Rice bran oil and cholesterol metabolism. *J. Nutr.*, 127: 521S, 1997.

116. Cara, L., Armand, M., Borel, P., Senft, M., Portugal, H., Pauli, A.M., Lafont, H., and Lairon, D. Long-term wheat germ intake beneficially affects plasma lipids and lipoproteins in hypercholesterolemic human subjects. *J. Nutr.*, 122: 317, 1992.

117. Dreher, M.L. The traditional and emerging role of nuts in healthful diets. *Nutr. Rev.*, 54: 241, 1996.
118. Fraser, G.E., Sabate, J., Beeson, W.L., and Strahan, T.M. A possible protective effect of nut consumption on risk of coronary heart disease. The Adventist Health Study. *Arch. Intern. Med.*, 152: 1416, 1992.
119. Fraser, G.E., Sumbureru, D., Pribis, P., Neil, R.L., and Frankson, M.A. Association among health habits, risk factors, and all-cause mortality in a black California population. *Epidemiology*, 8: 168, 1997.
120. Prineas, R.J., Kushi, L.H., Folsom, A.R., Bostick, R.M., and Wu, Y. Walnuts and serum lipids. *N. Engl. J. Med.*, 329: 359, 1993.
121. Hu, F.B., Stampfer, M.J., Manson, J.E., Rimm, E.B., Colditz, G.A., Rosner, B.A., Speizer, F.E., Hennekens, C.H., and Willett, W.C. Frequent nut consumption and risk of coronary heart disease in women: prospective cohort study. *BMJ*, 317: 1341, 1998.
122. Sabaté, J., Fraser, G.E., Burke, K., Knutsen, S.F., Bennett, H., and Lindsted, K.D. Effects of walnuts on serum lipid levels and blood pressure in normal men. *N. Engl. J. Med.*, 328: 603, 1993.
123. Kris-Etherton, P.M., Pearson, T.A., Wan, Y., Hargrove, R.L., Moriarty, K., Fishell, V., and Etherton, T.D. High-monounsaturated fatty acid diets lower plasma cholesterol and triacylglycerol concentrations. *Am. J. Clin. Nutr.*, 70: 1009, 1999.
124. Spiller, G.A., Jenkins, D.J., Cragen, L.N., Gates, J.E., Bosello, O., Berra, K., Rudd, C., Stevenson, M., and Superko, R. Effect of a diet high in monounsaturated fat from almonds on plasma cholesterol and lipoproteins. *J. Am. Coll. Nutr.*, 11: 126, 1992.
125. Spiller, G.A., Jenkins, D.A., Bosello, O., Gates, J.E., Cragen, L.N., and Bruce, B. Nuts and plasma lipids: an almond-based diet lowers LDL-C while preserving HDL-C. *J. Am. Coll. Nutr.*, 17: 285, 1998.
126. Morgan, W.A. and Clayshulte, B.J. Pecans lower LDL-cholesterol in normolipidemic individuals. *J. Am. Diet. Assoc.*, 98S: A82, 1998.
127. Turnbull, W.H. and Edwards, R.C. Walnuts and hazelnuts lower blood lipids [abstract]. *FASEB J*, 12: A507, 1998.
128. Curb, J.D., Wergowski, G., Abbott, R.D., Dobbs, J.C., Tung, J., Austin, M.A., and Marcovina, S. High monounsaturated fat macadamia nut diets: effects on serum lipids and lipoproteins [abstract]. *FASEB J*, 12: A506, 1998.
129. Edwards, K., Kwaw, I., Matud, J., and Kurtz, I. Effect of pistachio nuts on serum lipid levels in patients with moderate hypercholesterolemia. *J. Am. Coll. Nutr.*, 18: 229, 1999.
130. Kris-Etherton, P.M., Yu-Poth, S., Sabate, J., Ratcliffe, H.E., Zhao, G., and Etherton, T.D. Nuts and their bioactive constituents: effects on serum lipids and other factors that affect disease risk. *Am. J. Clin. Nutr.*, 70: 504S, 1999.
131. Farquhar, J.W. Plant Sterols: Their Biological Effects in Humans. In: *Handbook of Lipids in Human Nutrition* (Ed. Spiller, G.A.), CRC, FL, 1996, 101.
132. Relationship between absorption of cholesterol and serum plant sterols. *Nutr. Rev.*, 45: 174, 1987.
133. Nguyen, T.T. The cholesterol-lowering action of plant stanol esters. *J. Nutr.*, 129: 2109, 1999.
134. Jones, P.J. and Ntanios, F. Comparable efficacy of hydrogenated vs. nonhydrogenated plant sterol esters on circulating cholesterol levels in humans. *Nutr. Rev.*, 56: 245, 1998.

135. Rao, A.V. and Sung, M.K. Saponins as anticarcinogens. *J. Nutr.*., 125: 717S, 1995.
136. Amarowicz, R., Shimoyamada, M., and Okubo, K. Hypocholesterolemic effects of saponins. *Rocz Panstw Zakl Hig.*, 45: 125, 1994.
137. Rainey, C. and Nyquist, L. Nuts-nutrition and health benefits of daily use. *Nutr. Today.*, 32: 157, 1997.
138. Harland, B.F. and Oberleas, D. Phytate in foods. *World Rev. Nutr. Diet.*, 52: 235, 1987.
139. Shamsuddin, A.M. Inositol phosphates have novel anticancer function. *J. Nutr.*, 125: 725S, 1995.
140. Chung, K.T., Wong, T.Y., Wei, C.I., Huang, Y.W., and Lin, Y. Tannins and human health: a review. *Crit. Rev. Food Sci. Nutr.*, 38: 421, 1998.
141. Hebert, J.R., Hurley, T.G., Olendzki, B.C., Teas, J., Ma, Y., and Hampl, J.S. Nutritional and socioeconomic factors in relation to prostate cancer mortality: a cross-national study. *J. Natl. Cancer Inst.*, 90: 1637, 1998.
142. Cunnane, S.C., Ganguli, S., Menard, C., Liede, A.C., Hamadeh, M.J., Chen, Z.Y., Wolever, T.M., and Jenkins, D.J. High alpha-linolenic acid flaxseed (Linum usitatissimum): some nutritional properties in humans. *Br. J. Nutr.*, 69: 443, 1993.
143. Thompson, L.U., Robb, P., Serraino, M., and Cheung, F. Mammalian lignan production from various foods. *Nutr. Cancer.*, 16: 43, 1991.
144. Hirano, T., Fukuoka, K., Oka, K., Naito, T., Hosaka, K., Mitsuhashi, H., and Matsumoto, Y. Antiproliferative activity of mammalian lignan derivatives against the human breast carcinoma cell line, ZR-75-1. *Cancer Invest.*, 8: 595, 1990.
145. James, W.P., Duthie, G.G., and Wahle, K.W. The Mediterranean diet: protective or simply non-toxic? *Eur. J. Clin. Nutr.*, 43: 31, 1989.
146. Trichopoulou, A. and Lagiou, P. Healthy traditional Mediterranean diet: an expression of culture, history, and lifestyle. *Nutr. Rev.*, 55: 383, 1997.
147. Trichopoulou, A., Vasilopoulou, E., and Lagiou, A. Mediterranean diet and coronary heart disease: are antioxidants critical? *Nutr. Rev.*, 57: 253, 1999.
148. Kiritsakis, A. and Markakis, P. Olive oil: a review. *Adv. Food Res.*, 31: 453, 1987.
149. Visioli, F. and Galli, C. The effect of minor constituents of olive oil on cardiovascular disease: new findings. *Nutr. Rev.*, 56: 142, 1998.
150. Viola, P. and Audisio, M. Olive Oil and Health. (International Olive Oil Council, Madrid, Spain, 1987).
151. Thompson, L.U. Antinutrients and blood glucose. *Food Tech.*, 42: 123, 1988.
152. Craig, W.J. *The Use and Safety of Common Herbs and Herbal Teas*, Golden Harvest Books, Berrien Spring, MI, 1996.
153. Bruneton, J. *Pharmacognosy, Phytochemistry, Medical Plants*, Lavoisier, Paris, 1995.
154. Zheng, G.Q., Zhang, J., Kenney, P.M., and Lam, L.K.T. Stimulation of glutathione S-transferaxe and inhibition of carcinogenesis in mice by celery seed oil constituents. In: *Food Phytochemicals for Cancer Prevention I. Fruits and Vegetables* (Eds. Huang, M.J., Osawa, T., Ho, C.T. & Rosen, R.T.), American Chemical Society, Washington D.C., 1994, 230.
155. Hasler, C.M. and Blumberg, J.B. Phytochemicals: biochemistry and physiology. Introduction. *J. Nutr.*, 129: 756S, 1999.
156. Stoner, G.D. and Mukhtar, H. Polyphenols as cancer chemopreventive agents. *J. Cell. Biochem. Suppl.*, 22: 169S, 1995.

157. Nakatani, N. Chemistry of antioxidants from Labiatae herbs. In: *Food Phytochemicals for Cancer Prevention I. Fruits and Vegetables* (Eds. Huang, M.J., Osawa, T., Ho, C.T. & Rosen, R.T.), American Chemical Society, Washington, D.C., 1994, 144.

158. Ho, C-T., Ferraro, T., Chen, Q., Rosen, R.T., and Huang, M-T. Phytochemicals in teas and rosemary and their cancer-preventive properties. In: *Food Phytochemicals for Cancer Prevention II. Teas, Spices and Herbs* (Eds. Huang, M.-J., Osawa, T., Ho, C.-T. & Rosen, R.), ACS, Washington D.C., 1994, 2.

159. Kikuzaki, H. and Nakatani, N. Antioxidant effects of some ginger constituents. *J. Food Sci.*, 58: 1407, 1993.

160. Crowell, P.L. Prevention and therapy of cancer by dietary monoterpenes. *J. Nutr.*, 129: 775S, 1999.

161. Zheng, G.Q., Kenney, P.M., and Lam, L.K.T. Potential Anticarcinoenic Natural Products Isolated From Lemongrass Oil and Galanga Root Oil. *J. Agric. Food Chem.*, 41: 153, 1993.

162. Zheng, G.Q., Kenney, P.M., and Lam, L.K.T. Anethofuran, Carvone, and Limonene: Potential Cancer Chemopreventive Agents From Dill Weed Oil and Caraway Oil. *Planta Medica.*, 58: 338, 1992.

163. Zheng, G.Q., Kenney, P.M., Zhang, J., and Lam, L.K. Chemoprevention of benzo[a]pyrene-induced forestomach cancer in mice by natural phthalides from celery seed oil. *Nutr. Cancer,* 19: 77, 1993.

164. Petit, P.R., Sauvaire, Y.D., Hillaire-Buys, D.M., Leconte, O.M., Baissac, Y.G., Ponsin, G.R., and Ribes, G.R. Steroid saponins from fenugreek seeds: extraction, purification, and pharmacological investigation on feeding behavior and plasma cholesterol. *Steroids*, 60: 674, 1995.

165. Elson, C.E., Underbakke, G.L., Hanson, P., Shrago, E., Wainberg, R.H., and Qureshi, A.A. Impact of lemongrass oil, an essential oil, on serum cholesterol. *Lipids*, 24: 677, 1989.

166. Ishikawa, T., Suzukawa, M., Ito, T., Yoshida, H., Ayaori, M., Nishiwaki, M., Yonemura, A., Hara, Y., and Nakamura, H. Effect of tea flavonoid supplementation on the susceptibility of low-density lipoprotein to oxidative modification. *Am. J. Clin. Nutr.*, 66: 261, 1997.

167. Fuhrman, B., Buch, S., Vaya, J., Belinky, P.A., Coleman, R., Hayek, T., and Aviram, M. Licorice extract and its major polyphenol glabridin protect low-density lipoprotein against lipid peroxidation: in vitro and ex vivo studies in humans and in atherosclerotic apolipoprotein E-deficient mice. *Am. J. Clin. Nutr.*, 66: 267, 1997.

168. Nuttall, S.L., Kendall, M.J., Bombardelli, E., and Morazzoni, P. An evaluation of the antioxidant activity of a standardized grape seed extract, Leucoselect. *J. Clin. Pharm. Ther.*, 23: 385, 1998.

169. Kawakishi, S., Morimitsu, Y., and Osawa, T. Chemistry of Ginger Components and Inhibitory Factors of the Arachidonic Acid Cascade. In: *Food Phytochemicals for Cancer Prevention II. Teas, Spices, and Herbs.* (Eds. Ho, C.-T., Osawa, T., Huang, M.-T. & Rosen, R.T.), American Chemical Society, Washington D.C., 1994, 244.

170. Kleijnen, J. and Knipschild, P. Ginkgo biloba for cerebral insufficiency. *Br. J. Clin. Pharmacol.*, 34: 352, 1992.

171. Vibes, J., Lasserre, B., Gleye, J., and Declume, C. Inhibition of thromboxane A2 biosynthesis in vitro by the main components of Crataegus oxyacantha (Hawthorn) flower heads. *Prostaglandins Leukot. Essent. Fatty Acids.*, 50: 173, 1994.

172. Dorsch, W., Wagner, H., Bayer, T., Fessler, B., Hein, G., Ring, J., Scheftner, P., Sieber, W., Strasser, T., and Weiss, E. Anti-asthmatic effects of onions. Alk(en)ylsulfinothioic acid alk(en)yl- esters inhibit histamine release, leukotriene and thromboxane biosynthesis in vitro and counteract PAF and allergen-induced bronchial obstruction in vivo. *Biochem. Pharmacol.*, 37: 4479, 1988.

173. Fleming, T. (Ed.) *PDR for Herbal Medicines*, (Medical Economics Co, Montvale, NJ, 1998).

174. Lau, B.H.S., Adetumbi, M.A., and Sanchez, A. Allium Sativum (garlic) and atherosclerosis: a review. *Nutr. Res.*, 3: 119, 1983.

175. Kendler, B.S. Garlic (Allium sativum) and onion (Allium cepa): a review of their relationship to cardiovascular disease. *Prev. Med.*, 16: 670, 1987.

176. Kleijnen, J., Knipschild, P., and Ter Riet, G. Garlic, onions and cardiovascular risk factors. A review of the evidence from human experiments with emphasis on commercially available preparations. *Br. J. Clin. Pharm.*, 28: 535, 1989.

177. Srivastava, K.C. Onion exerts antiaggregatory effects by altering arachidonic acid metabolism in platelets. *Prostaglandins Leukot. Med.*, 24: 43, 1986.

178. Niukian, K., Schwartz, J., and Shklar, G. In vitro inhibitory effect of onion extract on hamster buccal pouch carcinogenesis. *Nutr. Cancer*, 10: 137, 1987.

179. Hu, J.F., Liu, Y.Y., Yu, Y.K., Zhao, T.Z., Liu, S.D., and Wang, Q.Q. Diet and cancer of the colon and rectum: a case-control study in China. *Int. J. Epidemiol.*, 20: 362, 1991.

180. Koch, H.P. and Lawson, L.D. (Eds.). Garlic. *The Science and Therapeutic Application of Allium sativum L. and Related Species*, Williams and Wilkins, Baltimore, MD, 1996.

181. Block, E. Flavorants from Garlic, Onion, and Other Alliums and their Cancer-Preventive Properties. In: *Food Phytochemicals for Cancer Prevention I. Fruits and Vegetables*, Vol. I (Eds. Huang, M.-J., Osawa, T., Ho, C.-T. & Rosen, R.T.), American Chemical Society, Washington D.C., 1994, 84.

182. Newall, C.A., Anderson, L.A., and Phillipson, J.D. Herbal Medicines. *A Guide for Health-Care Professionals*, The Pharmaceutical Press, London, 1996, 129.

183. Warshfasky, S., Kramer, R.S., and Sivak, S.L. Effect of garlic on total serum cholesterol: a meta-analysis. *Ann. Intern. Med.*, 119: 599, 1993.

184. Silagy, C.A. and Neil, H.A. A meta-analysis of the effect of garlic on blood pressure. *J. Hypertens.*, 12: 463, 1994.

185. Foushee, D.B., Ruffin, J., and Banerjee, U. Garlic as a natural agent for the treatment of hypertension: a preliminary report. *Cytobios.*, 34: 145, 1982.

186. Ali, M. and Thomson, M. Consumption of a garlic clove a day could be beneficial in preventing thrombosis. *Prostaglandins Leukot. Essent. Fatty Acids.*, 53: 211, 1995.

187. Orekhov, A.N. and Grunwald, J. Effects of garlic on atherosclerosis. *Nutrition*, 13: 656, 1997.

188. Koscielny, J., Klussendorf, D., Latza, R., Schmitt, R., Radtke, H., Siegel, G., and Kiesewetter, H. The antiatherosclerotic effect of Allium sativum. *Atherosclerosis*, 144: 237, 1999.

189. Berthold, H.K., Sudhop, T., and von Bergmann, K. Effect of a garlic oil preparation on serum lipoproteins and cholesterol metabolism: a randomized controlled trial. *JAMA,* 279: 1900, 1998.

190. Dausch, J.G. and Nixon, D.W. Garlic: a review of its relationship to malignant disease. *Prev. Med.,* 19: 346, 1990.

191. Lau, B.H.S., Tadi, P.P., and Tosk, J.M. Allium sativum (garlic) and cancer prevention. *Nutr. Res.,* 10: 937, 1990.

192. Lau, B.H., Woolley, J.L., Marsh, C.L., Barker, G.R., Koobs, D.H., and Torrey, R.R. Superiority of intralesional immunotherapy with Corynebacterium parvum and Allium sativum in control of murine transitional cell carcinoma. *J. Urol.,* 136: 701, 1986.

193. Belman, S. Onion and garlic oils inhibit tumor promotion. *Carcinogenesis,* 4: 1063, 1983.

194. Key, T.J., Silcocks, P.B., Davey, G.K., Appleby, P.N., and Bishop, D.T. A case-control study of diet and prostate cancer. *Br. J. Cancer.,* 76: 678, 1997.

195. You, W.C., Blot, W.J., Chang, Y.S., Ershow, A., Yang, Z.T., An, Q., Henderson, B.E., Fraumeni, J.F., Jr., and Wang, T.G. Allium vegetables and reduced risk of stomach cancer. *J. Natl. Cancer Inst.,* 81: 162, 1989.

196. Steinmetz, K.A., Kushi, L.H., Bostick, R.M., Folsom, A.R., and Potter, J.D. Vegetables, fruit, and colon cancer in the Iowa Women's Health Study. *Am. J. Epidemiol.,* 139: 1, 1994.

197. Sivam, G.P., Lampe, J.W., Ulness, B., Swanzy, S.R., and Potter, J.D. Helicobacter pylori — in vitro susceptibility to garlic (Allium sativum) extract. *Nutr. Cancer,* 27: 118, 1997.

198. Milner, J.A. Garlic: its anticarcinogenic and antitumorigenic properties. *Nutr. Rev.,* 54: S82, 1996.

199. Abdullah, T.H., Kirkpatrick, D.V., and Carter, J. Enhancement of natural killer cell activity in AIDS with garlic. *Dtsch. Ztschr. Onkologie.,* 21: 52, 1989.

200. Dirsch, V.M., Gerbes, A.L., and Vollmar, A.M. Ajoene, a compound of garlic, induces apoptosis in human promyeloleukemic cells, accompanied by generation of reactive oxygen species and activation of nuclear factor kappa *B. Mol. Pharmacol.,* 53: 402, 1998.

201. el-Bayoumy, K., Chae, Y.H., Upadhyaya, P., and Ip, C. Chemoprevention of mammary cancer by diallyl selenide, a novel organoselenium compound. *Anticancer Res.,* 16: 2911, 1996.

202. Niki, E., Noguchi, N., Tsuchihashi, H., and Gotoh, N. Interaction among vitamin C, vitamin E, and beta-carotene. *Am. J. Clin. Nutr.,* 62: 1322S, 1995.

203. Schardt, D. Phytochemicals: plants against cancer. *Nutrition Action Healthletter,* 21(3): 1, 1994.

204. Setchell, K.D. and Cassidy, A. Dietary isoflavones: biological effects and relevance to human health. *J. Nutr.,* 129: 758S, 1999.

15

VEGETARIAN DIETS AND DIETARY GUIDELINES FOR CHRONIC DISEASE PREVENTION: HOW MEATLESS DIETS CONFORM TO CURRENT RECOMMENDATIONS FOR HEALTHY EATING

Ella H. Haddad

CONTENTS

0-8493-8508-3/01/$0.00+$.50
© 2001 by CRC Press LLC

I. INTRODUCTION

It is generally recognized that habitual dietary patterns have profound effects on nutritional status, health, and longevity. Although the exact composition of the ideal diet is not fully known, increasing awareness of the role of diet in health and advances in scientific knowledge have prompted nutrition professionals and policymakers to periodically issue dietary advice and recommendations for the public. Concern about diet initially focused on the problems of hunger and inadequate nutrient intake, and dietary recommendations emphasized animal food sources such as meat and milk products for improving nutritional status. As patterns of disease shifted away from infectious and nutrient-deficiency diseases toward higher rates of chronic disease, dietary advice also changed. Dietary recommendations throughout the world currently promote a more simple vegetarian-like diet derived largely from plant food sources as being conducive to health.

One compelling reason for interest in plant-based and vegetarian diets comes from the rather consistent research findings that such diets as consumed in industrialized countries are accompanied by desirable long-term benefits. All-cause morbidity and mortality from a number of chronic conditions are lower in vegetarians than in non-vegetarians. This chapter provides an overview of how meatless and vegetarian diets agree with and conform to dietary guidelines and to recommendations for the primary and secondary prevention of chronic disease. In fact, implementation of the various guidelines can best be achieved by adopting plant-rich and vegetarian diets.

II. DIETARY GUIDELINES

Dietary guidelines are designed to provide advice for healthy individuals regarding diet and related life-style practices to promote healthful eating and reduce the risk of disease.[1] Dietary guidelines differ from nutrient standards such as the Reference Dietary Intakes (RDI) and Recommended Dietary Allowances (RDA),[2] or food guides such as the Food Guide Pyramid.[3,4] Nutrient standards define the reference points for average daily intake of essential nutrients; food guides provide a framework for selecting kinds and amounts of foods of different types that together provide a nutritionally adequate diet and dietary guidelines give advice on consumption of types of food or food component related to a public health concern. The guidelines are intended to be population-based recommendations for health promotion and disease prevention.

A. Overview

1. U.S. Guidelines

The dietary guidelines concept was first introduced by Atwater over a century ago. He indicated that food production at the time provided a relative excess of fats, meats, starch, and sugar, and recommended a diet that provided 33% of energy as fat and 15% as protein.[5] In the more recent history of dietary guidelines, a major step was achieved in 1977 when the U.S. Congress issued the landmark *Dietary Goals for the United States* after extensive hearings held by the Senate Select Committee on Nutrition and

Human Needs.[6] The decades after World War II were marked by a progression of thinking among nutrition scientists and policymakers from problems of hunger and nutrient adequacy to the role of diet as a controllable risk factor in chronic degenerative conditions such as heart disease, stroke, diabetes, and cancer that are the leading causes of death in the U.S.[7] The dietary goals report attributed these killer diseases to dietary and other life-style factors and established quantitative standards for what was considered to be a more optimum intake of total fat, saturated fatty acids, total carbohydrate, added sugars, cholesterol, sodium, and protein. The report generated much controversy among nutritionists and scientists about the proposed standards and goals.

First released in 1980, the *Nutrition and Your Health: Dietary Guidelines for Americans* booklet represented a joint effort by the Departments of Agriculture and Health and Human Services to promote the dietary recommendations addressed in the "goals" for which there was considerable consensus and which were deemed to have greatest potential benefit for public health.[8] The dietary guidelines were revised and reissued in 1985, 1990, and 1995. Most recently, in the year 2000, the fifth revision of the guidelines was released.[1] Meanwhile, there have been numerous scientific papers and research reviews that have provided the documentation and underlying scientific research needed to validate the guidelines. Most prominent, from the national perspective, were (1) *The Surgeon General's Report on Nutrition and Health* (1988) published by the Surgeon General's office,[9] and (2) the *Diet and Health: Implications for Reducing Chronic Disease Risk* (1989) document published by the National Academy of Sciences (NAS).[10] Table 15.1 compares the year 2000 *Dietary Guidelines for Americans with the Diet and Health* recommendations. The *Dietary Guidelines* substantially reflect the NAS *Diet and Health* recommendations and translate them into consumer-friendly language. Although the *Dietary Guidelines* statements are simple, concise and descriptive, much of the quantitative aspects of the *Diet and Health* recommendations are maintained in the more detailed instructions given in the guidelines booklet and in the *Food Guide Pyramid* advice.

Political legitimacy was achieved by the passage of the National Nutrition Monitoring and Related Research Act of 1990 (PL101-445), which established the guidelines as statements of federal nutrition policy and required the secretaries of Agriculture and Health to reevaluate and update (if needed) the guidelines every 5 years.[5] As official U.S. policy, they form the basis for all federal nutrition feeding programs and dietary guidance for the public. To encourage greater implementation, they are incorporated in the health promotion objectives of the *Health Objectives for the Nation* document.[11]

2. International Guidelines

The U.S. is not alone in issuing dietary guidelines. Most of the industrialized countries in the world, including Australia, Canada, Denmark, Ireland, Finland, France, Germany, Hungary, India, Israel, Italy, Japan, South Korea, Netherlands, New Zealand, Norway, Singapore, Sweden and the U.K., have their own sets of dietary guidelines. International organizations such as the World Health Organization (WHO) and the Food and Agriculture Organization, have also issued dietary guidelines. Comparisons among dietary guidelines from various countries have been published.[12,13] There is considerable consistency among the guidelines from many countries as well as those issued by study groups of the WHO and the U.S. Dietary Guidelines, especially with regard to recommendations pertaining to fat, saturated fat, carbohydrate, and fiber intake.[12]

B. Is the Vegetarian Diet Consistent with the Dietary Guidelines?

1. What Do Vegetarians Eat?

The vegetarian label encompasses a wide variety of dietary and life-style values and practices. For the purposes of this chapter, the term vegetarian refers to a diet that avoids flesh foods such as meat, poultry, and fish but may include dairy products or eggs. The term vegan applies to a diet composed entirely of plant foods. Vegetarian and vegan diets emphasize plant foods such as grains, legumes, nuts, vegetables, and fruits. Plant-rich diets are those that include a generous proportion of plant foods and relatively small amounts of animal foods, whether meat, poultry, seafood, eggs, or dairy products. Plant-rich diets such as those consumed by traditional populations in Mediterranean countries or the Far East are sometimes referred to as vegetarian-like diets.

It is difficult to establish an exact vegetarian pattern of intake. First, individuals and groups who adopt the vegetarian diet differ in their food intake and avoidance patterns. Second, there are no large-scale dietary studies with appropriate sampling and stratification techniques conducted on vegetarians. Recently, however, Messina and Messina[14] summarized the data obtained from more than 60 dietary studies conducted on vegetarians since the early 1950s. The studies reviewed encompassed various types of vegetarian eating styles, national as well as a number of international vegetarian groups, and included studies of individuals in different life-cycle stages such as childhood, adolescence, pregnancy, lactation and the elderly. The results consistently showed that vegetarians consumed less fat, saturated fat, and cholesterol and more polyunsaturated fat and dietary fiber than non-vegetarians in those studies.

Table 15.1 The Year 2000 Dietary Guidelines for Americans and the Diet and Health Recommendations

U.S. Department of Agriculture, US Department of Health and Human Services. Dietary Guidelines for Americans, 5th edition, 2000[1]	*Committee on Diet and Health, Food and Nutrition Board, National Research Council: Diet and Health 1989*[10]
Aim For Fitness	**Body weight**
• Aim for a healthy weight.	Maintain appropriate body weight. Balance food intake and physical activity.
Healthy weight: BMI 18.5 to 25	**Fat intake**
	Total fat 30% of calories or less
Overweight: BMI 25–30	Saturated fatty acids 10% of calories
Obese: BMI 30 and above	Polyunsaturated fatty acids 7% to 10% of calories
• Be physically active each day.	
Adults: 30 minutes of moderate activity most days	Dietary cholesterol less than 300 mg daily
	Concentrated fish oils not recommended
Children and teens: 60 minutes of moderate activity most days	**Food groups**
	5 or more servings of vegetables and fruits each day, especially green and yellow vegetables and citrus fruits
	Increase intake of starches and complex carbohydrates as breads, cereals and legumes. Increase of added sugars is not recommended
• Build A Healthy Base	**Protein intake**
Let the Pyramid guide your food choices.	Moderate, less than twice the RDA
Choose a variety of grains daily, especially whole grains.	Alcohol consumption not recommended
Choose a variety of fruits and vegetables daily.	For those who do drink, limit consumption to two standard drinks a day. Pregnant women and women attempting to conceive should avoid alcoholic beverages.
Keep food safe to eat.	

Table 15.1 The Year 2000 Dietary Guidelines for Americans and the Diet and Health Recommendations (Continued)

U.S. Department of Agriculture, US Department of Health and Human Services. Dietary Guidelines for Americans, 5th edition, 2000[1]	Committee on Diet and Health, Food and Nutrition Board, National Research Council: Diet and Health 1989[10]
•Choose Sensibly	• Salt intake
Choose a diet that is low in saturated fat and cholesterol and moderate in total fat.	• 6 grams sodium chloride (NaCl) per day or less
Choose beverages and foods to moderate your intake of sugars.	• Adequate calcium intake
Choose and prepare foods with less salt	• Dietary supplement intake Avoid taking in excess of the RDA.
If you drink alcoholic beverages, do so in moderation.	Adequate fluoride intake
•Food Guide Pyramid	
Bread, Cereal, Rice, Pasta Group (Grains Group):	
6–11 servings per day (especially whole grain)	
Vegetable Group:	
3–5 servings per day	
Fruit Group:	
2–4 servings per day	
Milk, Yogurt, Cheese Group (Milk Group):	
2–3 servings per day (preferably fat-free or low-fat)	

Not only does the macronutrient composition of vegetarian diets differ from those of non-vegetarians, but so too does the pattern of food group consumption. In vegetarian households, children and adults consume substantially more vegetables, fruits, legumes, and nuts than non-vegetarians.[15-17] Vegetarian Seventh-Day Adventists eat more whole grains, fruits, tomatoes, legumes, nuts, and plant-based meat substitutes than their non-vegetarian counterparts.[18]

Observations gleaned from descriptive studies of various vegetarian groups allow some generalizations about the diet.[14-18] Table 15.2 offers a qualitative description of the nutritional and food group patterns of

Table 15.2 Vegan, Vegetarian and Mediterranean Dietary Patterns compared to the Dietary Guideline Recommendations[14-18]

Dietary Guidelines	Vegan	Vegetarian	Mediterranean
Total fat ≤ 30% energy	⇓ ⇔ ⇑	⇓ ⇔ ⇑	⇑
Saturated fatty acids ≤ 10% energy	⇓	⇓	⇓
Monounsaturated fatty acids ≤ 10% energy	⇔ or ⇑	⇔ or ⇑	⇑
Polyunsaturated fatty acids ≤ 10% energy	⇔ or ⇑	⇔ or ⇑	⇔
Dietary cholesterol ≤ 300 mg per day	0	⇓	⇓
Protein (animal sources)	0	⇓	⇓
Protein (vegetable sources)	⇑	⇑	⇑
Fiber ~ 25 g per day	⇑	⇑	⇑
Whole grain breads and cereals: 6–11 servings per day	⇑	⇑	⇔
Fruits and vegetables: 5–9 servings per day	⇑	⇑	⇑
Meat, poultry, fish, dry beans, eggs, nuts group: 5–7 ounces per day			
Meat, poultry, fish	0	0	⇓
Eggs	0	⇓	⇑
Dry beans	⇑	⇑	⇑
Nuts	⇑	⇑	⇑
Milk, yogurt, cheese: 2–3 servings per day	0	⇔ or ⇓	⇓

⇑ higher intake, ⇔ similar intake, ⇓ lower intake, 0 avoided

vegetarian and plant-rich diets as compared with the recommendations of the Dietary Guidelines

2. Vegetarian Diets, Plant Foods, and the Guidelines

Modern-day vegetarians have, for more than 100 years now, advocated plant foods as being healthier. Meanwhile, scientific views on the relative proportions of plant and animal foods in healthful diets have markedly shifted since the introduction of the dietary guidelines. Food guides, nutrient standards, and dietary advice prior to the guidelines emphasized foods from animal sources (meat and dairy products) to prevent deficient intake of essential nutrients. The guidelines instruct the public to eat less energy, fat, saturated fat, cholesterol, etc. and more complex carbohydrates and fiber. As succinctly expressed by Marion Nestle[19] the principle sources of the eat-less foods (other than sugar, salt, and alcohol) are meat and dairy products, whereas the principal sources of the eat-more items are plant foods. It is important to note that the 1995 version of the guidelines included the statement: "Vegetarian diets are consistent with the *Dietary Guidelines for Americans* and can meet Recommended Dietary Allowances for nutrients."[20] To express this more accurately, the optimum diet as recommended by the guidelines emphasizes plant foods and substantially resembles the vegetarian diet. In fact, the dietary recommendations common among the advice promoted by various authoritative groups and countries can best be achieved by adhering to a largely vegetarian dietary pattern.

3. The Year 2000 Guidelines

The year 2000 guidelines encompass three categories designated as the ABCs for good health:

1. **A**im for Fitness statements emphasize healthy weight and physical activity.
2. **B**uild a Healthy Base statements promote the Food Guide Pyramid.
3. **C**hoose Sensibly statements reflect the traditional guideline recommendations.[1]

a. Aim for Fitness

The first message of the guidelines is intended to emphasize the importance of weight control and physical activity in disease prevention. Maintenance of a healthy weight reduces the risk of heart disease, type 2 diabetes, hypertension, stroke, and certain cancers. Most plant foods are bulky and low in calories. This property of high volume and low caloric density promotes fullness and satiety and reduces the likelihood of overeating. Vegetarians emphasize whole foods, especially whole-grain cereals, which are higher in dietary fiber than the refined varieties. Studies have consistently reported that vegetarians are, on the average, thinner than non-vegetarians when the average BMI is compared. Lower BMIs mean lower prevalence of obesity among vegetarians than in comparable groups.[21-23]

b. Build a Healthy Base

This message is intended to establish the food guide pyramid as the basis for food selection, to promote a variety of plant food consumption, and to address food safety issues. There is widespread consensus about the guideline to eat more and varied plant foods. Fruits, vegetables, whole grains, and legumes are significant sources of most essential nutrients such as complex carbohydrate, protein, essential fats, vitamins, and minerals. More importantly, they are exclusive sources of fiber, folate, vitamin C, carotenoids, and other phytochemicals. Numerous epidemiological studies show plant foods to be strongly associated with the prevention of chronic disease such as heart disease and cancer.[21,24-26] In the food guide pyramid, first grains, then fruits and vegetables, occupy the greatest amount of space at the base of the pyramid, sending the message that these foods are more important and should be consumed in greater quantities than foods higher up in the pyramid.

Dietary advice often includes an emphasis on consuming a variety of foods. It is more likely that a wide complement of needed nutrients will be obtained if a variety of items from each food group is selected. Recently, however, dietary variety per se has been linked to excessive consumption and increased body weight.[27] The 2000 *Dietary Guidelines* apply variety only to the consumption of plant foods, not to the myriad refined products found on supermarket shelves.

Earlier dietary guideline statements encouraged the consumption of complex carbohydrate and fiber. Because of the ambiguity of its definition, the term complex carbohydrate does not appear in the 2000 guidelines. The intake of fiber is emphasized as well as that of whole grain breads and cereals. Vegetarian diets traditionally include whole grain cereals and whole foods instead of white flour and refined products.[18]

c. *Choose Sensibly*

The third message reiterates the advice that first prompted the dietary goals, and addresses intake of fat, saturated fat, sugar, salt, and alcohol.

Total fat: Most dietary guidelines encourage a reduction in total fat intake to help lower the amount of saturated fat in the omnivorous diet and to facilitate weight control. The NAS report Diet and Health set the target of an average of 30% or less of calories from fat. Dietary guidelines have used expressions such as "reduce fat," "limit fat," or "choose a diet low in fat" in their statements. The fifth edition of the *Dietary Guidelines* employs the words "moderate in fat" to counteract the common misconception that low fat means no fat. Vegetarian diets are not intrinsically low in fat and can be planned to provide a range of fat intake. However, even when higher in fat, vegetarian diets are low in saturated fat.

Saturated fat: Much experimental and epidemiological evidence implicates saturated fatty acid intake as associated with high levels of blood cholesterol and increased risk of coronary heart disease.[28] High levels of blood cholesterol promote atherosclerotic lesions and thrombus formation. *The Diet and Health* report set the target of an average of 10% or less of calories from fat, and dietary guidelines consistently advise reductions in saturated fat intake. The greater the reduction in saturated fatty acid intake, the greater the lowering of total blood cholesterol and low density lipo-protein cholesterol (LDL). The major sources of saturated fat in the diet are foods of animal origin, such as dairy products, eggs, and meats. Diets based entirely on plant foods provide the lowest amounts of saturated fat. Vegetarian diets with moderate amounts of fat typically contain less than 10% of calories as saturated fat if low fat or non-fat dairy products are consumed, and less than 5% of calories as saturated fat if only plant foods are consumed.[29]

The dietary guidelines also address the intake of *trans* fatty acids, which may also be atherogenic. Since these are found mostly in partially hydrogenated vegetable oils, the guidelines recommend the consumption of oils and fats that have not been hydrogenated

Dietary Cholesterol. The dietary guidelines recommend a reduction in dietary cholesterol along with fat and saturated fat. Diet and Health sets a limit of 300 mg of dietary cholesterol per day. Dietary cholesterol, like saturated fat, is derived primarily from animal food sources or products made from them. Plant foods are devoid of cholesterol.

Sugar. Although sugar intake has not been directly linked to risk of disease except for dental caries, foods high in sugar and refined carbo-hydrates are high in calories and low in fiber and essential vitamins and minerals. Major sources of added sugar in the U.S. are beverages such as soft drinks, fruit ades, and sweetened drinks.[30] Foods with added sugar tend to replace more nutrient-dense items in the diet. An emphasis on fruit consumption rather than sweetened drinks can substitute for much of the added sugar in the diet.

Salt. Dietary guidelines for the public usually include a recommenda-tion to restrict sodium chloride intake based on the evidence, derived from epidemiological and clinical observations, for an association between dietary salt and blood pressure. Most salt is obtained from processed foods. Vegetarian and plant-rich diets based on whole or minimally refined food contain much less salt than is commonly consumed.

III.   DISEASE-SPECIFIC GUIDELINES

Dietary advice for persons with one or more risk factors for a particular condition, or those with an established disease, differ from national guide-lines, which target the population as a whole and focus on the prevention of chronic disease in essentially healthy persons. Such disease-specific guidelines are often issued as consensus statements or recommendations by health agencies, professional associations, and other authoritative groups. For example, the earliest advice linking diet and health came from the American Heart Association (AHA) in a series of position statements released periodically beginning in 1957.[5,31] Since then, numerous authoritative bodies and agencies have issued recommendations related to the secondary prevention and treatment of specific disease conditions.

A. Heart Disease Guidelines

Coronary Heart Disease (CHD) is the major cause of death in industrialized and emerging nations and is the most common and serious form of cardiovascular disease. Elevated blood lipids and related disorders of lipoprotein metabolism are implicated in the progression of atherosclerosis and subsequent obstruction of coronary blood vessels and development of atherosclerotic heart disease. Atherosclerosis is infrequently hereditary in origin and there is an extensive body of epidemiologic, laboratory, and clinical evidence of an association between diet and the incidence of CHD. Recent clinical trials provide evidence that reducing serum cholesterol levels through diet, drugs, or both decreases the incidence of CHD. Although much attention has been focused on the effect of dietary fat and cholesterol on blood lipids, diet may influence other steps in the pathogenic sequence leading to atherosclerosis or to a cardiac event. For example, dietary factors may influence the propensity toward thrombosis (essential fatty acids, omega-3 fatty acids), lipoprotein oxidation (antioxidant nutrients), and endothelial damage (folate), among others.[31,32]

1. Risk-Reduction Strategies

Millions of individuals in the U.S. and throughout the world have some manifestations of atherosclerotic disease and are at risk for a fatal or nonfatal myocardial infarction. From a public health perspective, it is most important to emphasize secondary prevention measures that reduce the likelihood of serious later illness. The AHA guidelines,[31] and the National Cholesterol Education Program (NCEP) Adult Treatment Panel II (ATP II),[32] recommend that cholesterol-lowering therapy be initiated in individuals with CHD if their LDL cholesterol level is more than 100 mg/dL. The guidelines confirm diet therapy as primary intervention for lowering cholesterol; drug therapy is reserved for persons who do not respond to diet, or who are high risk. High risk is defined as LDL cholesterol at baseline ≥ 130 mg/dL.

Dietary modifications for the management of elevated blood lipids do not differ much from the dietary guidelines. These diets limit total fat intake to 30% or less of total calories. Step I and Step II diets progressively restrict intake of saturated fat and cholesterol. Step I limits saturated fat to 8% to 10% and cholesterol to no more than 300 mg per day. Step II restricts saturated fat to 7% and cholesterol to less than 200 mg per day. Typical response to the diet in free-living individuals is a reduction in blood cholesterol of 3–10% for Step I and 5–15% for Step II.[32-35]

2. Low-Fat and Very-Low-Fat Diets

To obtain maximum reductions in cholesterol-raising nutrients, especially saturated fatty acids, low fat (≤ 20% of energy), and very low fat (≤ 10% of energy) diets have been tested by Connor, Pritikin, and Ornish, among others.[32,36] Such lower fat diets usually provide a greater percentage of energy from carbohydrate. Although these diets facilitate weight reduction and reverse advanced atherosclerotic lesions, their use remains controversial. In many individuals, reduction in total cholesterol and LDL cholesterol is accompanied by a decrease in high-density lipoprotein cholesterol (HDL) and often an increase in plasma triglycerides.[37] Unlike the data for LDL cholesterol and HDL cholesterol, which show strong, consistent, and opposing correlations with CHD risk, the evidence for an independent association between triglyceride concentrations and risk of heart disease is equivocal. There is, however, some indication that elevated blood triglyceride is an independent risk factor in certain subgroups such as older women and individuals with type 2 diabetes. On the other hand, the risk may be indirect and secondary to the decreased HDL cholesterol and increased levels of the highly atherogenic small-dense LDL cholesterol particles that accompany the rise in blood triglyceride levels.[38]

Hypertriglyceredemia secondary to low fat intake is not seen with lower energy or calorie content of diets, or when accompanied by weight loss.[39,40] It is also not seen if the diet is high in plant foods with ample whole grains and fiber, or among populations in developing countries consuming mostly unrefined plant-based diets containing low quantities of animal foods.[41]

3. High Monounsaturated Fat (Mediterranean) Diet

From a practical point of view, saturated fat in the diet can be replaced by either carbohydrate or by monounsaturated fatty acids. Substantial reductions in total cholesterol and LDL cholesterol can be obtained by substituting sources of saturated fat in the diet (meat, poultry, eggs, whole-fat dairy products) with foods rich in monounsaturated fatty acids (olive oil, canola oil, nuts). This dietary pattern is similar to that observed in some Mediterranean regions. The dietary pattern in those areas is associated with low risk for heart disease. Although moderately high in fat

(30–40% of kcals), the Mediterranean diet is relatively low in saturated fat and effectively helps lower LDL cholesterol levels without reducing HDL cholesterol or increasing plasma triglycerides. In the mind of nutritionists, the Mediterranean diet is one in which olive oil is the dominant fat and the diet includes plenty of vegetables (including legumes) cereals, fruits and vegetables, nuts, and small amounts of cheese, fish, and meat; or, it is a plant-rich vegetarian-like diet.[19]

4. Vegetarian Diets

The relationship between diet and coronary heart disease is more complex than one that simply considers the influence of dietary saturated fat and cholesterol on blood lipid levels. Processes such as plaque formation, thrombosis, endothelial function, and antioxidant status may be influenced by a number of dietary components and interactions. Vegetarian diets that include small amounts of non-fat or low-fat dairy products, or vegetarian diets based entirely on plant foods (vegan) may provide greater overall benefits that go beyond those obtained by simply reducing fat or saturated fat.

a. Vegetarian Diets and Heart Disease

Compared with non-vegetarians, vegetarians in Western countries have lower mean plasma cholesterol levels and lower mortality from CHD.[42,43] In a recent pooled analysis of five cohort studies from the U.S., Britain, and Germany, vegetarians had a 24% reduction in mortality from this disease.[43] It is suggested that much of the reduction in heart disease among vegetarians is due to the lower intake of saturated fat and cholesterol. The data shows that, among vegetarians, consumption of total animal fat and dietary cholesterol are strongly associated with CHD mortality. However, it is also likely that other foods commonly consumed by vegetarians in large amounts offer additional protective effects. Such foods are fruits, vegetables, whole grain cereals, legumes, and nuts. Dietary patterns that emphasize plant foods provide a unique set of nutritive and non-nutritive components such as plant protein, plant sterols, and phytochemicals, which may positively influence certain biological processes and reduce disease risk.

Fruits and vegetables. Recent cohort studies highlight the protective role of fruits and vegetables in CHD. A high fruit intake is associated with reduced risk for both coronary artery and cerebrovascular disease.[44] Oxidized lipoproteins are key in provoking inflammation and deposition of cholesterol in the vascular endothelium. Physiologically active components in fruits and vegetables such as vitamin C, carotenoids, and flavonoids may reduce the risk of heart disease by reducing the oxidation of cholesterol in the arteries.[45-48] Sulfur-containing compounds found in garlic, onions, and leeks help reduce blood cholesterol levels.[49] Trace minerals found in plants such as selenium, manganese, and copper enhance the activity of antioxidant enzyme systems and offer additional antioxidant protection.

Elevated blood homocysteine concentrations are toxic to endothelial cells and have been implicated as a risk factor for heart disease and other vascular disorders.[50] Cross-sectional studies have shown a strong inverse association between dietary folate, blood folate, and blood homocysteine concentration. Plant foods are rich sources of folate, and both the consumption of fruits and vegetables and folic acid supplements lower elevated blood homocysteine levels.[51,52]

Fruits, vegetables, and especially legumes are rich sources of soluble fiber. Eating foods high in viscous and soluble fiber significantly lowers blood cholesterol and LDL concentrations. Soluble fiber sources that have been especially effective are pectin, oat bran, and legumes in lowering total and LDL cholesterol.[53-57]

Whole grains. Epidemiological studies show that fiber intake, independent of fat intake, is associated with a reduced risk of heart attacks in men. The protective effect is due mostly to cereal fiber obtained from whole grains.[58] Consumption of whole grains is associated with reduced mortality in older women.[59] Whole grains contain a wide variety of possibly beneficial nutrients and other constituents that are lost in the refining process.

Nuts. Nuts, including peanuts, are considered by vegetarians to be an important component of their diet and a valuable source of energy, protein, and essential fat. This is in contrast to the general perception of nuts as snack foods or attractive ingredients in candies and cookies.

Two large cohort studies have shown that higher nut consumption reduced the risk for heart disease.[60,61] Clinical intervention trials have shown that substituting nuts for a portion of healthful diets results in lowering of plasma lipids in individuals with normal and elevated blood lipid levels.[62,63]

Legumes. Beans are a staple in vegetarian dietary patterns as a source of protein and essential nutrients such as iron, zinc, and folate. As a rich source of soluble fiber, bean consumption has been shown to lower blood lipids in hypercholesterolemic individuals.[53] Among carbohydrate foods, cooked beans exhibit the lowest glycemic load, and so have beneficial effects in blood sugar modulation, satiety, and weight control. Protease inhibitors, phytic acid, oligosaccharides, and saponins found in beans are being studied for their anti-cancer and anti-tumor properties.[56]

Plant protein. The type of dietary protein (plant or animal) may influence blood lipids and risk of cardiovascular disease. Clinical studies on human subjects have shown soy protein to lower blood cholesterol. The vegetable protein of legumes and nuts are rich in arginine and glutamine, amino acid regulators of vascular and cardiac function.

Dietary lipids. Recent research suggests that the influence of dietary lipids on blood lipids and coronary artery function is complex. Dietary saturated fatty acids and cholesterol are known to raise blood lipid. The major source of saturated fat and cholesterol in the diet is meats and dairy foods, whereas the fat of plants is mostly unsaturated. However, trans fatty acids produced during the partial hydrogenation of vegetable oils also adversely influence blood lipids. Monounsaturated fatty acids as found in olive oil, nuts, and avocados are rather neutral with respect to heart disease mortality. The optimal intake of polyunsaturated fatty acids and the ratio of omega-3 to omega-6 fatty acids remains controversial.

The impact of fatty acids on thrombosis is unclear. A higher proportion of omega-3 relative to omega-6 inhibits platelet aggregation and thrombus formation. Although fish consumption is somewhat protective, fish oil supplements may not provide a beneficial effect.[67] Omega-3 fatty acids are lower in erythrocyte, platelet, and serum phospholipids of vegetarians, especially vegans, who also show increased platelet aggregation compared with meat eaters.[68,69] Although potential sources of omega-3 fatty acids other than fish and marine animals exist in plant foods (walnuts, flaxseed, algae), they may not be consumed in adequate amounts by all vegetarians.

Dietary cholesterol. The impact of dietary cholesterol on altering blood lipids is small. The average change in plasma total cholesterol levels is 2.2 mg/dL for every 100-mg change in dietary cholesterol. Also, there is much variability among individuals in response to consuming dietary cholesterol.[70] Most individuals compensate for increases in dietary cholesterol by suppression of endogenous cholesterol production to maintain near-constant plasma cholesterol levels. Others are unable to compensate and demonstrate enhanced cholesterol absorption and increased plasma cholesterol with high dietary cholesterol intake.

Since dietary cholesterol is derived exclusively from animal foods, vegan diets are devoid of cholesterol, whereas vegetarian diets that include dairy products may contain some cholesterol, albeit at lower amounts compared with the general population.

Plant sterols. The main plant sterols present in the diet are sitosterol, stigmasterol, and campesterol. Plant sterols are poorly absorbed in humans and interfere with the absorption of dietary cholesterol. They have also been shown to increase LDL-receptor activity. Their effectiveness has been recently demonstrated in a trial in which participants consumed a margarine containing a sitosterol derivative (sitostanol) for a year and maintained a mean decrease of 10% in plasma cholesterol.[71]

Body weight. The favorable effect of vegetarian diets on blood lipids may be partially mediated through the effects of the diet on body weight. Weight loss lowers total cholesterol, triglyceride, and VLDL, and raises HDL. A metanalysis showed that an 11-lb weight loss was associated with a decline of 10 mg/dL triglycerides.[72]

b. The Vegetarian Diet as Intervention

The advantage of a vegetarian diet is that substantial reduction in lipid levels can be obtained without resorting to severe fat restriction. Controlled metabolic studies, in which vegetarian diets were fed to non-vegetarians, with crossover control to omnivorous diets, resulted in lower total and LDL cholesterol levels but no change in HDL levels.[73,74] This is in contrast to very low fat interventions, which result in reduced HDL cholesterol.

Can vegetarian dietary practices be used instead of angioplasty or bypass surgery to manage and reverse heart disease? Ornish et al. demonstrated in the Life-Style Heart Trial that major life-style changes that included a vegetarian diet (~10% energy from fat, <5% from saturated fat, and <100 mg cholesterol) retards progression of coronary plaques and promotes regression documented by angiography.[36] Total cholesterol was reduced by 24% and LDL cholesterol by 37%. What is not known at present is whether vegetarian diets with a moderate content of fat are similarly effective in reversing atherosclerosis.

B. Obesity Guidelines

The prevalence of overweight and obesity is reaching epidemic proportions nationally and worldwide.[75,76] In the U.S., 55% of adults aged 20 years and older are either overweight or obese. Overweight is defined as having a body mass index (BMI) of 25.0 to 29.9 kg/m²; and obesity as BMI equal to or greater than 30 kg/m². Similar trends are observed in children and adolescents with a doubling of the number of obese children from 20 years ago.[75] Obesity is a major risk factor for coronary heart disease, hypertension, type 2 diabetes, stroke, gallbladder disease, osteoarthritis, respiratory problems, and some cancers. In addition to the enormous health consequences that result in increased health care costs, there are significant social and psychological burdens for obese individuals and their families.[77]

1. Risk Reduction Strategies

It is generally recognized that overweight and obesity result from a complex interaction between genetic and environmental factors characterized by long-term energy imbalance due to a sedentary life-style and excessive caloric consumption. To promote healthful eating patterns and discourage dieting as such, dietary guidelines have focused on lowering fat and increasing carbohydrate intake as the population-based dietary strategy for the problem. Even though reducing fat intake was primarily a message to reduce saturated fat and lower blood cholesterol, it was considered to be a useful guideline for also addressing the obesity problem. Unfortunately, public awareness of the importance of reducing fat and increasing carbohydrate does not appear to have been accompanied by sufficient knowledge about how to successfully achieve this without increasing body weight. Whereas the percentage of dietary energy derived from fat has fallen steadily in the U.S. during the past 20 years, caloric intake and the rates of obesity have risen.

Because of the growing problem, the National Heart, Lung, and Blood Institute (NHLBI) recently initiated the Obesity Education Initiative.[78] Guidelines from the initiative's expert panel on the identification, evaluation, and treatment of overweight and obesity in adults emphasize that, although reducing dietary fat is a practical way to reduce calories, the strategy must be accompanied by caloric restriction to be effective in weight management. As shown in Table 15.3, the focus of the initiative is on dietary caloric reduction and increased physical activity.

2. Vegetarian Diets

Studies have consistently found that vegetarians are, on the average, thinner and have lower BMIs than non-vegetarians within the same cohort.[21-23] Adult populations that subsist on mostly vegetarian diets not greatly impacted by Westernization are often quite lean.[76] Low fat diets that adhere to the dietary guidelines and emphasize plant foods have been found to be effective in reducing weight without caloric restriction.[79]

The foremost advantage of the vegetarian diet in weight control is the emphasis on consumption of minimally processed foods derived mainly from plant sources. Such unadorned whole plant foods (grains, fruits, vegetables, legumes) can be consumed in relative abundance during weight loss interventions. Such ample quantity and variety is necessary to provide a wide complement of nutrient and non-nutrient substances found in plants and needed by humans. This high-volume, low-energy dietary pattern is vital for achieving fullness and satiety, as recently affirmed in the studies conducted by Bell and colleagues.[80]

Table 15.3   Dietary Guidelines for Weight Control*

Dietary Component	Guidelines
Energy	Food energy reduction to achieve a weight loss of 1 to 2 lbs per week
	Low-calorie diet (800 to 1,500 kcal per day), or
	A reduction of 500 to 1,000 kcal/day
Fat	
Total fat	30% or less of total calories
Saturated fatty acids	8% to 10% of total calories
Monounsaturated fatty acids	Up to 15% of total calories
Polyunsaturated fatty acids	Up to 10% of total calories
Cholesterol	< 300 mg per day
Protein	Approximately 15% of total calories
Carbohydrate	55% or more of total calories
Sodium chloride	Approximately 6 g per day
Calcium	1,000 to 1,500 mg
Fiber	20 to 30 g

*From the National Institute of Health's *Clinical guidelines on the identification, evaluation, and treatment of overweight and obesity in adults*, 1998.[78]

The physiological advantage of an emphasis on plant foods may also stem from the influence of these foods on blood sugar control, where there is renewed interest in the role of foods with a lower glycemic index. Whole foods and foods rich in unrefined starch and fiber produce a more blunted postprandial blood sugar response and effectively control hunger than those based on highly refined carbohydrate foods.

C. Hypertension Guidelines

High blood pressure is one of the most common health problems in industrialized countries. Among U.S. adults, about one fourth suffer from hypertension. Certain subgroups within the population, such as African-Americans and the elderly, exhibit a markedly greater prevalence of hypertension. Elevated blood pressure is a significant risk factor for stroke, end-stage renal disease, congestive heart failure, and sudden death.[81]

1. Risk Reduction Strategies

Dietary factors have long been known to affect blood pressure control and have been the subject of years of investigation to determine their specific roles in the prevention and treatment of hypertension. Current public policy expressed in the Dietary Guidelines recommends moderate sodium restriction for the entire population to prevent hypertension and stroke. In its 6th report, the National Institutes of Health (NIH) Joint National Committee on Detection, Evaluation, and Treatment of High Blood Pressure (JNC VI) outlines dietary and life-style modifications effective in the prevention and treatment of hypertension.[82] Dietary modifications that have been demonstrated as beneficial are shown in Table 15.4 and include:

- reducing dietary sodium consumption
- avoiding excessive alcohol intake
- restricting calories to reach an optimal weight if overweight
- increasing dietary potassium, calcium and magnesium

Table 15.4   Dietary Guidelines for Blood Pressure Management*

Aspect	Guidelines
Weight reduction	Caloric restriction and increased activity in individual with BMI** ≥ 27
Alcohol intake	Limit to 2 drinks*** per day for men; 1 drink per day for women
Physical activity	Moderately intense physical activity (40%–60% of maximum oxygen consumption) for 30–45 minutes on most days
Dietary Sodium	100 mmol/day (approximately 6 g sodium chloride or 2400 mg sodium)
Dietary potassium	90 mmol/day of potassium from food (approximately 3600 mg)
	Additional potassium from potassium salt-substitutes or supplements in hypokalemia
Dietary calcium	Adequate intake for health
Dietary magnesium	Adequate intake for health
Dietary fats	Reduce intake of dietary saturated fat and cholesterol for cardiovascular health
Tobacco avoidance	

*From the 6th report of the Joint National Committee on Detection, Evaluation, and Treatment of High Blood Pressure (JNC VI)[82]

**BMI is body mass index or weight in kilograms divided by height in meters squared

***A "drink" contains 15 ml of alcohol

2. The DASH Diet

As a result of increasing awareness of the impact and complexity of dietary interactions, The National Institutes of Health initiated a multi-center, randomized clinical trial called Dietary Approaches to Stop Hypertension (DASH) that examined the effects of the guidelines on blood pressure.[83] The subjects were randomized into one of three dietary treatment groups. The control group received a typical American diet with four servings of fruits and vegetables and half a serving of dairy products per day. The fruit and vegetable group received 8.5 servings of fruits and vegetables that provided increased magnesium and potassium, but the diet was otherwise similar to the control diet. The combination group received 10 servings of fruits and vegetables including legumes and nuts, and 2.7 servings of low-fat dairy products. The combination diet provided higher amounts of magnesium, potassium, and calcium. Sodium intake and body weight were kept constant for all groups. Both the high fruit and vegetable diet and the combination diet (fruit, vegetable and low-fat dairy) produced substantial reductions in blood pressure, with the combination diet being more effective.

3. Vegetarian Diets

Within populations, vegetarians exhibit lower blood pressure than non-vegetarians,[84,85] and replacing a mixed diet with a vegetarian diet reduces blood pressure in both normotensive and hypertensive individuals.[86] The effect has been shown in individuals who follow a lacto-vegetarian diet characterized by a relatively low intake of saturated fat, and high intake of fruit, vegetables, and other fiber-containing foods. High fruit and vegetable intake has been linked to low stroke mortality.[44,87] Vegetarian diets and dietary patterns that emphasize plant-based foods provide the best strategies for the prevention and control of high blood pressure. The beneficial effect of plant-rich diets could be due to type of fat (monoun-saturated and polyunsaturated), fiber, antioxidant vitamins, carotenoids, flavonoids, and mineral contribution of the diet, especially calcium, mag-nesium, and potassium.

D. Diabetes Guidelines

Diabetes mellitus is a chronic condition that contributes to disease and death worldwide. Type 1 diabetes occurs less frequently and results from an autoimmune destruction of the insulin-producing pancreatic beta cells. Type 2 diabetes is the more common disease. In the U.S., it is estimated that at least 90 to 95% of the 15 million persons with diabetes mellitus have type 2 diabetes. Complications from diabetes are serious and disabling. Diabetes is the leading cause of end-stage renal disease, lower-extremity amputations, and blindness in adults. Other complications include heart disease, stroke, hypertension, nervous system disease, dental disease, and complications of pregnancy.

The management of individuals with diabetes relies heavily on dietary control along with hypoglycemic agents and insulin. The goals of therapy are the optimization of blood glucose control and minimization of the risk of hypoglycemia in individuals treated with insulin, and the prevention or delay of the onset of chronic complications for all diabetics. Clinical trials have demonstrated the benefit of aggressive treatment to achieve glycemic control in delaying complications.[89]

1. Insulin Resistance

It is proposed that most individuals with type 2 diabetes have had a less severe abnormality of carbohydrate metabolism before progressing to diabetes.[90] The transition from normal glucose tolerance to type 2 diabetes in genetically susceptible persons involves manifestations described as insulin resistance, a condition in which body cells lose sensitivity to insulin action, and insulin-stimulated glucose disposal is compromised. Insulin resistance is associated with a metabolic syndrome characterized by a cluster of atherogenic risk factors including hyperinsulinemia, obesity with an abdominal pattern of distribution, some degree of carbohydrate intolerance, hypertension, and an abnormal blood lipoprotein profile of increased triglycerides and decreased HDL cholesterol. Other features of the syndrome include easily oxidized small LDL particles, heightened blood-clotting activity (plasminogen-activating inhibitor-1), and elevated serum uric acid concentration.

2. Risk Reduction Strategies

Despite the public health significance of type 2 diabetes, little is known about the dietary risk factors in the development of the disease.[91] Although genetic predisposition is a determinant of insulin resistance, diet and lifestyle are thought to play a role in the development of the syndrome. Animal studies suggest that a high-fat, high-refined carbohydrate, low fiber diet (typical Western diet) induces insulin resistance and precedes other aspects of the syndrome including obesity. Epidemiological studies of groups such as the Pima Indians have shown decreased prevalence with high-carbohydrate native diets, and increased with Westernized high-fat diets. Risk of diabetes has also been associated with low fiber intake and large glycemic response of foods.[92]

The negative effects are not limited to excess consumption but also to a sedentary life-style. The incidence of type 2 diabetes is lower in physically active persons than in those who are inactive. Physical activity enhances insulin sensitivity, decreases abdominal obesity, and may prevent the development of type 2 diabetes in susceptible persons.[93,94]

Current dietary recommendations for persons with diabetes shown in Table 15.5 are similar to those advocated for health promotion in the general populace. They hinge on diet, exercise, and weight loss. Recommendations to decrease caloric intake and increase energy expenditure are of primary importance for people with diabetes whose BMI > 25kg/m². The clinical disturbances of type 2 diabetes associated with obesity improve with weight reduction. To prevent the atherogenic complications of diabetes, the ADA guidelines have in the past advocated the restriction of total and saturated fat intake, and an emphasis on carbohydrates and dietary fiber. Recent findings that low fat diets tend to increase blood triglycerides and reduce HDL in diabetics have shifted the recommendations toward an individualized approach suggesting lower carbohydrate and higher monounsaturated fatty acid diets for diabetics whose blood triglycerides are high.[95]

3. *Vegetarian and Plant Rich Diets*

Although the evidence is not strong, vegetarians may have lower rates of type 2 diabetes.[96] There have been a number of large cohort studies that show an inverse association between incidence of diabetes and intakes of cereal grains and dietary fiber.[97-99] High risk of diabetes was associated with a large glycemic index of foods consumed by participants.[97] The glycemic index is an indicator of carbohydrates' ability to raise blood glucose levels. These relationships are physiologically substantiated by the clinical trials of J.W. Anderson and others, who demonstrated that a high carbohydrate, albeit high fiber, diet composed of low glycemic foods (whole grains, fruits, vegetables, legumes, nuts) decreased postprandial glucose and insulin concentrations, and improved insulin sensitivity.[100,101] Similar results were obtained recently with a low fat vegetarian diet that emphasized plant food.[102]

E. Cancer Guidelines

In the U.S., cancer is the second leading cause of death after cardiovascular disease and is responsible for one out of four deaths. Existing scientific evidence suggests that about one third of the 5,000,000 cancer deaths that occur in the U.S. each year are due to dietary and life-style factors, and another third can be blamed on cigarette smoking. The evidence also

Table 15.5 Dietary Guidelines for Type 2 Diabetes*

Component	Patient Characteristics	Guidelines
Energy	Overweight	Moderate caloric restriction to achieve moderate weight loss (5 kg to 9 kg)
		A reduction of 250 to 500 calories per day.
Protein	Normal renal function	10% to 20% of calories
	Nephropathy	$0.6 \text{ g} \cdot \text{kg}^{-1} \cdot \text{day}^{-1}$ to $0.8 \text{ g} \cdot \text{kg}^{-1} \cdot \text{day}^{-1}$
Total fat	Normal blood lipids	NCEP Step 1 diet ($\leq$ 30% calories fat)
	Elevated triglycerides or VLDL	>30% calories fat, mainly monounsaturated fat (10% to 15% of calories)
Saturated fat and cholesterol	Normal blood lipids	NCEP Step 1 diet (saturated fat 8% to 10% of calories, cholesterol <300 mg per day)
	Elevated LDL	NCEP Step 2 diet (saturated fat 7% of calories, cholesterol <200 mg per day)
Carbohydrate	Normal blood lipids	Approximately 50% to 60% of calories
	Elevated triglycerides or VLDL	< 50% of calories
Sugar (sucrose, fructose)		Moderate part of total carbohydrate
Fiber		20 to 35 g per day from soluble and insoluble fiber sources
Sodium	Mild to moderate hypertension	$\leq$ 2,400 mg per day
	Hypertension and nephropathy	$\leq$ 2,000 mg/day
Alcohol intake		Limit to 2 drinks** per day for men; 1 drink per day for women

*From the American Diabetes Association Nutrition recommendations and principles for people with diabetes mellitus. 1998. **A "drink" contains 15 ml of alcohol

indicates that, although genetics is a factor in the development of cancer, behavioral factors such as cigarette smoking, dietary choices, and physical activity can modify the risk of cancer at all stages of its development.[103] A recent report commissioned by the World Cancer Research Fund and the American Institute for Cancer Research (AICR), in which an exhaustive collection of the relevant worldwide research on this topic was reviewed, estimated that "recommended diets, together with maintenance of physical activity and appropriate body mass, can in time reduce cancer incidence by 30-40%." The AICR report specifically identified the preventive contribution of a diet rich in plant foods. This is of particular relevance to vegetarian diets which are based mostly or entirely on plant foods.[104]

1. Risk Reduction Strategies

Cancer development in man is a multistage process involving multiple steps and interactions. Habitual dietary patterns can influence cancer development in various ways and at different levels. For example, food may be the source of genotoxic or carcinogenic chemicals capable of forming DNA adducts and altering genetic material, or food components may act as tumor promotors and enhance the carcinogenetic process. On the other hand, food may contain a number of preventive substances that inhibit the development of tumors.

a. Carcinogens in Food

Carcinogens may occur naturally in the diet, such as the pyrrolizidine alkaloids that exist in some plants consumed as food or herbal remedies. Some foods may be contaminated either intentionally or unintentionally by harmful agents, possible pesticide residues, additives to food, or chemicals from packaging materials. Cancer-causing substances may be produced during food storage, cooking, or processing. Aflatoxins are carcinogenic metabolites produced by *Aspergillus flavus* and other molds if grains and peanuts are inadequately stored. Nitrosamines, polycyclic aromatic hydrocarbons, and oxidized lipids form during cooking or processing of various foods. In developed countries, vigilance by the food industry and government regulatory agencies has been effective in maintaining negligible levels of these contaminants in the food supply and in reducing the exposure of the public to such substances. Recently, however, a new class of potent genotoxic substances called heterocyclic amines has been identified in meat cooked at high temperatures.[104]

b. Meat and Heterocyclic Amines

Frequent consumption of cooked meats has been associated with an increased risk of colorectal, pancreatic, and urothelial cancer.[105,106] The charred surface of the meat contains heterocyclic amines such as dimethylimidazo quinoxaline (MeIQx), and phenylimidazo pyridine (PhIP), which are produced during frying, broiling, or cooking of meat and fish. These compounds are multi-site animal carcinogens and form DNA adducts in humans. Their metabolites are detected in various body tissues and fluids. The carcinogenic potential of heterocyclic amines may differ in individuals based on inherited variation (polymorphism) in genes that influence the activation or inactivation of dietary carcinogens.[107,108]

c. Dietary Modulators

Dietary factors that do not of themselves exhibit a genotoxic effect may modulate the carcinogenic response of caloric intake and dietary fat. Studies in laboratory animal model systems show the component of the diet with the most dramatic effect on cancer risk is caloric intake. Restriction of energy from carbohydrate, or carbohydrate and fat, inhibits a number of cancers and results in a considerably longer life span in the restricted than in the fully fed animals. Human epidemiological studies also provide strong support for the role of dietary energy and energy balance in cancer. Observations consistently indicate that increased body weight and obesity are risk factors for cancer, especially that of the colon, endometrium, prostate, and breast, whereas higher levels of physical activity are protective in the prevention of the same cancers.[104]

The role of dietary fat in cancer modulation has been extensively studied in animal models. In general, diets rich in polyunsaturated fat have enhanced the development of cancer more than saturated or monounsaturated fat. This effect has been attributed to the role of linoleic acid as an essential nutrient in tumor development.[105]

d. Protective Substances

Foods and dietary patterns may inhibit or retard the development of cancer. The classic animal studies of L.W. Wattenberg[110] first awakened the scientific community to the potential role of certain foods and their components in the prevention of cancer. Epidemiological studies demonstrated that diets containing higher amounts of plant-derived foods (fruits and vegetables) are associated with relatively low risk of cancer. Fruit and vegetable intake consistently lowered risk of a variety of tumors, especially epithelial cancers of the respiratory and GI tract (lung, esophagus, stomach, colon). Protective properties of plant foods can most likely be attributed to their rich composite of beneficial nutrients and biologically active compounds referred to as phytochemicals.

Fruits, vegetables, grains, legumes. Of the many studies on the topic of dietary pattern, the higher consumption of plant foods provides the best protection against the risk of developing cancer. The mechanism to explain the health benefits derived from eating plant foods and their relation to cancer is yet to be determined, but likely to be multiple in origin. There are many potentially anticarcinogenic substances in plant foods. Vitamin C, found in citrus and other fruits, and vitamin E in whole grains and nuts, are important antioxidants and may protect cell membranes and DNA from oxidative damage. Green leafy vegetables, legumes, and citrus fruit are sources of folic acid, which may have a protective role at the molecular level in cancer development. The sulfur-containing compounds in cabbage family vegetables (dithiolthiones, isothiocynates) and onion family vegetables (allyl sufides) enhance the activity of enzymes involved in detoxifying carcinogens and other *xebiotics* in the body.[111-114]

Carotenoids from food, not from supplements. Interest in carotenoids as anti-cancer agents were based on evidence from epidemiologic studies consistently suggesting that diets rich in fruits and vegetables are associated with reduced risk of cancer. Because of the strong supportive evidence from several animal models and cell culture systems,[115] it was assumed that the protective component in fruits and vegetables was the plant pigment beta-carotene. Studies also showed that higher blood concentrations of beta-carotene are associated with decreased risk for cancer, especially lung and stomach cancer.[116] In addition to beta-carotene, lycopene in tomato sauce has recently received attention for its role in preventing prostate cancer.[117]

The efficacy of beta-carotene as a chemo-preventive agent was tested in several large clinical trials. Results from two of these trials revealed that individuals at high risk for developing lung cancer (heavy smokers and asbestos workers) who use high-dose supplemental beta-carotene had an increased relative risk (18–23%) for developing lung cancer than control subjects. Provided as a high-dose supplement, beta-carotene may have a different effect than the same agent acquired in a food. Beta-carotene is only one of a large number of carotenoids and other phytochemicals found in fruits and vegetables. The chemo-preventive effect of whole plant foods seems to be greater than that of a single food component.[118]

Soy foods. Cancer of the breast is the most common cancer in women. Because genetics is believed to account for only 10–15% of cases, the search for environmental factors assumes considerable importance. Studies of Asian women suggest that those who consume a traditional diet high in soy products have a low incidence of breast cancer. Genistein, an isoflavone found in soy, is being examined as a possible protective factor for breast cancer. Exposure of immature rats to genistein promotes cellular differentiation, which results in a less active epidermal growth factor in adulthood and suppression in the development of mammary cancer in those animals.[119] The consumption of soy may also reduce the risk of prostate cancer incidence. In the Adventist Health Study, men with a high consumption of soy beverage were at reduced risk of prostate cancer.[120]

2. Vegetarian Diets

Vegetarians in developed countries show lower cancer mortality rates for certain cancer sites than non-vegetarians.[122-124] In several large cohort studies, the consumption of red meat was associated with a greater risk for colon cancer.[125] In the Nurses Health Study, animal fat intake was correlated to risk of breast cancer.[116] Among California Seventh-Day Adventists, colon cancer was 88% higher and prostate cancer 54% higher in non-vegetarians compared with vegetarians.[123] In the cohort studied, both red-meat and white-meat consumption increased the risk of colon cancer, whereas legume consumption had a protective effect. Vegetarian diets are associated with lower levels of mutagenic activity and reactive oxygen species (free radical formation) especially in the digestive tract.[127,128] This is possibly a consequence of higher fiber content and nutritive and non-nutritive antioxidants found in plant foods. Plant foods are rich in folate, a nutrient that is associated with lower colon cancer risk.[125]

The risk of fatal pancreatic cancer is also lower in vegetarian Seventh-Day Adventists, with significant protective association found for consumption of dried fruits, legumes, and vegetarian meat substitutes, some of which are derived from soy.[123]

a. Vegetarian Diets and the Cancer Guidelines

Nutrition guidelines to advise the public about dietary practices that reduce cancer risk are published by authoritative organizations such as the American Cancer Society.[103] Table 15.6 shows these along with the guidelines published by World Cancer Research Fund and the American Institute for Cancer Research.[104] The guidelines are consistent with vegetarian dietary practices. Vegetarians tend to be leaner than non-vegetarians. Their food patterns emphasize a variety of whole plant foods and the avoidance of meat intake as expressed in the cancer prevention guidelines.

IV. CONCLUSION

Recent decades have witnessed a major shift toward increased promotion of plant foods in thinking about dietary patterns conducive to health. The release of the dietary goal and guidelines initially produced great protest among nutrition scientists, suggesting that the recommendations were premature and the evidence lacking. Since then, scientific support has accumulated that plant foods contribute to preventing the occurrence and

Table 15.6   Dietary Guidelines for Cancer Prevention

Guidelines on Diet Nutrition, and Cancer Prevention (American Cancer Society)[103]	*Advice to Individuals (World Cancer Research Fund/American Institute for Cancer Research)*[104]
1. Choose most of the foods you eat from plant sources.	**Food Supply, Eating and Related Factors**
Eat five or more servings of fruits and vegetables each day.	1. Food supply and eating Choose predominantly plant-based diets rich in a variety of vegetables and fruits, pulses (legumes) and minimally processed starchy staple foods.
Eat other foods from plant sources, such as breads, cereals, grain products, rice, pasta, or beans several times each day.	2. Maintaining body weight Avoid being underweight or overweight and limit weight gain during adulthood to less than 5 kg (11 pounds).
2. Limit your intake of high-fat foods, particularly from animal sources. Choose foods low in fat. Limit consumption of meats, especially high-fat meats.	3. Maintaining physical activity If occupational activity is low or moderate, take an hour's brisk walk or similar exercise daily, and also exercise vigorously for a total of at least one hour in a week.
3. Be physically active: achieve and maintain a healthy weight. Be at least moderately active for 30 minutes or more on most days of the week. Stay within your healthy weight range.	**Food and Drinks** 4. Vegetables and fruits Eat 400-800 grams (15-30 ounces) or five or more portions (servings) a day of a variety of vegetables and fruits, all year round.
4. Limit consumption of alcoholic beverages, if you drink at all.	5. Other plant foods Eat 600-800 grams (20-30 ounces) or more than seven portions (servings) a day of a variety of cereals (grains), pulses (legumes), roots, tubers and plantains. Prefer minimally processed foods. Limit consumption of refined sugar.

Table 15.6   Dietary Guidelines for Cancer Prevention (Continued)

Guidelines on Diet Nutrition, and Cancer Prevention (American Cancer Society)[103]	*Advice to Individuals (World Cancer Research Fund/American Institute for Cancer Research)*[104]
	6. Alcoholic drinks Alcohol consumption is not recommended. If consumed at all, limit alcoholic drinks to less than two drinks a day for men and one for women
	7. Meat If eaten at all, limit intake of red meat to less than 80 grams (3 ounces) daily. It is preferable to choose fish, poultry or meat from non-domesticated animals in place of red meat.
	8. Total fats and oils Limit consumption of fatty foods, particularly those of animal origin. Choose modest amounts of appropriate vegetable oils.
	Food Processing
	9. Salt and salting Limit consumption of salted foods and use of cooking and table salt. Use herbs and spices to season foods.
	10. Storage Do not eat food which, as a result of prolonged storage at ambient temperatures, is liable to contamination with mycotoxins.
	11. Preservation Use refrigeration and other appropriate methods to preserve perishable food as purchased and at home.

Table 15.6 Dietary Guidelines for Cancer Prevention (Continued)

Guidelines on Diet Nutrition, and Cancer Prevention (American Cancer Society)[103]	Advice to Individuals (World Cancer Research Fund/American Institute for Cancer Research) [104]
	12. Additives and residues When levels of additives, contaminants and other residues are properly regulated, their presence in food and drink is not known to be harmful. However, unregulated or improper use can be a health hazard, and this applies particularly in economically developing countries.
	13. Preparation Do not eat charred food. For meat and fish eaters, avoid burning of meat juices. Consume the following only occasionally: meat and fish grilled (broiled) in direct flame; cured and smoked meats.
	14. Dietary supplements For those who follow the recommendations presented here, dietary supplements are probably unnecessary, and possible unhelpful, for reducing cancer risk.
	Tobacco Do not smoke or chew tobacco.

ameliorating the complications of heart disease, hypertension, obesity, diabetes, and cancer. People in industrialized economies could reduce risks for chronic disease if they increased their intake of fruits, vegetables, and grains in proportion to animal foods.

Biochemical, clinical, and epidemiological research has provided a solid biologic foundation for the health benefits of plant-based and vegetarian diets. Plant-based diets are bulkier, have lower caloric density, and promote decreased caloric intake and more appropriate body weights. Saturated fat from animal foods is a major culprit in atherosclerosis and heart disease. Plant foods are richer in beneficial omega-6 and omega-3 fatty acids, plant sterols, and natural antioxidants. Vegetables, legumes, and whole grain cereals modulate postprandial hyperglycemia and reduce the risk of type 2 diabetes. Consumption of fruits and vegetables reduces the risk of some cancers.

It was assumed that the benefits of vegetarian diets derived mainly from their avoidance of meat or dairy products, or both. Vegetarian dietary habits are distinguished not simply by their animal food avoidance but also by their greater and more varied provision of minimally processed plant foods, and, consequently, much of the positive health outcomes of the diet are now attributed to eating more plant foods. The Dietary Guidelines clearly promote eating more unrefined grains, fruits and vegetables and reducing the intake of saturated fat and cholesterol. Thus, there is much overlap between the guidelines and vegetarian eating patterns. Present knowledge suggests that diets rich in plant foods with small or minimal amounts of animal foods may be the remedy for modern life-style diseases.

REFERENCES

1. U.S. Department of Agriculture. Dietary Guidelines for Americans, 5th ed. Washington, D.C.: U.S. Government Printing Office, 2000.
2. Monsen, E.R. New Dietary Reference Intakes proposed to replace the Recommended Dietary Allowances. *J. Am. Diet. Assoc.*, 96, 754, 1996.
3. Welsh, S., Davis, C., and Shaw, A. Development of the food guide pyramid. *Nutr. Today*, 27, 12, 1992.
4. U.S. Department of Agriculture, Human Nutrition Information Service. The Food Guide Pyramid. Home and Garden Bulletin No. 252. U.S. Government Printing Office, Washington, D.C. 1992.
5. Welsh, S. Nutrient standards, dietary guidelines, and food guides. In: *Present Knowledge in Nutrition*, 7th ed. Ziegler, E. E., Filer, L. J. (Eds.), ILSI Press, Washington, D.C. 1996.
6. U.S. Senate Select Committee on Nutrition and Human Needs. Dietary goals for the United States, 2nd ed. Washington, D.C.: U.S. Government Printing Office, 1977.
7. Monthly Vital Statistics Report. Ten leading causes of death in the U.S. Hyattsville, MD: National Center for Health Statistics, 1997, 46:32-33.
8. U.S. Department of Agriculture and U.S. Department of Health, Education, and Welfare. Nutrition and Your Health: Dietary Guidelines for Americans. U.S. Government Printing Office, Washington D.C., 1980.
9. U.S. Department of Health and Human Services. Public Health Service. The Surgeon General's report on nutrition and health. Washington, D.C.: U.S. Government Printing Office, 1988. DHHS (PHS) Publication No. 88-50210.
10. Committee on Diet and Health, Food and Nutrition Board, National Research Council. Diet and Health: implications for reducing chronic disease risk. Washington, D.C.: National Academy Press, 1989.

11. Healthy People 2010 Objectives: Draft for Public Comment. Washington, D.C.: U.S. Department of Health and Human Services. Office of Public Health and Science, 1998.

12. Truswell, A. S. Dietary goals and guidelines: national and international perspectives. In: *Modern Nutrition in Health and Disease*, 9th ed. Shills, M. E., Olson, J. A., Shike, M., Ross, A. C. (Eds.), Williams and Wilkins, Baltimore, 1998.

13. Diet, nutrition, and the prevention of chronic disease. Report of a WHO study group. Technical report series no. 797, Geneva: WHO, 1990:180-181.

14. Applications. Aspen Publishers, Inc., Gaithersburg, 1996, 405-416.

15. Bull, N. L. and Barber, S. A. Food and nutrient intakes of vegetarians in Britain. *Human Nutr: Applied Nutr.*, 38A, 288, 1984.

16. Donovan, U.M. and Gibson, R. Dietary intakes of adolescent females consuming vegetarian, semi-vegetarian, and omnivorous diets. *J. of Adolescent Health*, 18, 292, 1996.

17. Haddad, E. H., Berk, L. S., Kettering, J. D., Hubbard, R. W., and Peters, W. R. Dietary intake and biochemical, hematologic, and immune status of vegans compared with non-vegetarians. *Am. J. Clin. Nutr.*, 70(suppl.), 586S, 1999.

18. Fraser, G. E. Associations between diet and cancer, ischemic heart disease, and all-cause mortality in non-Hispanic white California Seventh-Day Adventists. *Am. J. Clin. Nutr.*, 70(suppl.), 532S, 1999.

19. Nestle, M. Animal v. plant foods in human diets and health: is the historical record unequivocal? *Proc. Nutr. Soc.*, 58, 211, 1999.

20. U.S. Department of Agriculture. Dietary Guidelines for Americans, 4th ed. Washington, D.C.: U.S. Government Printing Office, 1995.

21. Dwyer, J. T. Health aspects of vegetarian diets. *Am. J. Clin. Nutr.*, 48, 712, 1988.

22. Caan, B. J., Van Horn, L., Bragg, C., Manolio, T. A., Kushi, L. H., and Liu, K. Meat consumption and its associations with other diet and health factors in young adults: the CARDIA study. *Am. J. Clin. Nutr.*, 54, 930, 1991.

23. Appleby, P. N., Thorogood, M., Mann, J. I., and Key, T. J. Low body mass index in non-meat eaters: the possible roles of animal fat, dietary fiber, and alcohol. *Int. J. Obesity*, 22, 454, 1998.

24. Ness A. R. and Powles, J. W. Fruit and vegetables and cardiovascular disease: a review. *Int. J. Epidemiol.*, 26, 1, 1997.

25. La Vecchia, C., Decarli, A., and Pagano, R. Vegetable consumption and risk of chronic disease. *Epidemiology*, 9, 208, 1998.

26. Willett, W. C. Convergence of philosophy and science: the Third International Congress on Vegetarian Nutrition. *Am. J. Clin. Nutr.*, 70(suppl), 434S, 1999.

27. McCrory, M. A., Fuss, P. J., McCallum, J. E., Yao, M., Vinken, A. G., Hays, N. P., and Roberts, S. B. Dietary variety within food groups: association with energy intake and body fatness in men and women. *Am. J. Clin. Nutr.*, 69, 440, 1999.

28. Chait, A., Brunzell, J. D., Denke, M. A., Eisenberg, D., Ernst, N.D., Franklin, F. A., Jr., Ginsberg, H., Kotchen, T. A., Kullar, L., Mullis, R. M., Nichaman, M. Z., Nicolosi, R. J., Schaefer, E. J., Stone, J. F., and Weidman, W. H. Rationale of the diet-heart statement of the American Heart Association. Report of the Nutrition Committee. *Circulation*, 88, 3008, 1993.

29. Haddad, E. H. Development of a vegetarian food guide. *Am. J. Clin. Nutr.*, 59(suppl.), 1248S, 1994.

30. Guthrie, J. F. and Morton, J. F. Food sources of added sweeteners in the diets of Americans. *J. Am. Diet. Assoc.*, 100, 43, 2000.

31. Krauss, R. M., Deckelbaum, R. J., Ernst, N., Fisher, E., Howard, B. V., Knopp, R. H., Kotchen, T., Lichtenstein, A. H., McGill, H. C., Pearson, T. A., Prewitt, T. E., Stone, N. J., Van Horn, L., and Weinberg R. Dietary guidelines for healthy American adults. A statement for health professionals from the Nutrition Committee, American Heart Association. *Circulation*, 94, 1795, 1996.

32. Adult Treatment Panel II. National Cholesterol Education Program: second report of the Expert Panel on Detection, Evaluation and Treatment of High Blood Cholesterol in Adults. *Circulation*, 89, 1333, 1994.

33. Denke, M. A. Cholesterol-lowering diets, A review of the evidence. *Arch. Intern. Med.*, 155, 17, 1995.

34. Caggiula, A. W., Watson, J. E., Kuller, L. H., Olson, M. B., Milas, N. C., Berry, M., and Germanowski, J. Cholesterol-lowering intervention program, *Arch. Intern. Med.*, 156, 1205, 1996.

35. McCarron, D. A., Oparil, S., Chait, A., Haynes B., Kris-Etherton, P., Stern, J. S., Resnich, L. M., Clark, S., Moris, C. D., Halton, D. E., Metz, J. A., McMahon, M., Holcomb, S., Snyder, G. W., and Pi-Sunyer, S. Nutritional management of cardiovascular risk factors. *Arch. Intern. Med.*, 157, 169, 1997.

36. Ornish, D., Scherwitz, L.W., Billings, J.H., Gould, K.L., Merritt, T.A., Sparler, S., Armstrong, W.T., Ports, T.A., Kirkeeide, R.L., Hogeboom, C., and Brand, R.J. Intensive life-style changes for reversal of coronary heart disease. *J. Am. Med. Assoc.*, 280, 2001, 1998.

37. Katan, M.B., Grundy, S.M., and Willett, W.C. Should a low-fat, high-carbohydrate diet be recommended for everyone? Beyond low-fat diets. *N. Engl. J. Med.*, 337, 563, 1997.

38. Austin, M.A. Plasma triglyceride and coronary heart disease. *Arterioscler. Thromb.*, 11, 2, 1991.

39. Schaefer, E. J., Lichtenstein, A. H., Lamon-Fava, S., McNamara, J. R., Schaefer, M. M., Rasmussen, H., and Ordovas, J. M. Body weight and low-density lipoprotein cholesterol changes after consumption of a low-fat ad libitum diet. *J. Am. Med. Assoc.*, 274, 1450, 1995.

40. Flynn, M. M., Zmuda, J. M., Milosavljevic, D., Caldwell, M. J., and Herbert, P. N. Lipoprotein response to a National Cholesterol Education Program Step II Diet with and without energy restriction. *Metabolism*, 48, 822, 1999.

41. Anderson, J. W. and Ward, K. Hypolipidemic effects of high-carbohydrate, high-fiber diets. *Metabolism*, 29, 551, 1980.

42. Key, T.J.A., Thorogood, M., Appleby, P. N., and Burr, M. L. Dietary habits and mortality in 11,000 vegetarians and health conscious people: results of a 17-year follow up. *Brit. Med. J.*, 313, 775, 1996.

43. Key, T.J.A., Fraser, G. E., and Thorogood, M. Mortality in vegetarians and non-vegetarians: detailed finding from a collaborative analysis of 5 prospective studies. *Am. J. Clin. Nutr.*, 70(suppl), 516S, 1999.

44. Gillman, M. W., Cupples, L. A., Gagnon, D., Posner, B. M., Ellison, R. C., Castelli, W. P., and Wolf, P. A. Protective effect of fruits and vegetables on development of stroke in men. *J. Am. Med. Assoc.*, 273, 1113, 1995.

45. Cook, N. C. and Samman, S. Flavonoids: chemistry, metabolism, cardio-protective effects, and dietary sources. *J. of Nutr. Biochem.*, 7, 66, 1996.

46. Knekt, P., Reunanen, A., Jarvinen, R., Seppanen, R., Heliovaara, M., and Aromaa, A. Antioxidant vitamin intake and coronary mortality in a longitudinal population study. *Am. J. Epidemiol.*, 139, 1180, 1994.

47. Gaziano, J.M., Manson, J.E., Branch, L. G., Colditz, G. A., Willett, W. C., and Buring, J.E. A prospective study of consumption of carotenoids in fruits and vegetables and decreased cardiovascular mortality in the elderly. *Ann. Epidemiol.*, 5, 255, 1995.

48. Kritchevsky, S. T., Tell, G. S., Shimakawa, T., Dennis, B., Li, R., Dohlmeier, L., Steere, E., and Heiss, G. Provitamin A carotenoid intake and carotid artery plaques: the atherosclerosis risk in communities study. *Am. J. Clin. Nutr.*, 68, 726, 1998.

49. Warshafsky, S., Kamer, R., S., and Sivak, S. L. Effect of garlic on total serum cholesterol: a meta-analysis. *Ann. Intern. Med.*, 119, 599, 1993.

50. Boushey, C. J., Beresford, S. A., Omen, G. S., and Motulsky, A. G. A quantitative assessment of plasma homocysteine as a risk factor for vascular disease. Probable benefit of increasing folic acid intakes. *J. Am. Med. Assoc.*, 274, 1049, 1995.

51. Nygård, O., Refsum, H., Veland, P.M., and Vollset, S. E. Major life-style determinants of plasma total homocysteine distribution: the Hordaland homocysteine study. *Am. J. Clin. Nutr.*, 67, 263, 1998.

52. Brouwer, I. A., van Dusseldorp, M., West, C. E, et al. Dietary folate from vegetables and citrus fruits decreases plasma homocysteine concentrations in humans in a dietary controlled trial. *J. Nutr.*, 129, 1135, 1999.

53. Anderson, J. W., Gustafson, N. J., Spencer, D. B., Tietyen, J., and Bryant, C. A. Serum lipid response of hypercholesterolemic men to single and divided doses of canned beans. *Am. J. Clin. Nutr.*, 51, 1013, 1990.

54. Glore, S. R., Treeck, D. V., Knehans, A. W., and Guild, M. Soluble fiber and serum lipids: a literature review. *J. Am. Diet. Assoc.*, 94, 425, 1994.

55. Jensen, C. D., Haskell, W., and Whittam, J. H. Long-term effects of water-soluble dietary fiber in the management of hypercholesterolemia in healthy men and women. *Am. J. Cardiol.*, 79, 34, 1997.

56. Messina, M. J. Legumes and soybeans: overview of their nutritional profiles and health effects. *Am. J. Clin. Nutr.*, 70(suppl.), 439S, 1999.

57. Jenkins, D. J. A., Kendall, C. W. C., Vidgen E., Mehling, C. C., Parker, T., Seyler, H., Faulkner, D., Garsetti, M., Griffin, L. C., Agarwal, S., Rao, A. V., Cunnane, S. C., Ryan, M. A., Connelly, P. W., Leiter, A. A., Vuksan, V., and Josse, R. The effect on serum lipids and oxidized low-density lipoprotein of supplementing self-selected low-fat diets with soluble-fiber, soy, and vegetable protein foods. *Metabolism*, 49, 67, 2000.

58. Rimm, E. B., Ascherio, A,, Giovannucci, E., Spiegelman, D., Stampfer, M. J., and Willett, W. C. Vegetable, fruit, and cereal fiber intake and risk of coronary heart disease among men. *J. Am. Med. Assoc.*, 275, 447, 1996.

59. Jacobs, D. R., Meyer, K. A., Kushi, L. H., and Folsom, A. R. Is whole grain intake associated with reduced total and cause-specific death rates in older women? The Iowa Women's Health Study. *Am. J. Public Health*, 89, 322, 1999.

60. Fraser, G. E., Sabaté, J., Beeson, W. L., and Strahan, T. M. A possible protective effect of nut consumption on risk of coronary heart disease. The Adventist Health Study. *Arch. Intern. Med.*, 152, 1416, 1992.

61. Kushi, L. H., Folsom, A. R., Prineas, R. L., Mink, P. J., Wu, Y., and Bostick, R. M. Dietary antioxidant vitamins and death from coronary heart disease in postmenopausal women. *N. Engl. J. Med.*, 334, 1156, 1996.

62. Sabaté, J., Fraser, G. E., Burke, K., Knutsen, S. F., Bennett, H., and Lindsted, K. D. Effect of walnuts on serum lipid levels and blood pressure in normal men. *N. Engl. J. Med.*, 320, 915, 1989.

63. Zambón, D., Sabaté, J., Muñoz, S., Campero, B., Casals, E., Merlos, M., Laguna, J., and Ros, E. Substituting walnuts for monounsaturated fat improves the serum lipid profile of hypercholesterolic men and women. A random crossover trial. *Ann. Intern. Med.*, 132, 538, 2000.

64. Bakhit, R. M., Klem, B. P., Essex-Sorlie, D., Ham, J. O., Erdman, J. W., and Potter, S. M. Intake of 25 g of soybean protein fiber alters plasma lipids in men with elevated cholesterol concentrations. *J. of Nutr.*, 124, 213, 1994.

65. Anderson, J. W., Johnstone, B. M., and Cook-Newell, M. E. Meta-analysis of the effects of soy protein intake on serum lipids. *N. Engl. J. Med.*, 333, 276, 1995.

66. Smit, E., Nieto, F. J., and Crespo, C. J. Blood cholesterol and apolipoprotein B levels in relation to intakes of animal and plant proteins in U.S. adults. *Br. J. of Nutr.*, 82, 193, 1999.

67. Stone, N. J. Fish consumption, fish oil, lipids, and coronary heart disease. *Am. J. Clin. Nutr.*, 65, 1083, 1997,

68. Agren, J. J., Tormala, M. L., Nenonen, M. T., and Hanninen, O. O. Fatty acid composition of erythrocyte, platelet, and serum lipids in strict vegans. *Lipids*, 30, 365, 1995.

69. Li, D., Sinclair, A., Mann, N., Turner, A., Ball, M., Kelly, F., Abedin, L., and Wilson, A. The association of diet and thrombotic risk factors in healthy male vegetarians and meat-eaters. *Eur. J. Clin. Nutr.*, 53, 612, 1999.

70. McNamara, D. J., Kolb, R., and Parker, T. S, et al. Heterogeneity of cholesterol homeostasis in man. Response to changes in dietary fat quality and cholesterol quantity. *J. Clin. Invest.*, 79, 1729, 1987.

71. Vuoristo, M. and Miettinen, T. A. Absorption, metabolism and serum concentrations of cholesterol in vegetarians: effects of cholesterol feeding. *Am. J. Clin. Nutr.*, 59, 1325, 1994.

72. Dattilo, A. M. and Kris-Etherton, P. M. Effects of weight reduction on blood lipids and lipoproteins: a meta-analysis. *Am. J. Clin. Nutr.*, 56, 320, 1992.

73. Masarei, J. R. L., Rouse, I. L., Lynch, W. J., Robertson, K., Vandongen, R., and Beilin, L. J. Effects of a lacto-ovo-vegetarian diet on serum concentration of cholesterol, triglyceride, HDL-C, HDL2-C, HDL3-C apoprotein-B, and Lp(a). *Am. J. Clin. Nutr.*, 40, 468, 1984.

74. Cooper, R, S., Goldberg, R. B., Trevisan, M., Tsong, Y., Liu, K., Stamler, J., Rubenstein, A., and Scanu, A. M. The selective lipid-lowering effect of vegetarianism on low density lipoproteins in a cross-over experiment. *Atherosclerosis*, 44, 293, 1982.

75. Kuczmarski, R. J., Carrol, M. D., Flegal, K. M., and Johnson, C. L. Overweight and obesity in the United States: prevalence and trends, 1960-1994. *Int. J. Obes.*, 22, 39, 1998.

76. Popkin, B. M., Paeratadul, S., Zhai, F., and Keyou, G. A review of dietary and environmental correlates of obesity with emphasis on developing countries. *Obes. Res.*, 3, 145S, 1995.

77. Must, A., Spadano, J., Coakley, E. H., Field, A. E., Colditz, G., and Dietz, W. H. The disease burden associated with overweight and obesity. *J. Am. Med. Assoc.*, 282, 1523, 1999.

78. U.S. Department of Health and Human Services, National Institutes of Health, National Heart, Lung, Blood Institute. Clinical guidelines on the identification, evaluation, and treatment of overweight and obesity in adults. The evidence report. Washington, D.C., 1998.

79. Sheppard, L., Kristal, A. R., and Kushi, L. H. Weight loss in women participating in a randomized trial of low-fat diets. *Am. J. Clin. Nutr.*, 54, 821, 1991.

80. Bell, E. A., Castellanos, V. H., Pelkman, C. L., Thorwart, M. L., and Rolls, B. J. Energy density affects energy intake in normal-weight women. *Am. J. Clin. Nutr.*, 67, 412, 1998.

81. Burt, V. L., Whelton, P., Roccell, E. J., Brown, C., Cutler, J. A., Higgins, M., Horan, M. J., and Labarthe, D. Prevalence of hypertension the U.S. adult population: results from the Third National Health and Nutrition Examination Survey, 1988-1991. *Hypertension*, 25, 305, 1995

82. Joint National Committee on Detection, Evaluation, and Treatment of High Blood Pressure. The sixth report of the Joint National Committee on Detection, Evaluation, and Treatment of High Blood Pressure (JNC VI). *Arch. Intern. Med.*, 157, 2413, 1997.

83. Appel, L. J., Moore, T. J., Obarzanek, E., Vollmer, W. M., Svetkey, L. P., Sacks, F. M., Bray, G. A., Vogt, T. M., Cutler, J. A., Windhauser, M. M., Lin, P-H., and Karanja, N. For the DASH Collaborative Research Group. A clinical trial of the effects of dietary patterns on blood pressure. *N. Engl. J. Med.*, 136, 1117, 1997.

84. Beilin, L. J. Vegetarian diets, alcohol consumption, and hypertension. Ann. NY *Acad. Sci.*, 676, 83, 91.

85. Melby, C. L., Goldflies, D. G., and Toohey, M. L. Blood pressure differences in older black and white long-term vegetarians and non-vegetarians. *J. Am. Coll. Nutr.*, 12, 262, 1993.

86. Margetts, B. M., Beilin, L. J., Vandongen, R., and Armstrong, B. K. Vegetarian diet in mild hypertension: a randomized controlled trial, *Br. Med. J.*, 293, 1468, 1986.

87. Keli, S. O., Hertog, M. G. L., Feskens, E. J. M., and Kromhout, D. Dietary flavonoids, antioxidant vitamins and incidence of stroke. The Zutphen Study. *Arch. Intern. Med.*, 154, 637, 1996.

88. The Expert Committee on the Diagnosis and Classification of Diabetes Mellitus, Introduction. *Diabetes Care*, 22 (Suppl. 1), S5, 1999.

89. The Diabetes Control and Complication Trial Research Group. The effect of intensive treatment of diabetes on the development and progression of long-term complications in insulin-dependent diabetes mellitus. *N. Eng. J. Med.*, 329, 997, 1993.

90. Barnard, R. J., Roberts, C. K., Varon, S. M., and Berger, J. J. Diet-induced insulin resistance precedes other aspects of the metabolic syndrome. *J. Appl. Physiol.*, 84,1311, 1998.

91. Manson, J. E. and Spelsberg, A. Primary prevention of non-insulin-dependent diabetes mellitus. *Am. J. Prev Med.*, 10, 172, 1994.

92. Swinburn, B. A., Boyce, V. L., Bergman, R. N., Howard, B. V., and Bogardus, C. Deterioration in carbohydrate metabolism and lipoprotein changes induced by modern, high fat diet in Pima Indians and Caucasians. *J. Clin. Endocrinol. Metab.*, 73, 156, 1991.

93. Helmrich, S. P., Ragland, D. R., Leung, R. W., and Paffenbarger, R. S. Physical activity and reduced occurrence of non-insulin-dependent diabetes mellitus. *N. Engl. J. Med.*, 325, 147, 1991.

94. Eriksson, K. F., and Lindgarde, F. Prevention of type 2 (non-insulin-dependent) diabetes mellitus by diet and physical exercise. *Diabetologia*, 34, 891, 1991.

95. American Diabetes Association. Nutritional recommendations and principles for people with diabetes mellitus. *Diabetes Care*, 21(Suppl 1), S32, 1998.

96. Snowdon, D. A. and Phillips, R. L. Does a vegetarian diet reduce the occurrence of diabetes? *Am. J. of Public Health*, 75, 507, 1985.

97. Salmerón, J., Manson, J. E., Stampfer, M. J., Colditz, G. A., Wing, A. L., and Willett, W. C. Dietary fiber, glycemic load, and risk of non-insulin-dependent diabetes mellitus in women. *J. Am. Med. Assoc.*, 227, 472, 1997.

98. Salmerón, J., Ascherio, A., Rimm, E. B., Colditz, G. A., Spiegelman, D., Jenkins, D. J., Stampfer, M. J., Wing, A. L., and Willett, W. C. Dietary fiber, glycemic load, and risk of NIDDM in men. *Diabetes Care*, 20, 545, 1997.

99. Meyer, K., Kushi, L. H., Jacobs, D. R., Slavin, J., Sellers, T. A., and Folsom, A. R. Carbohydrates, dietary fiber, and incident type 2 diabetes in older women. *Am. J. Clin. Nutr.*, 71, 921, 2000.

100. Anderson, J. W. Fiber and health: an overview. *Am. J. Gastroenterol.*, 81, 892, 1986.

101. Nuttall, F. Q. Dietary fiber in the management of diabetes. *Diabetes*, 42, 503, 1993.

102. Nicholson, A. S., Sklar, M., Barnard, N. D., Gore, S., Sullivan, R., and Browning, S. Toward improved management of NIDDM: A randomized, controlled, pilot intervention using a low-fat, vegetarian diet. *Prev Med.*, 29, 87, 1999.

103. The American Cancer Society. 1996 Advisory Committee on Diet, Nutrition, and Cancer Prevention. Guidelines on diet, nutrition, and cancer prevention: reducing the risk of cancer with healthy food choices and physical activity. *CA Cancer J. Clin.*, 46, 325, 1996.

104. Food, nutrition, and the prevention of cancer: a global perspective. Washington, D.C.: World Cancer Research Fund/American Institute for Cancer Research, 1997.

105. Gerhardsson de Verdier, M., Hagman, U., Peters, R. K., Steineck, G., and Overvik, E. Meat, cooking methods, and colorectal cancer: a case-referrent study in Stockholm. *Int. J. Cancer.*, 49, 520, 1991.

106. Turteltaub, K. W., Dingley, K. H., Curtis, K. D., Malfatti, M. A., Turesky, R. J., Garner, R. C., Felton, J. S., and Lang, N. P. Macromolecular adduct formation and metabolism of heterocyclic amines in humans and rodents at low doses. *Cancer Lett.*, 143, 149, 1999.

107. Augustsson, K., Skog, K., Jagerstad, M., Dickman, P. W., and Steineck, G. Dietary heterocyclic amines and cancer of the colon, rectum, bladder, and kidney: a population-based study. *Lancet*, 353, 703, 1999.

108. Roberts-Thomson, I. C., Butler, W. J., and Ryan, R. Meat, metabolic genotypes and risk for colorectal cancer. *Eur J. Cancer Prev.*, 8, 207, 1999.

109. Trichopoulou, A. and Lagiou, P. Worldwide patterns of dietary lipid intake and health implications. *Am. J. Clin. Nutr.*, 66(suppl), 961S, 1997.
110. Wattenberg, L. W. Inhibition of carcinogenesis by minor dietary constituents. *Cancer Res.*, 52, 2085S, 1992.
111. Steinmetz, K. A. and Potter, J. D. Vegetables, fruit, and cancer. I. Epidemiology. *Cancer Causes Control*, 2, 325, 1991.
112. Steinmetz, K. A. and Potter, J. D. Vegetables, fruit, and cancer. II. Mechanisms. *Cancer Causes Control*, 2, 427, 1991.
113. Block, G., Patterson, B., and Subar, A. Fruit, vegetables, and cancer prevention: a review of the epidemiological evidence. *Nutr. Cancer.*, 18, 1, 1992.
114. Zeigler, R. G., Taylor-Mayne, S., and Swanson, C. A. Nutrition and lung cancer. *Cancer Causes Control*, 7, 157, 1996.
115. Krinsky, N. I. Carotenoids and cancer in animal models. *J. Nutr.*, 119, 123, 1989.
116. Flagg, E. W., Coates, R. J., and Greenberg, R. S. Epidemiologic studies of antioxidants and cancer in humans. *J. Am. Coll. Nutr.*, 14, 419, 1995.
117. Giovannucci, E., Ascherio, A., Rimm, E. B., Stampfer, M. J., Colditz, G. A., and Willett, W. C. Intake of carotenoids and retinol in relation to risk of prostate cancer. *J. Natl. Cancer Inst.*, 87, 1767, 1995.
118. Pryor, W. A., Stahl, W., and Rock, C. L. Beta carotene: from biochemistry to clinical trials. *Nutr. Rev.*, 58, 39, 2000.
119. Lamartiniere, C. A., Zhang, J. X., and Cotroneo, M. S. Genistein studies in rats: potential for breast cancer prevention and reproductive and developmental toxicity. *Am. J. Clin. Nutr.*, 68(6 Suppl), 1400S, 1998.
120. Jacobsen, B. K., Knutsen, S. F., and Fraser, G. E. Does high soy milk intake reduce prostate cancer incidence? The Adventist Health Study (United States). *Cancer Causes Control*, 9, 553, 1998.
121. Chang-Claude, J. and Frentzel-Beyme, R. Dietary and life-style determinants of mortality among German vegetarians. *Int. J. of Epidemiol.*, 22, 228, 1993.
122. Key, T. J., Fraser, G. E., Thorogood, M., Appleby, P. N., Beral, V., Reeves, G., Burr, M. L., Chang-Claude, J., Frentzel-Beyme, R., Kuzma, J. W., Mann, J., and McPherson, K. Mortality in vegetarians and non-vegetarians: detailed findings from a collaborative analysis of five prospective studies. *Am. J. Clin. Nutr.*, 10(suppl.), 516S, 1999.
123. Mills, P. K., Beeson, W. L., Phillips, R. L., and Fraser, G. E. Cohort study of diet, life-style, and prostate cancer in Adventist men. *Cancer,* 64, 598, 1989.
124. Giovanucci, E. and Willett, W. C. Dietary factors and the risk of colon cancer. *Ann. Med.*, 26, 443, 1994.
125. Willett, W. C., Hunter, D. J., Stampfer, M. J., Colditz, G., Manson, J. E., Spiegelman, D., Rosner, B., Hennekens, C. H., and Speizer, F. E. Dietary fat and fiber in relationship to risk for breast cancer: an 8-year follow-up. *J. Am. Med. Assoc.*, 268, 2037, 1992.
126. Erhardt, J. G., Lim, S. S., Bode, J. C., and Bode, C. A diet rich in fat and poor in dietary fiber increases the in vitro formation of reactive oxygen species in human feces. *J. Nutr.,* 127, 706, 1997.
127. Johansson, G., Holmen, A., Persson, L., Hogstedt, B., Wassen, C., Ottova, L., and Gustafsson, J. A. Long-term effects of a change from a mixed diet to a lacto-vegetarian diet on human urinary and faecal mutagenic activity. *Mutagenesis*, 13, 167, 1998.

16

DEVELOPING A VEGETARIAN
FOOD GUIDE

Crystal Whitten

CONTENTS

I. INTRODUCTION

A food guide is a conceptual framework for selecting different kinds and amounts of foods. Food guides may also be viewed as evolutionary attempts to define an optimal dietary pattern within a time and cultural context. Food guides are accompanied by a graphic representation that translates current knowledge and dietary recommendations into food groups, serving sizes, and a range of recommended servings that provide a nutritionally adequate diet for healthy people older than 2 years. Science

0-8493-8508-3/01/$0.00+$.50
© 2001 by CRC Press LLC

based food guides rely on data from experimental and human research, balance studies, epidemiological studies, food consumption surveys, nutrition status reports, and food composition databases, as well as a variety of cultural influences and food availability. Food guides not only translate current knowledge into healthy food choices, but should be flexible and relevant to society. They may also reflect broader issues related to food consumption such as achieving optimal health, maximizing longevity, cultural preferences, economic status, fair import-export practices, environmental concerns, efficient use of land and water resources, genetic modification of foods, and humane treatment of animals.[1-5]

II. A PERSPECTIVE ON U.S. FOOD GUIDES

An in-depth discussion of the development of U.S. food guides has been recorded by others.[3-6] This discussion is limited to characterizing the balance of animal- and plant-based proteins during the 20th century. In the early 1900s, human life span was around 50 years of age and infectious disease was the leading cause of death. Also, malnutrition was widely documented among many young men registering for military service as well as those in lower socioeconomic groups. For most of the 1900s, food guides and recommendations emphasized planning meals around meat and dairy foods. Some of the biases in modern dietary guidance may have been derived from the wording of food groups, the order of words used to describe food groups, and the graphic illustration of food groups seen in these early publications. For instance, the words "meat" and "milk" have consistently been used to define major sources as well as specific sources of protein rich foods. These words focus the user on a narrow range of protein options, and, in industrialized nations, have ultimately defined the protein-rich food groups. A second bias introduced by food guides has been the ordering of words used to describe animal and plant sources of protein. Animal proteins, without exception, are always listed first, while plant proteins, when specifically mentioned as part of the food group, have always been listed last, after meat, poultry, fish, and eggs. In addition to the qualitative bias of words used to describe protein-rich foods, food guides have quantitatively favored selection of animal protein over vegetable protein. Regarding the recommendation for milk consumption, the first food guide recommended one serving of milk per day. This amount has increased to the present recommendation of two to three servings of milk, yogurt, and cheese per day. The quantitative recommendation for meat consumption has also gradually increased over the past century. Plant-protein sources were only specifically mentioned in three of the six food guides published in the last century. The first and only time plant proteins were identified as a separate group was in the second food guide, published in 1933.[6] This guide consisted of twelve food groups, four of which targeted protein-rich foods: milk; lean meat, poultry, fish; dry mature beans, peas, and nuts; and eggs. Only one serving per week of the plant-based protein group was recommended. An example of visual bias among the food guides is the Basic Four food groups graphic, used from 1956 to 1979. The Basic Four graphic emphasized animal-based food groups by the placement of four equal boxes depicting the milk and meat groups on top of the bread–cereal and vegetable–fruit groups. It becomes apparent that a cultural bias in favor of consuming animal-based protein-rich foods has contributed to government-sponsored nutrition guidance in the 20th century, even in the presence of mounting science-based evidence to the contrary.[6-16]

The goals of the early food guides were qualitative and targeted to achieve "variety, balance, and moderation," not necessarily health and longevity. In 1941, recommended dietary allowances (RDA) were released for nine nutrients: protein, iron, calcium, vitamin A, vitamin D, thiamin, niacin, riboflavin, and vitamin C. The concept of achieving a balance between protective foods and high-energy foods moved into a quantitative arena. To meet newly established nutrient recommendations, which were primarily based on nutrient balance studies of omnivores, the U.S. government continued to emphasize protein-rich foods such as animal and dairy foods. The emphasis on animal-based food products attempted to ensure adequate intake of the B vitamins, iron, and calcium.[4-6,14,17,18]

In 1977, the U.S. Senate Select Committee on Nutrition and Human Needs (the McGovern report) issued quantitative goals for the intakes of protein, carbohydrate, fat, fatty acids, cholesterol, sugars, and sodium. However, these dietary goals stirred controversy among experts and a variety of special interest groups and were ultimately rejected by the USDA. The report was perceived as being too aggressive in limiting nutrients such as protein. Chief among their concerns was the recommendation to lower energy intake from protein to 12%, down from 16%. The quantitative goals for all the aforementioned nutrients were rejected, in part, because some experts perceived that the diets developed to reflect the lower protein recommendation were too different from the standard American diet (SAD) and some felt there was a lack of rationale in support of consuming a lower protein level.[6,18]

Today, life expectancy has increased to around 80 years of age and most Americans battle chronic diseases, many that are a result of extended life span, life-style, and dietary factors. Results of ongoing research support increased consumption of naturally occurring protective substances such as fiber, antioxidant nutrients, and phytochemicals. At the same time, overwhelming evidence suggests that most people living in industrialized countries can lower their risk of chronic, degenerative diseases by decreasing consumption of total energy, fat, saturated fat, trans fatty acids, sodium, and sugar. Plant foods such as fruits, vegetables, legumes, nuts, seeds, and whole grains are nutrient dense and are the primary foods contributing and delivering protective substances to the body. Animal products such as milk, cheese, eggs, beef, poultry, and fish are rich in energy and many nutrients, but these products lack the balance of protective substances.

The U.S. Department of Agriculture (USDA) and the Department of Health and Human Services (DHHS) are departments of the U.S. government that continuously monitor and advance nutrition policy as relevant scientific data accumulate and as food-nutrient data bases expand. In 1992, the USDA released its most recent food guide with a graphic, the Food Guide Pyramid. The pyramid was the first food guide graphic to visualize relative importance and proportionality of food groups. It should be noted that only the graphic had been changed since 1984 with the adoption of the "Better Eating for Better Health" food guidance system. However, the pyramid food groups, recommended serving ranges, frequency, and serving sizes remain the same. In 1993, the Food and Nutrition Board (FNB) set into motion the adoption of the Dietary Reference Intakes (DRI), a more complete set of reference values including the Recommended Dietary Allowances (RDA), Estimated Average Requirements (EAR), Adequate Intakes (AI), and Tolerable Upper Intake Levels (UL). Ultimately, the DRIs will allow for greater flexibility in planning healthy diets for diverse groups and individuals. U.S. food guides have traditionally reflected nutrient adequacy, and it is only recently, with the adoption of DRIs, that the government has broadened its focus and factored the prevention of chronic disease into quantitative nutrient recommendations. This leaves a gap in U.S. nutrient recommendations and the USDA Food Guide Pyramid recommendations.[4-6,19-24]

In reality, the U.S. government tends to lag behind researchers and academia in developing and recommending nutrition policy. One explanation is that the U.S. government, and even some professional organizations, have accepted and continued to accept influence from a variety of food industry organizations. These influences ultimately amount to special interests and should be minimized if science-based research is to be accurately evaluated and reflected in government-sponsored nutrition policy.

Since the USDA Food Guide Pyramid was introduced in 1992, a number of pyramid graphics have emerged. Most are adapted versions of the USDA pyramid, while a few others have been developed to reflect healthy eating patterns of people from different geographic regions or special interest groups.[25-27] Parallel to government sponsored nutrition recommendations, professional and science-based organizations, as well as academic institutions, have made and continue to regularly revise recommendations regarding food and nutrient intake.[28-31] Many of these organizations have developed their own food guides with a graphic, using widely varying research outcomes. For example, the recommendations for meat consumption by the federal government, professional, and science-based or academic organizations varies by a factor of more than two. The USDA Food Guide Pyramid recommends 5 to 7 ounces of meat consumption per day; the National Cholesterol Education Panel's Step One and Step Two diets respectively include up to 6 and 5 ounces of meat consumption per day; and the National Cancer Institute recommends no more than 3 ounces of meat consumption per day. In contrast, the Loma Linda University Vegetarian Food Guide Pyramid recommends no meat consumption.[32] For many in the scientific and academic communities, questions continue to emerge regarding how outside commercial corporations and organizations exert an influence on nutritional recommendations made by both professional organizations and the federal government. The obvious trend of the scientific and academic communities is to recommend reduced consumption of animal-based protein. Most scientists agree that reducing consumption of animal products reduces total intake of fat, saturated fat, and cholesterol while it increases the intake of dietary fiber, antioxidants, and phytochemicals. These changes in the SAD have been shown to reduce risk of cardiovascular disease and many cancers. Most science-based and professional organizations have been willing to recommend reductions in meat intake, but no organization has recommended zero animal consumption for disease prevention. For example, it is well known that people substituting fish for red meat experience significant reductions in cardiovascular disease (CVD) risk. However, those completely eliminating meat and fish experience similar or slightly greater reductions in CVD risk. This, and many other similar examples, lead one to the conclusion that there is a gap between evidence-based knowledge and dietary guidance in the U.S. This gap in government-sponsored nutrition guidance continues to mislead the public about the type, frequency, and quantities of various foods that provide a healthful, protective diet and promote optimal health.[33,34]

III. PROMOTING A SCIENCE-BASED VEGETARIAN FOOD GUIDE

For the average consumer, selecting a nutritious dietary pattern is a daily challenge. Food processing and marketing, fast food, variety, quality, availability, cultural influences, work schedules, family structure, food-related beliefs, economics, and food habits all contribute to complex dietary patterns documented among industrialized countries. During the mid 20th century, research on vegetarian populations shifted from describing nutrient deficiencies to documenting health benefits related to consuming fewer animal prducts.[35-42] In 1987, in support of vegetarian dietary practices, the American Dietetic Association adopted a position statement on vegetarian diets stating that, "appropriately planned vegetarian diets are healthful, nutritionally adequate, and provide health benefits in the prevention and treatment of certain diseases."[43] Other professional and scientific organizations have also recognized the benefits of vegetarian diets as both disease-preventive and therapeutic diets. Similar efforts have also been undertaken to promote other cultural dietary patterns based largely on plant foods. In 1994, Oldways Preservation & Exchange Trust published the Mediterranean Food Guide Pyramid.[26] This represented a significant departure from the USDA Food Guide Pyramid by depicting the dietary patterns of the different Mediterranean regions and characterizing frequency of consumption of its 10 food groups as "daily," "weekly," or "monthly." In 1998, Oldways developed and published the Asian Food Guide Pyramid. Plant-based diets are not necessarily vegetarian diets. The hallmark of many plant-based dietary patterns is the generous consumption of fruit, vegetables, whole grains, legumes, nuts, seeds, and olive oil. There is low to moderate consumption of eggs, dairy products, fish, poultry, and red meat. The Oldways pyramids represent plant-based dietary patterns of healthy populations, not necessarily achievement of nutrient standards such as the FAO/WHO recommendations or DRIs.

In the 1980s, as more Americans became interested in improving their health and nutrition, those choosing to adopt a vegetarian diet increased in numbers. It became apparent that there was a gap in appropriate nutrition guidance for these individuals. In addition, many health and nutrition professionals were ill equipped to provide sound dietary guidance, expecially to more vulnerable groups such as children and pregnant or lactating women. Adding to the confusion around the safety of consuming a vegetarian diet was the lack of a homogeneous vegetarian dietary pattern. A wide variety of dietary patterns existed and continue to exist under the term "vegetarian." With this historical backdrop in mind, a small number of scientists and academicians specializing in vegetarian research recognized it was time to describe and promote healthy vegetarian principles on a broader scale, as well as giving due diligence to potential areas of concern. In the late 1990s, vegetarian dietary practices gained enough momentum to warrant international support and promotion.

IV. THE PROCESS OF DEVELOPING THE LOMA LINDA UNIVERSITY VEGETARIAN FOOD GUIDE

In 1995, an international group of scientists, academicians, and medical practitioners with expertise in vegetarian nutrition was identified to assist in the process of developing a *de novo* vegetarian food guide with a graphic. Emphasis was placed on selecting individuals who would represent diverse vegetarian traditions and practices. Those organizing the alliance were involved with program planning for the Third International Congress on Vegetarian Nutrition, scheduled in 1997.[35] At the two previous meetings of the International Congress on Vegetarian Nutrition in 1992 and 1987, there were numerous requests for tools to use in the nutritional guidance of vegetarians. Most health practitioners were using a vegetarian-adapted USDA food guide pyramid sans meat, published by the General Conference Nutrition Council (GCNC) of Seventh-Day Adventists.[25] This pyramid has been and continues to be useful for a large number of lacto-ovo-vegetarians, but it fails to address frequency and the full continuum of vegetarian philosophy related to the degree of excluding animal products from the diet.

The following considerations contributed to the formation of an alliance to develop a vegetarian food guide:

1. When proper guidelines are applied, vegetarian diets promote adequate growth and development, and meet the nutritional needs of healthy individuals throughout the life cycle.
2. Evidence-based research on the dietary patterns of vegetarian populations had been observed and described and the data were available in the scientific literature.
3. Epidemiological data on vegetarians in Western countries over the last 4 decades had documented lower risk for most chronic diseases, increased longevity, lower body weight, lower blood pressure, and improved overall health status of vegetarians.
4. Results of experimental clinical trials and epidemiological research indicated that those consuming higher levels of plant foods had reduced risk for several chronic diseases, while those consuming higher levels of meat and animal fat had increased risks.[32]

A diverse international alliance of people with expertise in vegetarian nutrition was identified. Next, each member received a letter of invitation and a Questionnaire to Aid in the Development of a Vegetarian Food Guide (Figure 16.1). Based on the initial responses, a draft of the food guide supporting script and possible graphic illustration formats were shared with the contributors. The group eventually met in person to discuss the issues and select a graphic format in a consensus-building process.

A. Principles for Planning Healthy Vegetarian Diets

Recurrent themes of the respondents' comments were refined to what were termed *Principles of Healthy Vegetarian Diets* (see Table 16.1). These

---

Questionnaire to Aid in the Development of a Vegetarian Food Guide

---

Instructions: Please fill out the following questionnaire by answering both the yes/no questions and also responding to the open-ended questions. Should you need additional space, include additional pages.

1. The following are several possible applications of a vegetarian food guide. Which one(s) are the most important? When in conflict, which one(s) should prevail?
    A. Develop a food guide for the person wanting to become a vegetarian.
    B. Develop an "ideal" vegetarian food guide.
    C. Develop a guide that is flexible and applicable to a range of vegetarian practices.
    D. Develop a vegetarian food guide to aid in the prevention of chronic disease.
    E. Develop a vegetarian food guide that meets the requirements of the RDA's.
2. Should this vegetarian food guide apply primarily to people in developed countries (Western societies) or also to developing countries?
3. What criteria would you recommend to define a food grouping (i.e., common nutrients, botanical classification, cultural preferences, etc.)?
4. What foods should be included in a vegetarian food guide?
5. What foods, if any, should be excluded from a vegetarian food guide?
6. What foods would you define as a separate grouping in a vegetarian food guide?
7. In developing a new vegetarian food guide, how should the RDAs be used to guide the process? For example, should the lowest RDA for calcium be used or the highest RDA level for calcium be used? Or maybe ignore the RDA and use more recent research?
8. In designing a vegetarian food guide, how should epidemiological data be used? How should nutrition studies be used? Which has greater weight? For example, researchers have identified groups of people who are at very low risk of chronic disease, however, diets of these groups may fail to meet the RDA standards in certain nutrient categories.
9. Should the vegetarian food guide be flexible in its design, including guidelines for total vegetarians, lacto-ovo-vegetarians, and other modifications, or should this committee focus on one vegetarian philosophy?
10. Should a point system be used to designate nutrient-dense foods?
11. What graphic format would be best utilized in developing a vegetarian food guide?

    ————Pyramid   _____Star   _____Pie/Plate/Wheel
    _____Column   _____Table of foods   _____Other

Figure 16.1   Questionnaire to Aid in the Development of a Vegetarian Food Guide.

principles represent the basis for food selection and meal planning for diverse vegetarian populations. The following is a summary of these concepts and the underlying rationale for their selection.

The first principle, "*consume a variety and abundance of plant foods,*" positively emphasizes the daily consumption of a variety of healthy,

Table 16.1   Principles of Healthy Vegetarian Diets

- Consume a variety and abundance of plant foods.
- Primarily consume unrefined, minimally processed plant foods.
- Consumption of dairy products and/or eggs is optional.
- Consuming a wide range of fat from plants is compatible with health.
- Consume a generous amount of water and other fluids.
- Pay attention to other healthy life-style factors

protective plant foods. Plant foods include: whole grains (e.g., wheat, rice, oats, barley, gluten- and grain-based products and beverages), legumes (e.g., peas, lentils, beans, soy-based products and soy beverages), vegetables, fruits, nuts, seeds, plant oils, sweeteners, herbs, and spices. In principle, the daily consumption of a variety of foods from all of the plant groups, in quantities to meet energy needs, can provide all of the nutrients needed by humans except for vitamins B_{12} and D. Diets providing ample plant foods are low in total and saturated fat, and are high in fiber, folate, antioxidant nutrients, and phytochemicals. Consumption of a variety of plants contributes thousands of substances that are protective, many of which continue to be described and quantified.

The second principle, *"primarily consume unrefined, minimally processed plant foods,"* highlights consumption of plant foods that contain more vitamins, minerals, and dietary fiber than their refined and highly processed counterparts. Although most vegetables, fruits, nuts, and legumes can be consumed with minimal refinement, this is not the case for foods derived from grains. Regular consumption of whole grains is associated with a lower risk of heart disease, some cancers, and diabetes. However, the food industry has reaped massive profits from refining grains to the point where many grain products must be fortified to replace some of the nutrients lost to processing. This aspect of food processing has robbed the consumer of achieving optimal nutrition by removing beneficial substances and, oftentimes, in addition to mandated fortification practices, adding back other less-than-desirable chemicals. However, not all aspects of food processing are deleterious. Food processing may play an important role in the enrichment of plant-based foods with vitamin B_{12}, calcium, vitamin D, and other nutrients. Plant-based food products enriched with specific nutrients may be nutritionally valuable adjuncts to a vegetarian diet. This aspect of food processing should be evaluated for long-term benefits among vegetarians. In general, a diet based on unrefined and minimally processed food is more likely to supply the optimal balance of protective substances needed to promote health and prevent disease.

The third principle, "*consumption of dairy products and/or eggs is optional*," recognizes that some vegetarians (i.e., vegans) opt to limit dairy products and eggs. The consumption of dairy products and eggs is not necessary to achieve RDAs, but is often practiced for convenience and practicality. Quantitatively, consumption of dairy products and eggs by vegetarians varies from infrequent to daily. Vegetarian diets that include dairy products, eggs, or both (i.e., lacto-ovo-vegetarian diets), easily provide all the nutrients required by healthy adults. In population studies, such diets have been shown to be healthful and promote longevity, with no need for routine nutrient supplementation. Because some dairy products are high in fat and saturated fat, it is preferable to emphasize nonfat and low-fat options. Consumption of eggs should be evaluated on an individual basis relative to health and economic status.

Vegans represent a sub-group of vegetarians who rely completely on plants to meet all their nutrient needs. This dietary pattern requires due diligence to several nutrients that may be inadequately consumed: vitamin B_{12}, vitamin D, calcium, and linolenic acid. This is particularly important for vulnerable groups such as growing children, pregnant or lactating women, and older adults.

The requirement for protein is easily met by vegans' consuming adequate amounts of plants such as legumes, lentils, peas, whole grains, nuts, and seeds. However, there is potential for inadequate protein intake when overall kilocalorie needs are not met. Long-term inadequate consumption of protein may lead to muscle wasting or extreme thinness, disturbances in GI function, and immune or neurological dysfunction.

Vitamin B_{12} is the only vitamin not found in the plant kingdom. It was isolated in 1948 and synthesized in 1963. This made it possible to consume a vegan diet that included vitamin B_{12} either in pill form (oral or sublingual), added in processing to other plant foods, or as an injection prescribed by a physician. All vegans need to identify a regular and reliable source of vitamin B_{12}, either as a supplement or a fortified plant-based food.

Vegans also need to plan for obtaining vitamin D, whether by regular exposure to sunlight or regular consumption of vitamin D-fortified plant-based foods. In the U.S., the principal dietary source of vitamin D is fortified cow's milk. Diets that exclude cow's milk may require a supplemental source of vitamin D. A non-food source of this vitamin is daily exposure of unprotected skin to sunlight. Inadequate exposure to sunlight is more likely to occur in northern latitudes and during the winter months. Those with inadequate exposure to sunlight and inadequate dietary intake of cow's milk should be advised to consume vitamin D-fortified plant foods such as breakfast cereals, soy- or grain-based beverages, energy bars, candy, and a variety of other foods.

Historically, those eliminating dairy products have had greater difficult meeting the calcium RDA. However, in addition to almonds and leafy green vegetables, options for consuming plant-based sources of calcium have expanded to include calcium-fortified products such as soy and grain beverages, orange juice, energy bars, candy, bread, and calcium-precipitated tofu. New food products containing significant amounts of calcium will continue to become available, allowing for convenient consumption of calcium. In addition to fortified food producs, a wide array of calcium supplements may offer reliable sources of calcium for vegetarians.

Linolenic acid is an essential fatty acid, primarily found in the following plant foods: flax seed, walnuts, soybeans, soybean oil, tofu, and canola oil. It is also found in minute amounts in green leafy vegetables and wheat germ. Vegans should plan for regular and adequate consumption of linolenic acid.

The fourth principle, *"consuming a wide range of fat from plants is compatible with health,"* refers to the many highly diverse vegetarian dietary patterns that have been described in the scientific literature. Significant sources of plant fats include nuts, nut butters, seeds, avocados, olives, soy, coconut, and plant oils. Vegetarian diets are frequently equated with low-fat cardiac diets and various therapeutic diets. Very low-fat vegetarian diets (i.e., 10–15% energy from fat) have proven helpful in therapeutic approaches to disease management. In general, vegetarian dietary patterns contain less saturated fat, cholesterol, and trans fatty acids.

The fat content of vegetarian dietary patterns may represent an additional philosophical difference among vegetarians. The fat content of both lacto-ovo and vegan dietary patterns can vary widely from a very low fat content (<20% energy from fat) to a mid range of fat content (20 to 30% energy from fat) to a higher range of fat content (>30% energy from fat). The vegetable oils food group was designated as optional to provide for the maximal adjustment of fat intake (see Figure 16.2). Placement of the vegetable oils food group could have been either below or above the optional line. However, vegans frequently prefer to consume primarily "whole" plant fats and tend to avoid highly processed forms of fat. Most vegetable oils are processed to some degree. Olive and nut oils are pressed and therefore not as processed as other vegetable oils. Those consuming foods from the core plant food groups will primarily consume intact plant fats such as nuts, seeds, avocado, olives, coconut, and soybeans.

In reality, the average total fat intake of vegetarians is difficult to characterize and varies widely (from 15 to 40% of daily energy). Currently, public health recommendations targeted at the general population are to limit total fat intake to <30% of energy intake. This recommendation is supported by data from Western populations, where most dietary fat comes from animal foods, animal fats, and processed, high fat, snack-type foods. It is unclear whether the same recommendations regarding fat intake

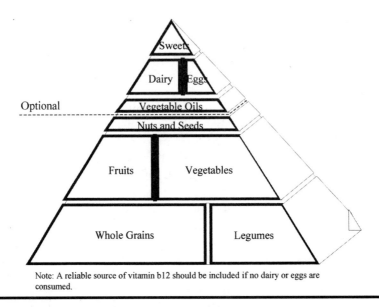

Note: A reliable source of vitamin b12 should be included if no dairy or eggs are consumed.

Figure 16.2   Loma Linda University Food Guide Pyramid.

should apply to vegetarians whose dietary fat consumption is primarily from unrefined plant fats. Among vegetarian populations, it appears that when energy intake is balanced with energy output, a whole range of fat intake, primarily from plant fats, is compatible with excellent health.

Fluid intake among vegetarian populations is higher when compared with the general population. The fifth principle, "*consume a generous amount of water and other fluids*," refers to the consumption of water, freshly prepared fruit and vegetable juices, and green and herbal teas. Green tea may represent an additional dietary source of antioxidants and phytochemicals in the diet not specifically mentioned in any of the plant food groups. Green tea, the least processed of all teas, has been consumed by plant-based Asian populations for nearly 5,000 years. Green tea provides a generous array of many antioxidants, including the flavonoids. Published reports suggest that the tradition of regularly consuming green tea may prevent or delay formation of tumors and reduce the risk of heart disease and stroke.[44-48] In summary, a generous intake of water and a variety of other fluids represents another characteristic of a healthy vegetarian dietary pattern.

The group discussed the inclusion of alcohol, but after careful evaluation of the available data, the following reasons formed the rationale for not including alcohol in the pyramid graphic and supporting document:

1. Most scientific data supporting the health benefits of vegetarian diets are from vegetarian populations that do not consume alcohol.
2. There is no evidence that adding alcohol to the diet of a low-risk vegetarian population will further lower the overall risk of chronic diseases.
3. The inclusion of alcohol may compromise acceptance of the food guide by a large segment of vegetarians. In addition, it should be noted that many of the protective factors identified in red wine can also be found in grape juice, which is considered part of the fruit group on the pyramid graphic.[49]

The sixth principle, *"pay attention to other healthy life-style factors,"* refers to healthy life-style practices seen among many vegetarians such as regular physical activity, frequent exposure to sunlight and fresh air, adequate rest, limiting prolonged exposure to stress, and avoidance of harmful practices such as smoking and excessive alcohol consumption. Diet is one of several behavioral factors that influence health status; other life-style factors should be addressed as well in the context of optimizing nutrition guidance and obtaining positive health outcomes.

B. Graphic Format of the Vegetarian Guide

The pyramid shape was chosen for its familiarity, flexibility, and current usage among consumers. Next, the principles of healthy vegetarian diets were used to guide identification and placement of the food groups. Beginning with the bottom of the pyramid, food groups were arranged in tiers based on ascending relative importance, proportionality, and frequency, and in such a way as to encompass the two most common vegetarian traditions: lacto-ovo and vegan. The food guide depicts nine food groups: whole grains, legumes, vegetables, fruits, nuts and seeds, vegetable oils, dairy, eggs, and sweets. The five major plant-based food groups (whole grains, legumes, vegetables, fruits, and nuts and seeds) form the vegan trapezoid. This lower portion of the pyramid illustrates the core plant food groups which, when consumed in adequate amounts, constitute the backbone of any healthy vegetarian dietary pattern (Figure 16.3). Some vegetarians will primarily use the trapezoid section for dietary guidance.

A line was drawn between the third and fourth tiers. Depicted above the line are the four optional food groups that may be added to the core plant food groups to meet the need for dietary guidance of lacto-ovo vegetarians. Depending on the philosophical values and health beliefs of individual vegetarians, one or more of the optional food groups (vegetable oils, dairy products, eggs, and sweets) may be included in the diet. The

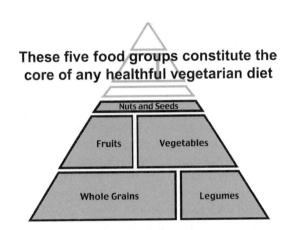

These five food groups constitute the core of any healthful vegetarian diet

Nuts and Seeds

Fruits | Vegetables

Whole Grains | Legumes

Figure 16.3 **Loma Linda University Vegetarian Food Guide Pyramid, Trapezoid bottom.**

consensus reached was that a line used to separate the core food groups from the optional food groups would facilitate the acceptance and use of the pyramid graphic by the majority of diverse vegetarians. It was also decided that a statement should appear on the graphic about the necessity of vitamin B_{12} supplementation for individuals consuming a strict vegan dietary pattern. The inclusion of fortified plant foods or foods from the dairy or egg food groups may facilitate the intake of selected nutrients, particularly vitamins B_{12} and D, but may also increase the consumption of total energy, saturated fat, and cholesterol.

Three of the healthy life-style factors documented among vegetarian populations are represented graphically outside the food pyramid. They include frequent exposure to sunlight, regular physical activity, and the abundant consumption of water and fluids. Positive dietary and life-style factors synergistically contribute to the health and longevity documented among vegetarians.

C. Number of Servings and Frequency of Food Groups

The pyramid format was initially a concept intended primarily for a scientific audience. Subsequent to the introduction of the vegetarian pyramid and supporting document at the Third International Congress on Vegetarian Nutrition, a sub group added numbers of servings to each of the food groups. These additions have provided health care professionals with a practical tool to aid in providing specific dietary guidance for vegetarians.[50]

Seven different cultural dietary patterns were characterized and analyzed: Western, Western fast food and meat analog, Hispanic, Mediterranean-

Italian, Mediterranean Middle Eastern, Asian, and Continental Indian. Multiple vegan and lacto-ovo-vegetarian dietary patterns were developed for each cultural variation. Except for the Western fast food and meat analog variation, menus were based on homemade meals. Initially, cultural menus were written only to reflect the actual food consumption patterns. Natives and cookbooks from each cultural tradition were consulted to ensure accurate representation of each dietary pattern. Target energy intakes for each cultural variation were set at 1600 kcal, 2000 kcal, and 2500 kcal. Initially, the 2000 kcal menus were developed and adjusted either upward or downward to achieve the target energy increments. The amounts of dairy or eggs included at the 2000 kcal level were not used to adjust energy intake.

After the cultural dietary patterns were completed and evaluated for accuracy, nutrient analysis was performed for each cultural variation using computerized nutrition software. Results of nutrient analysis indicated that all vitamins and minerals analyzed for (the exceptions were several trace minerals with three or more missing values) were at or above 90% of the RDA. Next, the number of servings for each food group was determined for each cultural variation and energy level. Using the multiple dietary patterns for each culture and energy level, the mean number of servings and standard deviations were determined. The standard deviations were used to determine a range of servings for each food group within a cultural dietary pattern. Not surprisingly, the range of servings for the core food groups was higher for all vegan cultural variations. The range of servings for each food group among the lacto-ovo dietary patterns were lower to allow for inclusion of more energy-dense foods from the dairy, egg, and sweets food groups.

In an attempt to simplify the application of the pyramid graphic, the vegan and lacto-ovo dietary patterns were merged to one set of ranges of servings (see Figure 16.4). Those consuming a primarily vegan pattern are advised to favor the upper serving numbers depicted in the trapezoid section. Those consuming a lacto- or ovo-vegetarian dietary pattern are advised to select the numbers of servings that correspond with the lower to middle range of servings. Energy intake may be adjusted by choosing a number from either the lower, middle, or upper range.

Standard serving sizes were chosen to allow the consumer to adjust calorie intake and meet nutrient needs (Table 16.2). It was important to use standard serving sizes to facilitate optimal use of the pyramid through the delivery of accurate dietary guidance and assessment. When properly planned, vegetarian diets provide adequate, if not optimal, nutrition for people at all stages of the life cycle as well as athletes and those seeking therapeutic results. However, those consuming a vegetarian dietary pattern limited in variety and quantity will find it more difficult to obtain the

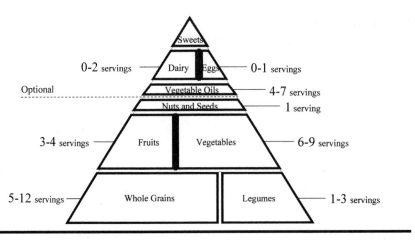

Figure 16.4   Loma Linda University Vegetarian Food Guide. Number of servings.

recommended nutrients and experience the positive health benefits ascribed to many vegetarians. As with any other dietary pattern, adherence to sound nutrition principles is important.

D. Vegetarian Food Groups

Whole Grains. Consumption of whole grains is emphasized in most dietary patterns around the world. Major whole grains include wheat, rice, and corn. Minor grains include oats, triticale, sorghum, and millet.[51,52] The term "whole grains" more accurately reflects minimally processed, optimal food choices such as whole grain breads, crackers, cereals, pasta, and rice. Placement of the whole grain and legume food groups on the bottom of the pyramid reflects the majority of plant-based dietary patterns seen around the world as well as the importance and proportionality of whole grains in the diet. Regular inclusion of whole grain foods in the diet is more likely to decrease risk of heart disease, some cancers, and diabetes, while regular consumption of refined grain food products does not appear to confer similar benefits. Refined grains are used more within industrialized, developed countries. Refining grain includes removing the endosperm and bran, hydrolyzing the starch, modifying size and texture, adding flavoring agents, and adding preservatives. In addition to the refining process, some lost nutrients may be replaced, which is known as enrichment. In the U.S., refined-grain bread is enriched with iron, thiamin, niacin, and riboflavin. More recently, U.S. policy has mandated that grain products should also be fortified with folate. Some breakfast cereals are highly fortified and one serving provides 100% of all the RDAs. However, these cereals may be highly refined, and while they are nutritious

Table 16.2   Loma Linda University Vegetarian Food Guide Pyramid: Suggested Number of Servings and Serving Sizes

Food Group	Number of Servings	Suggested Serving Sizes
Whole Grains	5–12	• 1 slice bread • 1/2 bun, bagel, muffin • 1/2 cup cooked cereal, rice, pasta • 3/4 cup flaked cereal • 1 1/2 cup puffed cereal
Legumes	1–3	• 1/2 cup cooked beans, lentils, peas • 4 oz tofu or tempeh • 1 cup soy beverage
Vegetables	6–9	• 1 cup raw vegetable • 1/2 cup cooked vegetable • 3/4 cup vegetable juice
Fruits	3–4	• 1 piece fresh fruit • 1 cup cubed fresh fruit such as melons, berries • 3/4 cup 100% fruit juice • 1/2 cup canned or cooked fruit
Nuts and Seeds	1	• 1 ounce nuts • 2 Tbsp ground nuts or seeds • 2 Tbsp seeds
Vegetable Oils	4–7	• 1 tsp vegetable oil
Dairy	0–2	• 1 cup milk or yogurt • 1 ounce cheese • 1/4 cup cottage cheese
Eggs	0-1	• 1 egg • 2 egg whites
Sweets		• Use sparingly

with respect to added nutrients, they do not contain the full spectrum of nutrients originally found in the whole grain version.[51-53] Nutrients common to whole grains include B vitamins, protein, fiber, iron, phytochemicals, and a number of trace and ultra trace minerals. Whole grains should be consumed daily.

Some vegetarians consume grains in the form of meat analogs primarily consisting of gluten. Gluten is the high-protein part of milled wheat. Gluten flour may be processed into different forms such as patties, balls, "burgers," and a variety of other shapes. Gluten is relatively high in protein, and is more comparable in protein content to legumes than whole grains. For example, one-quarter cup of gluten flour provides 14.5 grams of protein compared with one-half cup of pinto beans, which provides 7.9 grams of protein, and one-quarter cup of white flour, which provides 3.2 grams of protein.[54]

On average, half of the U.S. population is lactose intolerant; within the Asian, Hispanic, and African American communities, the percentage of lactose-intolerant persons is even greater. For this reason, among others, many people are turning to an ever-increasing variety of grain- and soy-based beverages as alternatives to cow's milk. For many adults, substituting a grain-based beverage for cow's milk poses no health risk. However, without proper dietary guidance, substituting a grain-based beverage for cow's milk may result in inadequate consumption of some nutrients among vulnerable groups such as children, teens, pregnant and lactating women, and some older adults. Traditionally, cow's milk has provided significant amounts of five important nutrients: protein, calcium, vitamin D, riboflavin, and vitamin B_{12}. Soy beverages are comparable to cow's milk in protein content, but levels of the other nutrients vary. Grain beverages provide riboflavin, but do not significantly contribute protein, calcium, vitamin D, and vitamin B_{12}. It is important to evaluate these nutrients before purchasing soy- or grain-based beverages. Unless fortified with protein, grain beverages may not be the best substitute for milk or soy beverages for children, teens, pregnant and lactating women, and older adults. Table 16.3 provides guidelines for evaluating the nutritional contributions of soy- and grain-based beverages.

Vegetarians typically consume almost twice as much dietary fiber as the average American. In the U.S., the average consumption of dietary fiber is 12 to 17 grams. Recommendations for fiber intake range from 20 to 35 grams, with intakes as high as 60 grams per day considered safe. Focusing on the regular consumption of whole grains will support a higher intake of dietary fiber.

Legumes, Lentils, Peas. In 1966, the average consumption of legumes in the U.S. was 1 gram per day, compared with Mediterranean populations, which consumed an average of 30 grams per day. In 1997, per capita consumption of legumes in the U.S. had jumped to almost 10 grams per day (excluding peanuts). Since 1966, Americans have gradually begun to embrace the legume, but consumption continues to lag behind that of many other countries.[55-57] In vegetarian dietary patterns, legumes are regularly consumed and often contribute to the main entree. Placement of the legume food group on the bottom of the pyramid with whole grains is consistent with many healthy vegetarian dietary patterns observed around the world. It is also consistent with the increased availability of legume products such as soy beverages, soy-based meat analogs, bean chips, and other legume-based products.

Legumes are botanically categorized as vegetables, but their nutrient contributions differ significantly from most vegetables. A half-cup serving of most legumes provides 7 grams of protein, which is roughly equivalent to 1 ounce of meat. Nutrients found in legumes, lentils, and peas include: protein, fibers, thiamin, folate, calcium, phosphorus, potassium, iron, phytochemicals, and many trace minerals. Legumes also contain the oligosaccharides raffinose and stachyose. which promote the growth of the beneficial bifido bacteria in the gut. The down side to consumption of oligosaccharides relates to methane production in the colon and, for some, excessive flatulence.[54-57]

Among legumes, the soybean possesses unique nutrient characteristics. Soybeans provide high-quality protein equivalent to animal protein. One-half cup of firm tofu provides almost 20 grams of soy protein. Soybeans uniquely protect against cardiovascular disease, cancer, osteoporosis, and menopausal symptoms.[58]

Soy beverages are legume based, but many food guides place them in the milk-dairy category. Soy beverages may be plain, flavored, defatted, or fortified. Taste and nutrient profiles, and the color and consistency of soy beverages vary from product to product. As previously stated, soy beverages are similar to cow's milk in protein content, but vary in calcium, riboflavin, vitamin D, and vitamin B_{12} content. See Table 16.3 for guidelines to use when evaluating soy- and grain-based beverages for nutrient desirability.

Meat analogs are now materializing in mainstream food markets around the world. Meat analogs are usually made from soy protein or gluten. Food manufacturers of meat analogs have been successful in imitating hamburgers, hot dogs, scallops, sausage, bacon, bacon bits, luncheon meats, and a variety of other meat counterparts. Nutrient content and degree of processing vary among products. Many are fortified with a number of nutrients, most notably vitamin B_{12}, making some products good food choices for vegans.

Vegetables. The distinction between vegetables and fruits has traditionally been a cultural one. Many foods considered to be vegetables are botanically classified as fruits. Vegetables can be sub categorized as: starchy, leafy green, orange-yellow, and sea. With the exception of starchy vegetables, most vegetables contain relatively little carbohydrate, and are abundant in vitamins, minerals, antioxidants, and phytochemicals. Consumption of vegetables may also provide a small amount of protein, fiber, calcium, iron, and trace nutrients. Vegetarians tend to consume the current minimum recommendation of vegetables.

Fruit. The fruit group includes not only fresh fruit, but frozen, dried, and canned fruit, and fruit juice. Fruits tend to be higher in carbohydrate than vegetables. Nutrient content varies, but most fruits provide fiber,

Table 16.3   Comparison Criteria for Evaluating Soy and Grain-based Beverages[20,21]

Nutrients	RDA/DRI	Soy and Grain Beverages	Nonfat Cow's Milk
KCAL	2,200–3,000 kcal/day	80 (65–160 kcal/cup)	86 kcal/cup
Protein	46 to 63 gram/day	2–10 gm/cup	
		Recommend 4+ gm pro/cup	8.4 gram/cup
Fat	15–30% total kcal/day	4 (0–6 gm/cup)	0.4 gram/cup
Calcium	1,000 to 1,200 mg/day	0–10 mg if not fortified	302 mg/cup
		Recommend 20% + DRI/cup	0 mcg if not fortified
Vitamin D	5–10 mcg/day	0 mcg if not fortified	
		Recommend 20%+ DRI/cup	
Riboflavin	1.1 to 1.3 mg/day	0.17 mg/cup	0.34 mg/cup
		Recommend 20% + DRI/cup	
Vitamin B_{12}	2.4 mcg/day	0 mcg if not fortified	0.93 mcg/cup
		Recommend 20% + DRI/cup	

Used with permission

vitamins A and C, B vitamins, minerals, antioxidants, and phytochemicals. Vegetarians typically consume the recommended amount of fruit.

Nuts and Seeds. Vegetarians consume more nuts and seeds than their omnivore counterparts. Unrefined plant sources of fat such as nuts and seeds are prominent in plant-based diets as well as many vegetarian dietary patterns. According to surveys, vegetarians consume more nuts and do so more frequently than non-vegetarians.[59,60] This is not a recent or a local phenomenon. In India, where there is a millennium of vegetarian tradition, peanuts and peanut oils are a prominent part of the diet.

Studies of some vegetarian populations in Western countries have shown daily energy intakes of up to 15% from nuts. Vegetarian Seventh-Day Adventists in California eat nuts more frequently than their non-vegetarian counterparts, and much more frequently than the general population. The Adventist Health Study reported that those consuming nuts ≥ five times per week lowered their risk of heart disease by 50%, and increased their life expectancy by several years compared with those who infrequently ate nuts.[59,60] Experimental trials have shown that specific nuts lower blood lipids. Similar beneficial effects have also been reported for olive oil, avocados, and other unrefined, fat-rich plant foods. A surprise finding was that those consuming nuts and seeds as part of their daily dietary pattern were more likely to maintain a desirable body weight. Because of their unique nutrient contributions and their inclusion among a variety of vegetarian populations, nuts and seeds are depicted on the pyramid as one of the five core plant-food groups.[61-63]

Nuts and seeds can be consumed whole, ground into a nut or seed butter, or as an ingredient. Regular consumption of several nuts such as almonds, coconuts, macadamias, pecans, and walnuts has been shown to have beneficial effects on reducing risk of various chronic diseases.[69-78]

Nuts and seeds are concentrated sources of nutrients. Nutrient content of nuts and seeds varies, but the spectrum of nuts and seeds provides fat, protein, fiber, B vitamins, vitamin E, vitamin A, iron, calcium, copper, magnesium, manganese, phosphorus, potassium, selenium, zinc, ultra trace minerals, and phytochemicals.

Seeds include flax, pumpkin, sesame, and sunflower seeds. A unique characteristic of flax seed and walnuts is their relatively high content of the essential fatty acid alpha linolenic acid (18:3). Vegetarians do not consume animal sources of the omega three fatty acids, docosahexaenoic acid (DHA) and eicosapentaenoic acid (EPA). Consuming plant sources of alpha linolenic acid such as one serving of flax seed, walnuts, Canola oil, and soybean products provides the precursor fatty acid needed for the synthesis of DHA and EPA in vegetarians.

Fats/Vegetable Oils. Fats can be categorized as animal or dairy fat (butter, sour cream, lard, mayonnaise, cream cheese), plant whole fat (avocado, olives, and coconut), vegetable and nut oils (processed, pressed) and hydrogenated or trans fatty acids (margarine, shortening, salad dressings). Plant fats such as avocado may also be culturally considered a vegetable, or botanically considered a fruit. Animal and hydrogenated fats generally contribute a greater amount of saturated fatty acids. Plant fats and vegetable oils contribute more monounsaturated and polyunsaturated fatty acids. Most plant fats and vegetable oils have been shown to have neutral to beneficial effects on the risk of CVD, while animal, hydrogenated, and trans fatty acids increase risk of CVD. Most scientists agree that monounsaturated fatty acids should contribute at least half of the total fat intake. Vegetarian dietary patterns are more likely to meet the recommendations for fat intake, including total fat and percentage of polyunsaturated, monounsaturated, and saturated fatty acids.

The title of vegetable oils best represented the fat category for healthy vegetarian populations. Animal-fat consumption by vegetarians is typically from dairy products and eggs. Food products containing hydrogenated fats represent less-than-desirable food choices, but can be considered part of the vegetable oil food group.

Milk/Dairy. Among vegetarians, there appears to be a continuum of intake of dairy products. Some vegetarians may consume a majority of protein not from meat, but from milk, cheese, yogurt, and cottage cheese. Other vegetarians consume little to no animal-based protein. Most vegetarians consume milk and milk products such as buttermilk, cheese, yogurt, kefir, and ice cream. In the U.S., dairy products supply 72% of calcium intake. Those drinking milk consume 80% more calcium than non-milk consumers. Additional nutrient contributions of milk include lactose, protein, fat, saturated fat, cholesterol, vitamin A, vitamin D, riboflavin, folate, vitamin B_{12}, magnesium, potassium, phosphorus, sodium, and a variety of other minerals. Since 1970, consumption of full-fat milk and dairy products has decreased, while consumption of low- to nonfat milk and dairy products is up. Cheese consumption has increased significantly. Low- to nonfat milk and dairy products are preferable to full-fat versions. Due to strong support from the dairy industry, consumption of dairy products is likely to continue. However, as more plant-based alternatives to dairy products continue to emerge, the consumer will be able to consume fewer animal-based products.

Eggs. Eggs provide inexpensive, high-biological-value protein, 5 to 6 grams of fat, and 213 mg of cholesterol. Egg whites contain no fat or cholesterol. Because of their nutrient profile, eggs are typically placed in the meat-substitute group, which also includes legumes, nuts, seeds, and tofu. This may confuse some, since the daily number of servings recommended for this group is usually between two and three. Most health professionals would not recommend this level of egg consumption. However, another option is to place eggs in a separate food group and provide appropriate recommendations relative to the health status of the individual. Placing eggs in a separate food group also provides for an easy distinction between vegan, lacto-vegetarian, ovo-vegetarian, and lacto-ovo-vegetarian dietary patterns.

Sweets. Sweets are typically combinations of two or more food groups. Most sweets contain sugar, refined flour, butter or margarine or oil, eggs, cream, and various other ingredients. Processed sweets often contain hydrogenated oils as well as oxidized cholesterol. Sweets or desserts should be consumed in moderation and should be limited when weight maintenance or weight loss is desired. In some cultures, the final course, or the dessert, is fresh fruit. Many living in industrialized countries could benefit by adopting this practice.

Miscellaneous Foods. Some foods commonly consumed by vegetarians are not easily categorized into a food group. Blackstrap molasses is a good source of calcium, magnesium, iron, and potassium. One tablespoon provides 170 mg calcium. Blackstrap molasses can be used in baking or added to foods. Vegans may also consume Red Star T6635 brand nutritional yeast as a reliable source of vitamin B_{12}, iron, and other B vitamins. Herbs and spices are beneficial plants that have been largely ignored by those providing dietary guidance. Herbs and spices provide concentrated sources of many vitamins, minerals, antioxidants, and phytochemicals. Parsley, cilantro, basil, coriander, turmeric, and many others have been shown to result in a variety of physiological consequences from anti-carcinogenesis to anti-thrombosis effects. Future consideration should be given to placing herbs and spices on a food guide.

V. CONCLUSIONS

Food guides will continue to evolve in an attempt to accurately represent healthy dietary paterns. Those involved in developing food guides will be compelled to review science-based outcomes and compare with current practices. By describing the ideal dietary pattern in broad general terms, academia, professional organizations, and governments should work together in developing and promoting healthier dietary patterns such as vegetarian and plant-based patterns. Efforts to characterize nutrient intake, dietary patterns, and the many additional healthy lifestyle characteristics of vegetarians should expand to include all ages across the life span, as well as those of different ethnicity. Attempts to provide current and useful nutritional guidance for vegetarians should be ongoing. Due diligence is also required to avoid unnecessary pitfalls related to nutrient deficiencies and disease states.

Additional issues the scientific community may address in future food guides could include, among others:

- plant-based foods offered at restaurant and fast food establishments
- enrichment or fortification of plant foods
- processing of plant foods
- combination plant foods
- energy requirements
- body weight issues among vegetarian groups
- culturally distinct plant foods
- genetically altered plant foods
- functional plant foods

Food guides are powerful educational tools and political statements. As the weight of scientific evidence tips in favor of diets based largely on plant foods, issues regarding the practical applications of vegetarian nutrition can no longer be ignored. The development of a vegetarian food guide that is flexible and useable by diverse vegetarian traditions, such as the one presented in this chapter, is useful to both consumers and health professionals.

REFERENCES

1. Gussow, J. Ecology and vegetarian considerations: does environmental responsibility demand the elimination of livestock? *Am. J. Clin. Nutr.* 1994;59: 1110S-1116S.
2. Nestle, M. Animal v. plant foods in human diets and health: is the historical record unequivocal? *Proc. Nutr. Soc.* 1999;58:211-218.
3. Messina, M. and Messina, V. The Dietitian's Guide to Vegetarian Diets. Gaithersburg, MD: Aspen Publishers, Inc., 1996.
4. Ziegler, E.E. and Filer, L.J., Eds. Present Knowledge in Nutrition, 7th ed. ISLI Press, Washington, D.C., 1996.
5. Shils, M.E., et al., Eds. Modern Nutrition in Health and Disease, 9th ed. Baltimore, MD: Williams & Wilkins, 1999.
6. USDA Food Guide Background and Development. U.S. Dept Agriculture, Miscellaneous Publication No. 1514, 1993.
7. Hunt, C.L. Food for Young Children. U.S. Dept of Agriculture, Farmers' Bulletin No. 717, 1916.
8. Hunt, C.L. A Week's Food for an Average Family. U.S. Dept of Agriculture, Farmers' Bulletin No. 1228, 1921.
9. Hunt, C.L. Good Proportions in the Diet. U.S. Dept of Agriculture, Farmers' Bulletin No. 1313, 1923.
10. Hunt, C.L. and Atwater, H.W. How to Select Foods. U.S. Dept of Agriculture, Farmers' Bulletin No. 808, 1917.
11. National Dairy Council. A Guide to Good Eating. Chicago: National Dairy Council leaflet, 1941.
12. Stiebeling, H.K. and Clark, F. Planning for Good Nutrition. In Food and Life: Yearbook of Agriculture, 1939.
13. Stiebeling, H.K. and Ward, M. Diets at Four Levels of Nutrition Content and Cost. U.S. Dept of Agriculture, Circ. No. 296, 1933.
14. U.S. Dept of Agriculture, War Food Administration. National Wartime Nutrition Guide, leaflet, 1943.
15. U.S. Department of Agriculture. Food for Fitness: A Daily Food Guide. USDA Leaflet No 424. Washington, D.C.: Agricultural Research Service, 1958.
16. U.S. Department of Agriculture. Food: the Hassle-Free Guide to a Better Diet. Home and Garden Bulletin No. 122.
17. U.S. Dept of Agriculture, Science and Education Administration. The Hassle-Free Guide to a Better Diet. Leaflet No. 567, 1980.
18. U.S. Senate Select Committee on Nutrition and Human Needs. Dietary Goals for the United States, 2nd ed. Washington D.C., U.S. Government Printing Office, 1977.
19. U.S. Dept of Agriculture, Human Nutrition Information Service. Developing the Food Guidance System for Better Eating for Better Health, a Nutrition Course for Adults. Human Nutrition Information Services, Admin. Rep. No. 377, 1985.
20. U.S. Dept of Agriculture. Human Nutrition Information Service. The Food Guide Pyramid. Home and Garden Bulletin No. 252, 1992.
21. U.S. Dept of Agriculture and U.S. Dept of Health and Human Services. Nutrition and Your Health: Dietary Guidelines for Americans, 4th ed. Home and Garden Bulletin No. 232, 1995.

22. Beaton, G.H. Recommended Dietary Intakes: Individuals and Populations. In: Shils ME, et al., Eds. Modern Nutrition in Health and Disease, 9th ed. Baltimore, MD: Williams & Wilkins, 1999;1705-25.

23. Truswell, A.S. Dietary Goals and Guidelines: National and International Perspectives. In: Shils M.E., et al., Eds. Modern Nutrition in Health and Disease, 9th ed. Baltimore, MD: Williams & Wilkins, 1999;1727-41.

24. American Heart Association, Nutrition Committee. Dietary Guidelines for Healthy American Adults. *Circulation.* 1988;77:721A-724A.

25. The Health Connection. The Vegetarian Food Pyramid. Hagerstown, MD. 2000 (catalog #24082)

26. Oldways Preservation & Exchange Trust. Mediterranean Diet Pyramid, 1994.

27. Oldways Preservation & Exchange Trust, Asian Diet Pyramid, 1998.

28. Cannon, G., Ed. Food, nutrition, and the prevention of cancer: a global perspective. Washington, D.C.: American Institute for Cancer Research, 1997.

29. Second Report of the Expert Panel on Detection, Evaluation, and Treatment of High Blood Cholesterol in Adults. National Cholesterol Education Program. National Institutes of Health, National Heart, Lung, and Blood Institute, NIH publication 93-3095, 1993

30. Vogt, T.M., Appel, L.J., Obarzanek, E., et al. Dietary Approaches to Stop Hypertension: rationale, design, and methods. J. Am. Diet. Assoc. 1999;99(8 suppl): S12-8.

31. Nicholson, A.S., Sklar, M., Barnard, N.D., et al. Toward improved management of NIDDM: a randomized, controlled, pilot intervention using a lowfat, vegetarian diet. Prev. Med. 1999;29(2):87-91.

32. Whitten, C., Haddad, E., Sabaté, J. Developing a vegetarian food guide pyramid: a conceptual framework. *Veg. Nutr.: Int. J.* 1997;1/1:25-29.

33. Key, T.J., Fraser, G.E., Thorogood, M., et al. Mortality in vegetarians and non-vegetarians: detailed findings from a collaborative analysis of five prospective studies. *Am. J. Clin. Nutr.* 1999; 70(suppl):516-24S.

34. Kromhout, D., Bosschieter, E.B., De Lezenne, Coulandere. The inverse relation between fish consumption and 20-year mortality from coronary heart disease. *N. Engl. J. Med.* 1985 May 9;312(19):1205-9

35. Vegetarian Nutrition, The Proceedings of a symposium held in Loma Linda, CA, March 24-26, 1997. Johnston P.K. and Sabaté, J., Eds. *Am. J. Clin. Nutr.,* September 1999, Vol. 70(suppl.), No. 3(S).

36. Johnston, P.K. (Ed.). Second International Congress on Vegetarian Nutrition. Proceedings of a Symposium held in Arlington, VA, June 28-July 1, 1992. *Am. J. Clin. Nutr.* 1994;59:1099S-1262S.

37. Fraser, G.E. Diet as primordial prevention in Seventh-Day Adventists. *Prev. Med.* 1999 Dec; 29(6 Pt2):S18-23.

38. Sanders, T.A. The nutritional adequacy of plant-based diets. *Proc. Nutr. Soc.* 1999 May;58(2):265-9.

39. Key, T.J., Fraser, G.E., Thorogood, M., et al. Mortality in vegetarians and non-vegetarians: a collaborative analysis of 8300 deaths among 76,000 men and women in five prospective studies. *Public Health Nutr.* 1998;1:33-41.

40. Snowdon, D.A. Animal product consumption and mortality because of all causes combined, coronary heart disease, stroke, and diabetes, and cancer in Seventh-Day Adventists. *Am. J. Clin. Nutr.* 1988;48(suppl):739-48.

41. Appleby, P.N., Thorogood, M., Mann, J.I., Key, T. The Oxford Vegetarian Study: an overview. *Am. J. Clin. Nutr.* 1999;70(suppl):525S-31S.

42. Trock, B., Lanza, E., Greenwald, P. Dietary fiber, vegetables, and colon cancer: a critical review and meta-analyses of the epidemiologic evidence. *J. Natl. Cancer Inst.* 1990;82:650-61.

43. American Dietetic Association Position Paper: Vegetarian Diets. *J. Am. Diet. Assoc.* 1997;97:1317.

44. Cao, G., Sofic, E., Prior, R.L. Antioxidant capacity of tea and common vege-tetables. *J. Agric. Fd. Chem.* 1996;44:3426-3431.

45. Dreosti, I. Bioreactive ingredients: antioxidants and polyphenols in tea. *Nutr. Rev.* 1996;54(11):S51-S58.

46. Kromhout, D., et al. Dietary antioxidant flavonoids and risk of coronary heart disease: The Zutphen Elderoy Study. *Lancet* 1993;342:1007-1011.

47. Zheng, W. et al. Tea consumption and cancer incidence in a prospective cohort study of postmenopausal women. *Am. J. Epidemiol.* 1996;144(2):175-182.

48. Keli, S.O., et al. Dietary flavonoids, antioxidant vitamins and incidence of stroke: The Zutphen Study. *Arch. Int. Med.* 1996;156:637-642.

49. Ninth Special Report to the U.S. Congress on Alcohol and Health from the Secretary of Health and Human Services June 1997. U.S. Dept Health and Human Services, Public Health Service, National Institutes of Health, and National Institute on Alcohol Abuse and Alcoholism. NIH publication No. 97-4017.

50. Haddad, E.H. Development of a vegetarian food guide. *Am. J. Clin. Nutr.* 1995;59:1248S-1254S.

51. Slavin, J.L., et al. Plausible mechanisms for the protectiveness of whole grains. *Am. J. Clin. Nutr.* 1999;70(suppl):459S-63S.

52. Kushi, L.H., Meyer, K.A., and Jacobs, D.R. Cereals, legumes, and chronic disease risk reduction: evidence from epidemiologic studies. *Am. J. Clin. Nutr.* 1999;70(suppl):451S-8S.

53. Ripsin, C.M., Keenan, J.M, Jacobs, D.R., Jr., et al. Oat products and lipid lowering: a meta analysis. *JAMA* 1992;267:3317-25.

54. Pennington, J.A.T. Bowes & Church's Food Values of Portions Commonly Used, 17th ed. Philadelphia, PA: Lippincott Williams & Wilkins, 1998.

55. Kushi, L.H., Meyer, K.A., Jacobs, D.R., Jr. Cereals, legumes, and chronic disease risk: evidence from epidemiological studies. *Am. J. Clin. Nutr.* 1999;70(suppl):452S-8S.

56. Messina, M. and Barnes, S. The role of soy products in reducing risk of cancer. *J. Natl. Cancer Inst.* 1991;83:541-6.

57. Anderson, J.W., Smith, B.M, and Washnock, C.S. Cardiovascular and renal benefits of dry bean and soybean intake. *Am. J. Clin. Nutr.* 1999;70(suppl):464S-74S.

58. Messina, M.J. Legumes and soybeans: overview of their nutritional profiles and health effects. *Am. J. Clin. Nutr.* 1999;70(suppl):439S-50S.

59. Phillips, R., Lemon, F., and Kuzma, J. Coronary heart disease mortality among Seventh-Day Adventists with differing dietary habits. *Am. J. Clin. Nutr.* 1978 Oct;31(10 Suppl):S191 -S198.

60. Sabaté J. Nut consumption, vegetarian diets, ischemic heart disease risk, and all-cause mortality: evidence from epidemiologic studies. *Am. J. Clin. Nutr.* 1999, 70(suppl):500S-503S.

61. Fraser, G.E., Sabaté, J., Beeson, W.L., and Strahan, M. A possible protective effect of nut consumption on risk of coronary heart disease. *Arch. Intern. Med.* 1992, 152:1416-1424.

62. Hu, F.B., Stampfer, M.J., and Manson, J.E., et al. Frequent nut consumption and risk of coronary heart disease in women: a prospective cohort study. *Br. Med. J.* 1998;317:1341-1345.

63. Dreher, M.L., Maher, C.V., and Kearney, P: The traditional and emerging role of nuts in healthful diets. *Nutr. Rev.* 1996;54:241-245.

64. Spiller, G.A., Jenkins, D.J.A., Cragen, L.N., et al. Effects of a diet high in monounsaturated fat from almonds on plasma cholesterol and lipoproteins. *J. Am. Coll. Nutr.* 1992;11:126-130.

65. Sabaté, J., Fraser, G.E., and Burke, K., et al. Effect of walnuts on serum lipid levels and blood pressure in normal men. *N. Engl. J. Med.* 1993;328:603-607.

66. Abbey, M., Noakes, M., and Belling, G.B., et al. Partial replacement of saturated fatty acids with almonds or walnuts lowers total plasma cholesterol and low-density-lipoprotein cholesterol. *Am. J. Clin. Nutr.* 1994;59:995-999.

67. Colquhoun, D.M., Humphries, J.A., and Moores, D., et al. Effects of a macadamia nut-enriched diet on serum lipids and lipoproteins compared to a low fat diet. *Food Aust: Off. J. Counc. Aust. Food Technol. Assoc. Aust. Inst. Food Sci. Technol.* 1996;48:216-222.

68. O'Byrne, D.J., Knauft, D.A., and Shireman, R.B. Low fat, monounsaturated rich diets containing high oleic peanuts improve the serum lipoprotein profiles. *Lipids* 1997;32:687-695.

69. Kris-Etherton, P.M., Yu-Poth, Sabaté, J., et al. Nuts and their bioreactive constituents: effects on serum lipids and other factors that affect disease risk. *Am. J. Clin. Nutr.* 1999;70(suppl):504S-511S.

70. Sabaté, J., et al. Effects of walnuts on serum lipid levels and blood pressure in normal men. *N. Engl. J. Med.* 1993;328:603-7.

71. Morgan, W.A. and Clayshulte, B.J. Pecans lower low-density lipoprotein cholesterol in people with normal lipid levels. *J. Am. Diet. Assoc.* 2000;100:312-318.

72. Edwards, K., et al., Effect of pistachio nuts on serum lipid levels in patients with moderate hypercholesterolemia. *J. Am. Coll. Nutr.* 1999 Jun;18(3):229-32.

73. Wolff, R.L., et al., General characteristics of Pinus spp. seed fatty acid compositions, and importance of delta5-olefinic acids in the taxonomy and phylogeny of the genus. *Lipids* 2000 Jan;35(1):1-22.

74. Wolff, R.L., Christie, W.W., and Coakley, D. The unusual occurrence of 14-methyldecanoic acid in Pinaceae seed oils among plants. *Lipids* 1997 Sep;32(9):971-3.

75. Macfarlane, B.J., et al. Inhibitory effect of nuts on iron absorption. *Am. J. Clin. Nutr.* 1988 Feb;47(2):270-4.

76. Padmakumaran Nair, K.G., Rajamohan, T., Kurup, P.A. Coconut kernel protein modifies the effect of coconut oil on serum lipids. *Plant Foods Hum. Nutr.* 1999;53(2):133-44.

77. Sindhurani, J.A. and Rajamohan, T. Hypolipidemic effect of hemicellulose component of coconut fiber. *Indian J. Exp. Biol.* 1998 Aug;36(8):786-9.

78. Kumar, P.D. The role of coconut and coconut oil in coronary heart disease in Kerala, south India. *Trop. Doct.* 1997 Oct;27(4):215-7.

V

GLOBAL ISSUES AND NON-NUTRITIONAL PERSPECTIVES OF VEGETARIAN DIETS

17

ENVIRONMENTAL IMPACTS OF MEAT PRODUCTION AND VEGETARIANISM

Lucas Reijnders

CONTENTS

0-8493-8508-3/01/$0.00+$.50
© 2001 by CRC Press LLC

I. INTRODUCTION

Food is taken partially from nature and is partially obtained by agricultural practices. In industrial countries, most of the food is provided through agriculture. Still, however, considerable amounts of food may come from natural sources. For instance, in the United States, an estimated 4.3 million metric tons of wild plants and animals are annually harvested.[1] Fish represent 80% of this harvest and the remainder consists of game, mammals and birds, nuts and berries.[1] In Europe, fish, wild fruits, and mushrooms augment the diet.

As it stands, on a weight basis, most of the harvest from nature in industrial countries concerns foods of animal origin. Fish are still largely caught in seas, rivers, and lakes. However, in industrialized countries, the source for meat derived from mammals and birds is overwhelmingly animal husbandry, although individual diets may have significant contributions from hunting. Food taken from nature may be more important outside industrial countries. For instance, for 740 African tribes investigated, 80% of the diet came from wild animals and plants.[1]

The provision of food is associated with environmental problems that are not uniformly defined. Here the term "environmental" relates to three partially overlapping matters: the use of natural resources, relation to living nature, and pollution. The relative environmental impacts of current practices underlying meat production and the provision of its vegetarian alternatives will be discussed in this chapter. It will emphasize average production practices in the industrialized areas of the world, such as Europe, North America, and Australia. It should be noted, however, that the actual practices involved vary substantially and may significantly deviate from the average. Moreover, one should realize that there may be substantial, or even vital, dependence on animal husbandry for crop production.

II. NATURAL RESOURCES

Fishing and hunting directly exploit natural resources. Several natural resources are used in agricultural production, the most vital being land and water. Energy resources, such as mineral oil, a number of metal ores, phosphate rock, and natural gas (which is used in fertilizer production), are also important. A matter for discussion is whether these resources are used optimally, and what, if any, effect current use will have on their future availability.

The natural resources that are involved in the provision of food may have different dynamics over time. Several of them, which include mineral oil, natural gas, phosphate rock, and metal ores, are formed in slow geological processes. Also, some "fossil" water stocks, such as the Ogallala Aquifer in the U.S., are included in this category.[2] Slow formation means that there are only very small additions to the recoverable stock of such natural resources. Such resources are usually described as virtually non-renewable.[2]

Other natural resources are characterized by substantial additions to the existing stock. Such resources are called renewable and include fertile soil, fish, ground and surface water.[2] Additions to fertile soil come from weathering and peat formation. Water resources are replenished by rain. Sometimes, substantial additions to the existing stock are conditional. For instance, additions to the stock of peat will occur only when water tables are sufficiently high and if a number of other factors are conducive to its formation. If these conditions are not met, there will be no addition to stock and there may even be a decrease due to oxidation of existing peat. Conditionality also applies for fish. Because the renewability of fish stocks is based on reproduction, the presence of a sufficiently large reproducing population of fish is a necessary precondition for its actual renewability.

Use of natural resources for agricultural purposes may have important implications for their future availability. When use leads to losses that exceed the addition to stock, future stocks will be reduced. So, for instance, if erosion exceeds the formation of fertile soil by weathering, future soil productivity could be negatively affected. Moreover, renewable resources, such as fertile soil, may be subject to other forms of quality loss. Compaction, salinization, and toxification of soils occur in practice and negatively affect their function as a natural resource. In fact, overexploitation and negative impacts of pollution are problems that may affect all renewable natural resources. Overfishing will reduce fish stocks in the near future. Extreme overfishing may lead to the extinction of fish species, and thereby to resource loss. Discharges of toxic substances can negatively affect the wholesomeness of fish.

Exploitation may also affect the future availability of virtually non-renewable resources. Large-scale burning of mineral oil and natural gas will have a negative impact on the availability of fossil carbon compounds for future generations. Using copper ores that do not significantly corrode and are recycled with high efficiency will have a negligible impact on future availability. On the other hand, the dissipative use of copper compounds as a feed additive for pigs will have a negative impact on future copper stocks.

The actual future impact of dwindling stocks of a number of natural resources in the future is a subject of heated discussion between opponents with very different points of view. While some maintain that there will be no problems due to the advances of science and the potential for substitution, others argue that the persistence of current rates of resource loss will sooner or later cause big problems. In view of the possibility that the latter view may be correct, the loss of natural resources associated with current practices in the provision of food will be discussed.

Obtaining food from nature is subject to the possibility of overexploitation, which may negatively affect its future availability. Hunting for food has been the main cause of a number of extinctions and near-extinctions of animals in the past centuries. Its victims include the Auroch (*Bos primigenius*), the European ancestor of domesticated cattle (extinct in 1627); the tarpan (*Equus caballus ferus*), the European wild horse that became extinct in 1851; and the Dodo (*Raphus cucullatus*), a large bird native to Mauritius that became extinct in the early 20th century due to hunting by white settlers.[1]

Currently, in many industrialized countries, hunting for food largely has evaded the threat of extinction to mammals and birds, although substantial negative effects of hunting on several species of migratory birds have been noted in Europe.[1] Gathering plants and mushrooms in industrial countries also has a limited effect on biodiversity.[2]

As it pertains to fishing, however, overexploitation of natural resources is a major problem. About 70% of the world's fish catch comes from marine areas.[3] The rest comes from aquaculture and freshwater fishing. Marine fish stocks are under heavy pressure in several areas of the world, including the North Atlantic and the seas adjacent to densely populated coastal areas in Asia. Currently, according to the Food and Agricultural Organization (FAO), 11 of the 15 main fishing grounds in the oceans and seas are overfished. In addition, overfishing is a problem for a number of freshwater systems.[3,4]

Agriculture uses several natural resources. In this chapter, attention will be focused on the agricultural use of, and the impact of animal production on, the following natural resources:

- land (fertile soil)
- energy resources (fossil carbon resources)
- water
- phosphates

A. Land

When considering the use of land, an important question that arises is whether the soil that produces animal feed is also suitable for the production of plants that may serve as human food. Buringh[5] estimated that about 22% percent of the earth's land area is, in principle, suitable for growing crops for human consumption. In 1984, roughly half that area was actually used for such crops and the rest was in use as pasture and for growing forest products.

There is also a much larger land area that is, practically speaking, unfit for growing crops that are edible to mankind, but is suitable for the growth of plants that may serve as a basis for pastoral farming. About 50% of the land surface falls in this category,[6] with about half of that located in the tropics and subtropics and the other half in temperate and cold regions. This area comprises mountain meadows, prairies, steppes, savannas, and halophytic areas.[6] Currently, pasture and range lands cover 3.1 × 10^9 hectares.[8]

Traditionally, crops edible to mankind were largely consumed by man. Animal feed consisted mainly of leftovers from processing and eating such crops. This has substantially changed. Increasingly, farm animals have become dependent on crops that may also serve as food for man. The crops involved are mainly grains and soybeans, with the latter belonging to the category of oilseeds.[7] Currently, the yearly worldwide per capita consumption of food grains is estimated at 201 kg, whereas its feed-grain equivalent is 144 kg.[8] In the U.S., yearly per capita food grain consumption is about 77 kg, whereas the corresponding feed-grain consumption is in the order of 663 kg.[8]

The explosive growth of soybean production from about 17 million tons in 1950 to 152 million tons in 1997 is largely due to the importance of soybeans in animal feed.[9] Even in China, where large quantities of soybean-derived products are for direct human consumption, by 1997 about 60% of soybean protein consumed went to animal feed.[9]

Feeding grains and soybean-derived produce to farm animals reduces the amount of protein and food energy (calories) ultimately available for human consumption, because much of the crop-derived proteins and calories is necessary for the sustenance of farm animals. Conversion efficiencies depend on the type of animal production.[6,10] In industrial countries, the ratio of edible energy over gross energy consumed is about 18% for a herd of pigs, 13% for a dairy herd, 10% for a broiler herd and 5% for a beef herd. For milk in the U.S., the protein conversion efficiency is about 31%, 27% for eggs, 18% for broiler production, about 9% for pork production, and 6% for beef production.[10] On average, 10 kg of plant protein in 1980 generated 1 kg of animal protein.[11] Since then, there has not been a significant change in conversion efficiencies.

Additionally, note the increase in aquaculture (farming of fish, mollusks, and shrimp). In 1996, aquaculture was estimated to generate 23.1 million kilograms of produce, strongly up from the 6.9 million tons in 1984.[9] Here again, grains are often used as feed. In feeding carnivorous species, marine fish are often used. It is estimated that, caloriewise, farming of herbivorous fish on grains has roughly the same efficiency as keeping chickens on grains.[9] Carnivorous species such as salmon and shrimp, on average, need 5 kilograms of fish for each kilogram of produce.[4]

Considering the natural resource land worldwide, somewhat over 50% of the area that is currently fit for growing plants that are edible for man in fact produces animal feed, partly composed of grasses, grains, and oilseeds. Because of the limited efficiency of turning animal feed into products that are edible by man, the overall land productivity of animal production, in terms of edible energy or protein, is low. The land involved in growing grains for animal production might have supported roughly five to 10 times as many people with a vegetarian diet.

1. Degradation of Arable Land

Another important aspect of land use is whether tilling and grazing practices are sustainable. Soils involved in crop production may be subject to processes like erosion, salinization, and compaction to such an extent that agricultural practices may prove to be unsustainable.[11]

Erosion is a major problem in growing crops. It affects the production of both food and animal feed. Strategies known as conservation tillage have been developed to curb erosion in crop production.[12] In the U.S., the adoption of conservation tillage has been relatively successful. In 1997, 37% of planted acreage was under conservation tillage.[12] Still, overall, there are substantial net losses of fertile soil in the main food- and animal-feed-growing areas of the world. In view of the relative efficiencies of providing calories and proteins that were pointed out above, net losses of fertile soil will, in all probability, be substantially larger for animal production, based on crops like grains and soybeans, than when the same or similar crops are directly used as food for man.

2. Degradation of Land Involved in Animal Husbandry

There are several ways in which animal husbandry may contribute to land degradation. A first possibility is the overstocking of range lands. Another unsustainable grazing practice may be found on peaty soils. Here, grass is often grown with lowered water tables and grazed by cattle and sheep. This leads to a rapid thinning of the peat layer.[2] Furthermore, increased erosion and loss of nutrients occur when woods on riverbanks are cleared so they can be converted into grasslands for animal husbandry.[13]

Many areas that are fit for sustainable extensive grazing are, in fact, overstocked. This, in turn, leads to land degradation — especially by compaction and erosion by wind and water. Oldeman[14] concluded in 1993 that, since 1945, 20 million square kilometers of land have been degraded by human activities. This is about 20% of the total vegetated area of the earth's land mass. 12.2 million square kilometers were found to be moderately or strongly degraded. Moderately degraded land (9.1 million square kilometers) has greatly reduced productivity, and strongly degraded land (3.1 million square kilometers) has no remaining agricultural function. About one third of the degradation noted by Oldeman[14] is due to overgrazing. In North America, the contribution of overgrazing to land degradation is 30%, and in Europe, it is 23%.[14-18] Relatively high contributions to land degradation by overgrazing were found by Oldeman[14] in Oceania (80%) and Africa (49%). In the mid-1980s, Perrens estimated that, in Australia, 55% of the dry land grazing area, totaling 4 million square kilometers, suffered from land degradation due to overgrazing and needed restorative measures.[18] Percentage-wise, this is still a relatively good score as far as dry range lands are concerned. The corresponding percentages for Africa, North, and Latin America are around 75%.[11] In the 1990s, the overall deterioration of land associated with grazing practices has, in all probability, increased over the values given by Oldeman.[14] In the mid-1990s, the annual rate of loss of agricultural soil, due to soil degradation, was still in the order of 5–6 million hectares.[15]

B. Energy Resources

Energy resources for agriculture are largely taken from the stock of fossil carbon compounds, which is virtually non-renewable.[2,19] Recently, the use of fossil carbon compounds for agricultural purposes has tended to grow faster than the overall energy use of economies.[20] By now, the use of fossil carbon compounds for the supply of food in industrial countries is very substantial. Mechanization, refrigeration, and the energy involved in providing inputs such as fodder, fertilizers, and pesticides substantially contribute to the energy intensity of agriculture.

There are considerable between-country differences of agricultural fossil-energy intensities. For instance, the fossil-energy input or subsidy in cultivated grassland ranges from 2–3 GJ/hectare in Australia and New Zealand to 70–80 GJ/hectare in Israel and the Netherlands, with the U.S. in an intermediate position.[20]

Generalizing the energy intensity of agriculture in industrialized countries would have a major impact on stocks of fossil fuels. If, for instance, the per capita use of fossil fuels for food supply currently used in the U.S. were to be extended all over the globe, and if the resulting energy demand were to be covered by mineral oil, known oil reserves would be depleted within 10 years.[21]

As it stands, the energy intensity of animal production in industrialized countries is much larger than the energy intensity of vegetarian alternatives such as grains, potatoes, and legumes.[9,10,20,21] To illustrate this, Table 17.1

Table 17.1 Estimates of Food Energy Output/Fossil Energy Input Ratios in the U.S.[9,10,20,21]

Product	Ratio Food Energy Output/Fossil Energy Input
Corn	2.7
Potato	2.2
Wheat	2.0
Beef	0.02–0.04
Pork	0.033

gives estimated food energy output/ fossil energy input ratios for the U.S. This table's data is mainly from the 1980s. However, given the relatively low prices for fossil fuels since 1985, it is not expected that the ratios given will have improved.

Data about energy efficiency in the European Union (EU) will probably be somewhat worse than those for the U.S. due to the higher intensity of agriculture that, energy-wise, tends to lead to diminishing returns.

There are also data pertinent to the energy efficiency of providing protein in the form of fish, meat, or shrimp. These are summarized in Table 17.2. In this table, for the sake of comparison data, estimates of the energy inputs of beef, eggs, and milk are added. Data are mainly from the 1980s, and again, in view of low energy prices, improvements in energy efficiency seem unlikely.

Table 17.2 Estimated Inputs of Energy/Gram Protein in kJ/Gram for a Variety of Animal Products[9,10,20]

Protein Source	Energy Input kJ/Gram Protein
Marine fish Europe	500
Marine fish NE USA	75
Fresh shrimp USA	1800
Carp East Asian polyculture	150–200
Salmon European monoculture	2000
Beef USA	>600
Eggs USA	350
Milk USA	200

There is and has been substantial discussion about the energy efficiency of current systems of agricultural production. From this, it is clear that major gains in energy efficiency are still possible.[19,20,22] However these gains do not substantially affect the relative energy intensities of meat and its vegetarian alternatives.

C. Water

Many water resources are currently under heavy pressure. Although water is abundant on earth, less than 1% of available water is fresh water suitable for most human uses, including agriculture. Also, available fresh water of good quality is not evenly distributed over the economies. The supply of good fresh water is increasingly becoming a regional problem. In some cases, this scarcity is even giving rise to political tensions, as exemplified in parts of the Middle East and Central Asia. Water-related political problems also seem to be brewing in the U.S. among southwestern states along the Colorado River. Therefore, water efficiency of food production may be a matter for considerable concern.[16]

The water intensity of animal production is much larger than the water intensity of crops. For instance, per gram dry weight, soybeans require about 0.75 liters of water.[6] Non-irrigated corn requires 0.6 liter, irrigated corn requires 1.4 liters and irrigated rice requires 4.7 liters.[8] For 1 gram dry weight in cattle production, on average, about 20 liters of water are required.[6,23] Using soybeans as a reference, available data suggest a water efficiency that is roughly 26 times better in soy production than in cattle breeding. Also, the quality of water resources suffers more from animal production than from growing crops. Section IV.B further explores this topic.

There is substantial technical scope for improving water efficiency in agriculture. However, it is not expected that the aforementioned water efficiency ratio of roughly 26 will be changed dramatically by implementing such improvements.

D. Phosphates

Currently, phosphate fertilizers derived from phosphate rock are frequently used in arable farming and on grasslands. Phosphate rock is formed by slow geological processes and may be considered virtually non-renewable. This means that business as usual will lead to a depletion of this resource.[2] It is estimated that, in a Western industrialized country like the Netherlands, phosphate rock input into meat production is at least six times larger than its equivalent in soya-protein production.[20]

Precision agriculture may substantially reduce the input of fertilizer derived from phosphate rock in crop production. In precision agriculture, the system for applying fertilizer is more precisely adapted to crop needs than in current agriculture. Phosphate present in animal manure will be less fit for inclusion in precision agriculture. This means that, upon the introduction of precision agriculture, there may be a relative shift in phosphate efficiency in favor of crop production.

III. RELATION WITH LIVING NATURE

Living nature provides mankind with a number of services that vary from useful to vital. The provision of food is only one of these services. Others include photosynthesis, pollination, recreation, cycling of substances, control of pests, genetic resources, the generation of non-food products, and pollution control. The total value of the services that nature generates is very hard to determine. Existing estimates are, however, in the same order as the gross world product.[15] Therefore, negative effects on nature should not be taken lightly.

Catching animals in the wild for food may have a substantial impact on living nature. It has already been pointed out in Section II that catching these animals in the wild has led to the extinction of some species. Currently, a number of species reductions are under way. For instance, mainly due to overfishing and the unintended catch of fish accompanying large-scale commercial fishing, in the past 25 years, populations of 102 freshwater species that were monitored have fallen by 45%, whereas monitored marine species declined by 35%.[4] Negative effects on fish species may in turn have effects on other species in the food web to which fish belong, such as fish-eating birds and mammals.

Negative impacts on living nature are also associated with agriculture. The expansion of agriculture has "rolled back" nature.[25–28] If nature is defined in terms of areas unaffected by mankind, one might even argue that nature has come to an end. By now, there probably is not any part of living nature on the earth that has remained completely unaffected by mankind's activities. However, if nature is defined as those areas not under direct human control, living nature, on land, still accounts for somewhat over 50% of photosynthesis ("primary production").[25] The rollback of nature has been accompanied by a substantial loss of biodiversity. The current rate of extinction is in the same order as, or exceeds, the rates of past mass extinctions. For instance, it has been estimated that in Europe, 11,000 native plant species have become extinct, whereas the corresponding number for the U.S is estimated to be on the order of 20,000.[1]

To a large extent, the diminution of nature is caused by replacement. When a wilderness is transformed into a meadow or a field where crops are grown, nature is largely replaced by culture. A smaller part of the rollback follows from the indirect effects of agriculture. For instance, to exploit new soy-growing areas in Brazil, rivers must be adapted to allow for the navigation of cargo, which, in turn, will affect river ecosystems.[29] Also, the use of pesticides in agriculture tends to have substantial effects on non-target organisms.[1] Another example concerns nitrogen fluxes that are generated by intensive animal husbandry and may have a strong impact on adjacent wild areas. Soils might be acidified or eutrophied (well fed). Eutrophication is likely to result in the loss of species diversity.[30] In European areas with a temperate climate, one often finds that the proliferation of brambles, stinging nettles, and grasses are favored by large nitrogen or phosphate fluxes. Following large additions of nitrogen compounds, heathlands with calluna (low shrubs such as heather) have been invaded by grasses such as *Deschampsia* and *Molina*.[30] Acidification of soils may contribute to the loss of vitality in trees.[9] In forests, loading with nitrogen compounds has led to the increased occurrence of pathogenic fungi, reduced levels of *Mycorrhizae* (symbiotic fungi), reduced diversity of undergrowth and reduction in the number of seedlings.[31] Also, the insect fauna in soils may change in reaction to nitrogen loading.[31] Furthermore, the replacement of nature with agriculture may change water tables and fluxes. In turn, such changes can lead to major changes in the biodiversity of adjacent areas.

The extent to which animal husbandry has an impact on living nature is strongly dependent on its precise modalities.

A. Animal Husbandry in Uncultivated Areas

At the low end of the impact spectrum, one may find very low density animal husbandry in uncultivated areas. Here, one can argue that biodiversity benefits. Grazing, for instance, creates new ecological niches that include new abiotic gradients that allow for the emergence of species that would have been absent when no grazers were present. When the density of grazers or other animals in uncultivated areas increases, this positive effect on biodiversity rapidly disappears. Overstocking, with its negative effects on biodiversity, occurs at apparently low densities of grazers. This is in line with the low density of vertebrates in natural systems in general, which on average does not exceed 0.03% of plant biomass.[18,20]

In "overstocked" and uncultivated areas, biodiversity is reduced. There is ample evidence of such reductions due to overstocking with grazing animals and pigs. When overstocking is extreme, deserts with strongly reduced biodiversity may emerge. In fact, in parts of Europe, such deserts were already created in prehistoric times.[32]

Currently, very low density grazing for food production is becoming increasingly rare, while overstocking has become more common. This is evidenced by, among other things, the desertification in the last 50 years of dry range lands (see Section I.A).

B. Animal Husbandry on the Basis of Agricultural Produce

To expand the number of animals on feed generated by cultivated areas, unspoiled nature is regularly replaced by cultivated land. Worldwide, there is a general shift in the nature of primary production (photosynthesis) on land. Natural primary production decreases. As pointed out before, its share in photosynthesis on land is probably still over 50%,[21] but, especially due to the expansion of agriculture, this may not last long. Because of its relative inefficiency in producing protein and calories, animal husbandry requires more land for a specified amount of food energy or protein than crop production. The actual amount is dependent on the precise nature of animal husbandry, but as discussed in Section I.A, roughly speaking, a fixed amount of meat protein requires five–ten times as much land as an equivalent amount of crop-based proteins. Thus, ceteris paribus, the expansion of animal husbandry based on cultivated arable land replaces five–ten times as much nature as does crop production that directly feeds mankind.

Extrapolation of American eating habits to countries where the current diet is more vegetarian may illustrate the impact of current practices in industrialized countries. If each Indonesian or Costa Rican had the same diet as the average American, and if the animal produce involved were to come from their own countries, the Indonesian and Costa Rican rainforests would be eliminated in a few years.[33] Replacement of nature by cultivated land strongly contributes to the much increased rate of extinction of natural species. [26–28] This, in turn, sharply reduces biodiversity.

There is also another possible effect on land of the loss of living nature. It has been argued by Huxley[34] and Lovelock[35] that nature plays a vital role in determining the composition of the atmosphere, and that it is instrumental in keeping this composition beneficial to mankind. If this hypothesis is true, a corollary may be that diminishing nature may sooner or later lead to a loss of this function. In fact, Lovelock,[35] in this context, has used the metaphor of burning one's skin. If the area of burnt skin surpasses a critical level of about 80%, death is inevitable because the internal homeostasis of the body is lost and vital organs fail. Whether Lovelock's hypothesis and metaphor are correct is presently uncertain. However, if they are correct, a further loss of wild areas would certainly be imprudent.

IV. POLLUTION

Pollution essentially refers to chemical, physical, and biological entities in the wrong place or in the wrong amounts. Its importance is related to associated negative impacts that are dose-dependent and often have a no-effect level. The negative impacts involved may directly affect human health. Also, pollution may have a negative impact on human activities like agriculture, on man-made structures, and on nature.

In practice, there is a wide variety of existing pollution problems, ranging from nuisance associated with excessive noise to global change caused by the increased atmospheric content of some trace gases, and from the discharge of bacteria that may cause infectious diseases to acid deposition.

Pollution comes in different types with varying geographical extensions. It varies from highly local (e.g., increased copper concentrations in soils originating in copper-rich manure) to truly global (e.g., increased climate forcing due to agricultural emissions of methane and dinitrogenoxide). In between, there are types of pollution that affect substantial areas of the globe, as exemplified by the eutrophication of river basins and adjacent parts of the seas by nitrogen and phosphorous compounds and acidification of soils associated with emissions of nitrogen compounds into air.

Table 17.3 charts the relative agricultural emissions of several compounds involved in pollution caused by Dutch meat production, compared with the production of an equivalent amount of soybean-derived produce. Pollution associated with growing plants that are eaten by meat-producing animals is included in the emissions caused by meat production.

Table 17.3   Relative Emissions Associated with Dutch Meat Production Compared with an Equivalent Production of Soya-Derived Products[24,32]

Compound Emitted	Emission Associated with Soya Derived Produce	Relative Emission Associated with Dutch Meat Production
Carbon dioxide	1	7
Copper	1	>100
Biocides	1	6
Acidifying compounds	1	>7

The compounds referred to in Table 17.3 are involved in a variety of environmental problems. Carbon dioxide is a "greenhouse gas," which is translucent to visible light but absorbs infrared radiation coming from the earth. Currently, its rising atmospheric concentrations are thought to be partly responsible for the global warming of the troposphere, the lowest part of the atmosphere (see also Global Air Pollution).

Copper may especially become a problem when there are large increases of its levels in soils. It is an essential element, but organisms may take up too much of it for their own good. What is too much is strongly dependent on the organism involved. Some species, including sheep and some varieties of earthworms, are relatively vulnerable to fairly moderate increases in soil concentrations of copper (also see IV.D).

Biocides are compounds that are used to control a wide variety of pests. Unfortunately, they also tend to have a negative effect on non-target organisms. Often, such negative effects remain confined to the vicinity of the point of discharge. However, some poorly degradable and relatively mobile biocides — such as some organochlorine pesticides — may have widespread effects that could, after use in temperate or (sub)tropical regions, extend even to the polar regions.

Finally, acidifying compounds, also known as "acid rain," are involved in acid deposition. Acid deposition may have negative effects on a number of materials and on biodiversity, which is particularly affected when critical loads are exceeded. Such critical loads are relatively low in poorly buffered lakes and soils. In practice, exceedance of critical loads occurs in parts of North America, Europe, and Asia, giving rise to the reduction of, and changes in, biodiversity.

Table 17.3 does not cover all important pollutants associated with agriculture. (Other important pollutants generated by agriculture are, however, examined in the following sections.) Moreover, for these pollutants, there is no deviation from the trend suggested by Table 17.3 that relative emissions associated with Dutch meat production are larger than those involved in soya-derived produce.[24,36]

In the following section, the direct polluting impact of animal production will be discussed in more detail.

A. Local Effects

Some of the compounds emitted due to animal husbandry are virtually immobile or have low mobility. For instance, copper compounds that are used as an additive to pig feed to enhance fattening are largely excreted with manure. Copper concentrations in pig feed may be as high as 175 mg/kg.[32] When manure resulting from pig farming is spread on soils, most copper is bound in the upper layer of the soil. When the application of pig manure is intensive, copper concentrations in the upper layer of the soil increase rapidly. In the Netherlands, where pig rearing is intensive, copper levels of up to 133 mg/kg have been found in soils.[33] Such large increases may have a negative effect on the number of earthworms that the soil can sustain. When copper concentrations exceed 60 mg/kg, populations of the earthworm *Lumbricus rubellus* may be negatively affected.[37,38] The increase of copper levels in topsoils will also lead to elevated amounts of copper in plants that are grown on soils treated with pig manure. This, in turn, may lead to problems associated with the consumption of those plants. Sheep are relatively vulnerable to increased concentrations of copper in their feed. An intake of 0.8 mg/kg body weight per day may lead to toxic effects in sheep, including death resulting from haemolysis.[36] When soil concentrations of copper are over 30 mg/kg, and the content of organic matter less than 5%, vulnerable varieties of sheep may be negatively affected.[36]

Another compound with relatively low mobility is phosphate. Phosphate excreted with manure is usually bound to soils. However, when manuring is intense and phosphate-binding capacity is very limited, as in sandy soils, soils may rapidly become saturated with phosphate. In this case, substantial amounts of "leaked" phosphate will emerge in ground and surface water.[39]

Other compounds that are emitted in animal husbandry are much more poorly bound to soils than are copper and phosphate. Specific examples include nitrogen and potassium compounds that rapidly leak into ground and surface water. Also, pesticides that are used in sheep dips, such as lindane, and veterinary medicines that are not readily degradable may turn up in ground and surface water.

The mobility of compounds dissolved in groundwater is limited. It usually does not exceed values on the order of millimeters a day. This means that initially, the near vicinity will be primarily affected. Particularly important in this context is the effect that groundwater pollution may have on wells that provide drinking water to man and animals. Strongly increased levels of nitrate (hotspots) may be found in wells close to dung heaps or fields that have been subject to intensive manuring. In the U.S., nitrate hotspots can be found in parts of the Midwest and in the sandhill regions of Nebraska.[18] In Europe, areas heavily involved in intensive animal husbandry such as France (Brittany), the northern part of Portugal, the Po area in Italy, and the Low Countries have strongly increased nitrate levels in groundwater. Such levels may have eutrophying effects (see Section III) and may be detrimental to human health. The risk of high nitrate levels is strongly associated with its conversion into nitrite. Nitrite reacts with hemoglobin and may give rise to the synthesis of carcinogenic nitrosamines in the digestive tract.[31,39] The World Health Organization (WHO) has established that an acceptable daily intake (ADI) for nitrite is 0.134 mg/kg body weight. With a 5% conversion in the human body, this would put the ADI for nitrate at 3.3 mg/kg body weight. Others have even proposed much lower ADIs.[39] Small children are especially vulnerable to increased levels of nitrate. On exposure to high levels (44.3–88.6 mg nitrate/liter), small children have been found to suffer from "blue-baby sickness" or cyanosis.[39] Also, several diseases of the stomach and kidneys may lead to increased vulnerability.[39] In view of such effects, the European Union (EU) has established a maximum level of 50 mg nitrate/liter of drinking water and a target value of 25 mg/liter. Such levels are often exceeded in groundwater near dung heaps and heavily manured sandy soils.[34,36]

Another local type of pollution may arise from the use of antibiotics in animal husbandry, particularly the use of antibiotics as a feed additive to prevent or limit microbial infection. The systematic use of antibiotics as feed additives favors the emergence of micro-organisms that are antibiotic resistant. For instance, it has been found that, in the vicinity of chicken farms using an antibiotic as an additive to chicken feed, resistance against vancomycin strongly increased.[39] This would especially be a problem when vancomycin resistance does not remain local but emerges in methicillin-resistant *Staphylococcus aureus*, against which vancomycin is currently the only effective antibiotic. More generally, the appearance of antibiotic resistance in infectious microorganisms that are important in veterinary and human medicine may be problematic.

B. Surface-Water Pollution

Over long periods, pollutants dissolved in groundwater may travel great distances. Thus, groundwater pollution might substantially contribute to the pollution of surface water, as many surface waters are partially fed by groundwater. Also, run-off from farmland and irrigation waters may contribute to the pollution of surface waters.

In surface water, pollutants may travel much faster than in groundwater. In rivers, speeds of tens of kilometers per day are not uncommon, a factor 10,000,000 faster than in groundwater. In view of this speed, it is clear that the pollution of river water may, geographically speaking, have a wide effect. This is especially significant when pollutants are not readily degraded in surface waters. Such riverine pollution may affect the downstream part of rivers and the lakes and seas into which river water is discharged.

An important effect of especially intensive animal husbandry is that substantial amounts of nitrogen, potassium, and phosphorous compounds may emerge in surface waters. Because nitrogen and phosphorous compounds are often limiting factors to primary production (such as algal growth) in natural waters, the emissions from animal husbandry may lead to eutrophication. Several negative effects are associated with eutrophic waters. For example, biodiversity in waters tends to decrease when oligotrophic waters become eutrophic. Also, eutrophic waters may sustain blooms of algae and dinoflagellates. This applies both to inland waters and parts of the sea near eutrophic rivers. The latter include the following areas in North America: Chesapeake Bay, Long Island Sound, and the Gulf of Mexico. In Europe, parts of the Baltic, North, and Adriatic Seas are affected.[16] Such blooms may include blue green algae and dinoflagellates that secrete toxins, thereby negatively affecting animals that live in these waters. Swimmers may also be negatively affected by algal and dinoflagellate blooms.

An illustrative example is the *Pfiesteria piscicide*, a dinoflagellate that has been implicated in a number of major fish kills along the coast of North Carolina.[40] *Pfiesteria* produces toxins that are also harmful to man. The growth of the toxic variant of *Pfiesteria* is stimulated by swine effluent spills.[40]

Toxic blue-green algae, which proliferate on eutrophication, include *Micocystis*. *Micocystis* secrete cyanotoxins and contain lipopolysacharidic compounds that may negatively affect swimmers, leading to gastrointestinal and skin complaints.[41] In extreme cases, algal blooms may be so intense that they lead to oxygen depletion. This could trigger the death of organisms dependent on the presence of oxygen, such as fish. An example is the so-called "dead zone" in the Gulf of Mexico, an area of many thousands of square kilometers of lifeless water, eutrophied by the Mississippi River.

Another contribution to water pollution that comes from animal husbandry concerns enteropathogens such as *Cryptosporidium* and *Giardia* species. Infections arise partially through the fecal–oral route from animals to humans, caused particularly by bathing in surface waters.[42]

C. Regional Air Pollution

Regional air pollution associated with animal husbandry, to a large extent, originates in the emissions of compounds from manure, formed under reducing anaerobic conditions. Particularly, the emissions of ammonia and reduced sulfur compounds are known to be important. While reduced sulfur compounds give rise to bad smells, ammonia compounds may contribute to eutrophication on deposition from air.[31] Also after deposition, ammonia tends to be partially converted into nitric acid and nitrous oxide (or dinitrogenoxide) by soil microorganisms. This, in turn, may give rise to elevated levels of nitrate in groundwater (see Section IV.A), acidification of soils, and the emission of nitrous oxide into air (see section IV.D).[39,43,44]

There may also be other significant emissions from livestock farming. This is suggested by the relatively high frequency of respiratory ailments such as asthma, in areas with high densities of farms involved in intensive animal husbandry.

D. Global Air Pollution

Animal husbandry contributes to global air pollution, and more specifically, increases the atmospheric trace gases that have a greenhouse effect. For greenhouse gases, like carbon dioxide and methane, the yearly increase in atmospheric concentration is currently 0.5% and nearly 0.4%, respectively.[45,46] For nitrogen dioxide, the increase is 0.25%/year.[45,46] As pointed out before, this increase induces an upward pressure on temperature near the earth's surface that, in turn, may lead to climate change. Animal husbandry also makes a small, indirect contribution to the deterioration of the ozone layer associated with the loss of chlorofluorocarbon refrigerants that are used in cooling and freezing animal products.

The contribution of animal husbandry to increasing concentrations of greenhouse gases mainly results from the emissions of carbon dioxide, methane and dinitrogen oxide. Carbon dioxide emissions are largely associated with the burning of carbonaceous fuels that are necessary for energy supply to animal production. As pointed out in Table 17.3, the carbon dioxide emission associated with Dutch meat production is seven times the carbon dioxide emitted in producing an equivalent based on soya protein. Methane emissions partly originate in the intestines of farm animals and partly in the anaerobic conversion of manure. Methane emissions from domestic livestock are estimated to be about 80 megatons/year with a range from 65–100 megatons.[45] Cattle and buffalo contribute about 80% to this emission.[45] Global methane emissions from manure and ruminants are estimated to be 85–130 megatons Carbon/year.[46] The overall anthropogenic emission of methane is 300–450 megatons Carbon/year.[45,46]

Dinitrogen oxide is formed by microorganisms converting nitrogen compounds generated by animal husbandry. Global dinitrogen oxide emissions from manure in 1990 were estimated at 1.0–1.1 Teragram N. out of a total anthropogenic emission of 2.6–4.4 Teragram.[44] Indirectly, animal husbandry gives rise to dinitrogenoxide emissions associated with growing crops for animal feed. These emissions are associated with the use of synthetic fertilizer and nitrogen-fixing by soybeans. This indirect emission associated with animal husbandry may be estimated at 0.5–0.7 Teragram N.[44]

V. CONCLUSION

The environmental effects of meat production and the production of meat equivalents based on crops was discussed, with an emphasis on practices in industrialized parts of the world such as North America, Europe, and Australia.

Overall, the conclusion from available data on the use of natural resources, impacts on wild areas, and pollution is that, on average, the negative environmental impact of meat production by animal husbandry on all dimensions of the environmental problem discussed tends to be much larger than that of its equivalent based on reference-crop (soybean) production. One should, however, keep in mind that, in practice, crop production is, to some extent, dependent on manure production generated by animal husbandry. Moreover, for organic farming, this dependence is overwhelming. Furthermore, as pointed out Section II.A, much agricultural land is unsuitable for cropping, but is fit for sustaining livestock farming. Also, there may be specific cases in which the environmental case against animal meat is not clear-cut at all. This, for instance, is exemplified by a case comparing meat from animals grazing on extensively stocked uncultivated areas with their nutritional equivalent in vegetables obtained from greenhouses.

It is harder to compare the environmental impacts of fishing with those of crop production. This is caused by the rather different nature of their respective impacts. To the extent that effects are more or less similar, on average, fishing seems to have a larger negative impact. However, crop production has a number of negative environmental impacts that fishing does not have. This leaves the outcome of the comparison between crop production and fishing dependent on the relative weights that one attributes to the environmental impacts involved. Since these are controversial, no verdict is given here on the relative environmental impacts of growing crops and fishing.

REFERENCES

1. De Groot, R. *Functions of Nature*. Wolters-Noordhoff, Groningen, 1992.
2. Reijnders, L. *Environmentally Improved Products and Production Processes*. Kluwer Academic Publishers, Dordrecht, 1996.
3. FAO. *Yearbook of Fishery Statistics: Catches and Landings*. Rome, 1996, 1998
4. WWF. *The Living Planet Report*. Geneva, 1999.
5. Buringh, H. Availability of Agricultural Land for Crop and Livestock Production. Food and Natural Resources. Pimentel, D. and Hall, C.W., Eds., Academic Press, San Diego, 1988.
6. Tivy, J. *Agricultural Ecology*. Longman Scientific, Harlow, 1990.
7. Pimentel, D., Oltenacu, P. A., Nesheim, M., Kummel, J., Allen, M. S., and Chick, S. Grass-fed livestock potential: energy and land constraints. *Science* 207: 843-848, 1980.
8. Kendall, H. W. and Pimentel, D. Constraints on the expansion of the global food supply. *Ambio.*, 23: 198-205, 1994.

9. Brown, L. R., Renner, M., Flavin, C. *Vital Signs* 1998. W.W.Norton and Company, New York, 1998.

10. Pimentel, D. and Pimentel, M. *Food, Energy and Society*. Edward Arnold, London, 1982.

11. Tolba, M. K. and El-Hholy, O. A. *The World Environment* 1977-1992. Chapman & Hall, 1992.

12. Uri, N. D. Energy and the use of conservation tillage in U.S. agriculture. *J. Energy Pol.*, 27: 299-306, 1999.

13. Ripl, W., Pokorny, J., Eiseltova, M., Ridgill, S. *A Holistic Approach to the Structure and Function of Wetlands and their Degradation*. IRWB Publications, 32: 16-35, 1984.

14. Oldeman, L. R. Global extent of soil degradation. *Soil Resilience and Global Land Use*, C.A.B., Wallingford (UK): 99-118, 1993.

15. United Nations Environmental Program. *Global Environmental Outlook*. Oxford University Press, New York, 1997.

16. World Resources Institute. *World Resources 1992*. Oxford University Press, New York, 1992.

17. Perrens, S. J. *Conversion of Forest Land to Annual Crops: Australian Experience*. RAPA Report 186, FAO Regional Office, Bangkok, 1986.

18. Schnoor, J. and Thomas, N. Soil as a Vulnerable Environmental System, In: *Industrial Ecology and Global Change*, Socolow, R., Ed.. Cambridge University Press, Cambridge, 1994.

19. Reijnders, L. The Factor X debate: Setting targets for eco-efficiency. *J. Ind. Ecol.* 2: 13-22, 1998.

20. Smil, V. *General Energetics*. John Wiley & Sons, New York, 1991.

21. Pierce, J. T. *The Food Resource*. Longman Scientific & Technical, Harlow UK, 1990.

22. Wilting, H. *An energy perspective on economic activities*. Ph.D. thesis, State University of Groningen, 1996.

23. Pagot, J. *Animal Production in the Tropics and Subtropics*. MacMillan, London, 1992.

24. DTO, *Spectrum van een duurzame voedselvoorziening*, Hagen en Stam, Den Haag, 1997.

25. Vitousek, P. M., Ehrlich, P. R., Ehrlich, A. M., and Matson, O. A. Primary production on land. *BioScience*, 36: 368-383, 1986.

26. Kaufman, L. and Malory, K. *The Last Extinction*. MIT Press, Cambridge (Mass.), 1986.

27. Raup, D. M. Biological extinction in earth's history. *Science*, 231: 1528-1533, 1986.

28. Wilson, E. O. The biological diversity crisis: a challenge to science. *Issues in Science and Technology* (fall): 20-29, 1985.

29. Buprawen, S. and Surupredo, A. Letter to H.H. *Apotheker*, Brasilia, 1999.

30. Schlesinger, W. Vulnerability of Biotic Diversity. In: *Industrial Ecology and Global Change*, Socolow, R., Ed., Cambridge University Press, Cambridge, 1994.

31. Van Duijvenbooden, W. and Matthijsen, A. J. C. M. *Integrated Criteria Document Nitrate*, RIVM, Bilthoven, 1989.

32. Ponting, C. *A Green History of the World*. Penguin Books, Harmondsworth, London, 1991.

33. Reijnders, L. Vegetarianism and the Environment, *Proc. World Veg. Congr.*, The Hague, 1994.
34. Huxley, A. *Physiography*, MacMillan, London, 1877.
35. Lovelock, J. E. *The Ages of Gaia*, Oxford University Press, Oxford, 1989.
36. Slooff, R. F. M. J., Cleven, J. A., Janus, J. A. and Ros, J.P.M. *Integrated Criteria Document Copper*, RIVM, Bilthoven, 1987.
37. Ma, W. Toxicity of copper to lumbricid earthworms in sandy agricultural soils amended with copper-enriched organic waste materials. *Ecol. Bull.*, 39: 53-56, 1988.
38. Klok, C., de Roos, A. M., Marinissen, J. C. Y., Baveco, J. M. , Ma, W. Assessing the impact of abiotic environmental stress on population growth in *Lumbricus rubellus*. *Soil Biol. and Biochem.*, 29: 287-283, 1997.
39. Copius Peereboom, J. W. and Reijnders, L. *Hoe gevaarlijk zijn milieugevaarlijke stoffen* 1 & 2, Boom, Meppel, 1991.
40. Springer, J. *NSCU Aquatic Botany Laboratoria Pfiesteria piscicide page*, www.pfiesteria.org/pfiest.html,1998.
41. World Health Organization. *Toxic Cyanobacteria in Water, a Guide to Public Health, Significance Monitoring and Management.* Geneva, 1999.
42. Medema, G. J. and Ketelaars, H. A. M. Betekenis van Cryptosporidium and Giardia voor de drinkwatervoorziening. *H2O*, 23: 699-704, 1995.
43. Bouwman, A. F., Fung, I., Matthews, E., and Hohn, H. Global analysis of the potential for dinitrogenoxide production in natural soils. *Global Biogeochem. Cycles*, 7: 557-597, 1993.
44. Kroeze, C. and Bouwman, A. F. Emissions of nitrous oxide. In: *Non-carbon-dioxide Greenhouse Gases*, van Ham, J., Ed. Kluwer Academic Publishers, Dordrecht, 1994.
45. IPCC, Climate Change 1995. *Impacts, Adaptations and Mitigation of Climate Change: Scientific-Technical Analyses.* Cambridge University Press, Cambridge, 1996.
46. Zwerver, S. and Kok, M. T. J. *Klimaatonderzoek*, RIVM, Bilthoven, 1999.

18

MEATLESS DIET: A MORAL IMPERATIVE?

Mark F. Carr and Gerald R. Winslow

CONTENTS

0-8493-8508-3/01/$0.00+$.50
© 2001 by CRC Press LLC

I.   INTRODUCTION: ADVOCATING VEGETARIANISM

For more than 20 years, noted philosophers, conservationists, and health advocates have aggressively called for people to embrace the vegetarian way of life. Over these years, the burden of proof has fallen upon the advocates of vegetarianism. In popular literature and obtuse philosophical treatises, the benefits of meat eating are increasingly questioned, and the harms are more and more evident. This includes harm to the creatures prepared for slaughter, the land on which they depend, and the people who eat their flesh. Advocates of vegetarianism argue that virtually no one and no thing is truly better off as a result of the modern-day meat industry.

Much has already been accomplished through the advocacy of vegetarianism. In general, vegetarianism is now more widely practiced and more socially accepted in America. Multiple studies show that advocates of vegetarianism are correct; it is a better way of life. And when we speak of vegetarianism as a "better way of life," we move beyond scientific investigation and summary reports to the realm of value. Arguments for vegetarianism often move beyond touting the health benefits of a meatless diet to ask questions of morality. Is it morally obligatory to adopt a vegetarian diet? In the face of overwhelming evidence from so many quarters, should it not be argued that there is a moral obligation to forgo meat eating?

Tom Regan, a prominent advocate for animal rights, helped to move the discussion of what some call "ethical vegetarianism"[1] into the realm of morality. In 1982, he wrote, "My belief is that a vegetarian way of life can be seen, from the moral point of view, to have a rational foundation. This is what I shall try to show...."[2]

Proponents of vegetarianism generally have very high expectations of their audience. They believe that, upon considering sound arguments, the audience should choose to become vegetarians. Indeed, Regan expressed confidence in the force and practicality of his rational argument for vegetarianism when he suggested that "most of those who should happen to read this essay will be leading lives that, if my argument is sound, ought to be changed in a quite fundamental way."[3] As with so many others, Regan was not simply seeking to present a strong case for vegetarianism. Rather, he was setting out to change lives — to change not just the way people think, but how they eat.

Recently, while visiting the department of nutrition and dietetics at the university where we work, one of the authors was waiting in the department lounge where students continued in their routine study and eating habits. Catching the eye of one student, he smiled and asked her about the program. Was it, he queried, an unwritten prerequisite that applicants be vegetarians for admission to program? The student seemed taken aback and did not immediately answer the question. Overhearing the query, the department's administrative assistant came around the corner to see who had dared voice such a question. "No," she and the student chimed emphatically together, "it is not."

Perhaps they were not vegetarians. But, if not, why not? Why would people who study such compelling evidence not become vegetarians? Are the arguments for a meat-free diet sufficiently weighty to produce both intellectual assent and behavioral change?

Puzzling over these questions invites consideration of the arguments in favor of vegetarianism. Most of these move beyond analysis of costs and benefits and toward advocacy of a moral obligation. While these arguments might be grouped in a variety of ways,[4] we have selected the following five categories.

A. The Health Argument

One of the oldest arguments is that a vegetarian diet is healthier than a carnivorous diet. This has been a particularly difficult argument to win in America. Given the widespread social presumption that meat protein is an essential element in the human diet and given the lack of scientific studies to prove otherwise, the burden of proof has fallen squarely on the shoulders of vegetarian health advocates. However, the scientific study of vegetarianism has shown that animal protein is not an essential element of our diet. Furthermore, certain studies show that the incidence of some diseases is significantly reduced for those who forgo meat in their diet.[5]

Some who approach the question from a Christian perspective argue that vegetarianism was God's "original diet." They point to the biblical story of Eden and the plenty that God provided Adam and Eve in the Garden. The fruits and nuts provided by the "green plants" were intended for those beings who had the "breath of life." On this view, people were designed to flourish without the use of flesh for food.

A second argument from the Christian perspective depends on the scientific evidence that the vegetarian diet is healthier for humankind. Because God intends our bodies to be the habitation of his Holy Spirit (1 Cor. 3.16–17 and 6:19–20), humans are obliged to live the most healthful lives possible. Thus, once it is understood that vegetarianism is a healthier diet and once this diet is possible, it becomes the morally preferable diet.

B. Animal Rights

Blending the language of utilitarian benefits with that of animal rights, some authors focus attention on ethical duties toward animals.[6] Crucial to this perspective is realizing the harm and suffering experienced by animals as a result of raising and killing them for food. It is considered immoral to cause such suffering merely to satisfy gustatory predilections. This should be evident once it is accepted that all sentient beings have both rights and intrinsic worth. Factory farming comes under special fire here because of the way in which animals are raised for human consumption. "Life" on the factory farm is really nothing more than an extended death. John Robbins captures the sense of outrage at the treatment of factory-farmed animals in the introduction to his successful book, *A Diet For a New America*:

> The suffering these animals undergo has become so extreme that to partake of food from these creatures is to partake unknowingly of the abject misery that has been their lives....We are ingesting nightmares for breakfast, lunch, and dinner....*It's not the killing of the animals that is the chief issue here, but rather the unspeakable quality of the lives they are forced to live.*[7]

Paul R. Amato and Sonia A. Partridge reveal the extent to which advocates of vegetarianism, coming from the perspective of animal rights, consider the issue to be of grave moral concern:

> Ethical vegetarians look forward to the day when factory farms will be totally eradicated. In the meantime, they see every decrease in the amount of suffering experienced by animals as a small moral victory.[8]

Again, the underlying desire of many who argue for animal rights is that their audience choose to become vegetarians. And there is evidence that they are succeeding. Among the studies that culminated in their book *The New Vegetarians: Promoting Health and Protecting Life*, Amato and Partridge identified 11 reasons that people choose the vegetarian life-style. At the top of the list was a "concern over animal suffering or a belief in animal rights."[9] Widespread and popular understanding of the language of rights makes this a particularly easy argument to accept. Sadly, however, the rights of unknown, unseen cows, chickens, and pigs are often over-ridden by the desires of the palate. Furthermore, both the philosophical foundations and the practical applications of the concept of rights continues to be difficult enough to establish for humans and thus, even more difficult for animals.

C. Environmental Concerns

The philosophical underpinnings for many who argue for vegetarianism out of concern for the environment were provided by Aldo Leopold's *A*

Sand County Almanac. Although Leopold was no vegetarian, his so-called "land ethic" fostered widespread awareness of the need to "think like a mountain."[10] Leopold's concern for matters of land conservation helped establish academic disciplines such as environmental philosophy and ethics and the now popular "deep ecology."[11]

At a more popular level, Jeremy Rifkin's *Beyond Beef* continues to bring awareness of environmental concerns associated with meat eating. Rifkin highlights the relationship between the cattle industry and the growing global environmental crisis, particularly as it relates to feeding the world's population. He charges that the "ecological devastation created by the burgeoning world cattle population exceeds many of the other more visible sources of environmental harm."[12]

Francis Moore Lappe's book *Diet for a Small Planet* should be read from the perspective of a concern for the environment. Although many readers would categorize her work as health promotion, it is equally powerful as an expression of environmental importance. Her now famous essay, "A Protein Factory in Reverse,"[13] brought attention to the massive amounts of earth's resources wasted by current agricultural practices. From the moral perspective, her work melds environmental advocacy with health promotion and what we refer to (in the following category) as "social evolution."

Despite the efforts of advocates like Rifkin and Lappe, and despite the huge success of their books, only a small number of people appear to change their diet as a result of environmental concerns. For example, Amato and Partridge's survey, noted above, found that only 5% became vegetarians out of concern for the environment.[14] Thus, while environmental ethicists urge more careful methods of land use and conservation, they rarely, if ever, explicitly refer to vegetarianism as a moral obligation.

D. Social Evolution

Under this rubric, we place a variety of authors and viewpoints that call for socio-political change. There is some overlap here with other categories. The work of Lappe, Singer, and Rifkin, for instance, should be considered in more than one category. For example, we include Lappe's work under this category because her concern is not simply with helping others to change their personal dietary habits, but with change in global dietary patterns. Note what she urges in the preface to the revised edition of *Diet For A Small Planet*:

> I had a more profound doubt ... what of the impact, what of the direction that I was suggesting for people's lives. Would the readers of my book become so interested in, even fixated

on, the nutritional nuances as to forget or neglect the *real message* after all?[15] (italics added)

What was the "real message" Lappe sought to spread? In this preface, she likens herself to the little boy who told the emperor he had no clothes. She wanted more than anything for her work to highlight how individual diet "relates each of us to the broadest questions of food supply for all of humanity."[16] With the publication of the revised and updated edition, she was particularly concerned, not only with making cooking and eating simpler and better, but fundamentally with the "political and social significance" of our dietary choices.[17]

Peter Singer, too, is rightly included under this argument. In his precedent-setting book, *Animal Liberation*, Singer equates his call for widespread vegetarianism with social reform movements of the past. The vegetarian life-style is a "form of boycott" very similar to other "great movements against oppression and injustice." South African apartheid, Caesar Chavez's work for farm laborers, bull-fighting in Spain, baby-seal harvests in Canada, slave trade, nationalistic wars, and the exploitation of children during the Industrial Revolution are among the socio-political events called as exhibits to which Singer compares the choice for vegetarianism.[18]

Jeremy Rifkin does not fail to make clear for his readers that his goal in presenting the evidence in *Beyond Beef* is not simply descriptive; his agenda calls for socio-political action:

> Moving beyond the beef culture is a revolutionary act, a sign of our willingness to reconstitute ourselves, to make ourselves whole .... The dissolution of the modern cattle complex and the elimination of beef from the diet of the human race portends a new chapter in the unfolding of human consciousness.[19]

E. Stewardship

The principle of stewardship provides the conceptual framework for the final category. John Robbins popularly portrays stewardship when he shares his dream for American society in his successful book *Diet For A New America*:

> It is the dream of a success in which all beings share because it is founded on a reverence for life. A dream of a society at peace with its conscience because it respects and lives in harmony with all life forms. A dream of a people living in accord with the laws of Creation, cherishing and caring for the

natural environment, conserving nature instead of destroying it. A dream of a society that is truly healthy, practicing a wise and compassionate stewardship of a balanced ecosystem.[20]

The notion of stewardship incorporates the concerns voiced by environmental ethicists and animal rights activists, as well. In the past, criticism was leveled at this argument because, it was said, this concept retains an anthropocentric obsession with tyrannical control over the rest of sentient and non-sentient life. Humankind's incessant striving for control and manipulation (sometimes wrongly understood as "stewardship") of our environment did, in fact, lead to widespread ecological devastation. But many advocates of stewardship have taken such criticism to heart and yet maintain an insistence that, as the only creature on earth with the rational capabilities to bring some management of both self and other, humankind must engage in stewardship. The renewal of a less anthropocentric notion of stewardship is one reason John Robbins can envision a stewardship that is "wise and compassionate."[21]

Andrew Linzey, writing of stewardship from a Christian perspective, urges a radical change in the way Christians have interpreted their relationship to the entirety of God's creation. Linzey challenges the traditional Christian notion that this world and all that is in it was made solely for the uplifting of humankind. Humans remain unique in the orders of creation, but this uniqueness grants no special status. In fact, this uniqueness urges a special duty upon humans to take up the role of "servant species." In this role as servant of all creation, stewards are to care for the creation just as God cares for it. Drawing upon the theological concept of a suffering God, Linzey proclaims:

> It cannot be sufficient merely to have a negative vision of what we should do to prevent suffering in the world. We need positive vision of how we can take upon ourselves the suffering of the world and transform it by the power of the Holy Spirit.[22]

Linzey insists that Christians must move beyond the notion that God suffers only when humans suffer. When we can fully accept the fact that "God suffers in all suffering creatures," we will be better able to accept our role as stewards.[23]

Aldo Leopold is largely responsible for the move away from anthropocentric understandings of stewardship from a non-Christian perspective. His "land ethic" urged a change in our role from one of "conqueror" of the "land-community" to one of "plain member and citizen of it."[24] While he used the outdated term "husbandry" to denote his idea of stewardship and conservation of the land, the idea was that "some art of management is applied to land by some person of perception."[25] His foundational works fostered what is now called environmental philosophy.

Paul Taylor, like Leopold, rejects an anthropocentric notion of stewardship in which humans manipulate our ecosystems to our own exclusive benefit. Taylor's idea of a "life-centered system of environmental ethics" still retains strong elements of the managerial or stewardship role for the human in this system. And his thoughts echo those of Leopold, who urged management by "some person of perception." As Taylor puts it:

> From the perspective of a life-centered theory, we have *prima facie* moral obligations that are owed to wild plants and animals themselves as members of the Earth's biotic community. We are morally bound (other things being equal) to protect or promote their good for their sake. Our duties to respect the integrity of natural ecosystems, to preserve endangered species, and to avoid environmental pollution stem from the fact that these are ways in which we can help make it possible for wild species populations to achieve and maintain a healthy existence in a natural state.[26]

Finally, William Aiken, writing as an environmental ethicist with attention to agricultural stewardship, speaks from a realistic perspective when he notes that "some intervention with natural ecosystems" is inevitable if we are to continue any form of agriculture needed to feed the earth's present population. The interaction he calls for is an expression of the principle of stewardship. He seeks to find a "form of agriculture which is sustainable, harmonious and compatible with conserving the stability and diversity of the ecosphere and which adequately supplies the food needs of people."[27]

The principle of stewardship understood in its reconstructed and less anthropocentric sense has the benefit of garnering widespread acceptance on the conceptual level. But for advocates of stewardship, as for the advocates of each of the other arguments, the audience is likely to give a simple response; namely, "Yeah, but...." Even in the face of a very tight argument, for this particular topic, respondents often retort, "Yeah, but I like meat." Advocates of the vegetarian life-style, however, are not simply engaging in their work with the goal of providing a sound argument. Recall Tom Regan's assumption that as a result of his argument, peoples' lives "ought to be changed in a quite fundamental way." The fact that more people have not chosen vegetarianism is puzzling.

II. MOVING BEYOND "YEAH, BUT..."

Each of the arguments noted above has enjoyed widespread acceptance in both philosophical and popular audiences, but the numbers of those who are choosing the vegetarian life-style are not reflective of these levels of acceptance. People are giving intellectual assent to the arguments while enjoying yet another hamburger. These great advocates of ethical vegetarianism have established the fact that meat eating is at least morally troublesome, even if the sense of obligation we feel as an audience has not brought about greater numbers of converts. It is true that vegetarianism is more acceptable now than it was 20 or 30 years ago, but why don't more people make this life-style change? And of those who do make the change, as Amato and Partridge's survey shows, why are they doing it largely out of concern for animals who suffer the cruel fate of human consumption?

A. Philosophical Argument, Personal Conviction, and Practical Action

Leopold was correct in his assertion that: "No important change in ethics was ever accomplished without an internal change in our intellectual emphasis, loyalties, affections and convictions."[28] Singer also knows that, all too often, there is a large gap between "intellectual conviction and the action needed to break a lifetime habit." Advocates do an admirable job of describing the moral problems associated with meat eating, but when we move beyond description to prescribing obligations and personal actions, we must have the hearts of the audience. Changes in personal practice often emerge more from the heart than the head. As Singer goes on to say, "There is no way in which a book can bridge this gap; ultimately it is up to the reader to put his convictions into practice."[29] Good arguments do not necessarily bring personal convictions to bear in life-style change.

The two most widely successful moral and philosophical arguments for vegetarianism emerge from the animal rights movement and the concern for the environment. Michael Allen Fox believes the weight of evidence that these two arguments provide should be taken as a "moral imperative" for vegetarianism. Yet he has been profoundly struck by the difference he finds in the dietary practices of the audience in each of these groups. The followers of animal rights are far more likely to be vegetarians than those in the environmental activist organizations. Fox draws on his meal-time experiences with each group as he involves himself in their various conferences and seminars. Invariably, animal rights groups insist on vegetarian meals at their meetings, while environmental groups receive just a few scattered requests from individuals for special meals at their meetings. He accuses environmentalists of either failing to "see the connections" between their intellectual arguments and the practice of vegetarianism, or of simply choosing to "ignore, bury, or rationalize them." Environmental ethicists, Fox postulates, have "more subtle, intellectualized ways of legitimating their choice." With Leopold and Singer, Fox recognizes that:

> Consistency in theorizing, and between theory and practice, is not just a purely "rational" value that philosophers cherish and that everyone should aim to realize; it is also a matter of seeing connections between what we believe, espouse and do, and that this in turn can lead us to a better understanding of what it means to minimize the harm that we cause by our choices and to live more lightly on the planet.[30]

Equally critical of many environmental groups, Sharon Bloyd-Peshkin charges that these groups have failed to "spread the 'V' word for fear of losing the 'M' words — members and money." Falling back on the hackneyed excuse that dietary practices are too personal, environmental groups have largely ignored the issue. Bloyd-Peshkin's observations about the issues environmental groups highlight and the methods used to do so further illustrate our point that the practical actions toward the vegetarian life-style will arise only as persons are moved emotionally, as well as intellectually.

As Bloyd-Peshkin analyzes the reasons that environmental groups are not as likely to be vegetarians, she reveals that it is not so much a sound argument that will persuade people to make difficult choices, but rather, it is the movement of people's emotions that brings concrete results. She quotes Alan Durning of Worldwatch Institute describing how his group understands this motivational process in its efforts to raise the ranks of their membership:

> The way you get members is to find egregious transgressions and get people mad about them. If it's a "big something," it is easier to drum up outrage. If it's "everybody needs to change a little bit," it's harder to get people excited.[31]

Bloyd-Peshkin is correct to note that "the environmental impact of meat eating is too indirect." One is not moved to give up meat in the checkout line at the grocery store. However, one is moved to outrage and action when confronted with the scenes of animal suffering and torture that precede the appearance of their flesh on the grocery store shelf. As Bloyd-Peshkin puts it, one is "far more likely to ... get mad about the industrial plant you pass on the way home; you see the filth coming out of its stack."[32]

B. David Hume and the Movements of Human Sentiment

Of course the realization that moral agents are moved more by emotion than reason is not a fresh revelation. David Hume's philosophical works highlighted this reality in the mid- to late-18th century. But the hegemony of rationalism in the morality of Western society has served to prejudice its philosophers from using appeals to emotion in the process of making moral arguments. The use of emotion in a moral argument is often derided as sappy sentimentality.[33]

David Hume refused to ignore the force of sentiment in the moral life of humankind. In fact, it is the sentiment, felt to be unique to humans of his day, that distinguishes human capability for living a moral life. It is the "sentiment of disapprobation" that we as humans "unavoidably feel on the apprehension of barbarity or treachery" that serves to pronounce such acts as criminal or immoral. Hume insists that human actions are never attributable to the "cool and disengaged" reason. Reason may convey "knowledge of truth and falsehood," but it will never serve to attach valuations of virtue and vice, the essence of morality. Furthermore, reason can never motivate a person to action. Sentiment is the "first spring or impulse to desire and volition." In Hume's view,

> The ultimate ends of human actions can never, in any case, be accounted for by reason, but recommend themselves entirely to the sentiments and affections of mankind, without any dependence on the intellectual faculties.[34]

Hume's most prominent and capable defender today, Annette Baier, summarizes this point for us: "For any motivation to action, and for any evaluative reaction, 'reason' must 'concur' with some 'passion'; the 'head' must work for the 'heart.'"[35] Thus, it is the cultivation and practice of these human sentiments that allow for the practical reality of living a moral life. Humans who inculcate the character traits or virtues of sympathy and compassion, among others, will live the moral life.

C. A Brief Personal Interlude

Recognizing that personal life-style change must engage both intellectual challenge and emotional involvement, we have asked ourselves how change came about in our own experience. We found that we could recount stories that profoundly affected our attitudes toward killing animals. We realized that these stories, and others like them, often give rise to reflection and to transformation. We recount two of them here to illustrate the point that humans may be more effectively motivated to alter life-style by a combination of intense experiences, which vivify the moral imagination, and by rational arguments, which give intellectual structure to convictions.

"The Rabbit's Squeal" (Carr)

A few magnificent evergreens towered over the old guest cabin where we had focused our attention. Dad, my brother Pete, and I were out on our first rabbit hunt at Grandpa's farm in Michigan. The rabbits that made their home among these trees were, according to Dad, particularly fast. Pete and I did not utter a word as we circled around the back of the cabin. We knew that if the rabbits heard us coming, they would run away too quickly to allow for a shot.

I readied my .20-gauge shotgun as we rounded the edge of the cabin. Dad came around the other side, and just as he reached my peripheral vision I saw a rabbit bolt for the underbrush at the edge of the yard. Nothing could have broken my concentration on that rabbit as I kept it in my visual range, as Dad had taught me. I knew that I'd have to get closer to shoot it with my shotgun so I crept closer, but before I had shortened the distance, the hunt was over. The shock wave from Dad's rifle rolled over me at the same instant that I saw the rabbit collapse. By the sound of the rabbit's squealing, I knew Dad's shot had not immediately killed it. The squeal was so intense and piercing we each hurried to the spot where it lay writhing in pain. Dad reached down and grabbed it by the hind legs, laid it out on the ground, put his foot on the rabbit's head and pulled. Blood spewed from the rabbit's body as its heart spent its final effort in sustaining life.

I'm sure I failed to hide the horror I felt. Dad must have seen it in my face, because what he said revealed his own need to justify his action in front of his two boys. "It's the quickest way to put it out of its misery," he said.

"The Pheasant's Feathers" (Winslow)

I was intensely proud of my new .12-gauge shotgun for which I had earned the money by picking string beans. My goal was to learn the art of hunting pheasants, Canadian geese, and other "game birds," so abundant in the Willamette Valley of my youth. My parents seemed confident that 14 was old enough for this activity.

The first outings with my friend Bob were unproductive. Despite our best efforts and the fact that Chinese pheasants can be slow and noisy when they begin flight, we missed every one. Mainly, we had long walks on damp, fall mornings, punctuated with a few moments of exciting, but inept shooting.

Finally, one weekend morning we went hunting with the "big guys," Bob's older brother and his friend. As the junior members, Bob and I were instructed to go to the far end of the cornfield and wait. The other two, with their German shorthaired retriever, would hunt in our direction. If they missed their targets, our job was to shoot the birds as they came flying in our direction.

And so it happened. A magnificent Chinese pheasant, a "rooster," flew up, was missed, and headed straight toward where I was crouched. I took aim and fired when it was just overhead. Feathers flew everywhere. The dog came running and fetched the largest part of what was left of the pheasant. It was nearly blown in two. But in what remained I could see the stunning white ring on the neck, the red and deep green feathers of the head, and the rich strips of the long tail feathers. Bob's brother took one look at the dead bird, pronounced it not worth taking home, and threw it in some blackberry brambles.

Covering disappointment and feigning bravado, I took one of the long feathers and stuck it in my hunting cap. Later, alone at home, I studied the feather. I could not erase the image of that colorful bird, minding its own affairs, and blown apart for no good reason. The irretrievable stupidity of it all overwhelmed me. I put the shotgun in the closet, sold it the following year, and never hunted anything again.

What does all this mean for the advocation of vegetarianism? More is required in the effort to move people toward change in their dietary habits. Good philosophical arguments do not make vegetarians. Moral sentiments, however, more often do. We are not recommending a traumatic hunting trip for all children so they can see just what has happened to the meat on their dinner plates. We are, however, encouraging the moral force of movements of the heart as an essential element of the argument for choosing the vegetarian life-style. This is one reason that advocates of animal rights have been more effective at gaining converts to vegetarianism. The hearts of the audience are moved through the written and visual representations of animals suffering. The audience is moved through sympathy and compassion toward actions that will lessen or eliminate the suffering.

III. ON THE VIRTUES OF VEGETARIANISM

A. Sympathy

Sympathy is one of a class of virtues often referred to as "other-regarding." The principal focus of this trait is the object of attention, but it presupposes a certain ability in the agent to engage in altruistic and empathetic dispositions. Thus, when other persons or beings are suffering, we are moved out of sympathy to respond in a fashion that would relieve their suffering. Following Hume, Edward F. Mooney writes that sympathy is "the 'mechanism' whereby we sorrow in the plight of others and are moved to respond benevolently."[36]

B. Compassion

Compassion is closely related to sympathy in that it also is other-regarding. Etymologically, its emphasis is upon a fellow feeling with the other; literally, to suffer with. There is a sense of shared community with other humans in this virtue and for advocating notions of steward-ship noted above, a sense also of an extension of this shared community to include all sentient and non-sentient beings. Like other virtues that involve engaging the emotions of the agent, compassion moves beyond a simple affective state to action. As Lawrence Blum notes, however, acting from the virtue compassion means that one will often act "very much contrary to one's moods and inclinations" because it is fundamen-tally other-regarding. Indeed, even when one's actions may not imme-diately eliminate the suffering of the other, it is "valuable to the sufferer for its own sake, independently of its instrumental value in improving" the lot of the other.[37]

IV. CONCLUSION

What practical effect will come from including the practice of sympathy and compassion with the intellectual arguments for vegetarianism? Our contention is that if we can move toward becoming a society in which these virtues are valued and practiced, we will see vegetarianism increase and meat eating decrease. These virtues will serve to move us beyond an intellectual assent to the arguments for the vegetarian life-style toward the actual practice of vegetarianism. Arguing a position similarly influenced by David Hume, the philosopher William O. Stephens suggests that,

> Compassionate persons who had to breed, raise and slaughter by their own hands the animals they would eat would be greatly disinclined to do so. The anguished cries, terrified struggles, and spurting blood of the farm animals would no doubt deter many people from cutting off the animals' heads in order to make a meal of them. The gory, visceral experience of slaugh-tering a breathing, feeling animal may trigger the sensitive person's latent compassionate impulse enough to make the prospect of a fleshly meal quite unappetizing.[38]

Having been moved to act upon our moral sentiments and actually become vegetarians, we are bolstered by the strength of the philosophical arguments for vegetarianism. Any single argument, or a combination of them, is able to provide the structured guidance for a socio-political position that urges vegetarianism, but they do not serve to bring converts to the vegetarian life-style.

A. Morally Praiseworthy Vegetarianism

Does the weight of the philosophical arguments serve to establish a moral obligation for vegetarianism? Does the added element of virtue insist that meat eaters should become vegetarians? And, if so, should society take the next step of prohibiting the production and consumption of meat?

Pressing for moral or legal obligations remains problematic even in the face of powerful arguments for vegetarianism. We can no more require people to be virtuous than we can require them to eat certain foods, particularly at this stage in our societal evolution. Perhaps the time will come when the environmental and socio-political crises human society faces on this planet will force policy makers to mandate such dietary practices. For now, we must settle for the notion that vegetarianism is simply morally praiseworthy. Advocates of vegetarianism can and should promote individual, national, and global dietary reform. There is an abundance of philosophical and popular moral reason to uphold and praise the vegetarian life-style. In fact, society praises people who have sympathy and compassion for others and sometimes even punishes those who fail to exhibit these traits.

For instance, our respective family members might well have worried about our moral development had we both laughed hysterically at the way our prey had died. If, thereafter, one of us had developed the practice of racing to the wounded rabbit to be the one who got to pull its head off, his father would rightly have been concerned for his development as a person. Likewise, if the other had developed an inner desire to use a shotgun at close range upon his prey, his family should have been concerned for his development. These intense emotional events, on the contrary, did a great deal to shape the way we appreciate and respond to the suffering of our fellow creatures.

Leopold once wrote that the task of creating more appropriate recreational activities for human society should focus on creating some receptivity in the "still unlovely human mind."[39] Taking our cue from Leopold, we submit that the task of creating vegetarians is a job, not of building tighter arguments in support of vegetarianism, but of building receptivity, sympathy, compassion, and character into the still unlovely human heart.

REFERENCES

1. "Ethical vegetarians" are not vegetarians who are morally upright persons. Rather, this term refers to vegetarians who choose this diet for ethical reasons. See the following for some discussion of the term and its implications: Paul R. Amato and Sonia A. Partridge, *The New Vegetarians: Promoting Health and Protecting Life*, New York: Plenum Press, 1989, p. 35ff; Andrew Linzey and Jonathan Webber, "Vegetarianism," *Dictionary of Ethics, Theology and Society*, New York: Routledge, 1996; Gotthard M. Teutsch, "Killing Animals: Reflections on the Ethics of Meat Eating," *Universitas* 2/1993, pp. 98-107.

2. Tom Regan, *All That Dwell Therein: Animal Rights and Environmental Ethics*, Berkeley: University of California Press, 1982, p. 4.

3. Ibid. Peter Singer, author of *Animal Liberation: A New Ethics for Our Treatment of Animals*, New York: Avon Books, 1975, also moves the question beyond the realm of simple concern for the treatment of animals when he says, on p. 165, that vegetarianism is "not merely a symbolic gesture.... Becoming a vegetarian is the most practical and effective step one can take toward ending both the killing of nonhuman animals and the infliction of suffering upon them."

4. William O. Stephens in "Five Arguments for Vegetarianism," *Environmental Ethics: Concepts, Policy, Theory*, Mountain View, CA: Mayfield Publishing Company, 1998, surveys arguments of the following types: Distributive Justice, Environmental Harm, Feminist, Moral Consideration for Animals, and Health. Jordan Curnutt, in proposing "A New Argument for Vegetarianism," *Journal of Social Philosophy*, vol. 28, no. 3, Winter 1997, pp. 153-172, treats only two "old" arguments, namely, Peter Singer's utilitarian argument and Tom Regan's rights-based argument. In the *Dictionary of Ethics, Theology and Society*, Andrew Linzey and Jonathan Webber include arguments from the following perspectives: Health, Spiritual or Ascetic, Ecological, and Animal-centered.

5. For a good introduction to one line of research that illustrates this point, see Fraser, G.E., "Associations between diet, cancer, ischemic heart disease, and all-cause mortality in non-Hispanic white California Seventh-Day Adventists," *American Journal of Clinical Nutrition*, 1999. Vol. 70 supplement; pp 5325-5385.

6. Peter Singer and Tom Regan are the two most prominent authors who fall under this category. Peter Singer's *Animal Liberation*, 1975 really served to move the advocating of vegetarianism into the moral realm. See the bibliography for a selection of the works of these two important authors.

7. John Robbins, *Diet For A New America*, Tiburon, CA: H. J. Kramer Inc., 1987, pp. xiv-xv.

8. Paul R. Amato and Sonia A. Partridge. *The New Vegetarians: Promoting Health and Protecting Life*, New York: Plenum Press, 1989, p. 264.

9. Ibid., p. 34.

10. Aldo Leopold, *A Sand County Almanac: With Essays on Conservation from Round River*, New York: Ballantine Books, 13th printing, 1978.

11. See Part Two of *Environmental Philosophy: From Animal Rights to Radical Ecology*, Michael Zimmerman and others, Upper Saddle River, NJ: Prentice Hall, 1998, pp. 165-262.

12. Jeremy Rifkin, *Beyond Beef: The Rise and Fall of the Cattle Culture*, New York: Dutton Books, 1992, p. 4.

13. See *Diet for a Small Plant*, rev. ed., New York: Ballantine Books, ninth printing, 1978, pp. 7-16.
14. Amato and Partridge, ibid.
15. Lappe, ibid., p. xviii.
16. Ibid.
17. Ibid., p. xix.
18. Singer, *Animal Liberation*, pp. 167-169, 189.
19. Rifkin, p. 291.
20. Robbins, ibid., p. xiii
21. A recent illustration of the popular usage of environmental stewardship is found in President Clinton's Saturday radio address of May 29, 1999. From the banks of St. Mary's River in northern Florida, Clinton referred to the years of effort that he and Vice President Al Gore have put into raising awareness of the need for "environmental stewardship." His comments reveal an assumption that Americans both understand and appreciate the notion of stewardship of the environment: "More than ever, the American people recognize the inherent value of pristine peaks, unspoiled beaches, clear and safe water. They believe in the value of environmental stewardship. I think all of us believe in the value of that stewardship." Radio Address of the President to the Nation, The White House, Office of the Press Secretary, Saturday, May 29, 1999.
22. Andrew Linzey, *Animal Theology*, Chicago: University of Illinois Press, 1995, pp. 58-59.
23. Ibid.
24. Leopold, ibid., p. 240.
25. Ibid., p. 293.
26. Paul Taylor, "The Ethics of Respect for Nature," in *Environmental Philosophy*, p. 72.
27. William Aiken, "Ethical Issues in Agriculture," in *Earthbound: Introductory Essays in Environmental Ethics*, Tom Regan, Ed. Prospect Heights, Illinois: Waveland Press, Inc., 1990. p. 249.
28. Leopold, ibid., p. 246.
29. Singer, ibid., p. 182.
30. Michael Allen Fox, "Environmental Ethics and the Ideology of Meat Eating," *Between the Species*, Summer 1993, p. 131.
31. Sharon Bloyd-Peshkin, "Mumbling About Meat," *Vegetarian Times*, October, 1991, p. 72.
32. Ibid.
33. Tom Regan reveals this disposition when he writes in *All That Dwell Therein*, p. 4, that it is possible to suppose that vegetarians, "suffer from a perverse sentimentality." That they "represent a way of life where an excessive sentimentality has spilled over the edges of rational action." Thankfully, Regan rejects this response, but he does ignore the force of sentiment as he proceeds with his effort to provide a "rational foundation" for vegetarianism.
34. David Hume, *An Enquiry Concerning the Principles of Morals*, reprinted from the edition of 1777, La Salle, Illinois: Open Court Publishing, 2nd ed., seventh printing, 1995, p. 134.
35. Annette Baier, "Hume, David," *Encyclopedia of Ethics*, New York: Garland Publications, 1992.
36. Edward F. Mooney, "Sympathy," *Encyclopedia of Ethics*.

37. Lawrence Blum, "Compassion," in *Explaining Emotions*, A. Rorty, Ed., Berkeley: University of California Press, 1980, p. 515.
38. Stephens, ibid., p. 299.
39. Leopold, ibid., p. 295.

BIBLIOGRAPHY

Aiken, W. and LaFollette, H. *World Hunger and Morality*, 2nd ed. Prentice Hall, NJ, 1996.

Aiken, W. and LaFollette, H., Eds. *World Hunger and Moral Obligation*. Prentice Hall, NJ, 1977.

Amato, P. and Partridge, S. *The New Vegetarians: Promoting Health and Protecting Life*. Plenum Press, NY, 1989

Boonin-Vail, D. The Vegetarian Savage: Rousseau's Critique of Meat Eating. *Environmental Ethics*, 15:75-84, Spring 1993.

Boyd-Peshkin, S. Mumbling About Meat. *Vegetarian Times*, October 1991.

Clarke, P.B. and Linzey, A., Eds. *Dictionary of Ethics, Theology and Society*. Routledge, NY, 1996.

Currant, J.A New Argument for Vegetarianism. *J. Social Philos.*, 28, No. 3:153-72, Winter 1997.

DesJardins, J. *Environmental Ethics: Concept, Policy, Theory*. Mayfield, Mountain View, 1999.

Fox, M.A. Environmental Ethics and the Ideology of Meat Eating. *Between the Species*, 121-32, Summer 1993.

Frey, R.G. *Rights, Killing, & Suffering*. Billing and Sons Ltd., Oxford, 1983.

Garner, R. *Animals, Politics and Morality*. Manchester University Press, Manchester, 1993.

Hillman, H. Applied Ethics: The Limits of Ethical Vegetarianism. *Free Inquiry* 18, No. 4:54-55, Fall 1998.

Hume, D. *An Enquiry Concerning the Principles of Morals*. Open Court Press, La Salle, 1966.

Kass, L.R. *Toward a More Natural Science: Biology and Human Affairs*. The Free Press, NY, 1985.

Leahy, M.P.T. *Against Liberation: Putting Animals in Perspective*. Routledge, NY, 1991.

Leopold, A. *A Sand County Almanac*. Oxford University Press, NY, 1966.

Linzey, A. *Animal Theology*. University of Illinois Press, Chicago, 1995.

Linzey, A. *Christianity and the Rights of Animals*. Crossroad Publishing Company, NY, 1987.

Linzey, A. and Regan, T., Eds. *Animals and Christianity: A Book of Readings*. Crossroad, NY, 1988.

Linzey, A. and Yamamoto, D., Eds. *Animals on the Agenda: Questions about Animals for Theology and Ethics*. University of Illinois Press, Chicago, 1998.

Moore Lappe, F. *Diet for a Small Planet*. Ballantine Books, NY, 1971.

Pierce, C. and VanDeVeer, D. *People, Penguins, and Plastic Trees*. 2nd ed. Wadsworth, NY, 1995.

Preece, R. and Chamberlain, L. *Animal Welfare and Human Values*. Wilfrid Laurier University Press, Waterloo, ON, 1993.

Regan, T. *All That Dwell Therein*. University of California Press, Berkeley, 1982.

Regan, T., Ed. *Earthbound: Introductory Essays in Environmental Ethics.* Waveland, IL, 1984.

Regan, T. and Singer, P., Eds. *Animal Rights and Human Obligations.* 2nd ed. Prentice Hall, NJ, 1976.

Reinhardt, M.W. *The Perfectly Contented Meat-Eater's Guide to Vegetarianism.* Continuum, NY, 1998.

Rifkin, J. *Beyond Beef: The Rise and Fall of the Cattle Culture.* Penguin Books, NY, 1992.

Robbins, J. *Diet for a New America.* Stillpoint, Tiburon, CA, 1987.

Rodd, R. *Biology, Ethics, and Animals.* Clarendon, Oxford, 1990.

Rosen, S. *Food for the Spirit: Vegetarianism and the World Religions.* First Bala, San Diego, 1990.

Sheth, T. and Sheth, T. *Why Be A Vegetarian?* Jain, Fremont, CA, 1973.

Singer, P. *Animal Liberation: A New Ethics for Our Treatment of Animals.* Avon Books, NY, 1975.

Singer, P. *How Are We to Live?* Prometheus Books, Amherst, NY, 1995.

Singer, P. *Practical Ethics.* Cambridge University Press, Cambridge, 1979.

Sterba, J.P. *Earth Ethics.* Prentice Hall, NJ, 1995.

Tester, K. *Animals and Society: The Humanity of Animal Rights.* Routledge, NY, 1991.

Teutsch, G.M. *Killing Animals: Reflections on the Ethics of Meat Eating.* Universitas, 2, 1993.

Zimmerman, M.E., et al., Eds. *Environmental Philosophy: From Animal Rights to Radical Ecology.* 2nd ed. Prentice Hall, NJ, 1998.

19

THE HISTORICAL CONTEXT OF VEGETARIANISM ,

James C. Whorton

CONTENTS

0-8493-8508-3/01/$0.00+$.50
© 2001 by CRC Press LLC

I. INTRODUCTION

The history of vegetarianism as a dietary movement has recently been condensed nicely, if inadvertently, in a Jumble, a type of word puzzle that appears in many American newspapers. In the Jumble, several words are presented with their letters rearranged, and the solver challenged to restore the scrambled words to their proper spelling. Certain designated letters in each reconstituted word must then be rearranged into new words to provide an answer to a picture riddle. In the Jumble under consideration, a man in a pith helmet is depicted up to his waist in a soon-to-be-simmering cauldron, nervously holding out a book titled *Good Nutrition*. The puzzle caption reads, "What the missionary had to convert the cannibals to."

The answer, of course, is vegetarianism, but the message of the puzzle is mixed. On the one hand, the text on nutrition implies that the truth of vegetarianism is derived from science; on the other, the man presenting the text is a missionary, an emissary from the church rather than the laboratory. He is attempting, furthermore, to "convert" his audience, to change their minds with moral appeals, instead of through scientific evidence and argument. In truth, for much of the history of vegetarianism in Western society, its proponents have behaved much like the missionary in the Jumble, presenting good nutrition more as a gospel than as a text, and striving to convert dietary heathen as much by preaching as by teaching.

A. The Fusion of Science and Morality in Vegetarianism

When, for example, the American Vegetarian Society was founded in 1850, the very first resolution adopted by its membership stated, "That comparative anatomy, human physiology, and...chemical analysis ... unitedly proclaim the position, that not only the human race may, but should subsist upon the products of the vegetable kingdom." The resolution that immediately followed, though, declared, "That the Vegetarian principle of diet derives its most ancient authority from the appointment of the Creator to man" in the Garden of Eden. The next two resolutions similarly claimed Biblical, as well as moral, sanctions for vegetarian diet.[1] Granted, many people today would agree that there are powerful moral, and perhaps religious, arguments to be made in support of vegetarianism. Nevertheless, modern nutritionists would take pains to keep morality separate and distinct from physiology, and not allow sentiment to dictate science.

Historically, vegetarians have not been so careful. For most of the past two centuries, their pronouncements of the nutritional superiority of a fleshless diet have been based less on independent science than on adaptations of science, directed by the faith that what is right morally must of necessity be right physically. This zealous fusion of moralism with nutrition unfortunately has given vegetarianism the reputation of fanaticism, and thus inhibited objective evaluation and recognition by mainstream nutritional science, as well as by the public at large.

II. VEGETARIANISM IN ANTIQUITY

The term vegetarianism was coined relatively recently — in the mid-1800s — when abstinence from meat began to take on the form of an organized movement. As a practice, however, it dates to quite early times in Western society, at least to Pythagoras, the Greek natural philosopher of the 6th century BC, who founded a religious community in southern Italy in which vegetarianism is supposed to have been part of the rule of life. Pythagoras' rejection of the eating of meat seems to have been based on the doctrine of the transmigration of souls: in Orphic tradition, the human spirit was reborn in other creatures. If so, animal souls were of the same quality as human souls, and animals thus of the same moral standing as people. Slaughtering an animal equated to murder, and eating it was akin to cannibalism.[2-3]

Additional justifications of vegetarianism on moral grounds were put forward by other writers in later antiquity. During the first two centuries of the Christian era, Ovid and Plutarch both spoke out against the killing of animals for food. It was "horrible cruelty!," the latter insisted, to "deprive a soul of the sun and light, and of that proportion of life and time it had been born into the world to enjoy" merely "for the sake of some little mouthful of flesh." Plutarch's essay "On Eating of Flesh," was, in fact, the most thorough condemnation of conventional diet to be penned before the Renaissance. Furthermore, while it was fundamentally a moral analysis, it did include physical arguments to complement the spiritual ones. Flesh foods, Plutarch maintained, were guilty of "clogging and cloying" the body, thereby making meat-eaters' "very minds and intellects gross." He seems also to be the first to offer an anatomical argument for vegetarianism as the natural human diet. "A human body no ways resembles those that were born for ravenousness," he observed, for it lacks fangs, claws and all the other predatory equipment of carnivores. Plutarch believed that meat was injurious to health because it brought on "grievous oppressions and qualmy indigestions" and "sickness and heaviness upon the body."[4]

III. VEGETARIANISM AND THE MEDIEVAL CHURCH

Plutarch had a final observation: "It is indeed a hard and difficult task ... to dispute with men's bellies, that have no ears."[5] The centuries that followed would only confirm his cynicism. In most people, the stomach does speak more loudly than the conscience, and it is deaf to pleas to deny self for the sake of others, particularly other species. The rise of Christianity to cultural dominance, moreover, did nothing to strengthen the voice of conscience with respect to animal welfare. There were vegetarian sects within the medieval church (like the Manichees, for example), but the orthodox position, presented by Aquinas, was that the human race was given dominion over the animal creation, and could use it as best served human needs. The ideal of kinship between people and animals that had been put forward by ancient vegetarians was overridden by Aquinas' principle that the possession of rationality was necessary for moral consideration to be extended to a creature.[6] To be sure, certain prominent churchmen —Saints John Chrysostom and Benedict, for example — did forswear the eating of flesh food; their motivation, however, was primarily the desire to suppress their own carnal appetites, rather than to show compassion for the animal creation.[7]

IV. 17TH- AND 18TH-CENTURY VEGETARIANISM

A. Thomas Tryon

It was not until the 1600s that any significant addition to the vegetarian polemic was made. But then one encounters, in the writings of Thomas Tryon, the most comprehensive brief yet, for the virtues of flesh-free diet (that an Englishman should revive vegetarianism was prophetic, for England would serve as the fountainhead of vegetarian thought well into the 19th century). Tryon, a dissenting religionist cum health reformer and sometime poet, was one of his era's better known commentators on the rules of right living, both the moral and physical. In *The Way to Health, Long Life and Happiness* (1683), he brought the two spheres together, asking

> How shall they but Bestial grow,
> That thus to feed on Beasts are willing?
> Or why should they a long Life know,
> Who daily practice KILLING?

Why they shall not know a long life, he proposed (offering the first clear mechanism for how flesh food injured), was because "nothing so soon turns to Putrifaction" as meat. In short, meat rots more quickly than vegetables, and "tis certain, such sorts of food as are subject to putrifie before they are eaten, are also liable to the same afterwards." In Tryon's reasoning, meat is highly putrescible, even after ingestion, and so must "breed great store of noxious Humours" (the humoral doctrine that ruled medical thought into the 1700s looked upon putrefied or noxious body fluids as the seat of disease). If not for the adoption of carnivorous diet, he concluded, "Man had not contracted so many Diseases in his Body."[8]

But the weight of Tryon's analysis was still on the immorality of killing animals for food. Slaughter had to be discountenanced, both because it inflicted suffering and death on "fellow creatures," and also because holy scripture indicated the original diet provided for the human race by God was meatless (Genesis 1:29). As a spiritual consequence, those who feed on meat will grow bestial in both mind and soul, while those who actually perform the butchering of animals will become so inured to pain that they will lose all feeling of tenderness toward their fellow man as well, and even sink into a life of crime. By the time his indictment was complete, Tryon had charged flesh-eating with so much sickness and vice that he could suggest that, if it were abandoned, society would soon lose any need for physicians or lawyers.

B. The 18th Century

The intertwining of the medical and the moral would remain central to the vegetarian rationale throughout the 18th century. During the later 1700s, moreover, each theme would take on additional import. More serious consideration of the moral implications of diet was encouraged by developments in two areas of thought in particular: physiology and religion. The former discipline had been made a subject of philosophical dispute in the mid-17th century by the physiological theories of France's René Descartes. Cartesianism posited that beasts were mere automata, utterly lacking in consciousness and sensation. That supposition had concentrated the attention of scientists and philosophers alike on the question of animal pain, and had provoked considerable debate over the moral implications of slaughter, vivisection experiments, and other uses of animals for human advantage.[9] But while it was generally agreed that Descartes was in error, that animals truly do experience pain, it was also suspected that their pain is not felt as keenly as humans', and maintained that, in any event, people are justified in using lower animals to realize their own desires.

During the 18th century, however, physiologists' investigations of the nervous system revealed close structural similarities between humans and other mammals, dramatically increasing the probability that brutes suffer pain as severely as people: "Answer me, mechanist," Voltaire sneered at the Cartesian physiologists; "Has nature arranged all the springs of feeling in this animal in order that he should not feel? Has he nerves in order to be unmoved?"[10] Concurrently, and especially in England, several intellectual currents were encouraging a feeling of closer relationship to animals.

The Enlightenment's promotion of the doctrine of natural rights and of humanitarian sympathy for the less fortunate encouraged a sharpened sensitivity to physical pain and abhorrence of cruelty that was sometimes being extended to the animal kingdom by the later 1700s. Jeremy Bentham, the founder of utilitarianism, expressed the new concern for animal welfare in his 1789 rejection of the argument that brutes do not have to be treated with kindness because they are not rational beings. "The question," he objected, "is not, Can they reason? nor, Can they talk? but, Can they suffer?" To be sure, the point was not necessarily an endorsement of vegetarianism; as Bentham noted, a butcher might give an animal a quicker and less painful death than it could expect from nature (one might draw from that argument that meat-eating was actually more humane than vegetarianism).[11] But in reality, butchers were not known for mercy, and every animal had a right — the word is Bentham's — to not be tormented. Limited as it was at this point, there was a notion of animal rights that was meanwhile being advanced at the same time by several other Enlightenment authors, some of whom included the right to not be used as food. Simultaneously, English religious thought was entertaining the possibility that animals possess souls and even have a heaven, thereby at least suggesting a condemnation of flesh-eating that would have made sense to Pythagoras.[12,13]

C. Evangelicalism

The most significant impact of religion on vegetarianism came from the English Evangelical movement. The product of John Wesley's determination to make Christianity a "social gospel," Evangelicalism was dedicated to alleviating the misfortunes of society's dispossessed through aggressive political action. Evangelicals, in fact, succeeded in motivating Parliament to enact legislation against the slave trade, child labor, Britain's barbaric penal code, and any number of other injustices. Not least among the Evangelicals' good works was a crusade for animal protection that attacked the mistreatment of creatures used for labor or sport, and resulted, in 1822, in Western society's first animal welfare legislation, a law to protect work animals from abuse.[14]

Vegetarianism greatly gained in appeal in this new climate, of course; and though it would remain the doctrine of a small and marginal group, vegetarian ranks did swell noticeably around the beginning of the 19th century. The literature of vegetarianism grew apace, no longer just an occasional treatise from an isolated eccentric, but a steady flow of works voicing outrage at the cruelty inflicted on innocent creatures. The title of the first major volume in the new genre expresses its moral and emotional animus perfectly: *The Cry of Nature*, John Oswald named his book, *Or, an Appeal to Mercy and to Justice, on Behalf of the Persecuted Animals* (1791). Romantic sensitivity to the beauty and purity of the world of nature gushed through such books. Oswald's frontispiece, for instance, shows a fawn that had been killed by a hunter shedding its blood upon the earth while its mother tearfully called on it to rise; an unclothed child of nature stood nearby, hiding her face in shame. "Come," Oswald invited, "approach and examine with attention this dead body. It was late a playful fawn, which, skipping and bounding ... awoke, in the soul of the feeling observer, a thousand tender emotions. But the butcher's knife hath laid low the delight of a fond dam, and the darling of nature is now stretched in gore upon the ground."[15]

V. THE 19TH CENTURY

A. Introduction of Physical Arguments for a Vegetable Diet

The moral hideousness of killing animals for food still dominated vegetarian discussions into the early decades of the 19th century. But the physical depravity of flesh food was hardly being overlooked, and by the middle of the century it would ascend to at least equal status with morality. Even Oswald recognized the unsuitability of meat for the human body. "Approach," he requested, urging readers to gaze upon the scene of carnage a second time; "Approach, I say, ... and tell me, tell me, does this ghastly spectacle whet your appetite? Delights your eyes the sight of blood? Is the steam of gore grateful to your nostrils, or pleasing to the touch, the icy ribs of death? ... or with a species of rhetoric, pitiful as it is perverse, will you still persist in your endeavour to persuade us, that to murder an innocent animal, is not cruel nor unjust; and that to feed upon a corpse, is neither filthy nor unfit?"[16] Filthy and unfit are moral terms, to be sure, but they have physiological connotations as well. The revulsion produced by the sight of blood and the smell of gore is not only an esthetic reaction; it is equally a physiological response to physical filth and physical unfitness, a recognition that the human body is not designed to receive such food as nutriment.

Increased attention to the nutritional, as opposed to the spiritual, aspects of vegetarianism was a reflection of the 18th-century Enlightenment's apotheosis of science as the indispensable method of investigation and proof. Though newly energized by the changing moral climate, vegetarianism still had to prove itself, nutritionally, if it hoped to make an impact on society's eating habits. Gaining nutritional legitimacy was actually a two-step process, the first being to demonstrate that humankind could live in health without consuming meat. It was recognized, of course, that many people went without meat by economic necessity, and were not dropping in their tracks. It was assumed, though, that such people did not live as healthfully or as long as those who enjoyed a complete diet. Meat was essential, according to general opinion, because it was most similar chemically to human muscle, so therefore must be more easily digested and assimilated than vegetable food, and provide greater strength and endurance. An all-vegetable diet, this thinking concluded, must be weakening, and surely self-preservation carried greater moral weight than kindness to other species. Two English physicians were particularly influential for demonstrating that vegetarianism was not, after all, a form of slow self-destruction.

The first was an 18th-century London practitioner, George Cheyne, one of the most widely read health writers of his day. Cheyne misspent his youth physically, attaining a weight of more than 400 pounds before turning to vegetarianism to undo the damage. Not only did he manage to return to a reasonable weight on his diet of milk and vegetables, but several other complaints that had nagged him for years disappeared as well. Through subsequent observations of "my own crazy Carcase," as well as of numerous patients, Cheyne became convinced that flesh food "shortens Life, begets chronical Distempers, and a decrepid Age."[17] His several guidebooks to health were the first to recommend vegetarianism almost exclusively for reasons of physical well-being, and to buttress claims of health with clinical cases.

William Lambe, another London practitioner, followed a similar course in the early 1800s. Although obesity was not a problem for him, he did relieve himself of longstanding illness by removing meat from his table. He then applied the diet to the care of his patients, and succeeded in curing, he believed, many cases of asthma, tuberculosis, and other chronic complaints, even cancer. In his 1809 report on these personal and clinical experiences, he submitted that "a strict vegetable regimen" was adequate for health, that meat was unnecessary, and that "what is unnecessary cannot be natural, [and] what is not natural cannot be useful."[18]

Lambe's characterization of meat as unnatural and useless influenced several individuals prominent in English society to convert to vegetarianism. Best known of all among these was the Romantic poet Percy Shelley, who in 1813 published an emotionally charged pamphlet titled "A Vindication of Natural Diet." More poetry than logic, it nonetheless did achieve a certain balance by assigning roughly equal weight to the moral and physical objections to flesh diet. On the one side, the bloody horrors of the French Revolution and the tyrannical excesses of Napoleon were blamed on the French taste for rare meat. But on the other, there was the assertion that Buonaparte's poor health, "his bile-suffused cheek ...," his wrinkled brow," were incontrovertible proof that he had not "descended from a race of vegetable feeders." Meat, Shelley declared bluntly, is "demonstrably pernicious." That was why flesh-eaters were incapable, for instance, of the "easiness of breathing" that vegetarians enjoyed, why they suffered "from that powerful and difficult panting now felt by almost everyone after hastily climbing an ordinary mountain."[19]

In point of fact, the uphill battle had to be fought by vegetarians, for not only was the weight of medical opinion still on the side of meat, but so too was public opinion and, even more importantly, popular taste: "the forbidding of animal food," Lambe had despaired, is "an injunction that sounds more unwelcome to English ears than any perhaps that could be given."[20] If flesh-eaters' habits were to be overcome, meat had to be transformed into a positive menace, demonstrated to be "pernicious" by more sophisticated physical arguments than anecdotal claims that flesh-eaters make poor alpinists. The elevation of physiology to a position of primacy in the ongoing formulation of a rationale for vegetarianism, however, was the work of American theorists rather than English or other European ones.

Vegetarianism was brought to the U.S. toward the end of the 1810s by William Metcalfe, an envoy of the Bible Christian Church. The first organization in modern times to make vegetarianism one of the requirements of membership, the Church had been founded in Manchester, England in 1807, by the Swedenborgian minister William Cowherd (the founders of modern vegetarianism might have been named by Dickens — in addition to Lambe and Cowherd, there was the latter's envoy to America, William Metcalfe, to complete an herbivore triumvirate). Though motivated in part by humanitarian sentiment, Cowherd had been equally impressed by the writings of Cheyne, and forbade his congregation meat (and alcohol, too) in large part for reasons of health.[21]

B. Sylvester Graham and Vegetarianism in America

The Bible Christians would continue in existence in England until the 1880s at least, but their greatest impact came early in the century and on American soil. Around 1830, while engaged in the business of organizing a New World branch of his church in Philadelphia, Metcalfe caught the attention of a Presbyterian minister-turned-temperance lecturer named Sylvester Graham. At the time, Graham was in the process of expanding temperance into an all-inclusive program of physical and moral reform, and Metcalfe's interpretation of the virtues of a vegetable diet was in perfect philosophical harmony with the American's own view of health behavior generally. Graham's popular health reform movement, the first stage of what would become an enduring tradition of hygienic extremism in America, was rooted in the belief that the laws of health were as much the dictates of God as the Ten Commandments and, therefore, the two sets of rules could not conflict: physiology had to be congruent with morality.

Acting from this certainty that any behavior that blemished the soul must also damage the body, Graham and his health reform followers bombarded the public of the 1830s–1850s with health injunctions against alcohol, extramarital sex, late night entertainments, and sundry other practices both hateful and hurtful; included among these, by necessity, was the consumption of meat.[22,23]

Graham hardly labored alone in erecting more extensive physiological supports for vegetarianism. Numerous health reformers contributed, most notably William Andrus Alcott, who in the late 1830s supplanted Graham as commander of health reform's forces. One of the most prolific self-help writers of the entire 19th century, Alcott authored a 1838 volume under the title *Vegetable Diet*, explaining in his subtitle that vegetarianism was *Sanctioned by Medical Men and by Experience in all Ages*; the book was intended, in short, to show that science corroborated Christian moral principles (or at least Alcott's interpretation of the spirit of compassion of the New Testament). Comparative anatomy was one of the sciences applied to the task, though the similarity of human teeth and intestines to those of herbivores had been pointed out by any number of earlier authors. The most up-to-date demonstration that meat is a poison, though, seemed to be supplied by the just-budding science of nutrition, and Alcott, Graham, and other health reformers mobilized an impressive array of entirely new nutrition-based arguments to prove their point.

The arguments were impressive for their quantity. Qualitatively, they were completely inadequate, scientifically invalid both because of the period's restricted understanding of nutrition and biochemistry, and because of health reformers' determination to squeeze science into the straightjacket of their moral preconceptions. The latter was facilitated by adoption of the pathological theories that had recently been formulated by French physician François Broussais, theories that credited all illness to excessive stimulation of body tissues, especially those of the digestive tract. Stimulation was already a loaded word morally: to the Victorian mind, arousal of carnal appetites and animal passions was the root of all evil. Broussais' pathology, in short, was the ideal foundation on which the health reform version of vegetarianism could be built. Consequently, stimulation arguments, too numerous to relate, were advanced by health reform apologists for vegetable diet throughout the antebellum period. One effort, for example, interpreted the famous *in vivo* digestion experiments performed in the 1820s by William Beaumont on a man with a gastric fistula, an opening (induced by a gunshot wound) from his thorax into his stomach. Beaumont's studies included measurement of the digestion times required by various foods, accomplished by tying food samples to a string, introducing them into the stomach, and retrieving them hourly for inspection. Beaumont's conclusion was that "generally speaking, vegetable aliment requires more time, and probably greater powers of the gastric organs, than animal."[24] Graham pounced on the observation, arguing that greater speed of digestion is clearly evidence of a more intense response by the vital powers to the stimulus of food. The more intense a response, he elaborated, the more intense the stimulus must be, so meat must be more stimulating — pathologically stimulating — than vegetables. Additional evidence existed in the feeling of warmth one experienced after a meal heavy in meat. A later generation would attribute the warmth to the specific dynamic action of protein, but for health reformers it was a "digestive fever" in which, according to Alcott, "The system ... is inevitably worn into a premature dissolution, by the violent and unnatural heat of an over-stimulated and precipitate circulation."[25] Meat even stimulated itself, decomposing (as Tryon had noted two centuries earlier) in much less time than vegetables. It followed that human flesh constructed from the excessively stimulated molecules of meat must also be less stable, more subject to decay. By Alcott's interpretation, that explained why vegetarians smelled better. "The very exhalations of the lungs," he asserted, "are purer, as is obvious from the breath. That of a vegetable-eater," he had determined, "is perfectly sweet, while that of a flesheater is often as offensive as the smell of a charnel-house. This distinction is discernible even among the brute animals. Those which feed on grass ... have a breath incomparably sweeter than those which prey on animals. Compare the camel, and horse, and cow, and sheep, and rabbit, with the tiger (if you choose to approach him)," he cautioned; "the wolf, the dog, the cat and the hawk. One comparison will be sufficient; you will never forget it."[26] Still more to the point, however, was the explanation that the unstable atoms of a carnivore's muscles must be subject to more rapid molecular turnover than a vegetarian's tissues, and hence subject to accelerated aging and premature death. The mechanics of life could be summed up simply: "A man may not inaptly be compared with a watch — the faster it goes, the sooner it will run down."[27]

The condemnation of fast living was a double entendre, for try as they might to present their ideas as concrete science, health reform vegetarians could never stop moralizing. Alcott, for instance, immediately followed his alarm over the "violent and unnatural heat" of a flesh-eater's digestive fever with the reminder that a vegetable diet is cooling, and "has a tendency to temper the passions."[28] Health reform comrade Russell Trall was even more anxious about untempered passions, warning that "no delusion on earth [is] so widespread [as] this, which confuses stimulation with nutrition. It is the very parent source of that awful ... multitude of errors, which are leading the nations of the earth into all manner of riotous living, and urging them on in the road to swift destruction."[29]

To their credit, health reform vegetarians balanced their thrilling flights of theory with down-to-earth demonstrations by cases. The proof of the theory, after all, was in the state of health of those who practiced it, and history could offer vital vegetarians aplenty in evidence. The first to be recognized, predictably, were the antediluvians, those earliest people whose simple diet kept them vigorous all the way to the end of their 900 years. But pagans could serve the cause as well, though surprisingly, it was pagan soldiers who were held up as paragons of hygiene, especially those of the Roman army, who had marched to their greatest victories on plain vegetable rations. The incongruity of the diet of gentleness and benevolence providing the strength for battlefield slaughter was missed by the health reformers in their excitement over the physical glory of the vegetarians of antiquity. Subsistence on vegetable food, according to an agitated Graham, was "true of all those ancient armies whose success depended more on bodily strength and personal prowess, in wielding warclubs and grappling man with man in the fierce exercise of muscular power, and dashing each other furiously to the earth, mangled and crushed and killed."[30] Recent, less brutal examples were more compelling and suitable, though. Alcott allotted nearly 200 pages of his book on vegetable diet to the presentation of testimonials, including such examples of pro- digious health as Amos Townsend, a graminivorous bank cashier who could "dictate a letter, count money, and hold conversation with an individual, all at the same time, with no embarrassment."[31]

C. Vegetarianism in Europe

American vegetarians' more pronounced orientation toward health impressed European counterparts, as is evident from the deliberations associated with the formation of the first national vegetarian organization. On September 30, 1847, meat abstainers from all parts of England con- vened in Ramsgate, Kent to found The Vegetarian Society. It was at this organizational meeting that the term "vegetarian" was minted, being taken from the Latin "vegetus": lively or vigorous. The founding members then pledged themselves "to induce habits of abstinence from the flesh of animals as food, by the dissemination of information upon the subject, by means of tracts, essays, and lectures." But when they next itemized the "many advantages" of a vegetable diet that would be disseminated through literature and lecture, the traditionally favored advantage, morality, was pushed to a subsidiary position; again, vigor was the emphasis, their list beginning with "physical" improvements. The Society's monthly, *The Vegetarian Messenger*, was launched 2 years later and accorded the physical the same prominence in its messages; by 1853, 20 physicians and surgeons were included among the organization's membership of more than 800.[32]

The new society's unorthodox philosophy attracted ridicule at once. Punch, for instance, reported that "a prize is to be given [by the Society] for the quickest demolition of the largest quantity of turnips; and a silver medal will be awarded to the vegetarian who will dispose of one hundred heads of celery with the utmost celerity."[33] Yet an organized movement of vegetarianism did spread with celerity, with American vegetarians quickly following the English lead and forming an American Vegetarian Society in 1850.

In the meantime, vegetarianism was following a similar development on the European continent. There, treatises such as *Thalysie: ou La Nouvelle Existence (Thalysie: or the New Existence)* by Jean Antoine Gleizes (1840), and *Pflanzenkost, die Grundlage einer Neuen Weltanschauung (Vegetable Diet, the Foundation of a New Worldview)* by Gustav von Struve (1861), slowly raised public awareness of the dietary alternative and attracted devotees; the first national organization of vegetarianism on the continent was established in Germany in 1866. Vegetarian journals and magazines appeared during the mid-century period, at first in England with the *Vegetarian Advocate* (1848) and the *Vegetarian Messenger* (1849), then continuing in the United States with the *American Vegetarian* (1851, published by the American Vegetarian Society). During the decade of the 1870s, vegetarian restaurants opened their doors in major European and American cities; London could boast of a dozen by the close of the century. Finally, the first international organization — the International Vegetarian Union — was launched in 1908.[34]

VI. THE 20TH CENTURY

A. Henry Salt

Great Britain and the United States remained the centers of vegetarian philosophy and practice into the 20th century. In the former, the cause of vegetable diet was promoted with particular eloquence by Henry Salt (Mohandas Gandhi, among others, pointed to Salt as the inspiration for his own vegetarianism). Author of numerous books calling for elimination of social injustices, Salt was nevertheless best known — most notorious — for his advocacy of *Animals' Rights*, the title of an 1892 volume that subjected every form of exploitation of the brute creation to criticism. There, and in his later *The Logic of Vegetarianism* (1899), Salt employed a thoroughly unsentimental approach to argue that philosophy and science alike required abstention from meat. Philosophy, his logic of vegetable diet, could not support the common assumptions that human beings have no moral relationship or obligation to other creatures, and that the killing of animals for food is a law of nature. That second belief had become a particularly common justification for meat eating in the years following Darwin's dramatization of nature's rule of survival of the fittest. The response of Salt, and other late-century vegetarians, was that cooperation among animals was as common a strategy for survival as competition, and that human cooperation with other species was positively enjoined by Darwin's demonstration that people were the descendants of animal ancestors: How could one defend the slaughter of creatures with whom humans shared a "bond of consanguinity?" (Just such a bond had, in fact, been suggested by Darwin himself in The Descent of Man, where he presented a sizeable body of evidence to show that "there is no fundamental difference between man and the higher mammals in their mental faculties.... The difference in mind between man and the higher animals, great as it is, certainly is one of degree and not of kind.")[35-37]

B. John Harvey Kellogg

Evolutionary kinship with livestock was a prominent element, as well, in the case constructed by America's most influential spokesman for vegetarianism in the early 20th century. John Harvey Kellogg placed greater emphasis on medical than on biological theory, and propounded what was clearly the period's most persuasive argument against the consumption of meat. Kellogg was bred a Grahamite, if not born one, by virtue of his family's membership in the Seventh-Day Adventist Church, an institution that gave allegiance to Graham's hygienic system on the basis of the divine, health-related visions experienced by spiritual leader Ellen White.[38] He also received training in hydropathy, an alternative system of medical practice that treated all conditions with applications of water, and exhorted all patients to abide by Graham's rules of health (Kellogg's mentor, and the leading figure in American hydropathy, Russell Trall, was a founding member and officer of the American Vegetarian Society, and the author of a work titled The Scientific Basis of Vegetarianism, 1860). Kellogg completed an orthodox program of medical training too, then, in 1875, returned to his native Battle Creek, Michigan to take over the directorship of a struggling hospital and health education facility operated by the Adventist Church. Not only did he quickly turn the Battle Creek Sanitarium into a thriving business, he transformed it into the most famous health institution in the country from the 1880s until World War II. As part of the Sanitarium's dietary program, Kellogg, assisted by his brother Will, invented a variety of meat substitutes and other vegetarian health foods, including the breakfast cereals that have immortalized the family name.[39,40]

Kellogg also lectured tirelessly, from coast to coast, and wrote voluminously. In addition to editing the popular periodical *Good Health*, he authored several dozen books, analyzing every aspect of personal health behavior from *The Evils of Fashionable Dress*, to *Plain Facts About Sexual Life*, to *Colon Hygiene*. The last subject, the health of the large bowel, represented Kellogg's most significant contribution to the updating of the nutritional argument for vegetarianism. Here, he worked through the dietary implications of one of the grand pathology fads of the turn of this century — intestinal autointoxication. In the 1880s, laboratory scientists had isolated several substances produced in the intestinal tract through the bacterial putrefaction of undigested protein. The compounds were determined to be toxic when directly injected into the bloodstream in animals, and it was quickly supposed that they might be absorbed from the colon into the human bloodstream and then circulated to play havoc throughout the body. Since these agents of self-poisoning were the result of bacterial activity, the theory of autointoxication could be seen as an extension of medical bacteriology. Thus, hanging onto the coattails of the germ theory, autointoxication swept into professional and popular awareness at the end of the 19th century.[41,42]

For Kellogg, the autointoxication theory provided enough ammunition to back several book-length attacks on meat eating. In such works as *Autointoxication or Intestinal Toxemia* (1918), *The Itinerary of a Breakfast* (1919), and *The Crippled Colon* (1931), he expounded time and again how the ordinary diet contained so much protein from its flesh components as to foster the growth and activity of proteolytic bacteria in the colon. As the microbes acted on undigested flesh food, the body would be "flooded with the most horrible and loathsome poisons," and brought to suffer headache, depression, skin problems, chronic fatigue, damage to the liver, kidneys, and blood vessels, and other injuries totaling up to "enormous mischief." Anyone who read to the end of Kellogg's baleful list must have been ready to agree that "the marvel is not that human life is so short and so full of miseries, mental, moral, and physical, but that civilized human beings are able to live at all."[43]

"Civilized" referred to the fiber content of the ordinary diet, too. Modern people, Kellogg chided, ate too concentrated a diet, with too little bulk to stimulate the bowels to action. A vegetarian diet, he added for the unaware, was high in roughage. Its other advantage was that it was low in protein. The high protein diet common to flesh eaters was ideal fodder for the putrefactive microorganisms of the colon, while its low fiber content slowed its rate of passage to a crawl that gave the microbes time to convert all unabsorbed protein to toxins. In the meat-eater's sluggish bowels, Kellogg believed, could be found "the secret of nine-tenths of all the chronic ills from which civilized human beings suffer," including "national inefficiency and physical unpreparedness," as well as "not a small part of our moral and social maladies."[44]

Morality could be merged with medicine in other ways. In *Shall We Slay to Eat*, Kellogg applied a bacteriological gloss to the age-old objection to the cruelty of slaughter. Reminding readers of the gentleness of unoffending cows and pigs (animals with whom humans were bound by evolution), Kellogg then forced them, Oswald-like, to gaze upon the "tide of gore," the "quivering flesh," the "writhing entrails" of the butchered animals, and to listen to their squealing and bleating as they died. What he counted upon ultimately to move his readers, though, was the abominable filth through which the tide of gore flowed. The Augean nastiness of the typical abbatoir (here nauseatingly detailed a year before Upton Sinclair's much more famous *The Jungle*) guaranteed that meat would be infested with every germ known: "Each juicy morsel," Kellogg revealed, "is fairly alive and swarming with the identical micro-organisms found in a dead rat in a closet or the putrefying carcass of a cow."[45,46]

The physical superiority of a meatless diet was demonstrated by the extraordinary success of vegetarian athletes. Indeed, as early 20th-century society became captivated by competitive sports, vegetarians turned to athletic conquest for practical proof of the nutritional advantages of their regimen. As a result, a remarkable record of vegetarian victories in all sports was compiled in the 1890s and early 1900s, from the cycling records established by England's perfectly named James Parsley, to the championships won by the tug-of-war team of the unfortunately named West Ham Vegetarian Society. Carnivore competitors refused to acknowledge vegetarians' athleticism, however, attributing their triumphs not to diet, but to the dedication and competitiveness bred by fanaticism.[47]

C. "The Newer Nutrition"

If full-fledged vegetarianism was still being taken lightly, the early 20th century did foster a new respect for the nutritional value of vegetables. Though few accepted vegetable foods as wholly sufficient for a healthful diet, all did come to see more vegetables as necessary to health. The critical development was the growth of understanding of vitamins over the first two decades of the century, accompanied by the realization that vitamin-rich fruits and vegetables were largely ignored at most tables. The most prominent representative of the so-called "newer nutrition," vitamin discoverer Elmer McCollum, estimated that, in 1923, "at least 90 per cent" of the food eaten by most American families was restricted to the old standards of white bread and butter, meat, potatoes, sugar, and coffee. His call for nationwide "dietary reform" aimed at educating and converting the public to replace much of the traditional diet with what he called the "protective foods." The resultant dietary education campaign truly made the 1920s the decade of newer nutrition, as of bathtub gin and jazz. Food educators bombarded the public through lecture, newspaper, magazine, textbook, and comic strip, and were gratified to see national consumption of fruits and vegetables increase markedly. (To note one of the more extraordinary examples, between 1925 and 1927 the spinach intake of schoolchildren in Fargo, North Dakota increased tenfold.)[48]

Public consciousness of the nutritional virtues of plant foods was not confined to vitamin awareness. Another dominant health theme of the 1920s was the lack of bulk in modern society's diet of refined and processed foods. Bulk foods were needed, of course, to prevent constipation, and ultimately autointoxication, still an unsettling threat in the public mind. Kellogg, Post, and other manufacturers of bran-containing breakfast cereals, fostered popular anxiety over torpid intestines with grossly exaggerated advertising warnings, giving the '20s as pronounced a fiber consciousness as any more recent decade. But there was also a disinterested promotion of a higher fiber diet, carried out by altruistic health reformers, some of them physicians and scientists. At the head of this group was Britain's arch enemy to autointoxication, the renowned surgeon Sir William Arbuthnot Lane. Convinced that the upright posture and soft life-style of civilized people weakened the colon and produced "chronic intestinal stasis," Lane surgically removed the colons of hundreds of patients during the 1910s in order to save them from autointoxication. The risks of surgery, as well as criticism from his professional colleagues, forced Lane to stop doing colectomies in the 1920s. But he remained convinced that constipation was the fundamental disease of civilization, and was responsible for a host of illnesses, including colon cancer and other neoplasms. Consequently, in 1926, he organized the New Health Society in London, and dedicated the last 17 years of his life to lecturing and writing on the dangers of intestinal stasis. Through Lane, the New Health Society and the magazine *New Health*, British and American consumers were repeatedly harangued about the importance of fruits and vegetables for maintaining bowel regularity and preventing more-serious diseases.[49]

A regular part of Lane's presentations was anecdotal reports of the relative freedom from autointoxication diseases enjoyed by the vegetarian populations of less developed nations. It was not until the late 1940s, though, after Lane had died and autointoxication had disappeared from orthodox medical theory, that epidemiological studies of so-called Third World cultures began to verify Lane's anecdotes by demonstrating statistical correlations between a high intake of dietary fiber and low incidences of hemorrhoids, gallstones, colon cancer, and various other "Western diseases."[50] Although some of the specific conclusions associated with the dietary fiber hypothesis have sparked debate, not to mention controversy, among nutritionists and other health scientists, fiber has been formally recognized as a necessary component of the diet, and the general public has clearly been impressed with the health benefits of a diet high in unrefined vegetable foods.

Highly publicized studies linking cholesterol and saturated fats with cardiovascular disease have similarly conditioned society to associate vegetarianism with health, and have motivated physicians and nutritionists to study heart disease and longevity in vegetarian groups such as Seventh-Day Adventists and Trappist monks. Those studies, conducted from the 1950s onward and too numerous to cite specifically, have largely confirmed what early 19th-century vegetarians initially proposed, that a vegetable diet not only is adequate to sustain health, but may actually improve it.[51,52]

D. The Revival of Animal Rights

Running parallel to the 20th-century growth of medical support for vegetarianism has been the expansion of the diet's moral rationale. Until recently, this argument has been directed, almost exclusively, at the pain inflicted on animals at the time of slaughter, and the injustice of depriving them of life. Some attention has been directed also to the discomforts endured by livestock being driven or transported to market; this issue was introduced into discussion in the mid-19th century, as animals began to be shipped in crowded boxcars and ship holds. But while both types of objections continue, criticism has broadened since the middle of this century to take in the treatment of animals throughout their lives. The transformation of farming into agribusiness included the adoption of economies of scale in stock raising, fostering a system of more-intensive rearing methods — "factory farming" — that confines animals in unnatural environments from birth. Ruth Harrison's 1964 *Animal Machines* first called public attention to the raising of chickens in overcrowded coops and the packing of pigs into "Bacon Bin" fattening houses. Photographs of veal calves penned in narrow wooden cages all the days of their short lives soon became a regular feature in vegetarian appeals (outdone in emotional impact only by the pictures of bludgeoned baby seals used in anti-fur advertisements). The maintenance of hens under similar conditions has encouraged lacto-ovo-vegetarians to give up eggs; some have abandoned milk products, as well, in protest of the dairy industry's practice of separating calves from their mothers soon after birth (and the subsequent transformation of those calves into veal). The ranks of vegans thus have grown considerably in the later 20th century (vegans are sometimes referred to as pure vegetarians, but there is some question about the applicability of the term, since the word "vegetarian" was coined to refer to a diet that includes eggs and milk). Even meat-eaters have been affected by the critique of factory farming, a sizeable number now selecting "free-range" animal products whenever they are available.[53]

Bentham's suggestion that slaughtering an animal for food rescues it from a more painful and protracted death in the wild has lost its cogency in the age of the factory farm; now an animal's entire existence might be seen as one long death. The morality of sentencing any creature to so wretched an existence has been raised to a higher level of discussion, moreover, by the animal rights movement of the last quarter century. Peter Singer's 1975 work, *Animal Liberation*, is the primary catalyst of the movement. The book is a work in which the heavily sentimental tone of traditional vegetarian moralism is set aside in favor of a rigidly philosophical analysis that recognizes animals as sentient beings, capable of experiencing pain and pleasure, and concludes that they should therefore be granted the same respect as humans in areas where their interests are affected. Many violations of those interests are attacked by Singer (and they are much the same as the ones assailed by Salt nearly a century before): the use of animals in experimental research, for example, and the raising of animals for fur. But because of the sheer numbers involved, the worst example of "speciesism," of moral discrimination purely on the basis of biological species, is the raising and killing of animals for food: "the most extensive exploitation of other species that has ever existed."[54,55] The most significant element in such exploitation, however, is regarded not as the unnatural conditions of life imposed on livestock, or even their physical suffering. Fundamental to the animals'-rights analysis is the affirmation of a right to life for every creature. Thus, even if the animal is allowed a free-range existence and slaughtered painlessly, the simple act of killing it for food constitutes an unjustifiable moral offense.

The arguments of Singer, Tom Regan, and other advocates of equal moral consideration for animals have elicited a serious response from the philosophy community. Over the past two decades, professional journals and conferences have given an extraordinary amount of attention to the issue of animal rights and its practical applications, including vegetarianism. To be sure, much of the reaction among philosophers has been critical, the Singer analysis being faulted on grounds of logic, and even attacked as a trivialization of civil rights, women's rights, and other movements promoting more moral treatment of fellow human beings.[56] Yet, a good bit of the discussion has been supportive, endorsing both the abstract proposition of an animal's right to life, and older sentiments, such as an intuitive appreciation that eating animals with whom people sense a bond of kinship is wrong.[57] Speciesism has acquired an odious taint as well, from the human exploitation of wild animals that has pushed many species to the brink of extinction, and by research on communication in other mammals that has strengthened our feeling of relation to the animal kingdom.

E. Environmentalism And Vegetarianism

Not only have the moral and medical defenses of a vegetable diet individually grown stronger over the 20th century, they have been buttressed in recent decades by environmental arguments. This is not an entirely new approach — 18th- and 19th-century vegetarians occasionally pointed out that less land would be needed for agriculture if people were fed on grain rather than meat. But with this century's rampant growth of population, the ceaseless conversion of arable land into housing tracts and strip malls, and the dramatic expansion of industry and spread of industrial pollution, degradation of the environment has become an object of grave scientific and public concern. As attention has been focused ever more sharply on the multitudinous threats to the fragile environment of our shrinking globe, the flesh diet has been recognized as a significant contributor to environmental decline. The ecology of meat eating was first explored thoroughly by Frances Moore Lappe, whose 1971 best-seller *Diet For a Small Planet* examined livestock farming's toll on the land, water, and air. Since Lappe, it has become commonplace for vegetarian literature to detail the soil erosion associated with the cultivation of livestock food crops; the excessive demands on water supplies to irrigate those crops; the pollution of waterways by field and feedlot runoff; the vast amounts of fossil fuel energy expended in raising meat animals; even the contribution to global warming made by the methane released into the atmosphere through cattle flatulence. Lately, the destruction of the tropical rain forest to provide more grazing land for beef cattle has been singled out as the flesh diet's greatest threat to the viability of "spaceship earth." And, in the end, ecology has returned to ethics. In the 20th-anniversary edition of *Diet for a Small Planet* (1991), Lappe concentrated her criticisms on the immorality of growing grain for the fattening of cattle while millions of people worldwide starve.[58]

F. Asian Influences on Vegetarianism

A final characteristic of contemporary vegetarianism is its joining of East and West. Westerners' fascination with Asian religious traditions (Hinduism, Buddhism and Jainism all encourage abstention from meat to some degree) has been an important stimulus to the growth of vegetarianism over the past 25 years, with vegetarian religious sects such as the International Society for Krishna Consciousness now being widely distributed through North America and Europe. So even as the scientific foundation for vegetarian nutrition expands and solidifies, converts come into the fold for reasons additional to physical health, and too often lack a sound understanding of nutritional principles. (Zen macrobiotic dieters, in particular, have become notorious for self-injury.)[59-61]

The history of vegetarianism is of considerable interest for its own sake, regardless of any applications it might have to the practical dietary questions of the present. History does offer a modest moral, nonetheless. By demonstrating the difficulty of separating science from sentiment in questions of humane diet, it validates the concern of modern-day nutritionists that the moral fervor that has long activated so many vegetarians has to be informed by cool-headed science. If the vegetarian missionary is to be kept out of hot water, he has to read and understand that text of good nutrition himself, and not just brandish it before his detractors.

REFERENCES

1. Proceedings of the American Vegetarian Convention. *American Vegetarian*, 1: 1, 1851.
2. Dombrowski, D. *The Philosophy of Vegetarianism*. University of Massachusetts Press, Amherst, MA, 1984.
3. Spencer, C. *The Heretic's Feast*. Fourth Estate, London, 1993.
4. Plutarch. Of eating of flesh. In: *Plutarch's Miscellanies and Essays*. 3, Goodwin, W., Trans., Little, Brown, Boston, 6-9, 14, 1898.
5. Plutarch. Of eating of flesh. In: *Plutarch's Miscellanies and Essays*. 3, Goodwin, W., Trans., Little, Brown, Boston, 10, 1898.
6. Aquinas, T. *Summa Theologiae. A Concise Translation*. McDermott, T., Ed., Eyre and Spottiswoode, London, 146, 188, 1989.
7. Dombrowski, D. *The Philosophy of Vegetarianism*. University of Massachusetts Press, Amherst, MA, 1984.
8. Tryon, T. *The Way to Health, Long Life and Happiness*. Sowle, London, 342-460, 1683.
9. Cottingham, J. "A brute to the brutes?": Descartes' treatment of animals. *Philosophy*, 53: 551, 1978.
10. Voltaire. *Philosophical Dictionary*. vol. 1, Gay, P., Trans., New York, 1962.
11. Bentham, J. *An Introduction to the Principles of Morals and Legislation*. Garden City, NY, 380-1, 1961.
12. Turner, J. *Reckoning with the Beast*. Johns Hopkins University Press, Baltimore, 1-14, 1980.
13. Stevenson, L. Religious elements in the background of the British anti-vivisection movement. *Yale Journal of Biology and Medicine*, 29: 125, 1956.
14. Turner, J. *Reckoning with the Beast*. Johns Hopkins University Press, Baltimore, 15-38, 1980.
15. Oswald, J. *The Cry of Nature*. Johnson, London, 22, 1791.
16. Oswald, J. *The Cry of Nature*. Johnson, London, 22-3, 1791.
17. Cheyne, G. *An Essay of Health and Long Life*. Strahan, London, xvi, 94, 1734.
18. Lambe, W. *Additional Reports on the Effects of a Peculiar Regimen*. Mawman, London, 172, 1815.

19. Shelley, P. *A Vindication of Natural Diet.* Pitman, London, 17-20, 1884.
20. Lambe, W. *Additional Reports on the Effects of a Peculiar Regimen.* Mawman, London, 130, 1815.
21. Forward, C. *Fifty Years of Food Reform, Ideal Publishing Union.* London, 7, 1898.
22. Whorton, J. 'Tempest in a flesh-pot.' The formulation of a physiological rationale for vegetarianism. *J. History Med. and Allied Sciences,* 32: 115, 1977.
23. Whorton, J. *Crusaders for Fitness.* The History of American Health Reformers, Princeton University Press, Princeton, NJ, 1982.
24. Beaumont, W. *Experiments and Observations on the Gastric Juice, and the Physiology of Digestion.* Allen, Plattsburgh, NY, 36, 1833.
25. Alcott, W. *Animal and vegetable food. Library of Health,* 4: 220, 1840.
26. Alcott, W. *Vegetable Diet: As Sanctioned by Medical Men, and by Experience in All Ages.* Capen and Lyon, Boston, 1838, 233-4.
27. Cambell, D. Stimulation. *Graham Journal of Health and Longevity,* 1: 290, 1837.
28. Alcott, W. Animal and vegetable food. *Library of Health,* 4: 220, 1840.
29. Trall, R. *The Scientific Basis of Vegetarianism.* Fowler and Wells, Philadelphia, 10, 1860.
30. Graham S. *Lectures on the Science of Human Life.* Vol. 2, Marsh, Capen, Lyon and Webb, Boston, 188, 1839.
31. Alcott, W. *Vegetable Diet: As Sanctioned by Medical Men, and by Experience in all Ages.* Capen and Lyon, Boston, 75-6, 1838.
32. Forward, C. *Fifty Years of Food Reform.* Ideal Publishing Union, London, 22, 33, 1898.
33. Anonymous. The vegetarian movement. *Punch,* 15: 182, 1848.
34. Forward, C. *Fifty Years of Food Reform.* Ideal Publishing Company, London, 102, 1898.
35. Salt, H. *Animals' Rights Considered in Relation to Social Progress.* MacMillan, London, 1892.
36. Salt, H. *The Logic of Vegetarianism.* London, 50, 1899.
37. Darwin, C. *The Descent of Man.* Murray, London, 74, 143, 1877.
38. Numbers, R. *Prophetess of Health. A Study of Ellen G. White.* Harper and Row, New York, 1976.
39. Schwartz, R. *John Harvey Kellogg, M.D.* Southern Publishing, Nashville, 1970.
40. Whorton, J. *Crusaders for Fitness: The History of American Health Reformers.* Princeton University Press, Princeton, NJ, 201-38, 1982.
41. Chen, T. and Chen, P. Intestinal autointoxication: a medical leitmotif. *J. Clin. Gastro.,* 11: 434, 1989.
42. Whorton J. Inner hygiene: the philosophy and practice of intestinal purity in western civilization. In: *History of Hygiene.* Proc. 12th Int. Symp. on Comp. Hist. of Med. — East and West, Kawakita, Y., Sakai, S., and Otsuka, Y., Eds., Ishiyaku Euroamerica, Tokyo, 1-32, 1991.
43. Kellogg, J. *Autointoxication or Intestinal Toxemia.* Modern Medicine Publishing, Battle Creek, MI, 131, 1918.
44. Kellogg, J. *The Itinerary of a Breakfast.* Modern Medicine Publishing, Battle Creek, MI, 87, 93, 1919.
45. Kellogg, J. *Shall We Slay to Eat?* Good Health Publishing, Battle Creek, MI, 145-67, 1905.
46. Kellogg J. *The Natural Diet of Man.* Modern Medicine Publishing, Battle Creek, MI, 107, 1923.

47. Whorton, J. Muscular vegetarianism: the debate over diet and athletic performance in the progressive era. *J. Sport Hist.*, 8: 58, 1981.
48. Whorton, J. Eating to win. *Popular concepts of diet, strength, and energy in the early 20th century, in Fitness in American Culture. Images of Health, Sport, and the Body, 1830-1940.* Grover, K., Ed., University of Massachusetts Press, Amherst, MA, 86-122.
49. Whorton J. Inner hygiene: the philosophy and practice of intestinal purity in western civilization, in History of Hygiene. *History of Hygiene. Proc. 12th Int. Symp. on Comp. Hist. of Med. — East and West.* Kawakita, Y., Sakai, S., and Otsuka, Y., Eds., Ishiyaku EuroAmerica, Tokyo, 1-31, 1991.
50. Trowell, H. *Western Diseases, their Emergence and Prevention.* Harvard University Press, Cambridge, MA, 1981.
51. Hardinge, M. and Crooks, H. Non-flesh dietaries. *J. Am. Dietetic Assoc.*, 43: 545, 1963.
52. Amato, P. and Partridge, S. *The New Vegetarians.* Plenum Press, NY, 10-15, 1989.
53. Harrison, R. *Animal Machines.* Stuart, London, 1964.
54. Singer, P. *Animal Liberation. A New Ethics for our Treatment of Animals.* Avon, NY, 92, 1975.
55. Regan, T. The moral basis of vegetarianism. *Can. J. Phil.*, 5: 181, 1975.
56. Francis, L. and Norman, R. *Some animals are more equal than others.* Philosophy, 53: 507, 1978.
57. Diamond, C. Eating meat and eating people. *Philosophy,* 53: 465, 1978.
58. Lappe, F. *Diet for a Small Planet.* Ballantine, NY, 1971.
59. Barkas, J. *The Vegetable Passion.* Scribner, NY, 157-64, 1975.
60. Akers, K. *A Vegetarian Sourcebook.* Putnam, NY, 1983.
61. Dwyer, J., Mayer, L., Dowd, K., Kandel, M., and Mayer, J. The new vegetarians. The natural high? *J. Am. Dietetic Assoc.*, 65: 529, 1974.

20

RELIGION, SPIRITUALITY, AND A VEGETARIAN DIETARY

Glen Blix

CONTENTS

0-8493-8508-3/01/$0.00+$.50
© 2001 by CRC Press LLC

I. INTRODUCTION

Since the dawn of civilization, there has been an inexorable intertwining of food and religion. The earliest of recorded history is rife with the interconnections. The plethora of cultures with their divergent practices and behaviors still share this one commonality, for humans seem incapable of separating nourishment of the body from sustenance for the soul.

Because the religions of civilization are legion, an attempt to recite the relationship of a flesh-free, plant-based diet with each one individually would not only be impossible but would also obscure the unifying and underlying principles they often hold in common. Religious justification of vegetarian practice has evolved in and through five distinct phases, and while it is possible to see these as progressive and sequential developments, there is also an argument to be made for their simultaneous elaboration. Each of these categories exists today and each can point to the antiquity of its origin. Each position has its strengths, as well as its weaknesses, and truth, as always, must be found by treading carefully the ridge that separates the abysses on either side.

The recorded history of humanity is but a few millennia old and, in the absence of a written record, much of the understanding of the ancient past must be left to inference, myth, and even conjecture. Clear delineation of vegetarian ideas and ideals is not evident until the 6th century before Christ. This was a period of time that seems to mark a turning point in the intellectual and spiritual development of humankind.[1]

Charles Potter in his book The Faiths Men Live By, comments: "What was there in the air in the sixth century BC? Did cosmic rays from some distant bursting sun strike this old earth and stir up genes and chromosomes of the sons and daughters of men so that they begat and brought forth geniuses — prophets and philosophers and founders of religions?"[2]

This ancient renaissance produced the early mystic Zoroaster in Persia, many of the major Hebrew prophets including Daniel, Eastern religious leaders such as Mahavira and Buddha, and the early Greek philosophers like Pythagoras. Although some may question the historicity of some of these individuals, it is the ideas traditionally ascribed to them that are of prime interest in this discussion. The dating used herein is open to some uncertainty, but there is considerable evidence that these philosophers were contemporaries. (Figure 20.1)

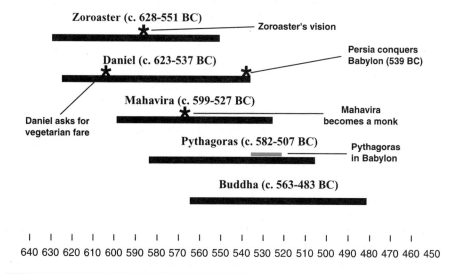

Figure 20.1 Overlapping lives of early religious vegetarians.

While these five notables are representative of the religious thought of the era, they are chosen primarily because of their incorporation of vegetarian principles into their religious practice and instruction. The various spiritual and religious tenets giving rise to the avoidance of flesh foods and the embracing of a plant-based diet are initiated and illustrated in the lives and teachings of these ancient philosophers.

Personal contact among these leaders of religious thought in the ancient world can only be conjectured, but given the pervasiveness of the Persian Empire, it is not inconceivable that at least the ideas were shared. These five magi provide a framework for the subsequent religious thought that has accompanied vegetarianism and are thus fittingly representative of the five phases of philosophical and religious vegetarian thought.

Although each of these philosophers has been chosen to represent a particular spiritual facet finding its expression in a vegetarian life-style, it must be understood that these principles were often simulta-neously present in the thought and action of both the leader and those who followed in his footsteps. Never did these principles develop in isolation, and the proximity of their originators in time and place undoubtedly argues for a cross-fertilization of ideas and practice. Instead, this division should be viewed as a somewhat arbitrary construct to assist in understanding these spiritual compo-nents of a vegetarian way of life.

II. THE RESPONSIBILITY FOR AND CARE TAKING OF NATURE

The initial religious construct justifying and compelling vegetarianism is that of caring for nature. This is expressed as a religious duty demanding a responsibility for nature in terms of preserving and maintaining its function. This stems either from a belief in a creator/originator who assigned this responsibility to humankind, or an understanding of nature itself as a deity demanding reverence and worship. In either case, the unnecessary destruction of both vegetative and animal life is seen as a violation of the principle. Although it can be argued that appropriate use of lower-order animals falls within responsible use, vegetarian adherents maintain that the destruction of animal life for human nourishment is unnecessary when sufficient plant sources are available. As a result, the use of lower-order animals for food is deemed a misuse, and even a sinful act because it violates the caretaking function. The inefficient and wasteful use of nature's resources in animal husbandry is a more recent expansion of this concept.

A. Zoroaster (c. 628–551 BCE)

The origination of this school of thought can be traced back at least as far as Zoroaster or Zarathushtra, the more accurate rendering of his old Persian name. This ancient mystic was the founder of Zoroastrianism, one of the world's oldest creed-based religions. Most of what is known of Zarathushtra is derived from the Gathas, or "divine hymns" that are ascribed to him.

He was most likely born near Azerbaijan in northern Persia.[3] As a youth, he was dismayed at the bloody animal sacrifices carried out by the priests and found it incongruous that the killing of helpless animals could in anyway be considered an act of worship worthy of the gods. Tradition holds that at the age of 30, Zarathushtra received a vision that marked the beginning of his prophetic calling. In it, a divine being instructed him that humans were to: "Consider yourselves no higher than anything else that is created. Plants and animals have kept themselves more pure than you have. Do not forget that you are to protect and look after them; in return they will help you."[4]

After years of struggle with the priests of the established cults, he found a champion in Vishtaspa, king of Chorasmia (thought to be the father of Darius I), in what is now western Turkistan. Thereafter, the religion preached by Zarathushtra prospered and was eventually adopted as the official state creed by the Medo-Persian Empire.

Zoroasterism existed in the Parthian and the second Persian Empire over a span of more than 1000 years, during which time the religion enjoyed great wealth and secular power. In the 7th century after Christ, the Arabs conquered Persia, and gradually Zoroasterians were reduced to a small minority, many having died for their faith. A persecuted few fled to India, settling primarily around Bombay, where their descendants, the Parsees, still live and practice. It is estimated that today some 200,000 subscribe to the religion and a vegetarian way of life.[5]

Zarathushtra taught a type of monotheism and saw good and evil as a continuous struggle within the human mind. The supreme deity, Ahura-Mazda, was regarded as the creator of all things and thus worthy of worship. Zarathushtra also believed that there was an afterlife very much like life on earth, however, this afterlife was available only to those who lived by God's eternal law. Bringing harm to nature was forbidden and any defilement of the soil or water was considered a violation of the creator's law. Life and matter were considered aspects of God's bounty and were therefore perfect. It was truly the first ecological religion. Because of these beliefs, Zarathushtra refused to eat meat.[6]

B. Ahimsa

The concept of ahimsa, loosely translated as "nonviolence," is a central element in most Eastern religions. While it is most often applied in a vegetarian sense to the sacredness of life, some Eastern religions, most notably the Jains, hold that the concept of ahimsa be extended to the well-being of the soil, water, and air.[7] Thus, ecological responsibility demands that only the most efficient use be made of these elements and that they not be exploited or damaged in any way. This is one of the principles that necessitates a vegetarian diet by its the adherents.

C. Christian and Jewish Ecological Responsibility

Vegetarian Christian and Jewish adherents find Biblical support for an ecological vegetarianism based on the dual obligations of loving their fellow humans and holding dominion over nature.

1. Loving One's Neighbor

Both the Old and New testaments of the Bible contain the command: "... thou shalt love thy neighbor as thyself" Leviticus 19:18, and "Love worketh no ill to his neighbor: therefore love is the fulfilling of the law," Romans 13:9 & 10.

This implies, among other things, the importance of performing actions that provide for a neighbor's health and well-being. In matters of diet, this would mean not only sharing the knowledge of the health benefits of vegetarianism, but also of circumscribing appetite and food choices in a way that will not deprive others' nourishment.

By Christ's own definition, a "neighbor" includes anyone in need. A Christian would thus be compelled to acknowledge that, in making dietary choices, consideration must be given not only to that which is most healthful and personally beneficial, but also to that which makes the most efficient use of available resources, particularly those in scarce supply. This responsibility extends, not only to earth's current inhabitants, but also to future generations, because the actions of today impact the food supply of tomorrow. The principle of neighborly love dictates that food and other choices be made so as not to negatively impact anyone's ability to meet nutritional needs, both now and in the future.

Christian and other vegetarian adherents point out that the rate at which the population is growing is alarming. Presently, there are over six billion inhabitants on earth — an increase from one billion only 150 years ago.[8] Looking ahead by about the same amount of time, assuming present growth rates, there will be 600 billion people on this planet by 2150. It will quite literally be impossible to feed this number. More than 90% of the population growth is occurring in the developing world, but at the same time, the industrialized nations are using 80% of the world's agricultural production.[9] A Cornell University study concluded that the world can support only 2 billion people at the standard of living now enjoyed by the U.S.[10] One of the major reasons for this is the heavy reliance on animal food products.

Unless steps are taken to both curb population growth and increase the available food in a voluntary and humane way, nature will do it in a cruel and vicious manner. This "natural" adjustment has already begun. Some 1.5 billion people are now living in absolute poverty and over 700 million are starving or severely malnourished.[11] Of these, 13 million die each year from the effects of malnutrition.[12]

Vegetarians assert that if food energy is harvested at the level of vegetative life, 12 to 25 times the number of individuals can be supported, as compared with food derived at the animal level.[13] Thus, for example, a milk and meat diet can support only 0.28 individuals per acre, while a rice and bean diet can provide nourishment to seven individuals on the same plot of land.

2. Dominion over Nature

The second principle is that of responsibility to and for the lower orders of life. The original command to Adam, in Genesis 1:28 of the Hebrew scripture, was to "have dominion" over nature: "And God blessed them, and God said unto them, Be fruitful and multiply, and replenish the earth, and subdue it: and have dominion over the fish of the sea, and over the fowl of the air, and over every living thing that moveth upon the earth."

For Jews and Christians, this divinely commanded responsibility is still in effect, having never been revoked. But as author Richard Schwartz points out,"Dominion does not mean that we have the right to conquer and exploit. Immediately after God gave people dominion over animals (Genesis 1:28), He prohibited their use for food (Genesis 1:29)"

Having dominion implies a responsibility for care taking and preservation. This extends to all living creatures, and apparently to the vegetative life as well, since Adam and Eve and, by extension, their descendants, were not only to "eat the fruit of the garden" but were also to "dress and keep it." While the Hebrew word abad, translated as "dress," implies making use of the garden, the word shamar, rendered "keep," refers to a guarding or protecting function.[14]

Many Christian and Jewish vegetarians insist that human nourishment must not come at the expense of nature, but rather must be in concert with it. This implies an obligation, not only to prevent the destruction of nature, but also for responsible and efficient husbandry, producing a conservation and preservation of the flora and fauna. Long before political correctness required it, Judao-Christian vegetarians felt bound by divine command to be ecologically responsible.

Their argument is persuasive. Over one third of all raw materials consumed — including fossil fuels — are devoted to the production of livestock.[15] Over 64% of the cropland[16] and 70% of the grain produced in the U.S. is used to feed livestock.[17] Feed grains are consumed at a rate of 1460 pounds per capita in the U.S., as compared with 255 pounds for the rest of the world.[18] More than half of all the water used in the U.S. goes to irrigate land to grow livestock feed.[19] Author Francis Moore Lappe notes that the amount of water required to produce just 10 pounds of steak equals an average family's water needs for an entire year.[20] The Rain Forest Action Network estimates that the production of a 4-ounce beef patty (for a hamburger) represents the destruction of 55 square feet of rainforest.[21] Two thousand years ago, tropical rainforests covered 5 billion acres of the earth's surface. In the intervening period, the creation of more farmland has destroyed half of this forest. Most of this destruction has happened in the past 200 years.[22]

Vegetarians of this persuasion argue that neighborly responsibility demands a curb on resource use. They maintain that, in providing food to the peoples of the world, a vegetarian diet is the only one that is unselfish.

A Christian's ecological responsibility is perhaps best summed up in a quote from Loren Wilkenson in her book *Earthkeeping: Christian Stewardship of Natural Resources*: "A concern, both for the world's poor and for the maintenance of the healthy diversity of the ecosphere, suggests that large-scale changes are needed in the diet to which most North Americans have been accustomed. Are we willing to reduce our own personal impact on the food production system, for reasons of economic and political survival? We, or our children, might have to. But for reasons of compassion, love and stewardly responsibility, not to mention for reasons of personal health, we might want to reduce our consumption. In either case, some sort of change in diet seems inevitable for North Americans in the near future. As Christians, we must determine whether that change will be forced upon us, or whether we will be leaders in effecting it."[23]

3. The Enhancement of Mental and Physical Faculties

The health of the body has not always been seen as a necessary adjunct to spirituality. In fact, asceticism devalues the physical body. Ironically, both bodily health and bodily mutilation are used to justify vegetarianism. Adherents who justify their vegetarianism on the basis of bodily health point out that mental health is impacted by physical health, and since the mind is the vehicle of spiritual communication, a healthy body will provide the sustenance and environment required by a healthy mind that, in turn, will be better able to communicate with divinity. This principle also applies to those who believe that the afterlife will be a continuation of a life similar to that now lived. Thus, the diet of Paradise will be similar to that which best promotes the health of mind and body here and now — a vegetarian regimen. Furthermore, since Paradise makes no provision for death, a flesh-based diet would be totally incompatible with a death-free afterlife.

4. Daniel (c. 623–537 BCE)

Daniel is, perhaps, the most controversial representative of vegetarian thought. Biblical scholars have long debated his existence because there is no extra Biblical evidence to support the scriptural accounts. Many have dated the Biblical records as originating some 400 years later than claimed. There is, however, no unanimity on this point and secular literature provides no evidence that he did not exist in the 6th century BCE.[24] Regardless of the historical accuracy of the actual individual, the principles enunciated by the Book of **Daniel** pertaining to vegetarianism still serve to characterize bodily health as one of the major religious reasons for a flesh-free lifestyle.

The Book of Daniel in the Hebrew scripture identifies Daniel as a Jewish captive taken by Nebuchadnezzar II (605–562 BCE), the Babylonian king, during his first Syrian campaign in 605 BCE when Jerusalem was also attacked.[25] As was the Babylonian custom, hostages from the nobility of the conquered peoples were retrained and instructed in the Babylonian schools, in an attempt to not only instill loyalty, but also to indoctrinate them in the religion and philosophy of the conquerors.

The first chapter of Daniel records what is, for all practical purposes, the first depiction of adherence to a vegetarian diet. Not wishing to partake of the food from the king's table, possibly due to the fact that it had first been presented to the Babylonian deities, but also perhaps due to its composition, four of the Hebrew captives asked for a modification. Daniel and his companions requested a diet composed of zeroim (things sown), in other words, food grown from seed — a plant-based diet. "Then Daniel said to the steward whom the chief of the eunuchs had appointed over Daniel, Hananiah, Mishael, and Azariah; 'Test your servants for ten days; let us be given vegetables to eat and water to drink.'"[26]

When an initial 10-day trial showed no noticeable deterioration, they were allowed to maintain their dietary preference for the remaining 3 years of their educational experience. At the conclusion of their education, they were found to have not only kept up with the other students, but also to have surpassed them in physical and intellectual attainment. "At the end of the time set by the king to bring them in, the chief official presented them to Nebuchadnezzar. The king talked with them and he found none equal to Daniel, Hananiah, Mishael, and Azariah; so they entered the king's service. In every matter of wisdom and understanding about which the king questioned them, he found them ten times better than all the magicians and enchanters in his whole kingdom."[27]

Daniel was advanced to the rank of advisor to the king and, as a result of his intellect, integrity, and an ability to interpret dreams, was held in very high regard by the royalty of Babylon. Even when he eventually retired, memory of his ability still lingered, and on the night of the Medo-Persian conquest of Babylon in 539 BCE, he was called to interpret yet another vision that announced the doom of the Babylonian Empire.

The Meads and Persians, having adopted Zoroaster's teachings, had high respect for anyone who interpreted dreams. Daniel's vegetarian diet would also have resonated with Zoroastrian principles and Daniel thus became a valued counselor in the Medo-Persian court, apparently serving as late as the third year of Cyrus the Great.[28] The principle of the connection of diet and mental state is even enunciated by Hippocrates, who, writing some 200 years later, claimed that, "beef causes exacerbation of melancholic disorders and is difficult of digestion."[29]

5. Vegetarian Christians and Health

For Christians, the makeup of diet follows the principle of treating the body as the "temple of God." In the Judao-Christian tradition, the Bible leaves little doubt that there is individual responsibility to maintain the body in a healthful state, as evidenced in such passages as 1 Corinthians 3:16 &17: "Know ye not that ye are the temple of God, and that the Spirit of God dwelleth in you? If any man defile the temple of God, him shall God destroy; for the temple of God is holy, which temple ye are."

This means treating it in a way that causes no defilement, but it also implies ingesting only that which will maintain it in the best of health and will contribute to mental acuity.

Interestingly, true scientific investigation exploring the health effects of a vegetarian diet has occurred only in the very recent past. Modern scientific evaluation of the effect of a plant-based regimen can be dated from the early 1950s, the most notable being the publication of research documenting the adequate nutritional status of vegetarians by Mervin Hardinge and Fredrick Stare.[30]

Since that time, numerous studies have shown that a plant-based diet is a healthier way to live. The Adventist Health Study, a prospective investigation of some 30,000 Californian members of the Seventh-Day Adventist church, found that, within that population, meat consumption was positively associated with all-cause mortality.[31] In looking at specific disease states, the researchers further reported that among food variables, total meat intake was the strongest risk factor for colon cancer.[32]

III. THE SACREDNESS OF LIFE

The ancients must have early observed that life was distinct from physical material. Death often occurred even when the body appeared intact and whole. Life was thus seen as something that empowered the body, a spirit that animated and gave rise to motion and consciousness. If this was true of humans, why might it not also be true of the beasts?

That life is sacred stems from two complementary belief systems; one maintains that each living creature possesses a soul or spirit that continues to exist and reinhabit another life form upon the death of the original creature. It appears that this doctrine originated in the religious thought of Egypt. There, the priests developed the notion that there existed a transmigration of souls from terrestrial, to marine, to bird, and finally to human form.[33] A vegetarian diet thus became the only one that would not result in the destruction of another ensouled being. This idea was further developed, particularly in eastern religious thought, to include a backward as well as a forward progression of a soul, depending on the quality of the current life. Premature death at the hands of a human would thus interrupt the process and possibly consign the soul to a lower life form than would have otherwise been the case.

The second reason for a vegetarian ideal from a sacred life perspective centers on the sentience of lower creatures. If the animal kingdom could experience emotion, particularly pain, suffering, fear, and deprivation, then causing such negative emotions would constitute a violation of that creature's life. This would be even more serious if death were to result.

This recognition of the pain experienced by lower-order animals causes the Greek philosopher Empedokles to cry out: "Alas that the pitiless day did not destroy me first, before I devised for my lips the cruel deed of eating flesh."[34]

While most Christian theologians have been reluctant to grant to the animal kingdom a soul similar to that held for humans, there has nevertheless been an increasing concern for the welfare of animals. While not necessarily believing in an in-dwelling animal soul, there is an increasing tendency to equate all life as being of equal value. Thus, vegetarian diets are necessary to avoid the taking of life. The earlier emphasis on a golden age where death does not occur easily gives rise to a fundamental belief in the sacredness of all life. This position holds that the destruction of one life to benefit another creates a hierarchy of values that is anathema to the creator's design where all life is of equal value.

A. Mahavira (c. 599–527 BCE)

Nowhere has the reverence for life been more profoundly stated or scrupulously practiced than by the Jains, followers of Mahavira, who was born in Kundapura near Vaishali about 599 BCE.

At the age of 30, Mahavira renounced all his wealth, property, wife, family, relatives, and pleasures. In a garden of the village Kundapura, at the foot of an Ashoka tree, no one else being present, after fasting 2 days without water, he took off all his clothes, tore out the hair of his head in five handfuls, and put a single cloth on his shoulder. He vowed to neglect his body and with equanimity to suffer all calamities arising from divine powers, people, or animals.

Mahavira's followers founded the Jainish religion, which today still maintains one of the strictest stands with regard to vegetarian principles.

B. Buddhist Thought

Buddha's insistence on the sacredness of all life also lent itself to a vegetarian lifestyle, even though he himself did not practice scrupulous vegetarianism. The major reason for Buddha's advocacy of non-violence and non-killing was centered in the concept of "mercy" toward all living things. Buddha taught that it was wrong to be the recipient of food that was prepared expressly for that individual through the slaughter of an animal. Eating the flesh of another living creature was a barbaric act if that animal had lost its life solely to provide that individual with food. With this also goes a belief in karma that mandates that all must eventually suffer the consequences of evil actions.[35] Buddha was pragmatic enough, however, to allow for eating meat if it had been already prepared for and by other non-believers who had no prior knowledge of the need and presence of himself or a follower.

Buddha's thought is probably best summarized in a poem said to be the only text actually written by Buddha himself.

> Creatures without feet have my love.
> And likewise those who have two feet;
> And those too, who have many feet.
> Let creatures all, all things that live,
> All beings of whatever kind,
> See nothing that will bode them ill.
> May naught of evil come to them.[36]

C. Hindu Philosophy

The Hindu philosophy adopted much from Buddhism. "For India's ancient thinkers, life is seen as the very stuff of the Divine, an emanation of the Source and part of a cosmic continuum. They further held that each life form, even water and trees, possesses consciousness and energy. Nonviolence, ahimsa, the primary basis of vegetarianism, has long been central to the religious traditions of India..."[37] The reincarnation of the soul makes it a sacred duty to avoid the killing and eating of any animal.

D. Christian Thought

Christians have been far less willing to see lower forms of life as anything more than mobile vegetables. There are, however, a few voices that call for a rethinking of that position. Dr. Andrew Linzey, professor of theology at Mansfield College, Oxford, U.K. and a passionate animal welfare activist, says, as well: "A God who remains passionless in the face of innocent suffering simply cannot be the Christian God. No theology which desensitizes us to suffering can be truly Christian theology."[38]

Even Christ himself commented that the Heavenly Father took note of, and was concerned with, the demise of even one sparrow.

Richard Dunkerly, an evangelical Christian, teacher, and writer states: "Of all people, Christians should not be the destroyers. We should be the healers and reconcilers. We must show NOW how it will be THEN in the Peaceable Kingdom of Isaiah 11:6 where 'the wolf shall lie down with the lamb... and a little child shall lead them.' We can begin now within our homes and churches by teaching our children respect and love for all of God's creation...by teaching them."[39]

E. Jewish Thinking

Jewish thinking has also, most often, seen the animal kingdom as little more than a source of food. But again, there are a few who challenge that view. Isaac Bashevis Singer, a noted contemporary Jewish vegetarian philosopher puts it bluntly, "When a human kills an animal for food, he is neglecting justice for his own hunger. Man prays for mercy, but is unwilling to extend it to others. Why should man then expect mercy from God? It's unfair to expect something that you are not willing to give. It is inconsistent."[40]

Even the Genesis account of permission to include animal flesh in the diet seems to contain a warning about misuse. "And surely your blood of your lives will I require; at the hand of every beast will I require it ...."[41]

The passage seems to have God saying, "If you kill needlessly I will require an accounting."

Count Tolstoi, the eminent Russian novelist, wrote: "The consumption of animal food is plainly immoral because it demands an act which does violence to our moral sentiments."

Commenting on the animal suffering caused by meat eating, Henry David Thoreau said, "Every creature is better alive than dead — men, moose and pine trees — and he who understands it aright will rather preserve it live rather than destroying it."

There is a growing awareness of the suffering endured by animals in the process of meat production. Over two thirds of the vegetarians surveyed by *Vegetarian Times* gave animal cruelty as a reason for their vegetarianism. Seven million Americans are members or supporters of animal protection organizations.[42]

In a recent *Los Angeles Times* poll, 47% of Americans said that they believed that animals are like humans in important ways in that they feel pain, act with altruism, communicate, and suffer fear.[43]

Death itself may not be the cruelest fate that animals raised for food suffer. Their short lives are often lived in discomfort and pain. Laying hens were the first to become "assembly line" components. Today over 95% of the eggs used in the U.S. come from these high tech factories where 250,000 to 5 million hens are raised indoors in crowded wire cages that are barely larger than their own bodies.[44]

The broiler business is little better. These birds have been so intensively bred for meat that they are now misshapen. Many cannot even walk or stand up. Genetic manipulation has also cut their growing time in half. These chickens now grow so rapidly that only 7 weeks elapse between hatching and their slaughter weight of 3 1/2 pounds.[45]

Probably the cruelest meat-raising practices are reserved for veal calves. Over a million of these animals are slaughtered each year.[46] Those not killed immediately for "drop veal" spend their short 4-month lives chained in tiny stalls, unable to exercise or even turn around.[47] This keeps their muscles underdeveloped so the meat is more tender.[48] Their diet is designed to produce anemia so as to keep their flesh pale.[49]

Dairy cattle fare little better. About half of this country's 11 million dairy cows are reared in confinement. The same is true for about 80% of the 95 million pigs raised for human food.[50]

The outcry against the cruelty of slaughter for food has a long history. Pythagoras found this one of the more compelling reasons for his vegetarian beliefs, as did his followers throughout the ages. He equated the slaughter of animals with murder and theorized that brutality toward animals bred violence toward humans.[51]

Ellen White, one of the founders of the Seventh-Day Adventist church first advocated a vegetarian diet in 1863.[52] But, apparently, she found it difficult to maintain and periodically continued to indulge in meat until 1894. It was a plea from a woman in Australia that finally made the impression that was needed to make vegetarianism a permanent commitment. In a letter to friends in the U.S., she wrote: "When the selfishness of taking the lives of animals to gratify a perverted taste was presented to me by a Catholic woman, kneeling at my feet, I felt ashamed and distressed. I saw it in a new light and I said, I will no longer patronize the butchers. I will not have the flesh of corpses on my table."[53]

Upton Sinclair in his novel *The Jungle* managed to, as he said, "hit America in the stomach." The problems he depicted were not only the cruelty to the animals, but also the cruelty displayed to the workers in the trade. Apparently little has changed since Sinclair's book was published in 1907. Eleanor Kennelly of the United Food and Commercial Workers Union says, "A meat-packing plant is like nothing you've ever seen or could imagine. It's like a vision of hell."[54] Federal statistics show that one in three of the 135,000 slaughterhouse employees in the U.S.

is injured each year, making it the country's second most dangerous occupation.[55]

IV. THE FOOD OF THE GODS AND THE DIET OF PARADISE

Common to virtually all religious doctrines is a belief in a deity or deities that transcend humankind in thought, power, and practice. Spirituality demands a supernatural constituent that is worthy of worship and often fear. This requires that there be a difference, as well as a distance between the human subject and the divine overlord. While the envisioned differences have often taken strange and grotesque forms, the gods have always been anthropomorphized to some extent. This allows for intellectual dialogue with humans and the possibility of human emulation. Central to almost all religious thought is the idea of achieving an oneness with the deity. While there may be argument as to whether this is a literal physical union or a more spiritual joining, it nevertheless implies a combining of human and divine attributes. Becoming godlike demands a change in behavior — not the least of which involves the choice of food. There seems to be in the collective conscience of humanity a remembrance of a time past when humans did commune with the gods. Equally universal is the desire to return to that blissful state. The ingestion of food was an obvious requirement for human life and it was logical and, in fact, necessary, to assume that the gods likewise required provender. But it was equally important to make a distinction between the nourishment required by humans and that required by a god.

A. Pythagoras (c. 582–507 BCE)

Pythagoras, with his orphic traditions, represents an early attempt at achieving a reunification with the gods. Pythagoras was born on the island of Samos about 582 BCE. Although he and his family were well off, they were at odds with Polykrates, the tyrannical ruler of the island. As a result, Pythagoras eventually left Samos and settled in southern Italy. Legend has it that he studied in Ionia, Israel, and Egypt. During his sojourn in Egypt, he was captured by the Babylonian invaders and spent some 13 years in Babylon, most likely around 530 BCE. This would have been immediately following the death of Daniel, but nevertheless in a close enough approximation to that era for him to have been influenced by Daniel's legacy. Tradition says that he explored from India in the East to Gaul in the West. He too saw dreams as divine revelations and adopted a vegetarian lifestyle that was emulated by his followers for hundreds of years. In fact, until the mid-19th century, vegetarians were termed Pythagoreans.

Pythagoras adopted and adapted Orphism, an older Greek religion. He saw earthly life as only a merciless round of pain and trouble (the product of evil). Although humans belong to the heavens and to the stars (as semi-gods), they were also bound to life by a cycle of death and rebirth. The goal of life was to escape from earthly existence and be released to eternal life. "Alas, what wickedness to swallow flesh into our own flesh, to fatten our greedy bodies by cramming in other bodies, to have one living creature fed by the death of another! In the midst of such wealth as earth, the best of mothers, provides, nothing forsooth satisfies you, but to behave like the Cyclopes, inflicting sorry wounds with cruel teeth! You cannot appease the hungry cravings of your wicked, gluttonous stomachs except by destroying some other life." — Ovid: *Metamorphoses*, translated by Mary M. Innes

The gods were not in need of the same foods on which humans subsisted. Hesiod, (c. 800 BCE), a poet of antiquity, described the dining habits of the gods: "immortals inhabiting the Olympian mansions feast ever on the pure and bloodless food of Ambrosia." Their beverage was the nectar of flowers.[56]

The French anthropologist Marcel Detienne continues:"The consumption of meat actually coincides with the offering to the gods of a domestic animal whose flesh is reserved for men, leaving to divinity the smoke of calcined bones and the scent of spices burned for the occasion. The division is thus clearly made on an alimentary plane between men and gods. Men receive the meat because they need to consume perishable flesh, of which they themselves consist, in order to live. Gods have the privilege of smells, perfumes, incorruptible substances that make up the superior foods reserved for the deathless powers."[57]

This concept is found numerous times in the Hebrew scripture. God is said to have "smelled a sweet savor" from the burnt offering presented by Noah following his deliverance from the Deluge (Genesis 8:21). Several passages in the Pentatuch refer to the required Jewish sacrifices as a "sweet savor unto the Lord."

To become godlike, godlike behavior is necessary. Since the gods live on "the nectar of flowers," and there was obviously no meat in that type of fare, it was also not the kind of substance that a human can live on. A compromise, however, was to eliminate meat altogether. Eating the flowers was almost as good as living on their nectar.

Ironically, it is possible that the offering of animal sacrifices first tempted humankind to taste animal flesh. The fire that invariably accompanied a sacrifice would leave at least a portion of the meat roasted. Since the gods did not consume the flesh, sampling that which remained after the fire had burnt out was most likely an irresistible temptation. Undoubtedly more than one supplicant tasted his oblation. Finding the flavor satisfying, it takes no great stretch of the imagination to see the indulgence extended to other non-ceremonial occasions.

The early biblical record of offerings to God indicated that vegetation was unacceptable and that only a blood offering would suffice. This original rejection of vegetable produce may have hastened the ascendancy of meat as a more desirable fare. Hebrew ritual actually made provision for the priests to obtain much of their nourishment in this way.

Although the 6th century BC marked the first written commentary on a meat-free diet, oral tradition places the introduction of such a regimen at a far earlier date. Those Jews and Christians alike who take a literal approach to scriptural interpretation believe that Genesis 1:29–31 indicates that the original diet given to both humans and animals was meatless. "Then God said, 'I give you every seed-bearing plant on the face of the whole earth and every tree that has fruit with seed in it. They will be yours for food. And to all the beasts of the earth and all the birds of the air and all the creatures that move on the ground — everything that has the breath of life in it — I give every green plant for food.' And it was so."

The Garden of Eden described in Genesis 1 and 2, with its harmony between man and beast and its plant-based diet, is not unique to Judao-Christian thought. The Roman historian and poet Ovid wrote that: "The first millennium was the Age of Gold, No brass-lipped trumpets called, nor clanging swords. Spring was eternal, and gentle breezes caressed the flowers with clear warm air. Fields were always fertile ... streams of nectar flowed forth.

No blood stained men's lips ... until some futile brain envied the lions' diet and gulped down a feast of flesh to fill his greedy guts."[58]

That a belief in a "Garden of Eden" existence is an almost universal characteristic is evident from the mythology of diverse cultures, literally from all over the world. The legends of a majority of cultures recall a time in the dim and distant past when the gods lived among men, and man and animals lived in peace and harmony because there was neither need nor desire to sacrifice animal life to appetite. Michael Mountain remarks: "The Cheyenne people of North America also spoke of an eternal springtime in which the original people roamed, innocent and free, before the coming of the age of flood, war, and famine. Northern European peoples celebrated the age of the Peace of Frodi, when there was no strife and a magical mill ground out peace and plenty. In South America, the legends of the Caribs of Surinam tell of a time when the trees were forever in fruit and the animals lived in perfect harmony so that the little agouti played with the fur of the jaguar. The Krita Yuga, or Perfect Age, of India, and China's Age of Perfect Virtue are said to have been a time without sickness, suffering, or war. And the creation stories of the Middle East all tell of a time when humankind lived at peace with nature and with God in a Garden of Eden, free of sickness or death and without need for labor or toil."[59]

Many cultures also have a tradition of a return to a "Golden Age" when all things will live in peace and harmony.[60,61] This is particularly true of Christian-Judaic philosophy that believes in an earth made new, where both man and animals revert to the Edenic state. "And the wolf also shall dwell with the lamb, and the leopard shall lie down with the kid; and the calf and the young lion and the fatling together; and a little child shall lead them. And the cow and the bear shall feed; their young ones shall lie down together: and the lion shall eat straw like the ox. And the suckling child shall play on the hole of the asp, and the weaned child shall put his hand on the cockatrice'den. They shall not hurt of destroy in my holy mountain saith the Lord: for the whole earth shall be full of the knowledge of the Lord, as the waters cover the sea" (Isa 11:9).

It is not hard to understand that attempts to hasten the return to this blissful state have provided the impetus for the adoption of a vegetarian lifestyle among many of the faithful. Even those who see this as a distant and heavenly reward may come to adopt a plant-based existence, in anticipation of the heavenly culture to which they fervently aspire and that they believe the afterlife will provide.

V. THE DENIAL OF THE FLESH

Self-denial is an important element of virtually all religious practices. It tends to assume two forms. One is that of an "otherworldly" detachment, such that the requirements for a literal physical life decline in importance, as the true believer comes closer to a oneness with the deity. The other position sees suffering and deprivation as a means to an end. If the body can be subdued and made to suffer, then perhaps the purer soul can gain the ascendancy and achieve the desired union with the divine.

A. Buddha (c. 563–483 BCE)

Buddhism, with its total lack of desire for material position, is a fitting representation of this principle. Buddha was most likely born in Lumbini, Nepal[62] about 250 kilometers southwest of Kathmandu. His given name was Siddhartha Gautama and, by the standards of his day, he grew up in luxury. His father was most likely a feudal lord who provided his family with all the comforts that his position and wealth could afford. In spite of this, the young man could not find peace, and on the eve of his 29th year, he left home and family to search for meaning in life. He joined a band of aesthetics and became a master at self-denial, including semi-starvation. He ate so little, one bean a day during one of his fasts, that "When I thought I would touch the skin of my stomach, I actually took hold of my spine."[63]

For almost 50 years, Buddha trudged from village to village with his followers, preaching his gospel of enlightenment, a religion of infinite compassion. His was, however, a religion of intense self-effort, believing that through intense labor, a devotee might breach the seemingly endless cycle of death and rebirth and attain enlightenment and a permanent end to suffering.

He enunciated four noble truths:

1. All who live suffer.
2. Suffering is due to desire.
3. Suffering will end when desires are repressed.
4. Moderation leads to an end of suffering.

Although Buddha eventually repudiated self mortification, his doctrine of eliminating discontent by minimizing desire results in many of the same practices. Where Buddhists see suffering as an inevitable happening that results from desire, many other religious philosophies have found virtue in the suffering itself — a sort of ecstasy in agony.

While there have always been vegetarians among the earth's population, most have chosen this way of life because of ecological necessity rather than dietary preference. Where and when it has been possible, flesh food has always been added to the diet. In general, diets without meat have been regarded as inferior and a deprivation. Meatless diets were, therefore, ideally suited to employment in the subjugation of the body, a concept that has been part of religious practice for millennia.

B. Jewish Asceticism

Many Jews, for similar reasons, eschewed meat following the destruction of the temple in AD 70. They felt it a sacrilege to eat flesh when they were not permitted to bring a similar animal as a sacrifice to God. Jewish folklore is filled with stories of abstinence from meat as a penance for violation of Hebrew law.

Rueben is said to have eaten no meat for 7 years following his indiscretion with Billah, his father's concubine, and likewise, Judah is credited with many years of similar abstinence following his encounter with Tamar.

C. Christian Asceticism

This concept infiltrated Christianity at an early date and became a necessary tenet of the Gnostic dualistic philosophy. This heretical school of Christian thought held that man is composed of two distinct and separate parts: the evil flesh and the pure spirit. In time, a variant of this philosophy permeated even the orthodox church. It was soon taught that a Christian's duty was to see to it that the spirit triumphed over the flesh. This made dietary restriction a rather common element in early Christian behavior. Meat was regarded as a food that symbolized worldly joy and pleasure, two emotions that a good Christian would avoid.

The 1st-century philosopher Philo maintained that God had forbidden the use of pork and shellfish because these were the most tasty of all meats and God wanted to curb pleasure and desire in His people. Vegetarianism took the restriction one step further and was seen as evidence of superior spirituality and humility.

This original Christian understanding of the relation of diet to religious piety was not confined to the early Christian era. It has found its place in each generation, with only minor modifications in its expression.

Grains and vegetables were regarded by the medieval world as animal food; only poverty compelled human beings to partake of such fare in place of meat. Meat, in fact, became a symbol of class status. The more frequently one dined on flesh, the more elevated his position in society. Samuel Johnson's definition of "oats" in his 1775 English dictionary reveals this bias and exposes his anti-Scot feeling. "Oats: a grain, which in England is generally given to horses but in Scotland supports the people."

Thus, if one wished to demonstrate humility and Christian commitment, abstinence from meat was an appropriate act. The substitution of vegetables for meat thus became an act of penitence.

This was rigorously enforced in the past. Within the Roman Catholic faith, from the Middle Ages though the 17th century, meat eating was forbidden on Fridays, some Saturdays and Lent. In fact, for devout Catholics, meat eating was forbidden on almost 180 days a year.[64] Vegetarianism survives today as a component of the asceticism practiced by monastic orders such as the Benedictine Trappist monks.

Prior to the beginning of the modern vegetarian movement in the early 1800s, this tendency toward the chastisement of the flesh was the primary motivation of those who devoted themselves to vegetarianism. A carryover of this attitude can be seen today in those who are prone to equate meat eating with sin. Christians of this persuasion practice a sort of "ecstasy of agony," designed to regain or maintain control of a continually wayward and sinful body.

The early Christian preoccupation with the evils of the flesh as a component of the previously mentioned dualistic philosophy has certainly been represented and practiced in modern vegetarianism. For this group, the main issue was that of bringing the body into subjection. Depriving the body of flesh food was seen not so much as a way to better health, but rather as a sort of modified fast, which, if nothing else, demonstrated to the world, as well as to God and self, that the purer spirit was in control of the evil body.

1. Modern Christian Vegetarianism

Diet, as a component of religiosity, is almost universally endemic. Its popularity waxes and wanes in direct relation to the strength of the religious commitment of the society. The New World proved to be no exception to this inclination. American religious fervor and its accompanying dietary prohibitions have displayed a rather cyclic pattern. Religious concern and fervor, which gradually built to a peak, was followed by a subsequent lessening of interest, finally ending in a cataclysmic event.[65]

These cycles have been so distinct and identifiable in American society that they have come to be termed "revivals" — a phenomenon that is a uniquely American contribution to the religious world. Revivalism differs from mere evangelism in that it connotes the evangelism of the masses by effective and charismatic preachers. Just as "conversion" is centered on the individual, "revival" is its equivalent applied to the group. Since its founding, America has experienced five such cycles.

1. The first of the religious revivals to affect the Americas was the Puritan Awakening (1600–1640) which eventually culminated in the English Revolution. While the colonies were not directly involved, they certainly did have an interest in the outcome.
2. The mid 1700s saw religious emphasis building to what has come to be termed "The Great Awakening." The Revolutionary War spelled the end of this phase.
3. This cycle was followed by a "Second Great Awakening," (1795–1835) characterized by William Miller and his contemporaries. This cycle climaxed in the Great Disappointment of 1844, but was actually ended by the Civil War.
4. The religious emphasis of the Victorian world (1875–1915), which followed the War Between the States, was ended by the "New Deal" society of FDR.
5. The present cycle of religious fervor (1950–1980) is just now beginning its decline.

These arousals of interest in religion were almost invariably accompanied by behavioral and lifestyle modifications, with diet often playing a major role. An individual who has experienced conversion or revival often feels that his life and behavior must somehow be changed. Thus, vegetarianism was often a behavioral adjunct of such revivals. This is particularly true of the last three of these cycles.

The health reformers of the 19th century saw vegetarianism as the ideal diet to control the body and mind and bring about harmony with their creator. Theirs was a pseudophysiological approach. They believed, for example, that since the "vital force" was less used by a vegetarian than by a meat-eater, it would be logical to conclude that a vegetarian would live longer since he would not have dissipated his vital force as rapidly as one who indulged in flesh food.

Their study of human anatomy convinced them that God had indeed designed man to be herbivorous. Vegetables provided more than enough of the essential nutrients and were not pathologically "simulating" like meat. Christian vegetarians were persuaded that they had indeed performed a service for humanity in bringing enlightenment to diet.

> Nature's dietetic laws lay hid in night
> Let vegetarians be to give us light
> Or in other words,
> Mankind in the dark ages were mostly carnivorous;
> But now the light shines, let us all be frugivorous.[66]

William Cowherd of Manchester, England is a characteristic example of this philosophy. In 1800, he convinced his Anglican "offshoot" congregation, The Bible Christian Church, to pledge themselves to abstain from alcohol and flesh food. In fact, the only requirement for membership in his congregation was evidence of abstinence from meat for a period of 6 months.[67]

Following Cowherd's death, the movement was exported to America by his son-in-law William Medcalfe, who, with a group of his parishioners, landed in Philadelphia in 1817 after an arduous voyage that saw considerable apostasy in matters of diet. While the group attempted to maintain its identity, it was never successful at convincing more than a handful to adopt its way of life. One convert to the dietary plan, if not the religious principles, was Sylvester Graham of graham-cracker fame. After visiting the church in 1829, he began to recommend a vegetarian diet. He succeeded in arousing the nation to his gospel of a simple diet. He proclaimed the virtues of a vegetable diet as one that would not "irritate the system" and that was more in tune with the design of the creator.

American notables like William and Bronson Alcott and Russell Trall, a "water cure" enthusiast, were among Graham's supporters and converts. In 1850, along with Medcalfe, they founded the American Vegetarian

Society. Graham's death at 56 caused some consternation among the faithful, but they were able to explain and apologize for his untimely demise. It was, they said, the result of a frail constitution and occasional lapses to the fleshpots.

Following the Civil War, the philosophy of the mortification of the body gave way to a more subtle form of chastisement. Led by individuals such as John Harvey Kellogg, vegetarianism came to be regarded as a method, not so much to subdue the body, but as a way to control the emotions and the mind, specifically the "animal passion." To believers, it was logical that the ingestion of animal flesh would confer upon the eater a temperament and character similar to that of the particular animal eaten, particularly in terms of its sexual nature.

Christian vegetarians of the most recent revival cycle are more apt to adopt their prohibition against meat on the grounds of responsible and unselfish service to humanity. While they readily acknowledge that they no longer see the abstinence from flesh food as a modified fast, and, in fact, may argue that the diet actually conveys health benefits, they see the necessity of condemning the excesses necessitated by meat production. They believe that true Christianity demands that they sacrifice to assist the less fortunate and that consuming a plant-based diet is a part of that responsibility. They are also intent on extending this need to prevent suffering to that of the animal creation as well.

VI. SUMMARY

Vegetarian philosophy and religious thought are not separate strands in the ribbon of human culture. Instead, they are perhaps an interwoven tapestry, with each better expressing the other than would have been possible individually. Religious thought seeks its expression in diet and diet reflects religious thought. Nowhere is this more evident than in vegetarian philosophy. The principles of vegetarianism cannot be adequately understood, except in the context of the religion of those practicing the lifestyle. The five spiritual principles outlined all have current adherents, and, more often than not, those who practice vegetarianism can point to a multiplicity of these spiritual rationales for their beliefs.

REFERENCES

1. Grun, B. *The Timetables of History*. Simon and Schuster, New York, 1975.
2. Potter, C.F. *The Faiths Men Live By*. pp. 64. Ace Books, New York, 1954.
3. *The World Book Encyclopedia*, Vol. 21. Field Enterprises Educational Corporation, Chicago, 1977.
4. Bernhardt, O.E. *Zoroaster: Life and Work of the Forerunner in Persia*. pp. 189. Grail Foundation Press, 1996.

5. Rosen, S. *Diet for Transcendence.* Torchlight Publishing, Badger, CA, 1997.
6. Mehr, F. *An Introduction To The Ancient Wisdom of Zarathustra.*
7. Berry, R. *Food for the Gods, Vegetarianism and the World's Religions.* Pythagorean Publishers, New York, 1998.
8. Blazar, J. Doomsayers of Overpopulation Sound a New Jeremiad. *Los Angeles Times*, June 7, 1994.
9. Ibid.
10. Ibid.
11. Hoop, J. *Champion of the Diversity of Life, an Interview with Peter H. Raven, 1994 Science Year.* World Book Inc., Chicago, 1994.
12. Woodwell, G. *Global Change*, 1993 Science Year. World Book Inc., Chicago, 1993.
13. Scharfenberg, J.A. *The Problems with Meat.* Woodbridge Press Publishing, Santa Barbara, 1982.
14. Strong, J. *The Exhaustive Concordance of the Bible.* Riverside Book and Bible House, Iowa Falls, ?.
15. The Environmental Impact of Meat vs. Vegetables. *Energy Times*, May/June 1994.
16. Ibid.
17. U.S. Dept. of Agriculture, Economic Research Service. *World Agricultural Supply and Demand Estimates*, WASDE-256. USDA, Washington, D.C., July 11, 1991.
18. Blazar, J. Doomsayers of Overpopulation Sound a New Jeremiad. *Los Angeles Times*, June 7, 1994.
19. Moll, L. Is There Such a Thing as a Humane Pair of Shoes? *Vegetarian Times*, January, 1989.
20. Rifkin, J. *Beyond Beef.* Dutton (Penguin Books), New York, 1992.
21. Metzger, M., Whittaker, C.P. *This Planet is Mine.* Simon and Schuster, New York, 1991.
22. Caulfield, A. Reporter at Large: The Rain Forests. *New Yorker,* Jan 14, 1985.
23. Wilkenson, L., quoted in Fox, M.W., Personal choice or ethical imperative. *Vegetarian Times*, January, 1987.
24. Ford, D. *Daniel.* Southern Publishing Association, Nashville TN, 1978.
25. Unger, M.F. *Archaeology and the Old Testament.* Zondervan Publishing House, Grand Rapids, MI, 1954.
26. Daniel 1: 11 & 12. *Revised Standard Version of the Holy Bible.*
27. Daniel 1:18-20. *New International Version of the Holy Bible.* Zondervan Bible Publishers, Grand Rapids MI, 1978.
28. Daniel 10:1.
29. Quoted in Messina, M. and Messina, V. *The Simple Soybean and Your Health.* pp. 9. Avery, Garden City Park, NY, 1994.
30. Hardinge, M.G., Stare, F.J. Nutritional studies of vegetarians. *J. Clin. Nutr.*, 2:73, 1954.
31. Snowdon, D.A. Animal product consumption and mortality because of all causes combined, coronary heart disease, stroke, diabetes, and cancer in Seventh-Day Adventists. *Am. J. Clin. Nutr.*, Sep;48(3 Suppl):739-48, 1998.
32. Singh, P. and Fraser, G. *Am. J. Epidemiol.*, 148:761-774, 1998.
33. Dombrowski, D.A. *The Philosophy of Vegetarianism.* University of Massachusetts Press, Amherst MA, 1994.

34. Wilkins, J., Harvey, D., and Dobson, M., quoted in *Food in Antiquity*. pp. 217. University of Exeter Press, Exeter, 1995.

35. Shywan, L.C. *Vegetarian Cooking, Chinese Style*. 1995.

36. Rosen, S. *Diet for Transcendence*. pp. 81. Torchlight Publishing, Badger CA, 1997.

37. Subramuniyaswami, S.S. Discussing Vegetarianism With a Meat-Eater: a Hindu View. *Hinduism Today*.

38. Linzey, A.A Gospel for Every Creature. *IVU News*, Issue 1-96.

39. Dunkerly, R. Hunting: What the Scripture says. *INROADS,* International Network for Religion and Animals, Number 14, Winter 1991.

40. Singer, I.J. In Rosen, S.,: *Food for the Spirit: Vegetarianism and the World Religions*. Bala Books, 1987.

41. Genesis 9:5.

42. Balzar, J. Creatures Great — and Equal? *Los Angeles Times*, December 25, 1993.

43. Ibid.

44. Pacelle, W. Bio-Machines: Life on the Farm Ain't What it Used to Be. *Vegetarian Times*, January, 1989.

45. Ibid.

46. Ibid.

47. Moran, V. Vegetarianism, the Ethics, the Philosophy, the Diet. *Vegetarian Times*, January, 1989.

48. Pacelle, W. Bio-Machines: Life on the Farm Ain't What it Used to Be. *Vegetarian Times*, January, 1989.

49. Moran, V. Vegetarianism, the Ethics, the Philosophy, the Diet. *Vegetarian Times,* January, 1989.

50. Pacelle, W. Bio-Machines: Life on the Farm Ain't What it Used to Be. *Vegetarian Times*, January, 1989.

51. Nicholson, G.P. Father of Vegetarianism: Pythagoras. *Vegetarian Times*, August, 1986.

52. White, E.G. *Counsels on Health*. Pacific Press Publishing Association, Mountain View CA, 1951.

53. White, E.G. Letter 73a, 1986, in F.D. Nichols, *Ellen G. White and her Critics*. Review and Harold Publishing Assn., Washington D.C., 1951.

54. Kerbs, A.V. *Heading Toward the Last Round Up: The Big Three's Prime Cut*. Prairie Fire Rural Action, Des Moines, June 1990.

55. Moll, L. Is There Such a Thing as a Humane Pair of Shoes? *Vegetarian Times*, January, 1989.

56. Spencer, C. *The Heretic's Feast: a History of Vegetarianism*. pp. 47. Fourth Estate Limited, London, 1993.

57. Detienne, M. *The Gardens of Adonis: Spices in Greek Mythology*, translated by Janet Lloyd. Princeton University Press, Princeton, NJ, 1994.

58. Ovid. *The Doctrines of Pythagoras*, translated by A.D. Melville. Oxford University Press, 1986.

59. Mountain, M. The Golden Age. *Best Friends Magazine*, July 1997.

60. Spencer, C. *The Heretic's Feast: A History of Vegetarianism*. Fourth Estate Limited, London, 1993.

61. Dombrowski, D.A. *The Philosophy of Vegetarianism*. University of Massachusetts Press, Amherst MA, 1984.

62. Gard, R.A. *Buddhism*. George Braziller, NY, 1962.

63. Smith, H. *The Religions of Man*. pp. 93. Harper and Row, NY, 1958.
64. Toussaint-Samat, M. *History of Food,* English Translation — Translated by Anthea Bell. Blackwell, London, 1992.
65. Gustad, E.S. *The Rise of Adventism*. Harper and Row, NY, 1974.
66. Thomas, E. For the American Vegetarian. *American Vegetarian*, 4: 131, 1854.
67. Unti, R. *Vegetarian Roots*. Vegetarian Times, April, 1990.

INDEX